D1543099

SPORTS MEDICINE

ORTHOPAEDIC SURGERY ESSENTIALS

SPORTS MEDICINE

ORTHOPAEDIC SURGERY ESSENTIALS

Adult Reconstruction
Daniel J. Berry, MD
Scott P. Steinmann, MD

Foot and Ankle
David B. Thordarson, MD

Hand and Wrist
James R. Doyle, MD

Basic Science and Oncology
Timothy A. Damron, MD
Carol D. Morris, MD

Orthopaedic Sports Medicine
Anthony A. Schepsis, MD
Brian D. Busconi, MD

Pediatrics
Kathryn E. Cramer, MD
Susan A. Scherl, MD

Spine
Christopher M. Bono, MD
Steven R. Garfin, MD

Trauma
Charles Court-Brown, MD
Margaret McQueen, MD
Paul Tornetta, MD

ORTHOPAEDIC SURGERY ESSENTIALS

SPORTS MEDICINE

Series Editors

PAUL TORNETTA III, MD
Professor
Department of Orthopaedic Surgery
Boston University School of Medicine;
Director of Orthopaedic Trauma
Boston University Medical Center
Boston, Massachusetts

THOMAS A. EINHORN, MD
Professor and Chairman
Department of Orthopaedic Surgery
Boston University School of Medicine
Boston, Massachusetts

Book Editors

ANTHONY A. SCHEPSIS, MD
Professor
Department of Orthopaedic Surgery
Boston University School of Medicine;
Director and Chief of Sports Medicine
Boston Medical Center
Boston, Massachusetts

BRIAN D. BUSCONI, MD
Associate Professor
Department of Orthopaedic Surgery
University of Massachusetts Medical School;
Chief, Division of Sports Medicine
UMass Memorial Medical Center
Worcester, Massachusetts

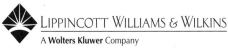
LIPPINCOTT WILLIAMS & WILKINS
A **Wolters Kluwer** Company
Philadelphia · Baltimore · New York · London
Buenos Aires · Hong Kong · Sydney · Tokyo

Acquisitions Editor: Robert Hurley
Developmental Editor: Grace R. Caputo, Dovetail Content Solutions
Managing Editor: Jenny Kim
Marketing Manager: Sharon Zinner
Manufacturing Manager: Ben Rivera
Project Manager: Fran Gunning
Production Services: Maryland Composition
Printer: Edwards Brothers

Copyright © 2006 by Lippincott Williams & Wilkins

530 Walnut Street
Philadelphia, Pennsylvania 19106 USA

351 West Camden Street
Baltimore, Maryland 21201-2436 USA

The publisher is not responsible (as a matter of product liability, negligence or otherwise) for an injury resulting from any material contained herein. This publication contains information relating to general principles of medical care which should not be constructed as specific instruction for individual patients. Manufacturer's product information should be reviewed for current information, including contraindications, dosages, and precautions.

Printed in the United States of America

Library of Congress Cataloging-in-Publication Data

Sports medicine / book editors, Anthony A. Schepsis, Brian D. Busconi.
    p. ; cm.—(Orthopaedic surgery essentials)
  Includes bibliographical references and index.
  ISBN 0-7817-5653-7
  1. Sports medicine. 2. Sports injuries.   I. Schepsis, Anthony A.
 II. D. Busconi, Brian D.   III. Series.
  [DNLM: 1. Athletic Injuries. 2. Sports Medicine.   QT 261 S76497
2006]
 RC1210.S6764 2006
 617.1′027—dc22

                                                        2005026374

The publishers have made every effort to trace copyright holders for borrowed material. If they have inadvertently overlooked any, they will be pleased to make the necessary arrangements at the first opportunity.

To purchase additional copies of this book, call our customer service department at (800) 638-3030 or fax orders to (301) 223-2320. For other book services, including chapter reprints and large quantity sales, ask for the Special Sales department.

For all other calls originating outside of the United States, please call (301) 223-2300.

Visit Lippincott Williams & Wilkins on the Internet: http://www.lww.com. Lippincott Williams & Wilkins customer service representatives are available from 8:30 am to 6:30 pm, EST, Monday through Friday, for telephone access.

10 9 8 7 6 5 4 3 2 1

To my late father, Anthony Sr., who always taught me to temper success with humility.
To my mother, Margaret, as well as to my beautiful children, Alexandra, Anthony, and Jesse.
And to my mentor, Dr. Robert E. Leach, an outstanding surgeon and educator,
who served as my role model.
—AAS

To my loving wife and best friend, Karolyn, whose patience, love, and understanding have been inspirational.
To our children, Liam and Aidan. You are the greatest joy and blessing in our lives. To my mom and dad,
Inez and Fred, whose sacrifice over the years has given me countless opportunities.
To June, a consummate professional. And to my mentors, especially
Dr. Arthur Pappas, for their encouragement, nurturing, and guidance.
—BDB

CONTENTS

Contributing Authors   ix
Preface   xv
Series Preface   xvi

SECTION I: SPECIAL ISSUES

1   **Pathophysiology of Muscle, Tendon, and Ligament Injuries   1**
   Paul Fadale, Eric Bluman, and Scott Allen

2   **Preparticipation Physical Examination   20**
   Vasilios Chrisostomidis, Brian D. Busconi, and
   J. Herbert Stevenson

3   **Sports Pharmacology: Drug Use and Abuse   32**
   Lee A. Mancini, Brian D. Busconi, and
   J. Herbert Stevenson

4   **Female Athletes   51**
   Julie Gill and Suzanne L. Miller

5   **Immature and Adolescent Athletes   61**
   Peter G. Gerbino

6   **Aging Athletes   81**
   Robert E. Leach

7   **Head Injuries   88**
   Robert V. Cantu and Robert C. Cantu

8   **Spinal Injuries   96**
   Christopher M. Bono, Marc A. Agulnick, and
   Mark G. Grossman

9   **Stress Fractures   105**
   Lee A. Mancini and Brian D. Busconi

10   **Soft-tissue Allografts   115**
   Joshua S. Hornstein

11   **Principles of Arthroscopic Surgery   126**
   Mark H. Getelman and Mark J. Albritton

SECTION II: MEDICAL ISSUES

12   **Medical Concerns of the Team Physician   135**
   Joseph Bernard, Philip Cruz, J. Herbert Stevenson,
   and Brian D. Busconi

13   **Dermatologic and Infectious Diseases   152**
   Matthew A. Pecci, Shawn M. Ferullo, Philip Cruz, and
   J. Herbert Stevenson

SECTION III: UPPER EXTREMITY

14   **Anatomy and Biomechanics of the Shoulder   169**
   Derek Plausinis, Laith M. Jazrawi,
   Joseph D. Zuckerman, and Andrew S. Rokito

15   **Physical Examination Tests for the Shoulder and Elbow   185**
   Robert J. Nicoletta

16 Shoulder Injuries in Throwing Athletes 200
    Andreas H. Gomoll, George F. Hatch, and
    Peter J. Millett

17 Anterior Instability of the Shoulder 214
    James Bicos, Augustus D. Mazzocca, and
    Robert A. Arciero

18 Posterior and Multidirectional Instability of the
    Shoulder 231
    Carlos A. Guanche

19 Disorders of the Rotator Cuff 244
    Alan S. Curtis and Abraham T. Shurland

20 Disorders of the Acromioclavicular and
    Sternoclavicular Joints 254
    Mark J. Lemos, Kelton Burbank, and
    Jennifer Taniguchi

21 Upper Extremity Nerve Injuries 268
    Richard M. Wilk

22 Elbow Injuries 285
    Anthony Schena and Ilya Voloshin

SECTION IV: LOWER EXTREMITY

23 Sports-specific Injuries of the Pelvis, Hip, and
    Thigh 320
    Brett D. Owens and Brian D. Busconi

24 Anterior Cruciate Ligament Injuries 333
    Vincent W. Chen, Robert E. Hunter, and John Woolf

25 Collateral Ligament Injuries of the Knee 348
    Andrew F. Arthur and Robert F. LaPrade

26 Posterior Cruciate Ligament Injuries 362
    Jeffrey A. Rihn, Paul Gause, Rick Cunningham, and
    Christopher D. Harner

27 Multiple Ligament Injuries of the Knee 376
    Gregory C. Fanelli, Daniel R. Orcutt, Justin D. Harris,
    David Zijerdi, and Craig J. Edson

28 Patellofemoral Disorders 391
    Beth E. Shubin Stein and Christopher S. Ahmad

29 Meniscal Injuries 402
    John A. Douglas and Nicholas A. Sgaglione

30 Articular Cartilage Injuries 418
    Tamara K. Pylawka, Richard W. Kang, and
    Brian J. Cole

31 Overuse Injuries of the Leg 430
    Kevin A. Nadel and Anthony A. Schepsis

32 Ankle Injuries 444
    Brian D. Busconi, Nicola A. DeAngelis, Heather Killie,
    and Timothy J. Marqueen

SECTION V: REHABILITATION

33 Rehabilitation in Sports Medicine 463
    Michael M. Reinold, Adam C. Olsen, and Kevin E. Wilk

34 Strength and Conditioning 476
    Stephen E. Lemos

Index 487

CONTRIBUTING AUTHORS

Marc A. Agulnick, MD
Attending Physician
Winthrop University Hospital
Mineola, New York
Clinical Assistant Professor
Department of Orthopaedics
SUNY Health Science Center at Stony Brook
Stony Brook, New York

Christopher S. Ahmad, MD
Assistant Professor
Department of Orthopaedic Surgery
Center for Shoulder, Elbow, and Sports Medicine
Columbia University
Attending Physician
Orthopaedic Surgery
Columbia University Medical Center
New York, New York

Mark J. Albritton, MD
Resurgens Orthopaedics
Fayetteville, Georgia

Scott Allen, MD
Fellow
Department of Orthopaedics
Brown Medical School
Providence, Rhode Island

Robert A. Arciero, MD
Professor
Co-Director, Sports Medicine Fellowship
University of Connecticut Health Center
Department of Orthopaedics
Farmington, Connecticut

Andrew F. Arthur, MD
Chief Resident
Department of Orthopaedic Surgery
University of Minnesota
Minneapolis, Minnesota

Joseph Bernard, DO
Assistant Professor
Department of Family Medicine
University of Massachusetts Medical School
Department of Family Medicine
UMass Memorial Medical Center
Worcester, Massachusetts

James Bicos, MD
JRSI Sports Medicine
St. Vincent Medical Center
Indianapolis, Indiana

Eric M. Bluman, MD, PhD
Chief, Orthopaedic Traumatology
Chief, Orthopaedic Foot and Ankle Surgery
Division of Orthopaedic Surgery
Madigan Army Medical Center
Ft. Lewis, Washington

Christopher M. Bono, MD
Assistant Professor
Department of Orthopaedic Surgery
Boston University School of Medicine
Attending Surgeon
Department of Orthopaedic Surgery
Boston Medical Center
Boston, Massachusetts

Kelton Burbank, MD
Attending Physician
Department of Orthopaedics
UMass Memorial Health Alliance
Leominster, Massachusetts

Brian D. Busconi, MD
Associate Professor
Department of Orthopaedic Surgery
University of Massachusetts Medical School
Chief, Division of Sports Medicine
UMass Memorial Medical Center
Worcester, Massachusetts

Robert C. Cantu, MD, FACS, FACSM
Medical Director
National Center for Catastrophic Sports Injury Research
Chapel Hill, North Carolina
Chief
Neurosurgery Service
Emerson Hospital
Concord, Massachusetts

Robert V. Cantu, MD
Assistant Professor
Department of Orthopaedic Surgery
Dartmouth-Hitchcock Medical Center
Lebanon, New Hampshire

Vincent W. Chen, MD
Associate
Pacific Orthopaedic Group
Alhambra, California

Vasilios Chrisostomidis, DO
Assistant Professor
University of Massachusetts Medical School
Worcester, Massachusetts

Brian J. Cole, MD, MBA
Associate Professor
Department of Orthopaedics and Anatomy
Rush University Medical Center
Chicago, Illinois

Philip Cruz, DO
Clinical Instructor
Department of Community and Preventive Medicine
Mount Sinai School of Medicine
Jamaica, New York
Director of Sports Medicine
Family Medicine
Jamaica Hospital Medical Center
Jamaica, New York

Rick Cunningham, MD
Orthopaedic Surgeon
Vail-Summit Orthopaedics and Sports Medicine
Vail, Colorado

Alan S. Curtis, MD
Assistant Clinical Professor
Department of Orthopaedic Surgery
New England Baptist Hospital
Boston, Massachusetts

Nicola A. DeAngelis, MD
Assistant Professor
Department of Orthopaedic Surgery
University of Massachusetts Medical School
Worcester, Massachusetts

John A. Douglas, DO
Orthopaedic Surgeon
Department of Surgery
Mountain West Medical Center
Tooele, Utah

Craig J. Edson, MS, PT, ATC
Department of Orthopaedic Surgery
Geisinger Medical Center
Danville, Pennsylvania

Paul D. Fadale, MD
Associate Professor
Department of Orthopaedic Surgery
Brown University Medical School
Chief, Sports Medicine
Orthopaedic Surgery
Rhode Island Hospital
Providence, Rhode Island

Gregory C. Fanelli, MD, FAAOS
Department of Orthopaedic Surgery
Geisinger Medical Center
Danville, Pennsylvania

Shawn M. Ferullo, MD
Sports Medicine Fellow
Boston University Department of Family Medicine
Boston University
Sports Medicine Fellow
Family Medicine
Boston Medical Center
Boston, Massachusetts

Paul Gause, MD
Resident Physician
Department of Orthopaedic Surgery
University of Pittsburgh
Pittsburgh, Pennsylvania

Peter G. Gerbino, MD
Instructor
Department of Orthopaedic Surgery
Harvard Medical School
Assistant
Department of Orthopaedic Surgery
Children's Hospital
Boston, Massachusetts

Mark H. Getelman, MD
Assistant Fellowship Director
Attending Physician
Southern California Orthopedic Institute
Van Nuys, California

Julie Gill, PA-C
Physician Assistant
Department of Orthopaedics
New England Baptist Hospital
Boston, Massachusetts

Andreas H. Gomoll, MD
Fellow in Orthopaedic Sports Medicine
Department of Orthopaedic Surgery
Rush University Medical Center
Chicago, Illinois

Mark G. Grossman, MD
Chief
Division of Sports Medicine
Department of Orthopaedics
Winthrop-University Hospital
Mineola, New York
Clinical Assistant Professor
Department of Orthopaedics
SUNY Health Science Center at Stony Brook
Stony Brook, New York

Carlos A. Guanche, MD
Southern California Orthopaedic Institute
Van Nuys, California

Christopher D. Harner, MD
Blue Cross of Western Pennsylvania Professor
Director, Section for Sports Medicine
Department of Orthopaedic Surgery
University of Pittsburgh
Pittsburgh, Pennsylvania

Justin D. Harris, MD
Resident
Department of Orthopaedic Surgery
Geisinger Medical Center
Danville, Pennsylvania

George F. Hatch III, MD
Assistant Professor
Department of Orthopaedic Surgery
University of Southern California/Keck School of Medicine
Assistant Professor
Department of Orthopaedic Surgery
USC University Hospital
Los Angeles, California

Joshua S. Hornstein, MD
Attending Physician
Trenton Orthopaedic Group
Mercerville, New Jersey

Robert E. Hunter, MD
Professor
Department of Orthopaedic Surgery
University of Arizona
Surgeon
Department of Orthopaedic Surgery
University Medical Center
Tucson, Arizona

Laith M. Jazrawi, MD
Assistant Professor
Department of Orthopaedic Surgery
NYU–Hospital for Joint Diseases
Director
Shoulder/Elbow Research Lab
NYU–Hospital for Joint Diseases
New York, New York

Richard W. Kang, BS
Research Assistant
Departments of Orthopaedic Surgery & Anatomy and Cell
    Biology
Rush University Medical Center
Chicago, Illinois

Heather Killie, MD
Resident
Department of Orthopaedic Surgery
University of Massachusetts Medical School
Worcester, Massachusetts

Robert F. LaPrade, MD, PhD
Professor
Department of Orthopaedic Surgery
University of Minnesota
Staff Consultant
Orthopaedic Surgery
University of Minnesota Medical Center

Robert E. Leach, MD
Professor
Department of Orthopaedic Surgery
Boston University School of Medicine
Editor Emeritus
American Journal of Sports Medicine
Boston, Massachusetts

Mark J. Lemos, MD, PhD
Associate Professor
Department of Orthopaedic Surgery
Boston University School of Medicine
Boston, Massachusetts
Director of Sports Medicine
Department of Orthopaedic Surgery
Lahey Clinic
Burlington, Massachusetts

Stephen E. Lemos, MD, PhD
Assistant Professor
Department of Orthopaedic Surgery
Boston University School of Medicine
Boston, Massachusetts
Staff Physician, Section of Sports Medicine
Department of Orthopaedic Surgery
Lahey Clinic
Burlington, Massachusetts

Lee A. Mancini, MD
Assistant Professor
Family Medicine and Community Health
University of Massachusetts Medical School
Worcester, Massachusetts

Timothy J. Marqueen, MD, VMD
Orthopaedic Surgeon
Colonial Orthopaedics
Colonial Heights, Virginia

Augustus D. Mazzocca, MS, MD
Assistant Professor
Department of Orthopaedic Surgery
University of Connecticut
Farmington, Connecticut

Suzanne L. Miller, MD
Clinical Instructor
Department of Orthopaedics
Tufts University
Orthopaedic Surgeon
New England Baptist Hospital
Boston, Massachusetts

Peter J. Millett, MD, MSc
Assistant Professor
Department of Orthopaedic Surgery
Harvard Medical School
Co-Director
Harvard Shoulder Service
Brigham and Women's Hospital
Massachusetts General Hospital
Boston, Massachusetts
Associate Surgeon
Steadman Hawkins Clinic
Vail, Colorado

Kevin A. Nadel, MD
Center for Orthopaedic Specialists
West Hills Hospital and Medical Center
West Hills, California

Robert J. Nicoletta, MD
Director, Total Sports Medicine
Department of Orthopaedic Surgery
Unity Health System
Rochester, New York

Adam C. Olsen, MPT, ATC
American Sports Medicine Institute
Physical Therapist
Champion Sports Medicine
Birmingham, Alabama

Daniel R. Orcutt, MD
Resident
Department of Orthopaedic Surgery
Geisinger Medical Center
Danville, Pennsylvania

Brett D. Owens, MD
Orthopaedic Surgeon
Orthopaedic Surgery Service
Keller Army Hospital
U.S. Military Academy
West Point, New York

Matthew A. Pecci, MD
Assistant Clinical Professor
Department of Family Medicine
Boston University School of Medicine
Director of Primary Care Sports Medicine
Department of Family Medicine
Boston Medical Center
Boston, Massachusetts

Derek Plausinis, MASc, MD, FRCSC
Shoulder and Elbow Surgery Fellow
Department of Orthopaedic Surgery
NYU–Hospital for Joint Diseases
New York, New York

Tamara K. Pylawka, BS, MS
Medical Student
Department of Orthopaedic Surgery
Rush Medical College
Chicago, Illinois

Michael M. Reinold, DPT, ATC, CSCS
Coordinator of Rehabilitative Research and Clinical
   Education
American Sports Medicine Institute
Coordinator of Rehabilitative Research and Clinical
   Education
Champion Sports Medicine
Birmingham, Alabama

Jeffrey A. Rihn, MD
Resident Physician
Department of Orthopaedic Surgery
University of Pittsburgh
Pittsburgh, Pennsylvania

Andrew S. Rokito, MD
Assistant Professor
Department of Orthopaedic Surgery
New York University
Chief, Shoulder and Elbow
Orthopaedic Surgery Service
Hospital for Joint Diseases
New York, New York

Anthony Schena, MD
Associate Professor
Department of Orthopaedics
Tufts University
Boston, Massachusetts
Staff Surgeon
Department of Orthopaedics
St. Elizabeth's Medical Center
Brighton, Massachusetts

Anthony A. Schepsis, MD
Professor
Department of Orthopaedic Surgery
Boston University School of Medicine
Director and Chief of Sports Medicine
Boston Medical Center
Boston, Massachusetts

Nicholas A. Sgaglione, MD
Associate Clinical Professor
Department of Orthopaedic Surgery
Albert Einstein College of Medicine
Bronx, New York
Chief, Division of Sports Medicine
Associate Chairman of Orthopaedics
North Shore University Hospital
Manhasset, New York

Beth E. Shubin Stein, MD
Instructor
Department of Orthopaedic Surgery
Weill Medical College
Cornell University
Assistant Attending Orthopaedic Surgeon
Sports Medicine and Shoulder Surgery
Hospital for Special Surgery
New York, New York

Abraham T. Shurland, MS, MD
Clinical Lecturer
Department of Orthopaedic Surgery
Tufts University School of Medicine
Boston, Massachusetts
Attending Physician
Orthopaedic Surgery Inc.
Melrose, Massachusetts

J. Herbert Stevenson, MD
Director, Sports Medicine Fellowship
Department Family and Community Medicine
University of Massachusetts Medical School
Fitchburg, Massachusetts
Director, Sports Medicine
Department Family and Community Medicine
UMass Memorial Medical Center
Worcester, Massachusetts

Jennifer Taniguchi, MD
Resident
Department of Orthopaedic Surgery
Boston University Medical Center
Boston, Massachusetts
Lahey Clinic
Burlington, Massachusetts

Ilya Voloshin, MD
Assistant Professor
Department of Orthopaedic Surgery
Boston University Medical Center
Boston, Massachusetts

Kevin E. Wilk, DPT
American Sports Medicine Institute
Founder and Clinical Director
Champion Sports Medicine
Birmingham, Alabama

Richard M. Wilk, MD
Assistant Professor
Department of Orthopaedic Surgery
Boston University School of Medicine
Boston, Massachusetts
Vice Chairman
Department of Orthopaedic Surgery
Lahey Clinic
Burlington, Massachusetts

John Woolf, MS, PT, ATC
Clinical Instructor
Department of Orthopaedic Surgery
University of Arizona
Tucson, Arizona

David Zijerdi, MD
Resident
Department of Orthopaedic Surgery
Geisinger Medical Center
Danville, Pennsylvania

Joseph D. Zuckerman, MD
Professor and Chairman
Department of Orthopaedic Surgery
New York University School of Medicine
Chairman and Surgeon in Chief
Department of Orthopaedic Surgery
NYU–Hospital for Joint Diseases
New York, New York

PREFACE

Sports medicine is an ever-changing and evolving field that encompasses many subspecialties. That being said, *Orthopaedic Surgery Essentials: Sports Medicine* will be valuable for many readers, including orthopaedic residents-in-training, primary care physicians with a special interest in sports medicine, and orthopaedic or family practice sports medicine fellows. Physician assistants, physical therapists, and athletic trainers, as well as any physician involved in the care of the athlete will find this volume beneficial as well. It is intended to serve as a comprehensive foundation of knowledge, provided in a quick, concise manner, and also as a guide for more focused and detailed reading in certain subject matters. Our aim is for the reader to have a solid base of comprehension of each subject as he or she proceeds through sports medicine training.

This volume is divided into five sections. Section I, Special Issues, begins with an essential basic science foundation and the pathophysiology of muscle, tendon, and ligament injuries. It considers the important subjects of preparticipation physical examination and drug use and abuse in sports. A chapter each is devoted to female, immature, and aging athletes. Also included within Section I are chapters from noted authorities regarding head and spinal injuries in athletes. Special chapters on stress fractures, soft tissue allografts, and arthroscopic surgery round out the section.

Section II, Medical Issues, concentrates on "nonorthopaedic" issues one might see in the sports medicine field, including internal medicine concerns, dermatologic conditions, and infectious diseases. Section III focuses on the upper extremity, particularly athletic injuries that involve the shoulder girdle and elbow, since hand and wrist injuries are covered in another volume in the *OSE* series. Section IV considers the lower extremity and includes pelvis, hip, thigh, knee, and lower leg injuries. The volume concludes with an important section on rehabilitation, strength training, and conditioning in sports medicine.

We would like to thank Robert Hurley and Eileen Wolfberg from Lippincott Williams & Williams, as well as Grace Caputo of Dovetail Content Solutions and Ashleigh McKown of Maryland Composition, for their invaluable assistance in making this publication possible.

Most importantly, we thank all of the contributing authors. Most of the senior authors of each chapter are noted authorities within the orthopaedic sports medicine field. The time and effort that they sacrifice from their busy practices and personal lives to make this publication possible are most appreciated.

Finally, we hope that you, the reader, find this volume helpful in building a foundation and expanding your knowledge in the ever-growing field of sports medicine.

SERIES PREFACE

Most of the available resources in orthopaedic surgery are very good, but they either present information exhaustively—so the reader has to wade through too many details to find what he or she seeks—or they assume too much knowledge, making the information difficult to understand. Moreover, as residency training has advanced, it has become more focused on the individual subspecialties. Our goal was to create a series at the basic level that residents could read completely during a subspecialty rotation to obtain the essential information necessary for a general understanding of the field. Once they have survived those trials, we hope that the *Orthopaedic Surgery Essentials* books will serve as a touchstone for future learning and review.

Each volume is to be a manageable size that can be read during a resident's tour. As a series, they will have a consistent style and template, with the authors' voices heard throughout. Content will be presented more visually than in most books on orthopaedic surgery, with a liberal use of tables, boxes, bulleted lists, and algorithms to aid in quick review. Each topic will be covered by one or more authorities, and each volume will be edited by experts in the broader field.

But most importantly, each volume—*Pediatrics, Spine, Sports Medicine,* and so on—will focus on the requisite knowledge in orthopaedics. Having the essential information presented in one user-friendly source will provide the reader with easy access to the basic knowledge needed in the field, and mastering this content will give him or her an excellent foundation for additional information from comprehensive references, atlases, journals, and on-line resources.

We would like to thank the editors and contributors who have generously shared their knowledge. We hope that the reader will take the opportunity of telling us what works and does not work.

—Paul Tornetta III, MD
—Thomas A. Einhorn, MD

PATHOPHYSIOLOGY OF MUSCLE, TENDON, AND LIGAMENT INJURIES

PAUL FADALE
ERIC BLUMAN
SCOTT ALLEN

SKELETAL MUSCLE

Embryology

Limb buds occur as early as the fourth week of development and consist of a core of mesenchyme covered by the apical ectodermal ridge. During limb bud growth, the proliferating mesenchyme gives rise to all of the skeletal rudiments. Myotome cells from the adjacent somites advance into the limb buds and give rise to the skeletal muscles. By the seventh week, distinct muscle formation has reached to the level of the hand and foot. The lower five cervical and first thoracic myotomes lie opposite the upper limb bud, whereas the second through fifth lumbar and upper three sacral myotomes lie opposite the lower limb bud. Branches of the spinal nerves that supply these myotomes reach the base of the limb bud and, as the bud elongates to form a true limb, the nerves grow into it.

After two months of development, establishment of neurocontacts with the developing skeletal muscle fibers will occur. This is critical for muscular development, with complete differentiation and function of the muscle fibers. Large motor neurons contact the developing motor fibers of the growing muscles and establish formation of the neuromuscular junctions. Voluntary control of skeletal muscle contraction is completed when myelination of the nerve fibers of the corticospinal tract is complete. Each muscle fiber is innervated by one nerve ending.

Normal Structure

Approximately 40% to 45% of the human body is composed of skeletal muscle. Skeletal muscle is a highly organized structure that is surrounded by well-defined fascial layers (Fig. 1-1). The individual muscle is surrounded completely by a fascial layer called the epimysium. From the epimysium, extensions of the surrounding fascia (perimysium) divide the muscle belly itself into multiple fascicles. Finally,

each fascicle is further subdivided into individual muscle fibers by the endomysium. The muscle fiber is the basic structural element of skeletal muscle. Skeletal muscle fibers range in size from 10 to 80 μm in diameter. Each muscle fiber is surrounded by a plasma membrane known as the sarcolemma. Immediately beneath the sarcolemma, along the periphery of the muscle fiber, are numerous cell nuclei. There can be several hundred nuclei for each centimeter of fiber length. Satellite cells lie along the surface of the muscle and are thought to be stem cells capable of regenerating muscle tissue in the event of injury. Individual fibers are made up of smaller subunits called myofibrils running the length of the muscle. At the end of the muscle fiber cell, membranes and collagen tissue collect into bundles to form muscle tendons. Muscle fibers are arranged either parallel or oblique to the long axis of the muscle. Oblique arrangements are commonly described as pennate, bipennate, multipennate, or fusiform.

Each muscle fiber is composed of hundreds to several thousand longitudinally oriented myofibrils. Myofibrils are composed of thick and thin protein filaments. The thick filaments (myosin) and the thin filaments (actin) provide the mechanical force during a muscle contraction by sliding past one another. In addition to myosin, the thick filaments are also made up of C-protein, M-protein, and titin. The thin filaments are anchored at one end by a protein structure called the Z-band, which is oriented at right angles to the filaments. These Z-bands occur at regular intervals along the length of the myofibrils and give skeletal muscle its striated appearance.

The sarcomere is the section of the myofibrils between two adjacent Z-bands (Fig. 1-2). Therefore, myofibrils are constructed of many sarcomeres linked end to end. Understanding the structure and function of the sarcomere is important because it is the basic unit of contraction. The sarcomere can be further divided into an A-band, which is a subunit containing the critical interdigitation of actin and

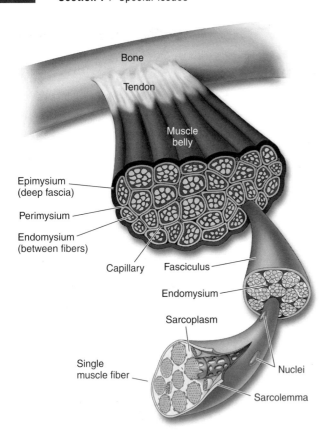

Figure 1-1 Macroscopic structure of skeletal muscle. (From McArdle WD, Katch FI, Katch VL. Essentials of Exercise Physiology, 2nd ed. Baltimore: Lippincott Williams & Wilkins, 2000.)

myosin filaments. In the middle of this A-band is the M-band, representing the middle portion of the thick filaments only. Another section, called the I-band, is made up of only actin; it does not interdigitate with the myosin molecules and therefore overlaps two successive sarcomeres where the actin molecules are anchored to the Z-bands. In the normal resting state, the thin filaments of the sarcomere are attached at either end to the Z-band and point toward one another. However, they do not touch or overlap. This creates a region in the middle of the sarcomere where the thick filaments are not overlapped by the thin filaments. This is called the H-zone.

The thick filaments are primarily composed of large proteins called myosin. On electron microscopic examination, these molecules look like long rods with two paddles attached at one end. These paddles are critical in forming the cross bridges between the thick and thin filaments. In a relaxed muscle, the paddles point toward the Z-bands. The actin in its normal state resides in the form of a double helix. Along the notches between the strands of actin are molecules of troponin and tropomyosin. These proteins enable calcium to regulate the contraction–relaxation cycle.

Elongation and growth of the muscle occur in both the muscle fibers and their associated tendons. Sarcomere length remains fixed throughout development. Additional sarcomeres are added to the muscle fibers to achieve longitudinal growth in the region of the musculotendinous junction.

The Motor Unit

Peripheral nerves enter skeletal muscle at the motor point. From there, the nerve cell axon branches many times. Skeletal muscle fibers are innervated by neurons entering the

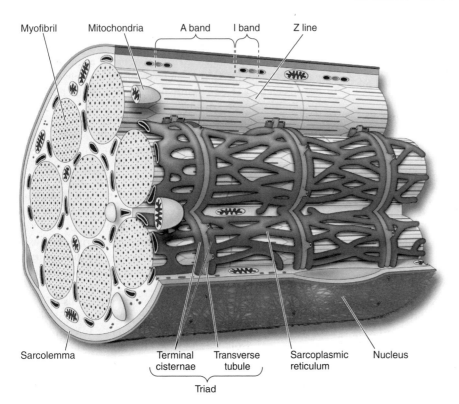

Figure 1-2 Microscopic structure of a skeletal muscle fiber. (From McArdle WD, Katch FI, Katch VL. Essentials of Exercise Physiology, 2nd ed. Baltimore: Lippincott Williams & Wilkins, 2000.)

muscle in a region called the endplate zone. The cell bodies of these neurons are located in the anterior horn of the spinal cord. Each motor neuron branches several times within the muscle and innervates a variable number of muscle fibers. However, each muscle fiber can be innervated by only one motor neuron. The motor unit is composed of a single motor neuron and all the muscle fibers it innervates. Muscle fiber type is related to its interaction with the singular motor nerve, as all muscle fibers in a single motor unit have the same metabolic and contractile properties (Fig. 1-3). The strength of a muscle contraction depends on the number of muscle fibers that are activated at the same time. As each motor neuron branches several times and innervates many muscle fibers, the central nervous system cannot activate a single muscle fiber, but most work through individual motor neurons in the activation of multiple muscle fibers comprising the motor unit. Therefore, the degree of control that is exerted on the strength of the muscle contraction in part depends on the number of muscle fibers comprising each motor unit that are activated. Powerful extremity muscles may contain more than 1,000 muscle fibers in each motor unit, whereas when fine control is required, the motor units may contain only a few muscle fibers. Smaller motor neurons usually innervate fewer muscle fibers and therefore have smaller motor units. Often, these neurons are activated first. If more power is needed, larger motor units are progressively recruited. This has been referred to as the size principle of motor control.

Different types of motor units—based on structural, metabolic, and functional variations—have been identified. Different classification schemes have been proposed. Muscles are able to function for a short time without oxygen by using the glycolytic pathway to generate adenosine triphosphate (ATP). Muscle fibers that generate high power over a short time have been called "fast-twitch," "white," or type II and make extensive use of this pathway. These muscle fibers release energy rapidly from ATP but regenerate energy stores slowly. Therefore, these muscles become easily fatigued. Fast-twitch motor units are generally larger and generate more strength. They have higher enzymatic activity for the phosphagen and glycolytic systems and are used predominantly during activities dependent on anaerobic energy. Type II motor units can be further subdivided. Most commonly, two main subgroups are considered. Type IIB motor units (or fast glycolytic motor units) have the fastest contraction time and are the least resistant to fatigue. This motor unit has the largest number of muscle fibers, the largest axon, and the largest cell body. Type IIA motor units are considered to be in between type I and type IIB groups. Contraction times and fatigue resistance profiles are between type I and type IIB, as both the oxidative and glycolytic pathways are well developed. Motor unit size is also intermediate. In contrast, muscle fibers that are active over a long period of time are considered "slow-twitch," "red," or type I. These fibers are rich in mitochondria and have a greater oxidative aerobic capacity. Type I motor units are resistant to fatigue. These motor units are often small and used in fine manipulations. In addition, they are the first fibers activated when lower levels of power are required.

Athletes have a special interest in knowing their distribution of motor unit types. Variations in muscle fiber type between individuals are common. A preponderance of one type over another may lead to a greater chance of success in a given sport. For example, power athletes or sprinters should benefit from higher concentrations of fast-twitch fibers within their muscles, whereas distance runners would benefit from having predominantly type I fibers. It is believed that the distribution of muscle fibers in any one individual is determined genetically. However, there is evidence for interconversion between type IIA and type IIB fibers. Certainly, during training, there is selective recruitment of the appropriate fibers that are best suited for specific athletic demands.

Muscle Contraction

Motor nerves to the motor unit are generally large, myelinated fibers. The nerve forms a synapse with the muscle at a specialized region known as the motor endplate (Fig. 1-4). Transmission of the impulse is not achieved by direct electrical transmission but requires a chemical transmission at the motor endplate. At the end of the neuron, there are fingerlike projections found between the membranes of the nerve and the muscle. These primary synaptic folds act to increase the area of membrane interaction between the nerve and muscle. The nerve terminal is rich in mitochondria and contains many synaptic vesicles that contain the neurotransmitter acetylcholine. The presynaptic and postsynaptic membranes are separated by a small (50 nm) synaptic cleft. In the muscle membrane are junctional folds containing acetylcholine receptors that mediate the action of the neurotransmitter and acetylcholinesterase, which acts to destroy the neurotransmitter.

When the motor neuron is stimulated, electrical impulses are propagated along the axon toward the neuromuscular junction. When the action potential arrives at the motor unit, the depolarization opens up calcium channels in the

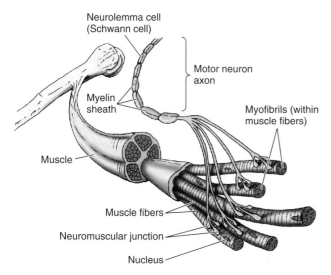

Figure 1-3 Structure of a skeletal muscle and a motor unit. The aggregate of a motor neuron axon and all muscle fibers innervated by it constitute a motor unit. (From Moore KL, Agur A. Essential Clinical Anatomy, 2nd ed. Philadelphia: Lippincott Williams & Wilkins, 2002.)

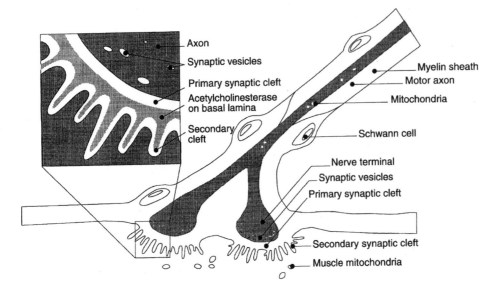

Figure 1-4   The motor endplate. (From Woo SL-Y, An KN, Frank CB, et al. Anatomy, biology, and biomechanics of tendon and ligament. In Buckwalter JA, Einhorn TA, Simon SR, eds. Orthopaedic Basic Science, 2nd ed. Rosemont, IL: American Academy of Orthopaedic Surgeons, 2000:581–616.)

axon terminal. This results in calcium becoming concentrated in the presynaptic nerve terminal. The sudden increase in the calcium concentration causes the vesicles to fuse with the terminal axon membrane and results in the release of acetylcholine into the synaptic cleft. This acetylcholine passes across this cleft and binds to a receptor molecule on the postsynaptic membrane. This results in the opening of channels to permit the influx of sodium ions and the efflux of potassium ions. The net effect is the depolarization of the muscle membrane and triggering of the muscle action potential. The acetylcholine is then rapidly hydrolyzed and deactivated by the enzyme acetylcholinesterase into choline and acetate. Breakdown products are then reabsorbed into the terminal axon to be used in the resynthesis of a new transmitter.

Pharmacologic manipulation of the neuromuscular junction is possible. Severe muscle weakness in the disease myasthenia gravis is the result of a shortage of acetylcholine receptors. Inhibition of the acetylcholinesterase enzyme with neostigmine and edrophonium can allow the acetylcholine molecules to have a longer life and a better chance to interact with receptors before they are broken down. Impulse transmission can be blocked by Curare, which binds to the acetylcholine receptors. Succinylcholine produces muscle relaxation by keeping the acetylcholine channels open for too long a period of time. This keeps the muscle membrane depolarized and refractory to further impulse initiation.

The muscle action potential is propagated along the entire length of the muscle fiber. Between the adjacent myofibrils are elements of the conducting pathway, called the sarcoplasmic reticulum-transverse tubule system. The T-tubules are internal extensions of the cell membrane, oriented perpendicular to the long axis of the cell and bring the action potential into the interior of the muscle fiber. These often lie at the level of the A- and I-band junctions. Calcium ions are held in high concentrations in the sarcoplasmic reticulum. When the adjacent T-tubule system is excited by a muscle action potential, calcium ions are released into the muscle cytoplasm and diffuse to the nearby

myofibrils. There, they bind strongly to troponin. This results in structural changes that allow actin to bind to the myosin cross bridges. This binding elicits a muscle contraction as ATP is hydrolyzed by myosin and the thick filaments slide past the thin filaments. The cross-bridging cycle occurs many times as the thick filaments release from the actin on the thin filament, return to their original configuration, create another cross bridge with conformational changes, and further shorten the muscle fiber (Fig. 1-5). This process may occur in rapid succession. The thick filaments pull toward each other and toward the center of the A-band, and the sarcomeres shorten or resist stretch. During a muscle contraction, the angle between the cross bridges and the rod portion of the myosin becomes more acute. This has been described as the sliding filament-swinging cross-bridges theory of muscle contraction. The sarcoplasmic reticulum contains a calcium pump that removes the calcium from the myofibrils at the end of a single contraction. When calcium is no longer available, tropomyosin undergoes a conformational change, thus preventing further cross-bridge formation.

Biomechanics

The tension response by muscle to a single nerve stimulus is called a muscle twitch. If a second contraction is elicited before the first one has relaxed, a stronger contraction results. As the stimulation frequency increases, the tension in the muscle also increases. When the frequency of activation is high enough, a continuous contraction (tetanus) will result. Involving more motor units can also increase the force of muscle contraction. This has been termed "recruitment." To increase the overall strength of muscle contraction, both the frequency of activation and the recruitment of more motor units are required.

The tension a muscle can generate is also dependent on the length of that muscle when the contraction begins. The Blix curve describes this important muscle length–tension relationship (Fig. 1-6). When a muscle is at its normal rest-

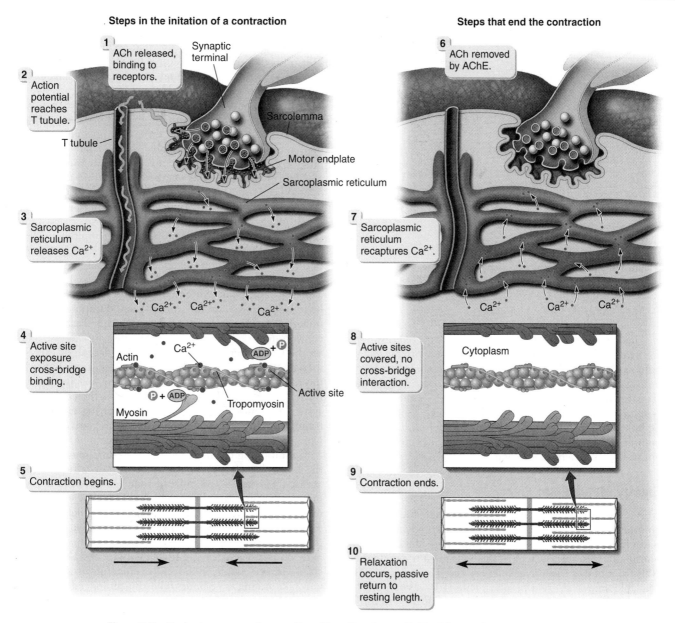

Figure 1-5 Excitation–contraction coupling. (From Premkumar K. The Massage Connection, Anatomy and Physiology, 2nd ed. Baltimore: Lippincott Williams & Wilkins, 2004.)

ing state and length, there is maximal overlap of the thick and thin filaments. This maximal overlap allows for the creation of maximum cross-bridging tension to be developed. Once a muscle is in a contracted position, the thin actin filaments impede one another. This interferes with cross bridging and effectively reduces the maximum tension that can be created. Conversely, stretching the muscle out to a point where the filaments have minimal cross-bridging contact also results in a weak muscle contraction. The maximum amount of force produced by a muscle is proportional to its cross-sectional area. Also, the total amount and speed of muscle shortening is proportional to the individual muscle fiber length.

Muscle contraction and function can be studied in different ways. An isometric contraction (same length) occurs when the muscle length is held constant and the resultant force is measured. In an isotonic contraction (same load), the muscle is activated to shorten against a constant load while muscle length changes with time are measured. Muscle can also be evaluated under isokinetic activation (same speed), in which the load accommodates to maintain a constant velocity of shortening or lengthening. When a muscle is activated, shortening of the sarcomeres results in force generation. The muscle will shorten (concentric action) if the resisting load is less than the force generated by the muscle. Conversely, the muscle will lengthen (eccentric action) if the resisting force is greater than that generated by the muscle. Muscles that are stimulated eccentrically can produce more work than muscles that are activated concentrically. No motion will occur if the forces are equal.

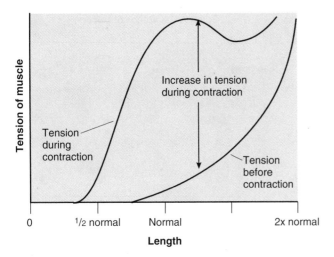

Figure 1-6 Blix curve length-tension diagram for a single sarcomere. (After Guyton AC. Textbook of Medical Physiology, 7th ed. Philadelphia: WB Saunders, 1986:128.)

The force generated by a muscle is transmitted through the myotendinous junction before integration into the distal tendon. This is a region of highly folded membranes, which increases the contact area and decreases stress. In this area, stresses are changed from tensile to shear. A well-developed basement membrane allows the muscle force generated to be linked to the collagen fibers of the tendon. Fibronectin, laminin, and type IV collagen are among the proteins present in the basement membrane.

Energy Metabolism

ATP is the immediate source of energy needed for muscle contraction. Once ATP is broken down into adenosine diphosphate (ADP)/adenosine monophosphate and inorganic phosphate(s) to release energy, the body must re-create the ATP from one of three available sources. The most readily available source is creatine phosphate (CP). When enzymatically broken down, the energy released is used to form ATP again:

$$ADP + CP + \text{creatine kinase} \rightarrow ATP + CP$$

This reaction is primarily used in high-intensity, short-duration activities such as sprinting, because the amount of energy available is limited. CP cannot be used directly by the muscle cells as a source of energy. Some athletes have used oral creatine supplementation in an attempt to maximize CP levels that may then promote greater muscle hypertrophy from resistance training.

Anaerobic glycolysis utilizing the hydrolysis of glucose is the second source of energy. Glucose is metabolized and releases energy to convert ADP to ATP, as well as forming lactic acid as a byproduct. Lactic acid buildup causes the symptoms of fatigue. This inefficient system is a limited source of energy and is used by the muscle when a lot of energy is needed for a relatively short period of time.

Aerobic glycolysis occurs when glycogen or triglycerides are completely broken down to carbon dioxide and water in the presence of oxygen. This process occurs in the mito-

chondria of the muscle cells. It is responsible for releasing the large amounts of energy needed for ATP resynthesis. A single molecule of glucose can yield 34 molecules of ATP. This is an excellent energy source for prolonged endurance type of activities. The amount of oxygen available to the cell is the limiting factor. Athletes whose diets are rich in carbohydrate have higher stores of glycogen and therefore may benefit from a higher energy production (carbohydrate loading). For most individuals, fat storage provides an abundant source of energy. Breakdown of free fatty acids can provide sufficient energy to convert large amounts of ADP to ATP. These fatty acids can be found within the muscle or mobilized from adipose tissue. It is unlikely that availability is a limiting factor in energy metabolism.

Although energy metabolism has been broken down into separate systems, most often, they occur simultaneously to provide working muscles the energy required for the formation of ATP. The different motor unit types have varying levels of enzymes required for both aerobic and anaerobic capacity. The body will emphasize the appropriate metabolic system based on the intensity and duration of activity undertaken. This variation has been described as the energy continuum. For example, brief high-intensity exercise relies on the CP system. If intensity falls and length of exercise increases, the anaerobic system is used more to replenish the required ATP. If the exercise intensity falls further and the length of activity continues to increase, then the aerobic system becomes most efficient for supplying energy. The training an athlete performs can significantly influence which pathways are chosen.

Conditioning has been described as the time it takes for the body to return to its pre-exercise state after vigorous activity. The lactic acid must be removed from the muscle, muscle glycogen must be replenished, phosphagen and ATP must be restored, and the remaining oxygen debt must be eliminated. Athletes benefit from warming down after competition because light exercise hastens the removal of the built-up lactic acid. Lost muscle glycogen can be resynthesized within a couple of hours after moderate exercise, but it may take as long as 48 hours following prolonged endurance activity. Muscle phosphagen store replacement occurs rather quickly. Oxygen debt recovery requires replenishing myoglobin with oxygen in the aerobic recovery of phosphagen stores, as well as recovery from the oxygen debt needed to assist the conversion of lactic acid. Conditioning can shorten all recovery times.

Response to Hormones

Hormonal manipulation of muscle has become a well-known concern in the sporting community. Insulin is a hormone secreted by the pancreas for the regulation of metabolism of food products. This hormone is considered anabolic because it increases glucose entry into the muscle cell and increases glycogen synthesis. Amino acid uptake is increased, resulting in protein synthesis, and protein catabolism is decreased. These effects are synergistic with growth hormone. Glucocorticoids oppose these actions by accelerating protein degradation and increasing the resulting amino acid release. Growth hormone, a product of the pituitary gland, increases amino acid transport into the muscle cell and stimulates protein synthesis, which results in increased muscle synthesis. Growth hormone also reduces glucose and protein metabolism by shifting metabolism toward the use of fatty acids. Synthetic human growth hormone has led to its increasing use as an anabolic agent. Testosterone has the main anabolic effect on muscle tissue. It increases protein synthesis while decreasing the rate of protein catabolism within the muscle. This results in an increase of the muscle size, weight, and strength. Another effect of testosterone is the expression of male sexual characteristics, including increased hair growth, voice deepening, and genital enlargement. Anabolic steroids were developed to decrease these "unwanted" characteristics. The benefit of these compounds to athletes has been to increase strength with an associated improvement in anaerobic performance. Although controversy remains in the medical literature on the effectiveness and safety of these compounds, competing athletes worldwide understand the possible gains in strength that are possible when used in conjunction with high-intensity exercise and an appropriate supporting diet.

Common Clinical Conditions

Muscle Training

Strength and Endurance Training
- Muscles have the capacity to respond significantly to both increasing and decreasing stimulation.
  - Atrophy may be quick and profound when appropriate stimulation of the muscle is removed.
  - Conversely, a progressively increasing resistance training program can result in significant muscle hypertrophy and strength gains.
  - This hypertrophy is more commonly seen in type II fibers than in type I fibers.
  - At the present time, it is still unknown whether this hypertrophy is the result of an increase in the size of the muscle fibers or an increased number of muscle fibers.
  - Either will result in an increasing amount of contractile proteins available.
- Strength training also improves the capacity for motor unit recruitment.
  - Untrained individuals may have as little as 60% of their muscle fibers firing simultaneously.
  - With an aggressive muscle strengthening program, greater than 90% of the muscle fibers become active.
  - With an increased capacity for motor unit recruitment and increased number of available contractile units, the targeted muscle will show increased strength and work capacity.
- A generalized recommendation for improving strength is to stress a muscle against a high resistance so that only several repetitions are possible before failure.
  - These high-intensity exercises often last less than a minute and rely on the CP/anaerobic glycolysis systems for ATP formation.
  - Highly conditioned athletes may have increased levels of stored phosphagens.
  - Conversely, training for endurance would require a lower muscle resistance so that many repetitions are required before muscle failure.
  - The critical point for endurance training is the appropriate supply of energy rather than hypertrophy of the muscle.
  - The cardiovascular system must supply enough oxygen to the muscles to allow the aerobic metabolism system to provide energy continually for the formulation of ATP.
  - The density of mitochondria within the muscle increases.
  - As the time of training progresses past 2 hours, fatty acids replace glycogen as the main fuel source.

Muscle Soreness
- Delayed-onset muscle soreness (DOMS) is common within 2 to 3 days after new or increased levels of exercise.
  - This is often associated with eccentric exercise.
- Clinically, athletes complain of soreness, swelling, stiffness, and weakness within the affected muscles after a particularly intense workout.
- Often, this will resolve itself within a couple of days, but if the insult to the muscle is severe enough, the soreness may last for 1 to 2 weeks.
- As the muscle adapts and responds to this level of stress, the occurrence of DOMS stops.
  - However, when the muscle is again pushed to new levels of stress, the DOMS may occur again.
- It is believed that the soreness is the result of intramuscular damage to the structural elements of the muscle.
  - Histologic analysis reveals Z-band streaming, A-band disruption, and malalignment of the myofibrils.
  - Fast-twitch type IIB fibers are most at risk.
  - There is associated connective tissue breakdown.
  - Most important, this injury is reversible.
- Some athletes will use this sense of DOMS as a guide to their training routine.
  - The theory is that the involved muscles become stronger and more resistant to damage from the initial inciting level of stress.
  - This adaptation allows for further muscle strengthening as the fragile fibers are replaced by stronger fibers that can resist further levels of stress.
  - Once there is no more muscle soreness, muscle growth slows, and a new level of stress is required to produce further muscle hypertrophy.

Cramping
- Some athletes are at risk for muscle cramps, and others appear to be immune.
  - The exact reason is unknown.
- The pathophysiology of muscle cramps is poorly understood.
- It appears that the muscle cramps are initiated from the motor nerves once they enter the affected muscle.
- The cramped muscle usually becomes symptomatic when it is in a shortened position.
- Unexpectedly, there will be a powerful and painful active contraction of the muscle.

- Usually, this can be interrupted by a forceful stretch of the affected muscle into an elongated resting position.
- Afterward, however, the muscle may remain with altered excitability.
- Athletes at risk often show fatigue from prolonged muscle use or dehydration.
- Treatment includes aggressive hydration, electrolyte replacement, stretching, and acclimatization.

Stretching

- Muscle stretching is part of nearly every exercise program.
- Proposed benefits of stretching include improved performance and reduced injury risk.
- The diminished stiffness and increased range of motion seen after stretching can be explained by the viscoelastic properties of the muscle.
- The tension developed in a stretched muscle diminishes over time, resulting in stress relaxation.
- Most stretching programs recommend a slow static stretching of the muscle.
- Ballistic movements should be avoided.
- This allows the electrical activity within the muscle to be quiescent and the stretching to be unopposed.

Muscle Injury

Muscle Strains

- Muscle strains are among the most common injuries sustained by athletic individuals.
- Rather than direct trauma, excessive force along the muscle can result in an anatomic disruption in the region of the musculotendinous junction.
  - Most commonly, this is from a significant eccentric muscle contraction.
- Muscle sarcomeres within a few millimeters of this junction appear more stiff than their more proximal counterparts and therefore at higher risk for failure.
- Incomplete tears are most commonly seen.
- Muscles that cross two joints appear clinically to be more at risk for this injury.
  - These include the lower-extremity hamstring, rectus femoris, and gastrocnemius muscles.
  - These muscles appear to have an increased length of their musculotendinous junction.
- Muscle healing has been described as occurring in three distinct phases.
  - Initially, there is inflammation with necrosis of the damaged muscle.
    - This allows for phagocytosis of the necrotic debris.
  - The second phase is characterized by protein synthesis from activation of the satellite cells that are myogenic precursors.
    - These cells differentiate into myotubules and muscle fibers.
  - In the last or final phase, there is maturation or remodeling of the repair tissue with a gradual return of the muscles' functional properties.
- Pharmacologic manipulation of this healing process with either oral anti-inflammatory medication or intra-

muscular corticosteroid injection has yielded conflicting results.
- Use of ultrasound as a therapeutic soft-tissue modality has also been tried.

Contusion

- Contusion is a common sports-related injury that can vary widely in its resulting symptomatology.
- In response to a blunt injury, a localized hematoma occurs and an inflammatory reaction begins.
- This repair process is regulated by growth factors and cytokines.
- The magnitude of these events is directly related to the level of trauma.
- Necrotic tissue is removed, and new muscle fibers are formed as myotubes fuse into mature muscle cells.
- Both muscle regeneration and scar occur at the site of injury.
- Although the injured athlete will place the injured muscle in a shortened and relaxed position to decrease pain, this may hamper recovery and delay rehabilitation because of the resulting muscle shortening and stiffness.
- Gentle mobilization of the muscle may result in a faster recovery of tensile strength.
- If the soft-tissue injury is severe enough, or if there is a history of previous muscle contusions, bone formation may occur in the muscle belly (myositis ossificans).
  - This condition may mimic osteogenic sarcoma.

Laceration

- Laceration of the muscle belly perpendicular to the long axis of the muscle results in denervation of the distal segment.
- Necrotic muscle at the injury site is removed by macrophages.
- New muscle cells appear from surrounding satellite cells forming myoblasts and muscle fibers.
- At the same time, there is a proliferation of connective tissue.
- This connective tissue fills the void left by the laceration and interferes with the ability of the muscle to return to its normal anatomic state.
- Therefore, recovery from a laceration is dependent on the magnitude of injury and relative location from nerve innervation.

Atrophy

- Immobilization results in muscle atrophy.
- Initially, there is significant and rapid muscle wasting with atrophy of the muscle fibers.
- The rate of protein synthesis in the muscle decreases within hours.
  - However, after this initial stage, the rate of loss lessens.
- Less cross-sectional muscle mass equates with less strength.
- Work capacity decreases and muscle fatigue increases with any applied stress.
- These changes are related to the length at which the muscle is immobilized.

- If a muscle is immobilized under some tension, these atrophic changes will be less than if the muscle is immobilized under no tension.
- This common clinical condition is seen in the lower extremity where an injured knee is braced in extension, placing the quadriceps mechanism under no tension and a hamstring musculature under tension.
- Quadriceps atrophy is seen to be greater than hamstring atrophy.
- Immobilized muscles also respond differently to passive stretch.
- If a muscle is immobilized in a shortened position, it will develop more tension in response to passive stretch.
- If the immobilized muscle is held in a lengthened position, it will develop less tension in response to passive stretch.

Malignant Hyperthermia

Malignant hyperthermia is an autosomal dominant abnormality of muscle. This process must be understood by orthopaedic surgeons because it most commonly develops after the administration of general anesthesia, although it may be triggered by other stimuli. During childhood, men and women appear to be equally at risk, but with advancing age, men appear more at risk. The peak incidence occurs at around 30 years of age. The pathophysiology of this disease appears to involve an abnormality in calcium transport of the cell membranes of the sarcoplasmic reticulum and mitochondria. A triggering event precipitates a leak of calcium from the sarcoplasmic reticulum resulting in a sustained actin–myosin combination that causes continued contraction and muscle rigidity. This results in the production of heat, metabolic acidosis, and carbon dioxide production with resulting respiratory acidosis. Protein denaturation results in a coagulopathy. If not appropriately treated, this process can result in death.

Diagnosis and Treatment

- An accurate history of family or personal anesthetic problems is the best method for preventing this disease.
  - However, a malignant hyperthermia event does not necessarily occur with the first exposure to anesthesia.
- Susceptible patients also tend to be healthy and athletic with large muscle masses.
- A history of leg cramping at night and exercise intolerance in hot weather may also provide insight into a possible at-risk individual.
- Conclusive testing can be achieved by muscle biopsy.
- Careful intraoperative monitoring is critical for the management of this disease.
- Early warning signs are nonspecific but include tachycardia, possible ventricular arrhythmias, and an unstable blood pressure.
- More worrisome is the finding of a combined respiratory and metabolic acidosis.
- Increasing temperatures of 1°C or more requires further investigation.
- If malignant hyperthermia is suspected, the surgical procedure and anesthetic are terminated as rapidly as possible.

- Medical management includes dantrolene sodium, which inhibits calcium release from the sarcoplasmic reticulum.
- Acidosis is corrected by hyperventilation with oxygen.
- Sodium bicarbonate may be required.
- Fluid management and a diuretic may be required to maintain urine output, which is important to clear away the products of muscle degradation.
- Accumulation of these degradation products could lead to renal damage.
- Surface cooling with an ice bag and cold intravenous fluids may also be helpful.

Compartment Syndromes

A rising pressure within a closed fascial space or muscle compartment defines a compartment syndrome. This rising pressure results in a reduced muscle capillary blood flow that is required for tissue viability. The local ischemia produced must be relieved by surgical decompression of the muscle compartment to prevent permanent muscle and nerve necrosis. Muscle microcirculation is compromised at tissue pressures of approximately 30 to 40 mm Hg. Practitioners must understand that the central arterial blood flow through the pathologic compartment is typically normal and results in normal peripheral pulses. In the right setting, one must be vigilant of the potential for this process to occur. Compartment syndromes are commonly described as occurring in two distinct clinical settings: the first with acute trauma resulting in immediate and unrelenting compartment swelling with the resulting compromise of capillary function and muscle/nerve necrosis, and the second in overuse situations (such as found in endurance athletes, where there are early symptoms related to microcirculatory embarrassment without serious progression and necrosis).

Diagnosis and Treatment
Acute Compartment Syndrome

- The first and most important symptom of an acute impending compartment syndrome is pain that is greater than would be expected from the primary problem.
- Pain with passive stretch of the muscles in the involved compartment is a common finding.
- Palpation of the involved compartment will often show greater than expected swelling and tenseness.
- Nerve ischemia manifests itself early on by an alteration of sensation.
- Most commonly, the patient will complain of paresthesia in the nerve distribution of the involved compartment.
- If untreated, this will be followed by a decreased sensation and then anesthesia in the nerve distribution. These are late findings.
- Even with a full-blown compartment syndrome, distal pulses are almost always palpable and normal unless there is a concomitant vascular injury.
  - Normal distal pulses therefore do not rule out a compartment syndrome.
- Many studies have been performed to help identify an exact compartment pressure measurement in which a compartment syndrome exists.

- The basic underlying premise is that, when compartment pressure measurements exceed 30 to 40 mm Hg, the microcirculation to that compartment will be occluded and nutrition to the soft-tissue structures will stop.
- Given the sometimes inaccurate and potentially poorly reproducible compartment pressure measurements, any patient with an appropriate clinical history and physical examination for a progressing compartment syndrome with impending permanent tissue damage should be considered for surgical decompression.

Chronic Compartment Syndrome

- Chronic or recurrent exertional compartment syndromes may be more common than acute compartment syndromes and are more difficult to accurately diagnose.
- Commonly, athletes will present with diffuse pain or aching over the anterior or lateral aspect of their lower leg.
- This pain is usually related to prolonged exercise, and it may be severe enough to cause the athlete to stop or reduce exercise.
- Symptoms may be unilateral or bilateral.
- Subjective complaints should be validated with objective elevated compartment pressure measurements to make this diagnosis.
- Sometimes these patients may have higher resting compartment pressures.
- To establish this diagnosis, athletes must have an abnormal pressure elevation during exercise and a slower return to their resting value at the end of the exercise.
    - Recommended pressure measurements for the diagnosis of chronic exertional compartment syndrome include a resting pressure higher than 12 mm Hg and a 1-minute recovery pressure above 30 mm Hg.
    - Also, diagnostic is if the 5-minute postexercise pressures are elevated above 20 mm Hg.
- Every effort should be made to pursue conservative management of this patient population.
- Anti-inflammatory medication, cross training, relative rest, rehabilitation, massage, soft-tissue release, and orthotics should be considered.
- Surgery should be considered only if an extended period of conservative management does not improve the athlete's symptoms.
- The physician must make sure that there are no other causes for the patient's subjective complaints.
- Elective fasciotomy of the involved compartments should then be considered.
- Appropriate realistic preoperative counseling is mandatory.

Tetanus

Tetanus is a potentially fatal disease caused by the exotoxin produced by *Clostridium tetani*. Tetanus is characterized by generalized skeletal muscle rigidity and convulsive spasms. It can occur after spores or vegetative bacteria gain access to injured tissue and produce the toxin locally. Because *C. tetani* is a noninvasive organism, the usual mode of entry is through a puncture wound or cut on an extremity during an athletic event. It is anticipated that extremity wounds are frequently contaminated with these spores, but the clinical manifestations of tetanus rarely develop. This is because the germination of spores occurs only when the oxygen tension is much lower than that of normal tissue. Toxin production in wounds is favored by necrotic tissue, foreign bodies, and associated infections that establish a low oxidation-reduction potential. The toxin produced may be transported to the central nervous system. There, the tetanus toxin attacks synaptic junctions to produce disinhibition. This results in generalized muscle rigidity from uninhibited afferent stimuli.

Diagnosis and Treatment

- The time between injury and the appearance of clinical manifestations is usually 14 days or less.
- Commonly, patients will present with complaints of pain and stiffness of the jaw, abdomen, or back.
- Swallowing may be difficult.
- Trismus (lockjaw) is the most common early manifestation of tetanus.
- Sustained contractions of the facial muscles produced a characteristic expression, termed *risus sardonicus*.
- As the disease progresses, minimal stimuli produce a more intense and longer lasting spasm.
- Respiration may be impaired.
- The diagnosis of tetanus is a clinical one.
- It is not dependent on bacteriologic confirmation, as cultures are positive in less than 50% of patients.
- Involved patients should be hospitalized and treated with tetanus prophylaxis, antibiotics, surgical debridement of the wounds, and administration of muscle relaxants, as well as generalized supportive measures.

TENDONS

Embryology

The embryological study of tendon development must be still considered to be in its infancy. Relatively little is known about the embryogenesis of tendons, compared with other musculoskeletal tissues such as muscle, cartilage, and bone. Tendons, like muscles, originate from mesoderm. More specifically, they arise from the lateral plate mesoderm. Although intimately functionally connected when mature, muscle and tendon are able to develop autonomously. One of the earliest steps in tendon embryogenesis is the formation of a mesenchymal lamina along the ectodermal basement membrane. Precursor cells then condense on the dorsal and ventral sides of this mesenchymal lamina to form the anlage that will eventually become the flexor and extensor tendons of the adjacent joints. Interestingly, although tendons are developmentally autonomous, subsequent muscle–tendon interaction is required to prevent tendon degeneration. Because tendons attain size and strength relative to the muscle mass and distance from insertion during growth and development, it is believed that tenocytes are responsive to the magnitude and direction of the load. Although the exact mechanism remains unknown, investigators have shown that isolated tendon fibroblasts respond to mechanical strains placed upon them. The role of specific proteins and the required pattern of expression for normal tendon development are just beginning to be elucidated.

Structure

Tendons link the motor units (muscles) to the bones so that joint motion is possible. They are generally cylindrical in shape with slight widening and flattening at the musculotendinous junction and their bony insertion. Notable exceptions are the rotator cuff tendons and pectoralis muscle tendons, which are flat and platelike at their insertions.

The predominant cell in tendons is the fibroblast. These fusiform cells are responsible for the production and maintenance of collagen and other proteins that confer the flexibility and tensile strength of tendons. Collagen is by far the largest constituent of tendons. Almost 90% of the dry weight is accounted for by collagen. Tendons are primarily composed of type I collagen, but they also contain small amounts of type III, type IV, type V, and type VI collagen. The primary structure of collagen is a three-amino acid residue-repeating pattern. Glycine is present every third amino acid on average, whereas proline and hydroxyproline each make up 15% of the molecule.

Proteoglycans are also present with decorin predominating, but biglycan, lumican, and fibromodulin have also been detected. Decorin is a sulfate-rich proteoglycan. Studies have shown it to bind collagen together along the length of fibrils, much in the way a rubber band holds a bunch of pencils together. It is believed to aid in the formation of the collagen fibrils. It has been postulated that decorin regulates fibril diameter, halting further accumulation past a certain point.

Proteoglycans are thought to regulate collagen fiber diameter, separate individual fiber bundles, and minimize the shear stresses fibers experience as they move relative to each other during normal function. Although tendons function under predominantly tensile loads, they do experience compressive loads as they pass around skeletal prominences and pulleys. Some of the pressures experienced in these regions are substantial, with measurements being reported in the range of 700 mm Hg. Glycosaminoglycan (specifically aggrecan) content in these regions is elevated relative to the rest of the tendon. This is probably a functional adaptation allowing for greater water content and resultant structural resiliency under compressive conditions.

The metabolic organization through which tendons maintain and repair themselves is just beginning to be understood. Although tenocytes initially appear to be spatially distinct within the matrix of the tendon, like osteocytes, they possess very long processes that form gap junctions to facilitate communications with other cells in their locale.

The microarchitecture of a tendon is hierarchical (Fig. 1-7). Microfibrils make up subfibrils which, in turn, make up fibrils. There are hundreds of these fibrils within each fascicle. It is these fascicles that make up the tendon itself. These fascicles are separated from one another by the endotenon. The endotenon is made of longitudinally oriented adventitia that is cell-poor. On the surface, and adherent to the tendon proper, is the epitenon. This diaphanous layer is composed of fibroblasts one to two cell layers thick.

Paratenon and Blood Supply

The blood supply to tendons is paramount in their healing and maintenance. This supply is from three sources: the perimysium, the periosteal insertion of the tendon, and the paratenon. The paratenon is, in turn, supplied by the surrounding tissues. Flexor tendons of the hand and wrist also have an additional blood supply. This is the mesotenon,

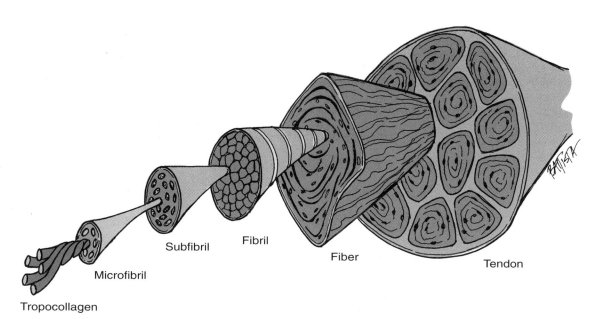

Microfibril

Subfibril

Fibril

Fiber

Tendon

Tropocollagen

Figure 1-7 Structural composition of ligament and tendon. (From Oatis CA. Kinesiology: The Mechanics and Pathomechanics of Human Movement. Baltimore: Lippincott Williams & Wilkins, 2004.)

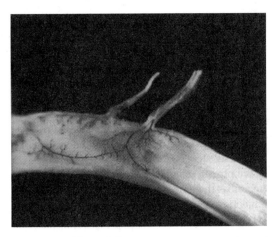
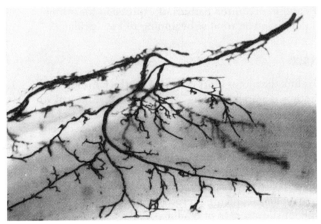

Figure 1-8   India ink preparation of vincula and blood supply to tendon. (From Garrett WE, Best TM. Anatomy, physiology, and mechanics of skeletal muscle. In: Buckwalter JA, Einhorn TA, Simon SR, eds. Orthopaedic Basic Science, 2nd ed. Rosemont, IL: American Academy of Orthopaedic Surgeons, 2000:683–716.)

which is condensed into the vincula on digital flexor tendons (Fig. 1-8).

Blood vessels are located within the epitenon and endotenon. The blood supply of the digital flexor tendons has been best studied. Blood is supplied in a segmental manner from four sources:

1. Intrinsic longitudinal vessels that are continuous with those in the palmar region of the tendon
2. Synovial folds in the proximal reflection of the tendon sheath
3. Vincula
4. Osseous insertions of the tendons

Both perfusion and diffusion contribute to nourishing the tendon. Avascular regions are believed to be supplied by diffusion.

Entheses

An enthesis is an insertion site and has been used to refer to locations where tendon, ligament, and joint capsules attach to bones. These are not just locations where these structures plug into bones, but rather highly organized tissues that prevent local stress concentration between two interfaces. Because tendon and bone have differing elastic moduli, transmission of a certain level of force across their junction would result in a stress concentration and possible damage to either or both tissues. Entheses have developed to dissipate stress away from these junctions.

Much of the function of the enthesis is performed by increasing the surface area of tendon insertion. If the area of an enthesis is too small, the stress generated by the tendon will be concentrated in a small area with resultant avulsion of the tendon from bone. To counteract this, many tendons fan out at their attachment sites (e.g., tibialis posterior tendon, which has attachment sites on all the bones of the tarsus, except the talus, and the proximal second, third, and fourth metatarsals). In addition to their morphology, entheses have unique compositions to aid in force dissipation at the tendon–bone interface. Traditionally, entheses

have been divided into two groups according to the character of their tissue at the tendon–bone interface. Generally, in the limbs, *fibrous* entheses are present at junctions located at the diaphyses of bone, whereas *fibrocartilaginous* entheses are typical of epiphyses or apophyses.

Sharpey's fibers are the perforating fibers that are present in fibrous entheses that anchor tendons to bone. Fibrous entheses can be classified into subgroups—periosteal and bony—according to their method of insertion. Periosteal fibrous entheses may become bony fibrous entheses with aging. This is necessitated by marked thinning or disappearance of the periosteum after completion of bony development. More research will be needed on fibrous entheses because this is the type of junction initially formed when surgical reattachment of tendon to bone is performed. This has obvious implications not only for tendon transfers but also for procedures such as rotator cuff, anterior cruciate ligament (ACL), and lateral ankle soft-tissue reconstructions.

More investigation has been done relating to fibrocartilaginous than fibrous entheses because fibrocartilaginous entheses are much more vulnerable to overuse injuries. These entheses have no periosteum at the attachment site. In this form of enthesis, there are four zones of tissue. From superficial to deep, these include the following: dense fibrous connective tissue, uncalcified fibrocartilage, calcified fibrocartilage, and bone. The fibrous layer is a fanning out of the tendon. The uncalcified and calcified fibrocartilage layers are avascular zones that are separated from one another by a calcification front that is represented by a basophilic line on stained sections. This is termed the *tidemark*. As with articular cartilage, this line represents the boundary between hard and soft tissues. If there is adjacent articular cartilage, the tidemark of the enthesis is contiguous with the tidemark of the joint, which is usually linear with minimal undulations. Although not technically Sharpey's fibers, there are fibers that continue from the tendon through the uncalcified fibrocartilage, tidemark, and calcified fibrocartilage. Unlike the tidemark, the junction between calcified fibrocartilage and bone is irregular and undulating. Anatomically, this is where the tendon ends and the bone begins.

Biomechanics

Ideally, tendons should have tensile strengths far higher than the maximal forces that the muscles with which they are contiguous can generate. In addition, they should be able to accommodate cyclic loading, as well as static loads without diminution of tensile properties, fatigue, or irreversible elongation. Tendons are anisotropic structures that demonstrate viscoelastic properties. They have the highest tensile strength of any soft tissue. There are two reasons for this fact. Collagen is the strongest fibrous protein in the body, and the linear arrangement of its fibrils is parallel to the direction of tensile force, making these structures ideally suited to resist tension. Strain rate–dependent lengthening is observed. As the elongation rate is increased, tendons appear stiffer. Because tendons contain a relatively larger proportion of collagen to ground substance than other musculoskeletal tissues, they demonstrate less viscoelasticity and more purely elastic properties than these tissues. The ultimate tensile strength of human tendons is 50 to 105 MPa. Elastic strain energy recovery upon unloading of tendons is 90% to 96% per cycle. The stress strain curve

observed for tendons is similar to those of other soft tissues (Fig. 1-9).

The short toe region results from the straightening of crimps in the fibrillar structure. This requires relatively small amounts of force, but because the fibers are already aligned in a parallel fashion, the region is truncated relative to other viscoelastic soft tissues. As with other substances, the slope of the linear region of the curve represents the elastic modulus of the tendon.

Exercise

Numerous animal models have been used to study the biomechanical effect of exercise on tendons. Many of the results have been conflicting. Ultrasonography of human tendon showed that the free tendon of the vastus lateralis was significantly stiffer in long-distance runners than in control subjects. A follow-up study revealed that the knee extensor tendons became stiffer with isometric training. The mechanism of this increased stiffness does not seem to be increased collagen concentration, an increase in collagen cross-links, or hypertrophy of the tendon itself. As alluded to later in this section, decreased fatigability may be an adaptive response that serves to prevent catastrophic damage associated with repetitive loading.

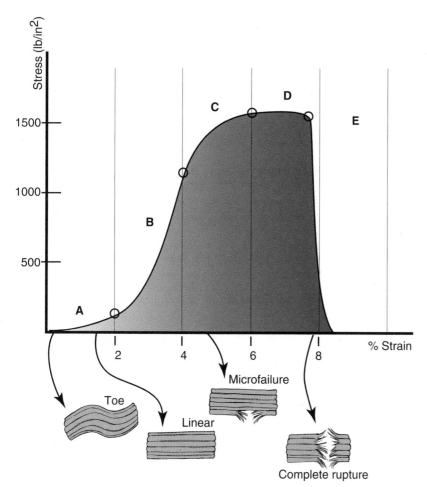

Figure 1-9 Stress–strain curve for a ruptured Achilles tendon. The five distinct regions are the toe region **(A)**, the linear region **(B)**, the progressive failure region **(C)**, the major failure region **(D)**, and the complete rupture **(E)**. (From Hendrickson T. Massage for Orthopedic Conditions. Philadelphia: Lippincott Williams & Wilkins, 2003.)

Biomechanical Effects of Aging

Fibrils vary in diameter and, as a function of age, anatomical site and exercise. Tendons from young animals have relatively small fibrils that fall within a unimodal distribution. As animals age, fibril diameters increase and generally segregate in a bimodal distribution. The stiffness and modulus continue to increase up until maturity and then levels off. Collagen cross-linking increases with age. The toe region of the stress–strain curve diminishes because crimps in the tendon diminish.

Tendon Injuries

Conditions that affect the tendons, as well as the manifestations of each, are diverse. The mechanisms and pathogenesis of these injures are also quite different. Tendinopathies may involve the tenosynovium, the peritenon, the tendon itself, or a combination of these structures. The initial condition may be inflammation of the peritenon secondary to overuse. If this inflammation becomes chronic, the tendon proper may become inflamed or hypovascular as a result of reduced perfusion through the peritenon. This induces degenerative changes in the tendon. The mechanism of injury has a direct impact on how these structures heal. Three main mechanisms of tendon injury are laceration, contusion, and tensile overload. Tensile overload may result in midsubstance tears, tears at the musculotendinous junction, avulsion from bone, or avulsion fracture of the bone at the insertion site.

One way in which these pathologies may be organized is by the acuity of their onset. Lacerations, contusions, tears, and avulsion from bone are the most sudden in their acuity. Although the treatment of these injuries may be similar, the reasons for their occurrence are quite different. Because most tendons can handle tensile forces greater than their accompanying muscles can generate, and greater than the sheer forces able to be withstood by the bones into which they anchor, midsubstance tears are uncommon. Musculotendinous junction tears or avulsion fractures are more common than midsubstance tendon injuries. Midsubstance tears of tendons require preexisting tendinopathy at or near the site of the tear. Failure that occurs only in collagenous material is due to the pulling apart of adjacent collagen molecules, not the breakage of tropocollagen molecules. Although within-the-hand and distal upper extremity lacerations constitute the majority of tendon injuries, degenerative-type injuries are more common in other anatomical locations.

Less acute in their onset are tendonitis, tendinosis, and enthesopathies. Tendonitis most commonly occurs as a result of overuse and is characterized by macroscopic or microscopic injury to collagen fibrils, tendon matrix, and the supporting microvasculature that results in inflammation and, secondarily, pain. Overuse tendon injuries account for a significant percentage of sports injuries. The ability to repair itself continually may be most important in preventing tendon overuse injuries. In simulating an in vivo loading pattern of the extensor digitorum longus tendon of the foot, the tendon was loaded to 20% of its failure stress. After the equivalent of 4 months of normal walking (approximately

300,000 cycles), the tendon failed. Because such tendon failure is not observed in vivo, repair and remodeling must be central to physiological maintenance of the tendon. It is enticing to speculate that overuse injuries of tendons may be due to reparative mechanisms that are not able to counterbalance the microtrauma associated with the inciting activity.

The histological appearance of *tendonitis* has been described as angiofibroblastic hyperplasia. The inflammatory cells present are not characteristic of other acute inflammatory conditions. *Enthesopathies* are defined as diseases that occur at the site of insertion of muscle tendons and ligaments into bone or joint capsules. *Tendinoses* are chronic degenerative conditions of tendons. More specific than chronic degeneration, *tendinosis* refers to intrasubstance degeneration without histologic or clinical signs of inflammation within the tendon. The morphologic changes evident in tendinosis include proliferation of fibroblasts, appearance of new capillary tufts, a decrease in collagen fibril diameter, and a more wavy orientation of the collagen fibers. Matrix components also show histologic changes. At the gross level, tendinosis shows thickened, condensed, and desiccated-appearing regions.

Histologically, tendinosis is characterized by interstitial microscopic failure of the tendon substance or central tissue necrosis with mucoid degeneration. Because inflammation may or may not be a part of this process, tendinosis may or may not be associated with symptoms.

Although tendonitis and tendinoses may be secondary to systemic disease, most cases result from overuse syndromes. These overuse syndromes all have some component of chronic inflammatory response that occurs in or around the tissue. A "tendinosis cycle" has been described in which tendinosis results from changes in the load experienced by tendons that are not compensated by adaptations of the cell matrix. Microtears occur through pathologic tendinous tissue and eventually result in tissue failure if there is not an adequate healing, reparative, or hypertrophic response.

Fluoroquinolones and Tendinopathy

Fluoroquinolones are a class of antibiotics that are bacteriocidal and function through disruption of bacterial DNA gyrase. Over the past decade, the increased use of fluoroquinolones in athletic individuals as antimicrobial chemotherapeutic agents has resulted in cases of fluoroquinolone-induced tendinopathies being reported in the literature. Frank ruptures have also been reported to occur. An increased relative risk of Achilles tendon disorders with standard use of these drugs has been epidemiologically demonstrated and is estimated at 3.2 times that of a control population. It appears that this increased risk is limited to those patients who are over 60 years of age. Concomitant use of these antibiotics with corticosteroids in those over 60 further increases the risk to 6.7 times that of a control population. It appears that the risk of tendinopathy is increased in those currently using the drugs and not those who have used them in the past.

Even limited doses in a rat model of fluoroquinolone-induced Achilles tendonitis resulted in degenerative alterations of the tenocytes. Electron microscopic findings include multiple vacuoles and vesicles in the cytoplasm that had developed as a result of swellings and dilatations of cell organelles. Cells not only lost normal cell–matrix interactions but also detached from the extracellular matrix.

Although the pathophysiologic effects these drugs have on tendons are not fully characterized, it is believed that the adverse effects are the result of altered tendon fibroblast metabolism. Culture of tendon fibroblasts with ciprofloxacin resulted in a 66% reduction in cell proliferation relative to control cultures. Collagen synthesis was also decreased by up to half of control values. Proteoglycan synthesis was also diminished. These studies also suggested that fluoroquinolones stimulate tendon matrix degradation by the upregulation of protease activity. At this point, it seems likely that fluoroquinolones not only decrease the synthesis of tendon structural components, but also accelerate the degradation of these components. Caution should be used when treating athletes with these medications.

Tendon Healing

Normal Healing Responses. Tendons pass through three phases in their healing process: the inflammatory phase, the fibroblastic phase, and the remodeling phase. These phases have characteristic cellular, temporal, and biomechanical patterns (Fig. 1-10).

- The first phase has been labeled *inflammatory phase* and occurs in the first week following injury.
  - It starts with the migration of macrophages from tissues surrounding the injury.
  - During this phase, the macrophages remove necrotic tissue and hematoma from the area of the injury, thereby preparing the tissue bed for reconstruction.
  - Collagenases and matrix metalloproteinases play a key role in removing not only collagen debris, but also matrix components from the site of injury.
- The second phase of the healing response is the *fibroblastic phase*.
  - Fibroblasts proliferate and begin to synthesize collagen and other proteins required for extracellular matrix construction at this time.
  - The fibroblastic phase is initiated approximately 1 week after injury, but collagen synthesis reaches a maximum 3 to 4 weeks after injury.
  - It is believed that the fibroblasts that drive this phase originate from locally resident cells of the perivascular tissues.
  - Revascularization at the site of injury is also initiated during the fibroblastic phase.
- The last phase is the *remodeling phase*.
  - The collagen fibers are originally oriented perpendicular to the long axis of the tendon.
  - At approximately 8 weeks after injury, the recently laid down collagen fibers are brought into orientation along the axis of the tendon.
  - It is during this period that adhesions may become more numerous and tenacious.
  - Older individuals have a lower metabolic activity within these structures that may be responsible for the diminished age-related tendon healing capacity observed.

Throughout tendon healing, there is a dynamic balance

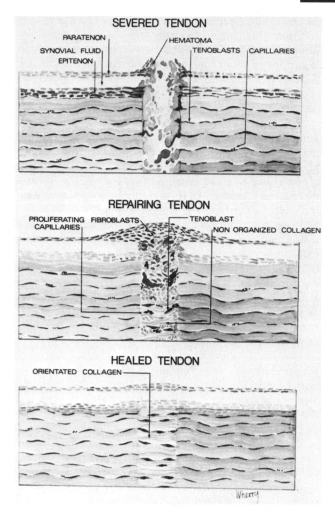

Figure 1-10 Sequence of events following tendon laceration. A hematoma forms between the tendon ends. Stimulated by chemotactic factors, inflammatory cells migrate into the hematoma, followed by blood vessels and fibroblasts. The fibroblasts synthesize a new matrix and then remodel the repair tissue to restore the structure and function of the tendon. Healing of the other dense fibrous tissues follows the same pattern.

between collagen breakdown and synthesis. Initially, collagenase activity and collagen breakdown predominate, but these levels diminish and become equal to the rising synthesis levels by 4 to 6 weeks after injury. After this time, synthesis and remodeling occur at a much greater rate than breakdown.

The biomechanical strength of surgical tendon repairs closely matches the histologic phases through which tendons pass during healing. During the inflammatory phase, there is a decrease in the tensile strength of the repair probably secondary to edema and tendon degradation. In the fibroblastic phases, there is an increase in strength that is furthered during the remodeling phase.

Investigations into the pathogenesis and normal healing responses of these conditions are both reliant on, and severely hampered by, the animal models used to study them. Most tendon, ligament, and capsular injuries result from acute trauma to the tissues or overuse syndromes. With the exception of lacerations, re-creating either acute or chronic soft-tissue injuries in laboratory animals is difficult to perform and standardize. Unlike the exquisite "knock-out" or "knock-in" recombinant techniques that have resulted in transgenic animals to model single molecular defect diseases, no elegant models for most tendon, ligament, and capsular disease amenable to repair are available.

In the past, there was debate as to whether healing of tendon injury was predominantly an intrinsic or extrinsic phenomenon. The extrinsic mechanism depends on fibroblasts and inflammatory cells entering from the periphery of the injury to effect repair of the tendon. The intrinsic mechanism involves migration of fibroblasts and inflammatory cells from within the tendon and epitenon. It is now believed that tendon healing involves both intrinsic and extrinsic mechanisms, with the latter predominating in the early phases and the intrinsic predominating in a more delayed fashion. Some hypothesize that an imbalance favoring the extrinsic mechanism leads to increased collagen content at the repair sight, as well as a suboptimal level of collagen organization. As a consequence, predominance of the extrinsic mechanism may result in scar formation and adhesions between the tendon and surrounding tissues.

Physical Modifiers to Tendon Healing. Tendon motion during healing has been shown to maximize the strength of repairs and excursion able to be obtained at the end of healing. As little as 2 mm of passive excursion at low levels of force is adequate to inhibit adhesion formation and promote healing. Increases of force and excursion beyond this do not accelerate the healing process. Repair of lacerated digital flexor tendons should be done within a few days of injury to maximize final tendon excursion and minimize the angular rotation of the repair.

Modulation of Adhesion Formation. A strong repair of a deficient tendon unit alone will not suffice to return the athlete to competition. In most cases, a repaired tendon must maintain a substantial amount of its excursive ability to maintain appropriate function. The ability to do this is dependent on the ability to achieve a strong repair at the injury site, as well as prevent adhesions from forming during the healing process. Adhesions can severely restrict tendon gliding after tendon healing has occurred. As previously described, it is believed that an overly aggressive extrinsic healing response results in the formation of these adhesions. Physical, pharmacologic, and biologic approaches have been used to combat this problem.

5-Flourouracil is a pyrimidine analogue that exerts its effects by causing thymidine depletion and disrupting RNA processing. The use of this pharmacologic agent to prevent tendon adhesions has been examined. At the sites of tendon repair, there is a less vigorous cellular response and a decrease in the local levels of transforming growth factor-β (TGF-β) which is a known potentiator of the fibrotic response. Fewer adhesions are observed histologically at repair sites.

Human amniotic fluid and hyaluronic acid membranes applied to the sites of suture-repaired tendons resulted in fewer adhesions relative to control groups. Although further work needs to be done to identify and isolate those factors responsible for the inhibitory properties of human amniotic fluid, the latter treatment may provide a currently available, cost-effective, and simply applied physiochemical barrier by which peritendinous adhesions can be minimized or prevented at repair sites.

Application of supraphysiologic temperatures to areas of tendon repair decreases the amount of peritendinous adhesions without adverse affect on gliding or strength of the treated tendons. Heat shock proteins limited the local inflammatory response and subsequent adhesion formation.

LIGAMENTS

Ligament sprains account for approximately 45% of musculoskeletal injuries and affect 5% to 10% of people up to age 65. Anatomically, ligaments connect bone to bone across an articulation. They function as joint stabilizers resisting forces applied to the joint while allowing joint motion. Other structures (including bone, cartilage, and tendons) contribute to joint stability by sharing the load across the joint. When ligaments are injured, forces they normally resist are shifted to the other structures. When the ligament does not heal properly, these structures are at risk for degeneration and failure. Thus, it is important to consider several biological, mechanical, and surgical factors to optimize functional recovery of the injured ligament.

Anatomy, Structure, and Biochemistry

Ligaments consist of cellular, extracellular matrix, and aqueous components. Cell types are fibroblasts, endothelial cells, and nerve cells. Fibroblasts are the primary cells in ligaments and are responsible for synthesizing extracellular matrix components, including collagen. The extracellular matrix is composed of 60% water and 40% collagens, elastin, proteoglycans, and noncollagenous proteins. Collagens are fibrillar proteins with high tensile strength composed of three polypeptide chains arranged in a helical pattern (tropocollagen) and covalently cross-linked together. Different combinations of polypeptide chains yield different types of collagen and higher levels of cross-linking between tropocollagen chains confers greater mechanical strength to the collagen and ligament. Collagen constitutes 70% to 80% of ligament dry weight. More than 90% of collagen found in ligaments is type I, approximately 10% is type III, and other types may be present in smaller concentrations. Ligaments contain a lower percentage of collagen than tendons. Elastin, a protein rich in glycine and proline, comprises less than 5% of dry weight in most ligaments. It is found in higher concentrations in flexible ligaments, such as the ligamentum flavum. Proteoglycans are composed of polysaccharide chains [glycosaminoglycans (GAGs)], which are connected to a protein core. They are negatively charged molecules that bind water and other positively charged ions. They form less than 1% of ligament dry weight. Most ligaments have higher GAG content than tendons. Two types of proteoglycans are found in ligaments: larger molecules with chondroitin and keratin sulfate GAG chains, and smaller molecules with dermatan sulfate chains. Proteoglycans serve to maintain ligament water content, organize the extracellular matrix, and interact with cellular elements. Noncollagenous proteins include fibronectin, a protein that allows cells to interact with the extracellular matrix.

Ligaments are relatively avascular, but they do contain small blood vessels originating at the ligament insertion sites. Cells contained within the ligament are maintained by this blood supply and through diffusion from the local aqueous environment. Nerve fibers have been noted in medial collateral ligament (MCL), and ACL specimens and are postulated to have proprioceptive, mechanoreceptive, and nociceptive functions.

Structurally, ligaments form cords, strips, and sheetlike structures that insert into bone on either side of an articulation. There are intra-articular and extra-articular ligaments. Their insertions have been described as direct or indirect based how the collagen fibers attach to bone. Direct insertions, such as the femoral insertion of the MCL or tibial insertion of the ACL, have ligament fibers passing directly into the cortex. This transition has been observed occurring over four zones: ligament, fibrocartilage, mineralized fibrocartilage, and bone. Indirect insertions, such as the tibial insertion of the MCL, have a broader area of insertion, superficial fibers that insert obliquely into the periosteum, and deeper fibers inserting via Sharpey's fibers forming the indirect insertion. Indirect insertions may be elevated off the bone without cutting the ligament itself, where direct inserting ligaments require cutting the substance of the ligament to detach it.

Biomechanics

Biomechanical properties of ligaments can be described in terms of the structural properties of the bone ligament bone complex and mechanical properties of the ligament substance. The structural properties of the bone ligament bone construct, which are influenced by ligament composition and insertion type, are tested with tensile stress and plotted on load-elongation curves. Stiffness is defined as the resistance of a structure to deformation, or the slope of the load-elongation curve. This curve has an initial low-stiffness toe region followed by a higher-stiffness linear region. This increase in stiffness has been attributed to the initial straightening of the undulating crimp pattern and nonuniform recruitment of the individual fibers as represented in the low-stiffness (and larger elongation) toe region of the curve. As the fiber bundles straighten and more fibers are recruited, stiffness increases. The ultimate load on the curve is where construct failure occurs. The slope may decrease before failure if individual fibers fail before the entire construct fails. Area under the curve is energy absorbed before failure.

The mechanical properties of the ligament—which are influenced by collagen composition, collagen fiber orientation, and interaction with the extracellular matrix—are tested with tensile stress and plotted on stress–strain curves. This slope of this curve is the elastic modulus. The tensile strength is the maximum stress before failure. The elastic modulus of the MCL is approximately twice as much as the ACL. The MCL has more densely packed fiber bundles per unit area with less crimp, or wave pattern, and greater fiber diameter than the ACL. Ligaments also display viscoelastic properties that reflect interactions of collagen and other extracellular matrix molecules: creep, stress relaxation, and hysteresis. It has been shown that preconditioning ACL grafts prior to reconstruction may reduce the amount of stress relaxation by approximately 50%, compared with ligament grafts with no preconditioning.

Many factors influence the biomechanical properties of ligaments, including biochemistry, immobilization, and aging. Stiffness, ultimate load, and energy absorbed at failure increase with age and skeletal maturity, which may be attributable to further tropocollagen chain cross-linking. As ligaments mature, the bone–ligament–bone construct failure sites change. Rabbit MCL testing has shown that younger rabbit ligaments fail by tibial avulsion and mature ligaments fail by intrasubstance ligament tears. Ligament immobilization causes intrasubstance and insertion site changes that alter structural properties. Insertion sites reveal disruption of deep fibers inserting into bone and osteoclastic activity that results in subperiosteal bone resorption. Mobilization causes slow reversal of these effects with ultimate load and energy absorbed at failure almost reaching control levels.

Injury and Healing

Ligament injuries are graded according to tissue damage and instability (Table 1-1). Extra-articular ligament healing passes through stages similar to general wound healing. An inflammatory phase is followed by a proliferative repair phase and, ultimately, a remodeling phase.

- The inflammatory phase, which usually occurs within 24 hours of injury, is characterized by release of inflammatory mediators, increased blood flow, and migration of inflammatory cells.
  - Immediately following ligament tear, the gap between the torn ligament ends is filled by hematoma.
  - Vasodilators and inflammatory mediators are released into the local environment causing increased blood flow, vascular permeability, and plasma fluid exudation, which are responsible for local tissue edema.
  - Factors released also stimulate inflammatory cell migration into the zone of injury.
  - Polymorphonuclear cells initially (and later, monocytes) are present in the injured tissue and release enzymes that breakdown necrotic tissue.
  - Macrophages phagocytose the necrotic debris.

TABLE 1-1 GRADING OF LIGAMENT INJURIES

Grade	Description
1	Ligament is stretched but remains intact and results in no instability
2	Partial tears that lead to mild instability
3	Complete tears that result in significant joint instability

- Within 3 or 4 days, capillary venules form new vascular buds, as endothelial cells are attracted toward the zone of injury by chemotactic factors.
- These cells begin to proliferate and ultimately form new capillary vessels, establishing blood flow in the forming granulation tissue.
- Toward the end of the inflammatory phase, fibroblast migration and proliferation begin.
- These cells will produce collagen, proteoglycans, and other matrix molecules that form the initial scar.

- The proliferative or repair phase is characterized by an increase in cells and matrix molecules.
  - Hematoma is replaced with highly cellular immature scar with limited tensile strength during this stage.
  - It starts within 48 to 72 hours of injury and continues over the next several weeks.
  - Fibroblasts proliferate in the granulation tissue filling the ligament gap.
  - New blood vessels are forming while fibroblasts synthesize matrix.
- The remodeling and maturation phase of ligament healing is characterized by a decrease in cellularity and vascularity, whereas organization of collagen and matrix increases.
  - This phase starts at several weeks after injury and may last longer than 12 months.
  - Cellular and vascular density also decrease to near-normal levels.
  - Ultimately, this phase results in a mature healed ligament with a greater volume of ligamentous tissue but with material properties that are less than normal uninjured ligament.

The mature healed ligament differs from normal tissue. It has less tensile strength, usually 50% to 70% of normal. Mechanical properties of healing intrasubstance MCL tears are inferior, but they have a larger cross-sectional area than the intact MCL. Although the healed ligament has lower tensile strength than an uninjured ligament, it does not usually result in alteration of joint function. This may be partially explained by the increased volume of the repaired tissue compared with the uninjured ligament.

Factors Influencing Ligament Healing

Factors that affect ligament repair include location and extent of injury, treatment type, immobilization, and systemic factors. Intrasubstance ligament tears of extra-articular ligaments appear to heal, resulting in a more functional ligament than in intra-articular, intrasubstance tears. This may be influenced by the synovial environment and decreased vascular ingrowth of the intra-articular ligaments. The extent of injury and multiple ligament involvement also impacts ligament healing. Combined ligament injuries have a worse prognosis than single ligament sprains. The torn MCL has some support from uninjured structures, including the ACL and joint capsule. When the ACL is torn in addition to the MCL, the knee is less stable and MCL healing quality is diminished.

Direct suture repair of collateral ligaments decreases the injury gap that would be filled with scar tissue and may increase initial structural strength by 10% to 30%. Repair of collateral ligaments in ACL-deficient knees did not improve structural strength. This is likely caused by the instability of the ACL injury leading to increased strain on the MCL. Suture repair has not been shown to ultimately affect increases in ligament strength, laxity, or stiffness.

Immobilization results in decreased collagen production, disorganization of collagen fibrils with decreased matrix remodeling, decreased mechanical and structural properties, and bone resorption at ligament insertion sites. Prolonged joint immobilization may also result in damage to the articular surface, changes in the osseous geometry, and inducement of joint adhesions.

Early controlled motion applied with low stress on injured ligaments results in improved scar stiffness and strength without compromising scar length. Extreme loading results in repair tissue disruption and may delay or prevent healing. Totally unloading a ligament also diminishes healing and results in decreased collagen fibril diameter and decreased ligament mechanical properties. The positive effect of early motion is likely mediated by local mechanical effects on fibroblasts, as well as effects on blood flow and inflammation. Movement may be responsible for stimulation of collagen synthesis and increased matrix remodeling, resulting in increased scar mass with increased tensile strength. Ligament mobilization has been reported to increase the ultimate load of the healed tissue. Increased scar formation appears to occur when injured ligaments are mobilized within weeks of injury. Later mobilization stimulates scar remodeling but may not result in increased scar mass. Short-term immobilization for pain control, followed by early mobilization, will provide optimal results. Clinical studies suggest that controlled motion favorably affects MCL healing and knee function. Current recommendations for isolated MCL injuries include controlled early range of motion as soon as pain subsides. The goal is to avoid aggressive movement that will cause excessive disruptive force across healing ligament. Early controlled motion is also important after ACL reconstruction because it had been shown to minimize capsular contractions that lead to joint stiffness and have a positive effect on articular cartilage.

Systemic factors have an impact on the local healing environment. Endocrine abnormalities may lead to altered collagen and proteoglycan synthesis causing decreased mechanical strength. Diabetes, vascular disease, and infection may prolong the inflammatory stage.

FUTURE DIRECTIONS

New techniques utilizing growth factors, gene therapy, and stem cell therapy may enhance quality of ligament healing. Growth factors are small peptides that bind to cell surface receptors and stimulate various cellular functions, including protein synthesis and cellular feedback loops. Growth factors—such as TGF-β, vascular endothelial growth factor, platelet-derived growth factor, basic fibroblast growth factor, and insulinlike growth factor—have been shown to be elevated at various stages of ligament and tendon healing. These factors are involved with chemotaxis of fibroblasts and inflammatory cells to the injury site; they stimulate cell proliferation and angiogenesis, as well as matrix molecule synthesis. Manipulation of these factors may lead to improved ligament healing. Gene therapy, transferring growth factor genes in viruses or liposomes, is under investigation to improve delivery of growth factors to injury sites. Mesenchymal stem, or progenitor, cells implanted into injury sites may be a source for cell types necessary for the healing process.

SUGGESTED READING

Amadio PC. Tendon and ligament. In: Lindblad WJ, ed. Wound Healing: Biochemical & Clinical Aspects. Philadelphia: WB Saunders, 1992:384–395.

Beiner JM, Jokl P. Muscle contusion injuries: current treatment options. J Am Acad Orthop Surg 2001;9:227–237.

Benjamin M, Evans EJ, Copp L. The histology of tendon attachments to bone in man. J Anat 1986;149:89–100.

Beynnon BD, Johnson RJ, Fleming BC. The science of anterior cruciate ligament rehabilitation. Clin Orthop 2002;402:9–20.

Buckwalter JA, Cooper RR. Bone structure and function. Instr Course Lect 1987;36:27–48.

Buckwalter JA, Woo SL. Basic science and injury of muscle, tendon, and ligaments. In: Drez D, ed. Orthopaedic Sports Medicine: Principles and Practice. Philadelphia: WB Saunders, 2003:39–49.

Cheung K, Hume P, Maxwell L. Delayed onset muscle soreness: treatment strategies and performance factors. Sports Med 2003;33:145–164.

Denborough M. Malignant hyperthermia. Lancet. 1998;352:1131–1136.

Fraipont MJ, Adamson GJ. Chronic exertional compartment syndrome. J Am Acad Orthop Surg 2003;11:268–276.

Francois RJ, Braun J, Khan MA. Entheses and enthesitis: a histopathologic review and relevance to spondyloarthritides. Curr Opin Rheumatol 2001;13:255–264.

Frank CB. Ligament healing: current knowledge and clinical applications. J Am Acad Orthop Surg 1996;4:74–83.

Frank CB, Hart DA, Shrive NG. Molecular biology and biomechanics of normal and healing ligaments—a review. Osteoarthritis Cartilage 1999;7:130–140.

Garrett WE Jr, Best TM. Anatomy, physiology, and mechanics of skeletal muscle. In: Dimon S, ed. Orthopedic Basic Science. Rosemont, IL: American Academy of Orthopaedic Surgeons, 1994:97–118.

Huard J, Li Y, Fu FH. Muscle injuries and repair: current trends in research. J Bone Joint Surg Am. 2002;84:822–832.

Johnson RJ, Beynnon BD, Nichols CE, et al. The treatment of injuries of the anterior cruciate ligament. J Bone Joint Surg Am 1992;74:140–151.

Lieber RL, Friden J. Morphologic and mechanical basis of delayed-onset muscle soreness. J Am Acad Orthop Surg 2002;10:67–73.

Molloy T, Wang Y, Murrell G. The roles of growth factors in tendon and ligament healing. Sports Med 2003;33:381–394.

Noonan TJ, Garrett WE Jr. Muscle strain injury: diagnosis and treatment. J Am Acad Orthop Surg. 1999;7:262–269.

Reider B, Sathy MR, Talkington J, et al. Treatment of isolated medial collateral ligament injuries in athletes with early functional rehabilitation. A five-year follow-up study. Am J Sports Med 1994;22:470–477.

Silva MJ, Boyer MI, Gelberman RH. Recent progress in flexor tendon healing. J Orthop Sci 2002;7:508–514.

Williams RJ III, Attia E, Wickiewicz TL, et al. The effect of ciprofloxacin on tendon, paratenon, and capsular fibroblast metabolism. Am J Sports Med. 2000;28:364–369

Woo SL, Debski RE, Zeminski J, et al. Injury and repair of ligaments and tendons. Annu Rev Biomed Eng 2000;2:83–118.

Woo SL, Vogrin TM, Abramowitch SD. Healing and repair of ligament injuries in the knee. J Am Acad Orthop Surg 2000;8:364–372.

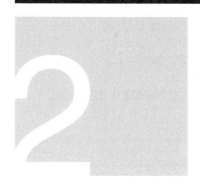

PREPARTICIPATION PHYSICAL EXAMINATION

VASILIOS CHRISOSTOMIDIS
BRIAN D. BUSCONI
J. HERBERT STEVENSON

Thirty-five million children and young adults participate in organized sports in the United States. There are 3.5 million injuries per year as a result. The preparticipation physical examination (PPE) is designed to be specific for athletic endeavors. Sporting events create specific concerns of which physicians need to be aware. Different sports create different injuries that medical personnel must be prepared to treat; for example, in football, trauma is more common when compared with cross-country running, in which overuse injuries are more common. The PPE will vary from a focused exam to an extensive workup depending on the sport, strenuousness of activity, or level of competition.

Nurse practitioners, physician assistants, and physicians may perform the PPE. Primary care physicians should consult specialty physicians when a problem requires further expertise. Conversely, when specialists perform screening examinations, they should contact a generalist regarding issues outside of their expertise.

OBJECTIVES

The primary goal of the PPE is to make sure that athletes are safe—to ensure the patient's health rather than to disqualify athletes. The examiner has a chance to detect current injuries that may require rehabilitation prior to the season beginning. In addition, the physician has the opportunity to detect life-threatening conditions that may preclude a person from participating in certain or all athletics. The PPE also addresses legal and insurance requirements, as well as fulfilling many schools' requirements. Finally, it gives the physician the chance to develop a rapport with the athlete.

TIMING

Ideally, the PPE should be performed 6 weeks prior to preseason practice. This time interval allows for the diagnosis and treatment of potential problems before the beginning of the season. Appropriate rehabilitative plans may be instituted with the goal of returning the athlete to his or her sport and having missed no practices or game time. Because scheduling the PPE in the midsummer may be difficult, one may consider performing evaluations at the end of the preceding school year. The responsibility of reporting injuries or illnesses that occur in the time between the PPE and start of the season falls on the athlete. This information may then be relayed to the athletic trainer or directly to the team physician.

FORMAT

Office-based PPE

The office-based PPE is performed in a private setting during a time that is convenient for both the patient and the health care provider. One person does the entire physical examination in contrast to the station-based examination, which requires multiple examiners. This has the advantage of maintaining continuity of care for the patient since it is performed by the athlete's personal or primary care physician in the office setting. There is added benefit if the physician already knows the patient because medical records are complete and the risk of "abnormalities falling through the cracks" decreases. In addition, athletes may feel more comfortable discussing sensitive issues, such as alcohol and drug use, birth control, and sexually transmitted diseases.

There are some disadvantages to the office-based approach, including increased cost to the athlete and availability of appointments. The large influx of patients in a fixed amount of time may overwhelm an already busy office practice.

Station-based PPE

This format consists of a series of "stations," each one devoted to a single part of the history or physical examination. The patients proceed in a stepwise fashion from one station to the next until all are completed. At checkout, the entire file is reviewed to make sure all appropriate information has been obtained, as well as to determine medical clearance.

The advantage to this system is that a large number of people may be screened in a relatively short period of time since there are multiple stations with multiple physicians. The disadvantages of this include a lack of privacy and fragmented care. Additionally, this requires a large number of trained medical providers to man the various stations.

Single Physician Assembly Line

This consists of multiple medical providers who perform the complete exam, often in the training room or locker room. This defrays some of the cost that is incurred when an athlete has to go to a physician's private office. This may be more personal to the athlete since one physician performs all the components of the PPE. A major disadvantage includes not having sufficient personnel trained to perform the complete exam.

MEDICAL HISTORY

In a PPE, the history plays a predominant role. A complete history can usually identify 60% to 75% of the problems affecting a patient. The history provides details regarding health problems and injuries, allowing the physician to focus on problem areas. A standard questionnaire may be used with further investigation during the assessment.

Recent or Chronic Injury or Illness

- It is important that the physician is aware of any injuries that have occurred recently.
- This also helps stimulate the athlete's memory so that a complete history can be done.

Hospitalizations and Surgeries

- Questions about recent medical care will alert the physician to previous serious medical problems, as well as assess if current medical or surgical problems are properly being cared for.
- Athletes who have had recent surgery will need appropriate review of results and status of any rehabilitation if indicated.

Medications

- An athlete's medication list allows the doctor to determine if chronic medical problems are being managed appropriately (anticonvulsants, insulin, asthma, and cardiovascular agents). More importantly, coaches and trainers may be alerted to potential adverse effects and drug interactions.
- Asking specifically about over-the-counter (OTC) drug use is important because of its high prevalence. Organizing bodies, including the National Collegiate Athletic Association (NCAA) and the International Olympic Committee, restrict many common OTC medications.
- It is crucial to ask about nutritional supplement use, including vitamins, protein supplements, amino acids, as well as the use of ergogenic aids, such as anabolic steroids.

Allergies

- Any allergic reactions to medications should be recorded, and care should be given to make sure they are not inadvertently administered to the patient.
- Any reaction to insect bites or stings should be noted so that appropriate medications are available (subcutaneous epinephrine).
- Any history of exercise-induced urticaria or anaphylaxis should be noted and prepared for.
- Ultimately, it is the athlete who is responsible for being prepared with allergy medications, though trainers or physicians may choose to carry them as well.

Cardiovascular

- Most sudden deaths in athletes under the age of 30 are due to a structural defect in the heart. A careful history should be taken to uncover those at risk.
  - A history of syncope or presyncope might be a clue to hypertrophic cardiomyopathy, dysrhythmias, or valve problems.
  - Chest pain with activity could be a sign of atherosclerotic disease (unusual under the age of 30).
  - Shortness of breath with exertion may indicate val-

vular problems, structural disease, or pulmonary disease.

- Palpitations may signify dysrhythmias or conduction abnormalities.
- For these problems, one may want to conduct further tests prior to clearance.

- A history of heart murmur or elevated blood pressure should alert the physician to a possible cardiac problem and may also require further evaluation.
  - Some cardiac problems are familial, so a careful family history should be obtained from the patient.
  - Any patient who was denied clearance previously for a cardiac issue should be thoroughly investigated prior to clearance.
- Any history of anabolic steroid or illicit drug use, particularly cocaine, may damage the heart and increase the risk of sudden cardiac death in athletes.

Skin

- Infectious dermatologic conditions—such as impetigo, herpes simplex, and molluscum contagiosum—are some of the primary concerns during review of an athlete's dermatologic history. This is especially important in contact sports or in sports where spread of an infection is possible through a fomite such as a mat or helmet.
- It is also important to note acne because it may be exacerbated from equipment.
- The physician should take a moment to emphasize the importance of sunblock for athletes who play outdoor sports.

Neurologic

- Any history of head injury, seizures, concussions, burners/stingers, or "pinched nerves" requires further scrutiny.
  - It is important to note whether symptoms occur with exertion or from trauma.
  - Any history of loss of consciousness, significant concussion, or repetitive concussion should prompt further inquiry, including the number of episodes, loss of memory, and length of full recovery.
  - If the patient is still experiencing symptoms, one should consider a referral to a neurologist or someone skilled in caring for such athletes.
- Burners/stingers occur as a result of trauma to the brachial plexus or cervical nerve roots and may present as unilateral numbness or tingling that may persist for several minutes (but rarely permanently).
  - A proper history should include the number of episodes and what has been done for treatment until the present. Athletes with such a history should be referred to coaches or athletic trainers for instruction on neck and upper extremity strengthening, protective equipment, and instruction of proper technique in tackling.
- Cervical spinal cord neurapraxia with transient quadriplegia is an uncommon entity that may result from trauma.
  - Usually, the patient will complain of burning pain,

numbness or tingling, and weakness or paralysis of all four extremities.
  - Recovery is usually within 15 minutes, although some cases gradually resolve over 36 to 48 hours.
- Positive findings in the history may direct further testing—such as radiographs or magnetic resonance imaging (MRI)—to rule out instability or other anatomical problems prior to clearance.

Heat Illness

- Heat-related disorders represent a spectrum of disease ranging from exercise-associated cramps to heat exhaustion to heat stroke.
- Often, heat illness is recurrent, so a detailed history may be helpful in preventing it in the future.
- Certain substances, such as caffeine, methylphenidate, or antihistamines, may predispose to heat illness.
- Pre- and postexercise weights are helpful to determine hydration status and help with pre-event hydration.
- Proper acclimatization is important in preventing heat illness and should be stressed to athletes.

Pulmonary

- Exercise-induced asthma is a commonly overlooked diagnosis, and an attempt should be made to identify it at the PPE.
- Athletes will often describe feeling "winded" or "out of shape," despite appropriate training. Some will complain of chest tightness or obvious wheezing. These symptoms may be related to cold weather or seasonal allergies.
- Treatment with albuterol prior to athletic activity will relieve many of these athletes' symptoms.
- One may consider formal pulmonary function or pre- and postexercise peak flow testing to make the diagnosis.

Eyes and Vision

- It is important for the physician to be aware of any eye injuries or surgeries that an athlete has had in the past.
- If an athlete wears glasses, one must ensure that the frames and lenses are safe for use in competition.
- It is important to assess if any athletes are "functionally one-eyed" (as determined by the American Academy of Ophthalmology) because their best-corrected vision is less than 20/40 in one eye.
- Anisocoria should be documented so a baseline of pupillary size is documented in case of head injury.

Musculoskeletal

- The musculoskeletal history should focus on injuries to muscles, bones, or ligaments and, as such, they should be recorded by the physician. This includes fractures, dislocations, instability, subluxations, sprains, or strains.
- Treatments including physical therapy, braces, and sur-

gery should be reviewed with the athlete, and plans for rehabilitation (if necessary) should be instituted.

- If the athlete has any current complaints or injuries, a thorough workup may be instituted immediately, including radiographs and lab work as the physician sees fit.

Gastrointestinal

- A history of mononucleosis is an important piece of information since the athlete is at increased risk of splenic rupture in the time following diagnosis.
- Any history of vomiting or diarrhea may put an athlete at risk for heat illness.

Genitourinary

- A testicular exam should be performed on male athletes, and time should be taken to instruct patients on the self-testicular exam for screening of testicular cancer.
  - Absence of one testicle, undescended testes, and inguinal hernias may be detected on examination.
- The female genitourinary exam is not performed routinely as part of the PPE and, if warranted, it should be conducted in a private setting.
- The use of Tanner staging reflects skeletal maturity but is not recommended as a routine part of the PPE.

Protective Devices

- A special pad or brace will alert the physician to any problems that the athlete may have forgotten to mention. Examples include a special neck roll for an athlete who has experienced multiple brachial plexus injuries in the past or a knee brace to protect against a previous knee injury.
- Athletes should wear a mouth guard if they have orthodontia, whether or not it is required by their sport.

Eating Disorders

- Because of the prevalence of eating disorders and their impact on the athlete's health, it is important to determine if an athlete is exhibiting any signs of disordered eating. This refers to any unhealthy behavior resulting in calorie deprivation, whether it is through poor food choices, self-induced vomiting, or use of laxatives or diuretics.
  - Females are more likely to engage in such behaviors.
- Disordered eating is often more common in sports with weight classes, such as wrestling or rowing, or sports in which leanness is emphasized, such as in track and field or gymnastics.
- A nonthreatening way to ascertain information about the presence of an eating disorder is to ask an athlete, "How much would you like to weigh?" or "Are you happy with your weight?"
- It is important to determine whether the athlete has lost any weight and, if so, whether it was accidental or intentional.

- The physician should look for any signs of bulimia or anorexia, including skin changes, oral ulcerations, and decreased tooth enamel.
- Asking about any history of stress fractures, menstrual irregularity, and excessive exercise habits may alert the doctor to the "female triad" (amenorrhea, osteopenia, and disordered eating).
- Disordered eating can be a difficult problem and often requires a multifaceted approach—including referral to a nutritionist or dietitian, psychologist, and primary care physician—if feasible. It is important to provide an ideal weight range and close follow-up.

Psychosocial Concerns

- The use of drugs and other illicit substances, such as ergogenic aids, is prevalent in the United States.
- Alcohol intake is rampant across college campuses, as well as in high schools. The PPE is an opportunity to explain the potential adverse effects of alcohol on the body, as well as its impact on athletic performance.
- Smokeless tobacco is the most commonly used tobacco product by athletes, particularly in baseball players. It is known to cause oral neoplasms, among other mouth disorders.
  - The NCAA has banned the use of tobacco by game personnel, as well as student athletes.
  - The United States Olympic Committee (USOC) has not banned it because tobacco use provides no competitive advantage.
- Illicit drugs such as cocaine or marijuana are illegal, as well as harmful to the athlete. They do not aid athletic performance. Intravenous drug use exposes the athlete to diseases such as hepatitis and human immunodeficiency virus (HIV).
- Performance-enhancing agents are a major concern in competition and often have hazardous side effects. The PPE provides an opportunity for the physician to discuss such issues.
- Anabolic steroids, such as testosterone, may be ingested orally or intravenously and are used to gain an advantage.
  - Side effects include liver disease, testicular atrophy, gynecomastia, menstrual irregularities, and sudden cardiac death.
  - The NCAA, USOC, and various other organizations ban these supplements.
- Nutritional supplements are used to increase energy stores and decrease fatigue. These include, but are not limited to, vitamins, minerals, amino acids, and electrolyte solutions.

Immunizations

- Vaccinations are an important health care maintenance issue that can be addressed at the PPE. Although delinquent immunizations are not grounds for disqualification, they do allow the physician to set up appropriate follow-up.
- Most schools have certain immunization requirements that must be met before the student may matriculate.

- The Centers for Disease Control and Prevention can be accessed to provide a recommended vaccination schedule.

Menstrual History

- For female athletes, a detailed menstrual history should be obtained regarding amenorrhea or oligomenorrhea.
- Amenorrhea may be described as *primary* (absence of menarche by age 16) or *secondary* (missing three consecutive periods in a previously menstruating female). Either may require a referral to the primary care physician or gynecologist.
- Although irregular menses is not uncommon in athletes, irregular menses or amenorrhea may be due to an underlying eating disorder.
  - One should rule out pregnancy prior to attributing this condition to poor nutrition or excessive exercise, as seen in the female triad.
- This is also an opportunity for health care maintenance regarding self-breast examination, Papanicolaou testing, and a frank discussion regarding prevention of transmission of sexually transmitted diseases, as well as the prevention of unwanted pregnancies.

PHYSICAL EXAMINATION

A variety of PPE forms are available on the Internet, or use of an institutional or statewide form may be required.

General

- Recording the height and weight of an individual may help determine if there are any underweight or overweight athletes.
  - Underweight individuals may be questioned about eating habits or recent weight loss.
  - Those who are overweight may be counseled on a proper diet and exercise routine.
- One may consider body fat analysis as part of the PPE, though it must be cautioned that it is sometimes difficult to determine what the ideal body fat is for every athlete in a given sport.

Head, Eyes, Ears, Nose, and Throat

- Examination of the head, eyes, ears, nose, and throat may begin with testing of visual acuity using a standard Snellen chart.
  - Vision should be at least 20/40 in each eye.
  - Appropriate eye protection should be worn if the athlete has any history of significant eye trauma or surgery.
- Anisocoria (asymmetry of pupil size) should be documented so there is a baseline for the athlete. This may become important in the event of head injury.
  - Make sure that this information is readily available to the entire training staff.
- The rest of the examination is to evaluate for pathology

in the athlete, including—but not limited to—a deviated nasal septum, a perforated or scarred tympanic membrane, oral ulcers, or decreased enamel as seen in bulimia.

Cardiovascular

- Examination of the heart should begin with obtaining a blood pressure reading from the athlete.
  - It is important to use the appropriately sized blood pressure cuff, and multiple readings may be required.
  - If blood pressure remains elevated, despite multiple readings, one should refer the athlete to his or her primary care physician, as well as discuss the use of stimulants such as caffeine or nicotine that may contribute to elevated blood pressure. This is not necessarily grounds for restricting athletic participation, however.
- Auscultation of the athlete's heart should occur in the sitting and supine position listening for any murmurs, irregular heartbeats, or extra heart sounds (S3 or S4). Various maneuvers can be performed to clarify the murmur type.
  - Special attention should be paid to the murmur of hypertrophic cardiomyopathy because it is the most common cause of sudden cardiac death in the United States among young athletes. This murmur will decrease in intensity with squatting (as venous outflow decreases) and will increase in intensity on standing or if the athlete does an abdominal "crunch" (increased outflow obstruction).
  - Systolic murmurs grade 3/6 in severity or greater, all diastolic murmurs, and any murmur that increases in intensity with Valsalva should be evaluated further before clearance with an electrocardiogram, echocardiogram, and exercise stress test.
- If any other testing is required, one should consider referral to a cardiologist.

Pulmonary

- The pulmonary exam should focus on good air movement with clear lung fields.
- Findings such as crackles, rhonchi, and wheezes are pathologic and may require further workup or treatment.
- Exercise-induced asthma may not be evident on physical examination.

Abdomen

- Examination of the abdomen is done with the athlete supine and relaxed.
- Abdominal masses, organomegaly, and abdominal pain may require further workup prior to clearance.
- Rarely may an abnormal kidney be palpated on examination.

Genitourinary

- Palpation of the male genitalia should reveal two descended testicles.
  - Any testicular masses, hernias, or irregularities should be noted.
  - Absence of a testicle or presence of an undescended testicle requires counseling because there is an increased risk of testicular loss due to contact sports that is reduced, but not removed, with the use of a protective cup.
- The self-testicular exam should be described and performed monthly because young males are at increased risk for testicular cancer. If there are any questions, the patient may be referred to his primary care physician.
- The female genitourinary exam is not routinely done in the PPE.

Dermatologic

- The skin should be examined for any signs of contagious infection, including herpes simplex, fungal infections, carbuncles, impetigo, and scabies that may preclude participation.
- Suspicious nevi should be noted and referred for removal.

Musculoskeletal

- The goal of the musculoskeletal examination is to determine whether an athlete has any strength deficits, atrophy, or instability that may require rehabilitation or preclude the athlete from participation.
- The type of examination depends on both the examiner and the athlete.
  - If the athlete is asymptomatic and denies any previous injury, it may be reasonable to perform a generalized musculoskeletal screening examination.
  - If the athlete has a current problem or previous injury, it may be prudent to perform a joint-specific examination.
  - History alone is 92% sensitive in detecting significant musculoskeletal injuries.

Generalized Examination

- The generalized exam can quickly assess instability, range of motion, and strength.
- The exam should begin with inspection of the athlete while he or she faces the physician. Ask him or her to do the following:
  - Move the neck in flexion, extension, rotation, and side-bending.
  - Shrug the shoulders against resistance from the physician (trapezius strength).
  - Move the shoulders in internal and external rotation (range of motion).
  - Flex and extend the elbow.
  - Pronate and supinate the elbow (range of motion).
  - Clench the fist and spread the fingers (range of motion).

- Next, ask the athlete to turn and face the other direction, away from you.
  - Check back extension (spondylolysis), flexion, rotation, and side-bending (range of motion).
  - Assess the lower extremities for alignment and symmetry.
  - Ask him or her to "duck walk" for four steps and assess the motion of the hip, knee, and ankle.
  - Finally, ask the athlete to stand on his or her toes and then the heels (calves).
- Any abnormalities on this exam should prompt a joint-specific exam of the area in question.
  - The joint-specific exam requires more time and expertise, though it does give the physician more information than the generalized musculoskeletal exam.
  - There is no evidence that this examination has a higher yield in the asymptomatic athlete than the general screen.

Complete Examination

- The complete examination includes inspection and range-of-motion testing of the spine, neck, shoulders, elbows, wrist, hands, hips, knees, ankles, and feet. Appearance and symmetry should be noted.
- The examination should be done in a stepwise fashion in the same order every time so that no part of the exam is omitted.

Spine

- Note alignment and test for range of motion in flexion, extension, rotation, and side-bending, noting any asymmetry or complaint of pain.
- Evaluate the thoracolumbar spine for kyphosis/scoliosis and evaluate the scapulae for any asymmetry.
- Finally, check range of motion in flexion, extension, side-bending, and rotation of the lumbar spine. Note any increase or decrease in lumbar lordosis.

Lower Extremity

- Examination of the lower extremity begins with the hip exam.
  - Inspect the athlete while standing, noting the level of the iliac crests bilaterally.
  - Have the athlete lie down and evaluate flexion and internal and external rotation of the hip.
- The knee exam begins with inspection, followed by palpation for any effusion, ecchymosis, contusion, or deformity.
  - The normal knee range of motion is 0 to 140 degrees; any decrease may be an indication of underlying pathology.
  - The ligamentous exam is often performed next to assess stability of the knee.
- Place the patient's knee in 20 degrees of flexion and stabilize the femur with one hand as the other pulls the tibia anteriorly. Compare the injured side to the unaffected side for excessive anterior motion, as well as presence of a firm "end point."
- This is the *Lachman test,* and when performed properly, it is very sensitive and specific for injury to the anterior cruciate ligament.

- To evaluate the medial and lateral collateral ligaments, place the knee in 20 to 30 degrees of flexion and apply a valgus stress (to evaluate the medial collateral ligament) and a varus stress (to evaluate the lateral collateral ligament). Assess for pain or laxity with this testing. Once again, it is important to compare the affected side with the unaffected side.
- The *anterior and posterior drawer tests* are used to evaluate the anterior collateral ligament and the posterior cruciate ligament, respectively.
- Bend the athlete's knee to 90 degrees, and then sit on the patient's foot. Place your hands on the tibial plateau and push posteriorly (posterior drawer test) and pull anteriorly (anterior drawer test), looking for excessive motion or no firm end point.
- While the knee is bent at 90 degrees and the foot flat on the table, check for joint-line tenderness both medially and laterally. The *McMurray test* is a very sensitive and specific test for meniscal tears. If there is a pain or a pop felt along the joint line, there may be a tear of the respective meniscus.
- Examination of the ankle involves inspection while the athlete is standing and sitting.
  - Palpation of any effusion or tenderness may be indicative of underlying injury.
  - Strength, dorsiflexion (20 degrees), and plantarflexion (40 degrees) should be assessed.
  - Ligamentous laxity may be assessed by the anterior drawer test (pulling on the heel while stabilizing the tibia looking for anterior motion with the foot in 20 degrees of plantar flexion) and the talar tilt test (inversion of the calcaneus with respect to the tibia). Excessive motion, compared with the other side, should trigger further evaluation.
- Examination of the feet should focus on cavus or planus deformity. Either may affect the athlete's performance by playing a role in lower extremity overuse problems, such as medial tibial stress syndrome.
  - Other deformities, such as bunions, may become painful in athletic footwear and should be noted.

Upper Extremity
- Examination of the upper extremity begins with inspection of the shoulder, looking for any asymmetry while the athlete is in the upright position.
  - Range of motion in abduction, adduction, flexion, and internal and external rotation should be assessed.
  - Strength testing is done in the same planes of motion.
  - The rotator cuff is assessed with the aforementioned strength testing, as well as with the *empty can test*. The patient abducts the arms to 90 degrees, flexes them to 30 degrees, and points the thumbs downward while actively resisting the physician. This specifically isolates the supraspinatus.
  - To detect impingement, passively flex (*Neer test*) and abduct (*Hawkins test*) the shoulder, which will recreate the patient's symptoms.
  - Laxity in the glenohumeral joint is assessed by pulling the arm inferiorly (sulcus sign) and by the *load*

and shift test for anterior instability, as well as the *apprehension and relocation tests*.
- Potential labral tears may be assessed by the *crank test*, as well as the *active compression test*.

Neurologic

- A detailed neurologic exam is required in athletes with a history of burners/stingers, herniated disc, or concussions.
- Testing involves evaluation of strength in the upper or lower extremities and evaluation of deep tendon reflexes.
- In addition, the cranial nerves and cerebellar and cognitive function should be tested if there is a history of head injury. Abnormalities may warrant further workup and a referral to a neurologist prior to clearance.

LABORATORY INVESTIGATIONS

- Laboratory screening is sometimes performed on certain diseases that are prevalent in a given area. A high prevalence is necessary for the test to have a good yield, even if it is highly sensitive and specific.
- Urinalysis is sometimes performed on athletes looking for asymptomatic proteinuria or glucosuria, which would signify renal or metabolic abnormality, including diabetes.
  - This has not been substantiated in any studies, and urinalysis is not currently recommended as part of the PPE.
- Hemoglobin and ferritin tests may be considered as screening tools for anemia. The results may be difficult to interpret in an athlete, however, particularly if he or she has no symptoms. For example, the increased plasma volume in athletes falsely lowers the concentration of hemoglobin, resulting in pseudoanemia. In addition, the use of ferritin does not necessarily predict who will develop true anemia, and those who take supplemental iron do not necessarily see an improvement in performance.
  - These tests are therefore not essential parts of the PPE.
- Cholesterol screening may be performed in an athlete if there is a significant familial history of hypercholesterolemia.
  - It is not routinely recommended in young individuals and, as such, need not be done routinely on the PPE.

SPECIAL TESTING

- Sudden cardiac death is an extremely rare but tragic event with far-reaching ramifications to the medical community. It often results in unrealistic pressures on the medical community to detect and prevent these deaths in the future. This is the reason for such a comprehensive cardiac history and examination in the athlete.

- Some have proposed the use of electro- and echocardiogram to screen all asymptomatic individuals as part of the PPE. However, the use of an electrocardiogram to screen for cardiac problems has never been proven useful. In addition, there is a wide variability of "normal" electrocardiograms in athletes ("athlete's heart").
  - The use of an echocardiogram may be useful in screening for structural abnormalities but is cost-prohibitive.
  - As such, these tests are recommended only if abnormalities are detected in the history or physical examination and not as part of the routine PPE.
- Asthma may be readily diagnosed with the use of pulmonary function testing (PFT).
  - Exercise-induced asthma may not be easily assessed with PFTs because they are performed at rest. The physician must maintain a high index of suspicion. Exercise PFTs may be performed but can usually only be done at large university centers.
  - There is currently no evidence that PFTs should be performed routinely as part of the PPE.

CLEARANCE

- The physician makes the final decision on whether the athlete may participate in sports.
  - He or she may decide that no athletic participation is allowed, that the athlete may participate after certain conditions are met, or that the athlete may participate in athletics. The last category may be further broken down into participation in events based on classification by contact or strenuousness of the activity.
  - Only 0.3% to 1.3% of athletes are denied clearance during the PPE, and only 3.2% to 13.5% require further evaluation.
- Classification of sports by contact allows for risk stratification based on potential for injury. High-impact collision sports, such as football and ice hockey, have an increased potential for injury than do low-impact sports, such as tennis (Box 2-1).
- Classification by strenuousness is important for any athlete who may have pulmonary or cardiac diagnoses.
  - Sports vary widely in how they stress the athlete's body.
  - They are categorized by the dynamic and static demands they place on the athlete. Those with high static or dynamic demands may be inappropriate for certain athletes (Box 2-2).
- Regardless of the type of evaluation done, it is important that coaches and trainers understand restrictions in participation or further workup in the athlete.
  - Communication should be maintained with the athlete and his or her parents so that there are no misunderstandings.
  - Documentation of clearance or need for rehabilitation may be provided using the attached standard PPE form. This may then be distributed to the school, as well as to the parents of the athletes.

BOX 2-1 CLASSIFICATION OF SPORTS BY CONTACT

Contact/Collision
- Basketball
- Boxing
- Diving
- Field hockey
- Football (tackle, flag)
- Ice hockey
- Lacrosse
- Martial arts
- Rodeo
- Rugby
- Ski jumping
- Soccer
- Team handball
- Water polo
- Wrestling

Limited Contact
- Baseball
- Bicycling
- Cheerleading
- Canoeing/kayaking (white water)
- Fencing
- Field events (high jump, pole vault)
- Floor hockey
- Gymnastics
- Handball
- Horseback riding
- Racquetball
- Skating (ice, inline, roller)
- Skiing (cross-country, downhill, water)
- Softball
- Squash
- Ultimate Frisbee
- Volleyball
- Windsurfing/surfing

Noncontact
- Archery
- Badminton
- Bodybuilding
- Bowling
- Canoeing/kayaking (flat water)
- Crew/rowing
- Curling
- Dancing
- Field events (discus, javelin, shot put)
- Golf
- Orienteering
- Power lifting
- Race walking
- Riflery
- Rope jumping
- Sailing
- Scuba diving
- Strength training
- Swimming
- Table tennis
- Tennis
- Track
- Weightlifting

Modified from the American Academy of Pediatrics. Medical conditions and sports. Pediatrics 1994;94:492–493.

BOX 2-2 CLASSIFICATION OF SPORTS BY STRENUOUSNESS

High-to-moderate Dynamic and Static Demands
- Boxing
- Crew/rowing
- Cross-country skiing
- Cycling
- Downhill skiing
- Fencing
- Football
- Ice hockey
- Rugby
- Running (sprinting)
- Speed skating
- Water polo
- Wrestling

High-to-moderate Dynamic and Low Static Demands
- Badminton
- Baseball
- Basketball
- Field hockey
- Lacrosse
- Orienteering
- Table tennis
- Race walking
- Racquetball
- Soccer
- Squash
- Swimming
- Tennis
- Volleyball

Low Dynamic and High-to-moderate Static Demands
- Archery
- Auto racing
- Diving
- Equestrian events
- Field events (jumping, throwing)
- Gymnastics
- Karate or judo
- Motorcycling
- Rodeo
- Sailing
- Ski jumping
- Water skiing
- Weight lifting

Low Dynamic and Static Demands
- Bowling
- Cricket
- Curling
- Golf
- Riflery

Modified from the American Academy of Pediatrics. Medical conditions and sports. Pediatrics 1994;94:492–493.)

- Cardiovascular abnormalities require an understanding of the demands of the sport, as well as the risk to the athlete prior to making a decision on clearance.
  - The guidelines established by the 26th Bethesda Conference cover the major cardiac abnormalities, including mitral valve prolapse, hypertrophic cardiomyopathy, hypertension, and dysrhythmias. One

should follow these guidelines and, if any further questions remain, one should consider a referral to a specialist.

- Acute illness may be grounds for temporary disqualification in the athlete.
  - Cases should be addressed individually based on symptoms. It is important to consider any risk to the individual athlete, as well as any risk to any teammates.
  - American Academy of Pediatrics guidelines disallow participation during febrile illness and with all but mild diarrhea. This decreases the risk of dehydration and heat illness.
  - One may summarize the decision for clearance with the adage, "if symptoms are present from the neck up (i.e., sore throat, nasal congestion, mild headache) and there is *no fever,* then the athlete may participate."
- Bloodborne pathogens are of concern in athletics, especially hepatitis and HIV.
  - Hepatitis B virus and hepatitis C virus are spread via sexual contact, exposure to blood or blood products, and contamination of open wounds or mucous membranes.
- There has been one documented case of spread in high school sumo wrestlers in Japan in 1982.
- Hepatitis does not have a higher prevalence in athletics.
- Infection with hepatitis B virus or hepatitis C virus should be viewed as any other viral illness. Athletes may be able to participate, as long as clinical symptoms such as fatigue and abdominal pain are not interfering. Cases should be assessed individually.
  - HIV is spread in the same manner as hepatitis.
- HIV transmission has never been conclusively documented in any sporting activities.
- The health status of the individual should be taken into account prior to clearance. HIV infection alone does not disqualify an athlete from participation. The type of athletic activity, strenuousness of activity, and risk of transmission to other athletes should all be considered.
- One must stress that confidentiality should be maintained in all such cases.
- Dermatologic conditions—such as herpes simplex, impetigo, or scabies—may preclude participation in certain sports (contact).
  - This is especially important in sports that require the use of mats, such as gymnastics and wrestling, as well as in sports in which equipment is shared, such as baseball.
  - Play may resume once the infection has cleared or is no longer contagious.
- If pregnancy is suspected, clearance for collision sports should be withheld pending appropriate testing or clearance given by the physician after pregnancy.
- Ovarian injuries are unlikely in sports, so that a female with only one ovary need not be restricted from activity.
- Menstrual disorders are not usually grounds for disqualification and may be further investigated after clearance is granted.
  - Amenorrhea should raise the concern for the "female athletic triad," and a frank discussion regarding

disordered eating should follow. Athletic activity should be restricted if there is evidence of compromised performance, significant weight loss, or risk to the athlete. The road to recovery is often a lengthy one, requiring multiple disciplines to work in concert.

- Functionally, one-eyed athletes (vision in one eye less than 20/40) should not participate in athletics with a high risk of eye injury when eye protection cannot be worn. Loss of the remaining "good eye" from injury can be devastating.
- Previous eye surgery or history of retinal detachment requires a referral to an ophthalmologist prior to clearance.
- Organomegaly may stem from various causes and may present a concern in athletes, especially those in contact sports. It is important to determine what is causing the problem so that appropriate treatment is instituted.
- Hepatomegaly may stem from a neoplasm or infection, such as mononucleosis. If the liver edge is palpable distal to the rib cage, it is at increased risk for injury.
    - Even though hepatic rupture is rare, the athlete with hepatomegaly should not be allowed to participate until it has been resolved.
- Athletes with splenomegaly may not participate in athletics because of increased risk of splenic rupture until it has resolved. This is not limited to contact sports because there have been reports of splenic rupture while engaged in nonstrenuous activity.
    - The physician may consider the use of ultrasound to follow organ size since the physical exam has a low sensitivity for detecting organomegaly.
- Athletes with a history of heat illness are at greater risk for recurrence.
    - The physician must try to determine any predisposing factors and keep it from happening again. Repeated occurrences may be due to medicines, medical conditions, poor acclimatization, or the environment.
    - Prevention should focus on appropriate hydration throughout activity, proper conditioning, and avoiding medications, such as antihistamines or stimulants.
    - Clearance may be restricted to participation under temperate conditions.
- Diagnosis of an inguinal hernia does not necessarily disqualify an athlete from athletics. It may intermittently cause pain and affect performance but is emergent only if it becomes incarcerated.
    - One may consider a surgical referral because the patient will inevitably require treatment in the future.
    - Cases should be assessed individually.
- An athlete with kidney abnormalities, such as a solitary kidney, may be at increased risk for rupture in contact sports. The actual risk is small, but the consequences, such as transplantation or dialysis, are quite severe.
    - One may consider a referral to a specialist prior to clearance to make sure the remaining kidney is normal and does not show any evidence of hydronephrosis or other abnormalities. If the kidney is normal,

the athlete should be counseled on the risks and then allowed to make his or her own decision in conjunction with family members or guardians.

- Athletes with the diagnosis of asthma may participate, provided it is well controlled with medication.
    - Athletes with poorly controlled asthma need to be seen by their primary care physician or pulmonologist and have their condition stabilized before participation.
    - Exercise-induced asthma may be difficult to assess in the PPE but may be treated with a trial of beta-agonist medication.
    - If symptoms do not resolve themselves, one may consider an exercise test with pulmonary function testing or a methacholine challenge to rule out exercise-induced asthma.
- Severe pulmonary dysfunction, such as in an athlete with cystic fibrosis, is justification for referral to a specialist for further testing prior to clearance.
- Testicular disorders, such as a solitary testicle or undescended testes, do not necessarily disqualify an athlete. There is no consensus on whether or not an athlete with only one testicle may participate in contact sports. The actual incidence of injury resulting in orchiectomy in sporting events is quite low.
    - The use of a protective cup, though cumbersome and uncomfortable, may decrease risk of injury. Ultimately, the risk of injury should be explained to the athlete, who may then make the decision on wearing protection.
    - Undescended testes should be thoroughly evaluated secondary to the increased risk of carcinoma, and decision making is similar to that of the athlete with a single testicle.
- Commonly, athletes may present with a medical history significant for concussions or burners/stingers.
    - Athletes with burners/stingers may be cleared if they are currently asymptomatic and there are no abnormalities on physical examination.
    - Consider cervical spine radiographs to evaluate for instability or an MRI to evaluate for spinal stenosis if the burners/stingers are recurrent.
    - Use of protective padding may be instituted.
    - If the athlete has a history of neurapraxia with transient quadriplegia, consider referral to a specialist to rule out structural abnormalities. If there are structural abnormalities, the athlete should not participate in contact sports. Cases should be individually assessed.
- Concussions occur an estimated 250,000 times per year in football alone.
    - A generally accepted and clinically useful definition is a traumatically induced alteration in mental status.
    - Classification and severity of concussion are rated by various systems, but there is no universally accepted system on concussion grading, as well as return to play.
    - The concern in allowing a player with a concussion to return to play is termed "second impact syndrome." This syndrome refers to the catastrophic re-

sults, including elevated intracranial pressure and brain swelling, that may occur when a player with a concussion injures his brain again.
- Players may return to play once their neurologic symptoms have subjectively resolved, there are no deficits on physical or neurological examination, and physical exertion does not cause a relapse in symptoms.
- In an athlete with a history of multiple concussions, one may consider a referral to a neurologist prior to clearance.
- There is very little literature regarding risk of participation for athletes with convulsive disorders.
  - In those with poorly controlled seizure disorders, clearance should be withheld for contact sports or any sports that are potentially hazardous to the athlete (e.g., scuba diving and motor racing) until appropriate medications are administered.
- Referral to a neurologist for further testing and treatment of uncontrolled seizures should be considered.
- Athletes may compete in athletics that pose no risk to themselves or others.
  - In athletes who have well-controlled convulsive disorders, clearance may be granted for participation in all types of athletics.
    - If there are any concerns, or the athlete competes in a high-risk sport, consider referral to a specialist for further testing.
    - Determination of clearance for those with musculoskeletal injuries requires evaluating multiple factors but is often dependent on determining that the joint has full range of motion, is stable, and has near full strength (>85% to 90%).
  - Clearance also hinges on the type of injury, as well as the sport that the athlete is involved in.
  - Protective padding or taping may protect the athlete while allowing him or her to compete.
  - If the athlete has an injury that does not allow him or her to compete safely, clearance should not be granted until appropriate measures are taken.
  - Important factors to assess for on examination when dealing with sprains, strains, subluxations, and overuse injuries include the presence of an effusion, decreased range of motion, decreased strength (<85% when compared with the unaffected side), ligamentous instability, and inability to complete functional testing. If these are present, one should consider further testing or a referral to a specialist prior to clearance for athletic activity.

MEDICOLEGAL ISSUES

- The issue of clearance for participation in athletics is not uncommon.
- When an athlete is not cleared for participation in a certain sport, he or she may seek a second opinion in hopes of gaining clearance for their desired sport.
- Under the Rehabilitation Act of 1973 and the Americans with Disabilities Act of 1990, the athlete may have the right to participate against medical advice.

- If the physician is contemplating disqualification of an athlete, it may be prudent to consider a referral to a specialist to determine risk of injury.
  - Such information should be passed along to the athlete and his or her parents/guardians. It is important to document clearly such discussions.
- If, despite the risks, the athlete decides to participate against medical advice, one may consider having the athlete or guardian sign an exculpatory waiver to indicate clearly that the risk has been explained and that the athlete still wishes to compete.
  - In such a document, the athlete promises not to sue the physician or school, thereby releasing them from liability.
  - A concern with this course of action is that the validity of such a document may vary from state to state, and some wonder whether this will actually protect the physician or institution from lawsuits.
  - Cases should be handled individually; consider legal counsel based on the circumstances of the case.
- There have been allegations of sexual improprieties against providers while performing the PPE.
  - The greatest risk of such claims appears to come from the mass station-based format.
  - In addition, athletes may not expect a thorough examination during the PPE. The physician should explain the extent of the examination, supply an appropriate environment, and use discretion.
  - Consider the use of chaperones in appropriate circumstances.
  - Consistency in the exam is important, as well as in attire of the athletes.
  - The use of common sense should protect the physician from such accusations.
- The liability of providers performing the PPE on a volunteer basis has received increased scrutiny.
  - Some states have taken measures to protect volunteer examiners under "Good Samaritan" statutes.
  - Physicians need to be aware of their state's laws and proceed accordingly.
  - To be protected under such statutes, the physician may not receive money or services in exchange for their time.

SUGGESTED READING

American Academy of Pediatrics, American Academy of Ophthalmology. Protective eyewear for young athletes. Pediatrics 1996;98:311–313.

American Academy of Pediatrics, Committee on Sports Medicine and Fitness. Medical conditions affecting sports participation. Pediatrics 1994;94:757–760.

26th Bethesda conference: recommendations for determining eligibility for competition in athletes with cardiovascular abnormalities. January 6–7, 1994. Med Sci Sports Exerc 1994;26(suppl):S223–S283.

Caine DJ, Broekhoff J. Maturity assessment: a viable preventive measure against physical and psychological insult to the young athlete? Phys Sportsmed 1987;15:67–80.

Calabrese LH, LaPerriere A. Human immunodeficiency virus infection, exercise and athletics. Sports Med 1993;15:6–13.

Cantu RC. Guidelines for return to contact sports after a cerebral concussion. Phys Sportsmed 1986;14:75–83.

Cantu RC, Voy R. Second impact syndrome: a risk in any contact sport. Phys Sportsmed 1995;23:27–34.

DiFiori JP. Overuse injuries in children and adolescents. Phys Sportsmed 1999;27:75–89.

Dorsen PJ. Should athletes with one eye, kidney or testicle play contact sports? Phys Sportsmed 1986;14:130–138.

Edwards SE, Glover ED, Schroeder KL. The effects of smokeless tobacco on heart rate and neuromuscular reactivity in athletes and nonathletes. Phys Sportsmed 1987;15:141–147.

Feinstein RA, Colvin E, Oh MK. Echocardiographic screening as part of a preparticipation examination. Clin J Sport Med 1993;3:149–152.

Feinstein RA, La Russa J, Wang-Dohlman A, et al. Screening adolescent athletes for exercise-induced asthma. Clin J Sport Med 1996;6:119–123.

Ferenchick GS, Adelman S. Myocardial infarction associated with anabolic steroid use in a previously healthy 37-year-old weight lifter. Am Heart J 1992;124:507–508.

Gallup EM. Law and the Team Physician. Champaign, IL: Human Kinetics Books, 1995:76–77, 80–81.

Gomez JE, Landry GL, Bernhardt DT. Critical evaluation of the 2-minute orthopedic screening examination. Am J Dis Child 1993;147:1109–1113.

Herbert DL. Professional considerations related to the conduct of preparticipation examinations. Sports Med Stand Malpract Rep 1994;6:33, 35–36, 49, 51–52.

Kashiwagi S, Hayashi J, Ikematsu H, et al. An outbreak of hepatitis B in members of a high school sumo-wrestling club. JAMA 1982;248:213–214.

Kelley JP, Nichols JS, Filley CM, et al. Concussion in sports: guidelines for the prevention of catastrophic outcome. JAMA 1991;266:2867–2869.

Linder CW, DuRant RH, Seklecki RM, et al. Preparticipation health screening of young athletes: results of 1268 examinations. Am J Sports Med 1981;9:187–193.

Magnes SA, Henderson JM, Hunter SC. What conditions limit sports participation? Experience with 10,540 athletes. Phys Sportsmed 1992;20:143–160.

Maron BJ, Bodison SA, Wesley YE, et al. Results of screening a large group of intercollegiate competitive athletes for cardiovascular disease. J Am Coll Cardiol 1987;10:1214–1221.

McKeag DB. Preseason physical examination for the prevention of sports injuries. Sports Med 1985;2:413–431.

Peggs JF, Reinhardt RW, O'Brien JM. Proteinuria in adolescent sports physical examinations. J Fam Pract 1986;22:80–81.

Rupp NT, Guill MF, Brudno DS. Unrecognized exercise-induced bronchospasm in adolescent athletes. Am J Dis Child 1992;146:941–944.

Sallis RE, Jones K, Knopp W. Burners: offensive strategy for an underreported injury. Phys Sportsmed 1992;20:47–55.

Smith DM, Kovan JR, Rich BSE, et al. Preparticipation Physical Evaluation, ed. 2. Minneapolis: McGraw-Hill, 1997.

Squire DL. Eating disorders. In: Mellion MB, ed. Sports Medicine Secrets. Philadelphia: Hanley and Belfus, Inc, 1993:136–141.

Tanner SM. Preparticipation examination targeted for the female athlete. Clin Sports Med 1994;13:337–353.

Taylor WC III, Lombardo JA. Preparticipation screening of college athletes: value of the complete blood cell count. Phys Sportsmed 1990;18:106–118.

Torg JS, Glasgow SG. Criteria for return to contact activities following cervical spine injury. Clin J Sport Med 1991;1:12–26.

Van Camp SP. Sudden death in athletes. In: Grana WA, Lombardo JA, eds. Advances in Sports Medicine and Fitness. Chicago: Year Book Medical Publishers, 1988:121–142.

SPORTS PHARMACOLOGY: DRUG USE AND ABUSE

LEE A. MANCINI
BRIAN D. BUSCONI
J. HERBERT STEVENSON

HISTORY

In the Beginning

For as long as there have been athletes, there has been the search for any advantage to succeed in competition. Believing that it would give them greater strength and power, Aztec warriors used to eat the hearts of their defeated enemies. The Chinese, more than 5,000 years ago; the Babylonians and Egyptians, more than 4,000 years ago; and the ancient Greeks, more than 2,500 years ago, all used various herbs to try to enhance athletic performance. The Greeks also tried to create the optimum diet for achieving athletic excellence. Ancient Greek athletes would consume strychnine found in seeds from the *nux vomica* plant. Strychnine was a known poison, but it was also believed to be a central nervous system (CNS) stimulant, and the Greek athletes thought it gave them an additional edge over their rivals. The Greek Olympic athletes felt that eating a known poison was worth the risk if it brought victory and immortality in the games, which would ensure immortality in history. Even thousands of years ago, athletes were pushing the en-

velope by endangering their health and breaking the rules. In fact, in 300 B.C., three Olympic athletes were banned from competition because they were found to have ingested a combination of mushrooms and animal protein. The word *ergogenic* comes from the Greek words *ergon* (meaning "work") and *gennan* (meaning "to produce"). In other words, an ergogenic aid is a substance that produces work.

Modern Times

At the turn of the 20th century, strychnine reappeared and was used by marathon runners in the first modern summer Olympics. Cyclists drank brandy before races in hopes of improving performance times. In Europe, in 1935, a major breakthrough came in terms of performance enhancement: androgenic anabolic steroids. Initially, steroids were used on starvation victims to help restore a positive nitrogen balance. The anabolic component was later developed to try and avoid the unwanted androgen side effects. In the 1950s, an American physician, Dr. J. Ziegler, created methandrostenolone, more commonly recognized as Dianabol. Dianabol was highly anabolic, with much fewer androgenic side effects than previous steroids. At the time, Ziegler was also a physician for the U.S. Olympic athletes and encouraged the athletes to use Dianabol. He believed at the time that he was aiding the athletes' training routines, unaware of the many harmful effects of steroid use.

INTERNATIONAL OLYMPIC COMMITTEE

With the use of steroids becoming more widespread in the athletic arena, the International Olympic Committee (IOC), in 1968, released its first list of banned substances. The Olympic games in Montreal, in 1976, were the first games to test for anabolic steroids. Over the years, the list has been expanded and refined; in 1984 blood doping was added, diuretics and β-blockers became part of the list in 1985, and in 1989, peptide hormones [such as human chorionic gonadotropin (hCG), adrenocorticotropic hormone, human growth hormone (hGH), and erythropoietin (EPO) were included].

The Current Landscape

In the 1990s, two important pieces of legislation changed the sports pharmacology landscape. The first, the Nutrition Labeling and Education Act, was passed on November 8, 1990. The purpose of this act was to change the nutritional labels on the sides of all food products. The goal was to make labels clearer to understand and to make sure the labels contained daily reference values and U.S. Recommended Daily Allowances (RDAs). The Dietary Supplement Health and Education Act was the other major legislation. It was passed on October 25, 1994, and remains the subject of much controversy. This act enabled supplement companies to market products as nutritional aids and not as drugs. This meant that the U.S. Food and Drug Administration (FDA) did not have the power to regulate supplements and gave the supplement companies freedom to market their products as long as they did not make medical claims. The supplement industry is a booming business. In 1994, it was a $8.3 billion industry. In 1999, it grew to $14 billion and, over the next few years, it is expected to reach $40 billion. With so many products flooding the market, now more than ever, team physicians need to learn about ergogenic aids and must be able to talk to their athletes and patients about risks and benefits. It is the goal of this chapter to discuss most of the major drugs, ergogenic aids, nutritional supplements, and recreational drugs being used by athletes today.

STEROIDS AND PROHORMONES

Testosterone

Testosterone is the forerunner of modern-day steroids. In 1849, Dr. A. Berthold discovered that implanting testicles in the abdomen of roosters had the effect of reversing castration. Building off Berthold's research, Dr. C. Brown-Sequard in 1889 at the age of 72, injected a unique concoc-

tion into himself. He proclaimed to the scientific community that this injection made his mind sharper, his body stronger, and his spirit more energetic. What was in this injection? A liquid extract of ground-up guinea pig and canine testicles. Later, in 1905, Brown-Sequard theorized that vital organs secreted substances within the body that exerted specific effects on the body, and the discovery of hormones was made.

Actions

Testosterone is the primary male hormone in the body. It has both anabolic and androgenic effects. Testosterone is formed in the body from cholesterol through a series of reactions. There are several pathways that lead to the formation of testosterone from cholesterol. One way is from dehydroepiandrosterone (DHEA) being converted into androstenedione and then testosterone. Another way is DHEA to 5-androstenediol and then testosterone. Yet another is DHEA to androstenedione, to 4-androstenediol, and then testosterone. Knowledge of the cholesterol to testosterone pathway is important because most synthetic anabolic steroids and prohormone supplements are based on tinkering with the various compounds in this pathway. The principal active metabolite of testosterone is 5α-dihydrotestosterone (DHT). DHT has a much higher affinity to androgen receptors than testosterone. Also, it is important to note that androstenedione can be converted to estrone instead of testosterone and continue on to form estradiol. Not only can androstenedione end up forming estradiol, but testosterone itself can be changed to estradiol.

Proven Performance Effects

The ergogenic effects of testosterone have been used for the greater part of the 20th century. At the 1936 Olympic Games, athletes used testosterone. There have been numerous studies that have proven that exogenous testosterone supplementation can increase lean body mass (LBM), decrease body fat, and increase strength and power. Testosterone has been shown to allow an athlete to perform greater volumes of work in each training session, to perform more sessions each day, and to recover more quickly from each session. Testosterone can be taken as a pill (75 to 100 mg qd), as an injection (200 to 250 mg qd), as a transdermal patch, or as a skin cream.

Adverse Effects

Exogenous testosterone use is associated with a host of dangers for an athlete. The androgenic effects include premature baldness, facial acne, body acne, and an increase in cardiovascular disease. In men, there is also a decrease in sperm production, a decrease in testicle size, and an increase risk of prostate cancer. The testosterone metabolite DHT, because of its high androgen receptor affinity, significantly contributes to these effects. Besides the serious health risks to an athlete taking testosterone, there are also the legal risks. The National Collegiate Athletic Association (NCAA), IOC, U.S. Olympic Committee (USOC), and various other governing sports bodies have banned testosterone use, which is tested by measuring the ratio of testosterone to epitestosterone (T:E ratio) in an athlete's urine. A normal

T:E ratio is 1:1, but the illegal supplementation cutoff value is 6:1.

Summary
- Testosterone has proven positive effects on athletic performance, as well as dangerous health risks.
- It is illegal to use testosterone.

Steroids

The first synthetic steroids were created in the 1950s. In 1953, nandrolone—one of the first steroids—was produced. Nandrolone and its two major metabolites, 3-norandrosterone and 2-noretiocholanolone were found to be more anabolic than testosterone. In 1959, oxymetholone and stanozolol were created. Today, some of the most used steroids are deconate, oxandrolone, oxymetholone, stanozolol, and nandrolone.

Actions

Steroids are believed to have a variety of effects on the human body. They are thought to have an anticatabolic effect. Steroids compete with glucocorticoids for glucocorticoid binding sites, leading to a decrease in the concentration of cortisol in the body. Cortisol is one of the major stress hormones that rise as exercise intensity increases and leads to increased muscle breakdown. Steroids prevent muscle breakdown associated with exercise. Besides anticatabolic effects, steroids are more often associated with their anabolic effects. Steroids cause nitrogen retention by forming an androgen–receptor complex. This complex is transported to a nucleus of a muscle cell, where it binds to complementary regions on DNA. This leads to activating transport RNA and increased protein synthesis, which leads to increased muscle growth.

Steroids have effects on other tissues in the body, including stimulating erythropoiesis and causing increased bone marrow activity, increasing hemoglobin, and increasing reticulocyte count. They also create larger, stronger bones by stimulating osteoblast production, thus increasing levels of 1,25-dihyroxy vitamin D, and producing bone matrix proteins.

Testosterone in the body can be converted to a highly androgenic metabolite (DHT) or to estradiol (an estrogen). Neither of these conversions is beneficial. Increased estradiol levels lead to feminization of male sex traits, such as gynecomastia and a higher-pitched voice. The term *aromatization* describes the conversion of steroids into estradiol. New generations of steroid manufacturers are always trying to find ways to prevent aromatization. Testosterone is converted into DHT by the enzyme 5α-reductase with the aid of androgen receptors. DHT causes male pattern baldness, an increased risk in prostate cancer, and many other androgenic side effects. Because testosterone, the original steroid, has both anabolic and androgenic effects, all synthetic steroids have both effects as well, but to varying degrees. New generations of steroids have attempted to have a decreased affinity for androgen receptors in favor of increased anabolic activity. Another important term is *C-17 alkylation.* This refers to the concept that the number 17 carbon in a steroid is capable of becoming a 17α derivative or a 17β

ester of testosterone. This difference is important because esterification makes the steroid more fat soluble, delays absorption in the blood, and can be metabolized in the liver. Injectable steroids are 17β esters or non-17α-alkylated steroids. Oral steroids are 17α-alkylated steroids and resist metabolism in the liver. This means a smaller dose of steroids are required orally to produce an equal effect, but it also means that 17α-alkylated steroids are much more hepatotoxic. The term *cycling* applies to athletes using steroids for a period of several weeks, usually 6 to 12, and then stopping usage for another period of time. *Stacking* refers to athletes using several different steroid agents all at the same time. *Pyramiding* means gradually increasing the dose of steroids over a period of time.

Proven Performance Effects

When castrated animals were given steroids, the result was an increase in nitrogen retention and increased lean muscle mass. In rats given steroids, the effects were an improvement in recovery after exercise, an increase in force generating, and improved recovery time from muscle contusions. Steroids have a variety of medicinal uses: to treat hypogonadism, to provide palliative care in breast cancer, to treat angioneurotic edema, and to treat acquired immune deficiency syndrome (AIDS)–related cachexia. Studies have shown that oxandrolone leads to hypertrophy of the diaphragm. This causes increased expiratory and inspiratory muscle strength, as well as an increase in pulmonary vital capacity. An increase in lean body mass occurs after taking steroids. One study on the effect of steroids showed that males taking steroids gained an average of 19.9 kg body weight and increased their maximum bench press by 47%. Muscle biopsies of athletes taking steroids showed an increase in both the average muscle fiber size and the number of muscle fibers. Although there is overwhelming evidence to show that steroids increase muscle mass, decrease body fat, increase strength, and decrease recovery time, there are not significant data to show that steroids improve aerobic performance.

Adverse Effects

Steroids have significant documented health risks on a variety of organ systems. They have proven CNS effects, including increased aggression, mood swings, and increased sexual arousal. Steroid users are significantly more likely to have a major mood disorders (mania, hypomania, or major depression) than nonusers. Steroids also have profound effects on skin, such as oily hair, oily skin, alopecia, increased sebaceous cysts, striae distensae, and facial and back acne. They cause premature closure of bone growth center, which leads to stunted growth in young steroid users. Another musculoskeletal effect of steroid use is an increased incidence of tendon ruptures as a result of excessive loads placed on tendinous insertion points. The effects of steroids on one's liver are also quite profound. Liver function tests (LFTs) find increased levels of aspartate aminotransferase, alanine aminotransferase, lactate dehydrogenase, alkaline phosphatase; and peliosis hepatis, which is the development of blood-filled cysts in the liver. If these cysts rupture, it is a life-threatening matter. Steroid use increases the risk of developing liver cancer. Exogenous steroids create numerous reproductive and endocrine changes in a user's body.

In males, steroids cause feedback inhibition along the hypothalamic-pituitary-gonadal axis. High levels of steroids cause the body to decrease production of luteinizing hormone and follicle-stimulating hormone, thus causing secondary hypogonadotrophic hypogonadism. This results in a decrease in mean testicular length, a decrease in sperm count, a decrease in sperm mobility, a decrease in sperm density, and an increase in infertility but no change in libido. The aromatization of steroids in males also causes gynecomastia and an increased risk of prostate cancer. In women, steroids cause hirsutism, voice deepening, clitoral hypertrophy, a decrease in breast size, amenorrhea, and male pattern baldness. In males, discontinuing steroids leads to a reversal of all the testicular and spermatogenic changes, but the changes in a female steroid user's body are irreversible. The cardiovascular system is also affected by exogenous steroid use. An increase in total cholesterol levels, an increase in low-density lipoprotein (LDL) levels, a decrease in high-density lipoprotein (HDL) levels, and a decrease in triglyceride levels are all well documented in steroid users. Steroid users experience cardiac hypertrophy and hypertension and are at increased risk for stroke or myocardial infarction. Injection of steroids also leads to an increased risk of exposure to human immunodeficiency virus (HIV), hepatitis B, and hepatitis C.

Although steroids have medical benefits that extend beyond the athletic field, the dosages of steroids used are much lower than those used by athletes for performance enhancement. For example, the recommended dose of Dianabol is 2.5 to 5.0 mg/day; however, one study showed that athletes using Dianabol were consuming 6,000 mg in a 2-week period, well above the recommended dose. It is important to emphasize to athletes that many of the dangerous effects of steroids can be reversed by discontinuing usage. LFT results, show that cholesterol levels, and cardiac hypertrophy return to normal, hypertension disappears, and the risks of stroke and myocardial infarction are decreased. However, it is not known whether the long-term risks of developing prostate and liver cancer remain increased.

Between 4% and 12% of high school males have used steroids. Use in NCAA athletes is 14% to 20%, and the number is higher for professional athletes. Steroid users have also been shown to be twice as likely to use tobacco, three times more likely to use marijuana, four times more likely to use cocaine, and ten times more likely to use amphetamines. They may consume three times as many alcoholic drinks in a week than nonusers. This self-reported study showed that, of the athletes who used steroids, 70% had gotten into a fight, 45% had gotten injured, 44% had performed sexual misconduct, and 41% had run into trouble with the law. These results have raised the question of whether steroids should be considered a gateway drug. For a summary of the adverse effects of steroids, see Box 3-1.

Summary

■ In 1988, the Anti-Drug Abuse Act prohibited distribution of anabolic steroids. The law made it illegal for physicians to prescribe steroids to enhance an athlete's performance.

BOX 3-1 ADVERSE EFFECTS OF STEROID USE

CNS
■ Increased aggression
■ Mood swings
■ Increased sexual arousal
■ Increased major mood disorders

Dermatologic
■ Oily hair and skin
■ Alopecia
■ Striae distensae (stretch marks)
■ Acne on the face and back
■ Increased sebaceous cysts

Musculoskeletal
■ Premature closure of growth plates
■ Increased risk of tendon ruptures

Liver
■ Increased LFTs
■ Peliosis hepatis (blood-filled liver cysts)
■ Increased risk of liver cancer

Men
■ Gynecomastia
■ Increased risk of prostate cancer
■ Decreased testicle size
■ Decreased sperm count
■ Decreased fertility

Women
■ Hirsutism
■ Voice deepening
■ Clitoral hypertrophy
■ Decrease in breast size and amenorrhea
■ Male pattern baldness

Cardiac
■ Increased total cholesterol, LDL, triglycerides
■ Increased risk of stroke
■ Decreased HDL
■ Increased risk of myocardial infarction
■ Hypertension

Immunologic
■ Increased risk of HIV
■ Increased risk of hepatitis B
■ Increased risk of hepatitis C

HDL, high-density lipoprotein; HIV, human immunodeficiency virus; LDL, low-density lipoprotein; LFT, liver function test.

■ Anabolic steroids were classified as a schedule III agent in 1990—the same category as amphetamines, opium, and morphine.
■ Possession of steroids is a federal offense, carrying 1 year in prison, a minimum $1,000 fine, or both.
■ Selling steroids is a federal felony carrying a 5-year prison term, a $250,000 fine, or both.
■ The IOC, NCAA, the National Football League (NFL), Major League Baseball (MLB), the National Hockey League (NHL), and the National Basketball Association (NBA) all have steroids on their banned substance lists.
■ Urine tests for steroids focus on the T:E ratio, using the

6:1 cutoff. Probenecid, epitestosterone, and ethacrynic acid are just some of the masking agents taken by steroid users.

■ Although steroids have been proved to enhance aspects of athletic performance, they have serious health risks and are prohibited and illegal.

Androstenedione

Actions

When people today hear the word "andro," the image that comes to mind is Major League Baseball's record home run season of 1998 and the ensuing supplement scandal. Androstenedione is a steroid precursor to testosterone. It is synthesized in the testes but can be made from DHEA peripherally. Variants of androstenedione that can be found as prohormones in supplements include 5-androstendione, 4-androstenediol, 5-androstenediol, 19-norandrost-4-enedione, 19-norandrost-5-enediol, and 19-norandrost-4-enediol. All are alleged to increase serum levels of testosterone. By increasing serum testosterone, exogenous androstenedione supplementation has been touted to increase strength, decrease body fat mass, and increase muscle mass.

Proven Performance Effects

No study has yet shown that androstenedione increases strength or improves athletic performance, but decreases in testosterone have resulted from androstenedione use. It has been hypothesized that there is a down-regulation of endogenous testosterone production in the face of exogenous androstenedione supplementation.

Adverse Effects

Androstenedione in males increases serum levels of the feminizing hormones estrone and estradiol. This can lead to gynecomastia. A decrease in serum levels of HDL has also been shown, which can increase the risk of coronary artery disease. No data exist on the long-term adverse effects of supplementation with androstenedione.

Summary

■ A review shows that androstenedione has no effect on strength, athletic performance, or LBM.
■ In males, it increases the levels of female hormones and decreases HDL.
■ It has been shown to cause a positive urine test for the anabolic steroid nandrolone.
■ As of February 2005, all prohormones—including androstenedione—have been banned by the FDA.

Dehydroepiandrosterone

DHEA is a main precursor of male and female sex hormones, which are produced in the adrenal glands. DHEA is converted first into androstenedione and ultimately to either testosterone or estradiol. DHEA is a weak androgen that can be changed in tissue to testosterone and DHT. There are two forms of DHEA, an unconjugated form and a stronger conjugated sulfate. DHEA has also been found in wild yams and in the seeds of the Austrian Pine.

Actions

DHEA supplemented in rats leads to decreased body fat, decreased cholesterol levels, and increased insulin sensitivity. One important physiologic difference between rats and humans is that DHEA is not produced in rat adrenal glands. It was believed that DHEA would lead to increased levels of growth hormone and insulin-like growth factor 1 (IGF-1), which would lead to increased muscle mass. Also, DHEA was thought to have an anticatabolic, accelerating recovery by counteracting the effects of glucocorticoids. Exercise has been shown to cause a rise in DHEA levels, with the half-life of DHEA at 25 minutes and conjugated sulfate DHEA at 10 hours.

Proven Performance Effects

Whereas animal studies have shown DHEA supplementation leads to decreased fat mass, decreased obesity, and increased muscle mass, the results in human studies are not as conclusive. No studies have shown any increase in strength, aerobic performance, or other ergogenic effects.

Adverse Effects

Doses of up to 1,100 mg/day of DHEA lower HDL levels, cause irreversible gynecomastia in men, increase estrone and estradiol levels, and increase risk of coronary artery disease. There have been case reports, but no studies, showing that DHEA causes voice deepening, virilization, hair loss, and hirsutism in women, as well as causes irreversible gynecomastia in men. The long-term effects of DHEA are unknown, but it is believed they include increased risks of breast, uterine, and prostate cancer.

Summary

■ In 1985, the FDA stopped the marketing of DHEA as a weight-loss product.
■ It is banned by the IOC.
■ For athletes, a dose as small as 50 mg/day for 3 days is enough to change that critical T:E 6:1 ratio.
■ The evidence is clear that DHEA does not have ergogenic effects, has proven side effects, and has unknown but serious long-term risks; thus, it is banned in Olympic competition.
■ As of February 2005, all prohormones, including DHEA, have been banned by the FDA.

Tribulus Terrestris

Tribulus terrestris is an herbal compound found in both the puncture vine and the caltrop fruit. It supposedly acts as a luteinizing hormone in the body, stimulating the production of endogenous testosterone, and thereby causing an anabolic effect. It has been shown to increase circulating levels of luteinizing hormone and testosterone in men who were infertile. Improvements on body composition and strength performance have not been seen, however. There are no reported side effects or toxic doses in humans taking *Tribulus terrestris*.

Summary

■ *Tribulus terrestris* clearly has not been examined as extensively as DHEA, androstenedione, testosterone, or anabolic steroids.

■ It is not ergogenic, but it shows no known side effects for athletes taking this supplement.

ANTIESTROGENS

This is a class of drugs and supplements whose primary use is not anabolic but rather to block some of the unwanted effects of anabolic steroid use. Some of the more commonly known antiestrogen agents that athletes use are tamoxifen, Clomid, Cytadren, human chorionic gonadotrophin (hCG), and resveratrol.

Clomiphene Citrate (Clomid)

Clomid is a triphenylethylene. Classified as a selective estrogen receptor modulator, Clomid has tissue-specific effects. It is antiresorptive on bone and is most widely used as a treatment of infertility, as it stimulates ovulation in women. It is an antiestrogen at the level of the pituitary gland because it stimulates the release of follicle-stimulating hormone from the pituitary.

Tamoxifen (Nolvadex)

Tamoxifen is widely known as a treatment in breast cancer, specifically estrogen-receptor positive breast cancer. Its antiestrogen effects are important in steroid users because it blocks aromatization, the conversion of testosterone to estrone and estradiol in the body. Tamoxifen prevents the development of gynecomastia in steroid users. It may also increase fat loss.

Aminoglutethimide (Cytadren)

Aminoglutethimide is used in the treatment of metastatic breast cancer. Like tamoxifen, it blocks aromatization and the production of adrenal steroids. It is used as a hardening agent, increasing muscle size and definition.

Human Chorionic Gonadotrophin

This hormone is taken by steroid users to reverse testicular shrinkage after completing a steroid cycle.

3,4,5-Trihydroxystilbene (Resveratrol)

Resveratrol is a stilbene, a naturally occurring phenolic compound found in mulberries, peanuts, and in the skins of grapes. It is associated with increased levels in wine, specifically red wine, and has a variety of positive effects on the human body. Resveratrol is well known for decreasing LDL levels, the risk of coronary artery disease, platelet aggregation, and coagulation. It also has been shown to inhibit lipid peroxidation, which produces free radicals. It is an antioxidant that prevents cell injury and death, as well

as the inhibition of tumor development. It also competes with 17β-estradiol for the binding site on estrogen receptors, functioning as an antiestrogen agent blocking the unwanted feminizing side effects of steroid use.

Adverse Effects

In the literature, there are no reported side effects or adverse effects of using tamoxifen, resveratrol, Cytadren, or Clomid.

Summary

■ Antiestrogens do not have performance-enhancing effects, but they are used to deal with some of the unpleasant and unwanted side effects of steroid consumption.

■ Because of their association with steroid use, these supplements are banned from the IOC and other sports governing bodies.

BANNED OR RESTRICTED DRUGS

Human Growth Hormone

Human growth hormone (hGH) is produced in the anterior pituitary gland by cells called somatotropes. The effects of hGH on the body are mediated by IGF-1. hGH is converted in the liver to IGF-1s. IGF-1s has an anabolic effect, increasing uptake of amino acids, increasing transcription and translation, and producing more protein.

Actions

Human growth hormone (hGH), also called somatotropin, has a host of roles in the body. It stimulates protein synthesis, increases tissue growth by increasing nitrogen retention, and inhibits glucose utilization by promoting lipolysis. Other functions include increasing cardiac output, increasing sweat rate, increased wound healing, increased bone formation and bone mass, increased LBM, decreased fat mass, and improved thermal homeostasis.

Proven Performance Effects

With endogenous hGH responsible for many beneficial functions in the human body, it was theorized that exogenous hGH could enhance athletic performance. In individuals who are growth hormone-deficient, supplementation with hGH led to increased muscle mass, increased muscle strength, increased LBM, and decreased fat mass. This anabolic effect of exogenous hGH supplementation on growth hormone–deficient patients lasted for 5 years after discontinuing supplementation. Muscle fiber-type ratios were also altered, as exogenous hGH increased the percentage of type II fast-twitch fibers and decreased type I slow-twitch fibers. Another medical use for exogenous hGH is in malnourished, elderly patients. Somatotropin decreases with age, as body fat percentage rises and LBM decreases. Supplementing hGH can lead to decreased body fat and increased LBM. Supplementation with hGH for only a few weeks can markedly increase bone and collagen turnover for several months.

An athlete using hGH may experience no increase in

strength and no effect on athletic performance even while gaining an increase in whole-body protein synthesis and LBM and having decreased in body fat.

Adverse Effects

Exogenous hGH supplementation poses significant health risks. Elderly patients supplemented with hGH had an increased incidence of myalgias, arthralgias, and edema. The edema is caused by increased sodium and water retention. Supplementation increases left ventricular hypertrophy, hypertension, increased insulin resistance, and increased lipoprotein A, which is associated with increased cardiovascular risks. Increased IGF-1s is linked to lung and colorectal cancer. Excessive exogenous hGH also leads to acromegaly. During the 1990s, hGH was often extracted from cadaver pituitary glands; this led to the development of Creutzfeldt-Jakob disease, a bovine spongiform encephalopathy, in seven patients.

Summary

- Exogenous hGH in healthy athletes does not lead to any strength or performance advantage.
- Only the injectable form of hGH has any effects on the human body, since orally the hGH molecule is too big to be absorbed in the gastrointestinal tract.
- It does appear to increase LBM and decrease body fat.
- There are clear health risks from healthy individuals taking medically recommended doses of hGH, and athletes have been found to take nearly 20 times the maximum dose.
- One reason athletes take hGH is that currently there is no way to detect it through a urine drug test.
- It is banned by the IOC, NCAA, and other sports governing bodies.

β_2-Agonists

Actions

Salbutamol, terbutaline, and Clenbuterol are all β_2-adrenergic receptor agonists. Salbutamol is a short-acting drug used in the treatment of respiratory disease as a bronchodilator. Terbutaline is a tocolytic agent used in pregnancy to stop uterine contractions during preterm labor. Clenbuterol is another bronchodilator used in the treatment of asthma. Clenbuterol can be inhaled, injected, or taken orally. Salbutamol is used in the cattle industry as an anabolic agent, as it increases cattle size. Of the β_2-agonists, Clenbuterol is the most widely used in athletic competition. It is considered a stimulant and a weight-loss aid. This is because of brown adipose thermogenesis. Brown adipose tissue is fat tissue in the body that contains large arterioles with a high number of red blood cells. Brown adipose cells have mitochondria that create energy. Because there are β_2-adrenoreceptors in brown adipose tissue, Clenbuterol can stimulate activation of these receptors, which causes brown adipose thermogenesis.

Proven Performance Effects

Large doses of Clenbuterol cause an increase in LBM and a decrease in fat mass in animals. Oral or injected Clenbut-

erol of 20 μg twice a day showed an increase in quadriceps force in orthopaedic patients. Administration of salbutamol to cyclists improved pulmonary function but did not have any effect on performance. There are no studies that show β_2-agonists have any effect on strength and performance.

Adverse Effects

Clenbuterol caused subjects to have tachycardia, increased headaches, muscle tremors, heart palpitations, and muscle cramps. In rats, Clenbuterol caused cardiac hypertrophy. There have been reports of withdrawal symptoms when athletes stop taking Clenbuterol.

Summary

- The IOC has banned any form of Clenbuterol.
- It has a long plasma half-life and a slow urinary excretion rate. The average urine level of Clenbuterol after supplementation is >10 μg/L. The IOC considers a positive test for Clenbuterol at a urine level of 2 μg/L.
- Although Clenbuterol is banned in any form, terbutaline and salbutamol are allowed as inhalants but not for systemic use. If an athlete is taking inhaled salbutamol or terbutaline, the athlete must have a note from his or her physician stating the medical necessity.
- β_2-agonists have little or no ergogenic effects, are banned for systemic use, and carry serious side effects.

Diuretics

Diuretics are drugs that cause the body to lose water. Diuretics have several different classes, and each class has its own mechanism of action. Loop diuretics like furosemide (Lasix) are some of the most potent. Other classes are potassium-sparing, like spironolactone; thiazide, like hydrochlorothiazide; carbonic anhydrase inhibitors, like acetazolamide (Diamox); and osmotic diuretics, like mannitol. Diuretics are used in sports in which athletes need to make specific weight classes, like wrestlers and weightlifters. Bodybuilders often use diuretics to rid themselves of extra water weight before a competition to appear more defined. Diuretics increase the volume of urine, enabling the athlete to urinate out excess weight. Studies of athletes consuming doses of furosemide ranging from 40 to 126 mg led to increased weight losses ranging from 2% to 4% body weight. The diuretic effect of furosemide did not lead to the athletes becoming dehydrated, but running and cycling times for distances of 1,500 m to 10 km were longer. The diuretic effect leads to impaired aerobic endurance since it decreases plasma volume by 8% to 10% and decreases cardiovascular function.

Diuretics decrease aerobic performance and decrease time until exhaustion for an athlete. Diuretics also cause hyperthermia, muscle cramps, cardiac arrhythmias secondary to electrolyte shifts, decreased cutaneous blood flow, and dizziness. A decrease in upper body strength was also found in athletes after diuretic use.

Summary

- Diuretics do work in enabling an athlete to lose a few pounds and make a weight class, but they also have serious side effects.

■ Diuretics are banned by the IOC because they can also serve as a masking agent for steroids.

β-Blockers

β-Adrenergic blockers, such as propranolol (Inderal), serve to block β_1- and β_2-receptors. In times of increased psychological stress, the body releases epinephrine and norepinephrine. This leads to increased anxiety, elevated heart rate, and increased hand tremors. β-Blockers serve to block these β-adrenergic receptors and block the effects of epinephrine and norepinephrine. β-Blockers affect exercise performance by suppressing maximum heart rate, reducing Vo_{2max}, and interfering with the utilization of substrates for conversion into energy. β-Blockers have a special niche as an ergogenic aid. Used in shooting and archery events to reduce anxiety and to steady tremors, they slow an athlete's heart rate to produce a calmer environment. β-Blockers improve pistol performance and shooting accuracy. They impair aerobic and anaerobic sports performance, however, and can cause drowsiness, fatigue, nausea, weakness, hypotension, and fainting episodes.

Summary

■ For most athletes, β-blockers are counterproductive to their training and performance.

■ For those unique shooting and archery sports, β-blocker use has been banned since 1986.

■ The events for which the IOC has prohibited β-blocker use are modern pentathlon, sailing, synchronized swimming, figure skating, ski jumping, diving, equestrian, bobsled, luge, freestyle skiing, archery, and 11 shooting events.

Erythropoietin and Blood Doping

EPO is a natural hormone secreted by the kidney to stimulate formation of red blood cells. In renal failure, the body has decreased production of erythropoietin, thereby causing a decreased red blood cell count. Recombinant human erythropoietin is used in renal failure to correct anemia. Darbepoetin (Aranesp) is another agent used in chronic renal failure. Blood doping occurs when blood is taken out of an athlete, stored, and then later reinfused into an athlete prior to a competition, creating increased packed red blood cell volume. Recombinant human erythropoietin is administered two to three times per week—whereas darbepoetin has a three times greater half-life—21 hours intravenously, and 49 hours subcutaneously, so it only needs to be given once a week.

The effects of blood doping are well documented, including increased red blood cell volume, aerobic power, and endurance. EPO use has been shown to increase power, Vo_{2max}, hemoglobin, time to exhaustion in males, and decreased maximum heart rate. By increasing hemoglobin, EPO increases oxygen-carrying capacity, decreases ratings of perceived exertion, and significantly increased Vo_{2max}. Because EPO and blood doping create erythrocythemia, they cause increased blood viscosity, hypertension, seizures, thromboembolic events, and stroke. Blood doping also carries the risk of exposure to HIV, hepatitis B, and hepatitis C.

Summary

■ EPO and blood doping have known performance-enhancing effects, as well as known dangers to use.

■ Blood doping was banned by the IOC in 1990.

■ It is also banned by the Fédération Internationale de Football Association, the NFL, and the NCAA.

■ The Union Cycliste Internationale has set a maximum hematocrit level cutoff of 50%, and the Fédération Internationale de Ski has set a maximum hemoglobin level of 18.5 g/dL.

SPORTS SUPPLEMENTS

Table 3-1 is a summary of some popular supplements used by athletes.

Creatine

Creatine was first discovered in 1832 by the scientist M. E. Chevreul. He named it for the Greek word for "flesh," because creatine is a compound found in animal protein, including red meat, chicken, fish, and other sources. Creatine is a tripeptide consisting of arginine, glycine, and methionine. The body requires about 2 g/day. Nearly all of the 2 g/day is supplied from a well-balanced diet; the rest the body makes in the liver, pancreas, and kidney. Creatine is found in all of the body's tissues including the liver, the heart, the kidneys, the testes, and the brain. However, more than 95% of creatine is found in skeletal muscle. One third of creatine is found as a free-form compound; the rest is bound to a phosphate group.

Actions

Creatine is involved in adenosine triphosphate (ATP) synthesis. In cells, creatine phosphate combines with adenosine diphosphate and is converted into ATP and creatine by the enzyme creatine kinase. Ingested creatine levels peak in the body from 60 to 90 minutes after oral intake. By increasing the levels of creatine, this leads to greater resynthesis of creatine phosphate by 12% to 18%. Creatine phosphate is the body's primary immediate source of ATP. During intense anaerobic exercise, ATP is consumed in the first 10 seconds. The more ATP that is available, the more strength and power a muscle can produce, and the longer an athlete can maintain higher maximum power output. Creatine also serves to buffer the muscle pH by using a hydrogen ion to resynthesize ATP. This delays muscle fatigue and shifts an individual's lactate threshold. Creatine also increases whole-body nitrogen retention, increases water retention at the cellular level, and increases myofibrillar protein synthesis.

Proven Performance Effects

Creatine is one of the most recently studied supplements, with nearly 100 scientific studies having been done, the vast majority of which within the past 10 years. Most cre-

TABLE 3-1 POPULAR SUPPLEMENTS

	Supplement				
	BCAAs	Creatine	Glucosamine and Chondroitin Sulfate	Glutamine	HMB
Definition	Essential amino acids = leucine, isoleucine, and valine	Tripeptide = arginine + glycine + methionine	Two major compounds found in healthy cartilage	Conditionally essential amino acid	Metabolite of leucine
Mechanism of action	Found in high levels in skeletal muscle	ATP synthesis	Unknown	Increases rate of muscle glycogen resynthesis Buffers the pH of skeletal muscle during intense exercise	Preserves lean body mass Enhances recovery
Proven effects	Decrease muscle breakdown Increase protein synthesis	Increases lean body mass Increases strength and power	Symptomatic relief from osteoarthritis Decrease progression of osteoarthritis	Increases muscle glycogen stores after exercise	Increases lean body mass Decreases muscle breakdown
Adverse effects	None reported	GI distress—diarrhea	None reported	None reported	None reported

ATP, adenosine triphosphate; BCAA, branched-chain amino acid; GI, gastrointestinal; HMB, β-hydroxy-β-methylbutyrate.

atine studies use a dose that consists of a loading period of anywhere from 4 to 7 days of 20 g/day, followed by a maintenance dose of 5 g/day for the rest of the study length. Chronic resistance training has been shown to produce gains in LBM of up to 1 kg/month. One-week supplementation with creatine can produce 1 to 2 kg of LBM. Creatine use has been associated with a larger LBM gain and significantly greater increase in strength than carbohydrate supplementation or use of a combination of carbohydrates and protein. Combining creatine supplementation was shown to lead to a greater increase in lean muscle mass when compared with placebo and creatine alone. Combining creatine with protein supplementation led to a 10% increase in muscle mass and strength gains when compared with protein alone. The strength and LBM effects lasted even 4 weeks after creatine use was discontinued. Creatine supplementation increases lean muscle mass by 0.36% per week over placebo or about a 2.2 kg increase in LBM over a 6- to 8-week period.

It has been well documented in the literature that creatine increases maximal strength. Although the evidence supports the fact that creatine supplementation does improve strength, some studies have not found this to be the case. One study of college football players found no difference in 1RM squat, anaerobic muscle endurance, body fat loss, or LBM between placebo and two different methods of creatine dosing.

Creatine also has an ergogenic effect on high-intensity, repeated sprints. In looking at 61 studies of creatine supplementation on running, swimming, or rowing sprints lasting less than 30 seconds, 45 studies found statistically signifi-

cant evidence of creatine improving athletic performance. Creatine supplementation seems to aid in recovery of creatine phosphate stores in recovery periods less than 6 minutes but has no added benefit in periods of 6 or more minutes. Single bouts of high-intensity cycling and swimming have shown no benefit from less than 1 week of creatine supplementation, but high-intensity repeated efforts have shown improved performance with creatine versus placebo. In short sprints from 6 to 30 seconds in length, there is an average improvement of 1% over placebo with creatine supplementation. In a sprint that may last only 25 seconds, a decrease in time of 1% equals 0.25 seconds—at the world-class level, this is a huge difference since medals can be won or lost in 0.01 seconds.

Creatine's effect on longer anaerobic and aerobic endurance events is debated, with some studies showing improvement and others showing no improvement. For longer-distance endurance events, the extra LBM from muscle and water retention may slow runners and swimmers down.

Adverse Effects
The major reported side effect of creatine versus placebo has been an upset gastrointestinal system. Other studies have shown no difference between the side effects in the creatine and placebo groups. There have been case reports of increased muscle cramping, believed to be the result of creatine's ability to bring water into the cell. Because creatinine is a major breakdown product of creatine, there has been concern about how creatine ingestion may affect renal function. It has been shown that increased consumption of creatine does lead to an increase in serum creatinine levels.

One study examining creatine supplementation over a 4-year period found no adverse reactions, no change in cholesterol levels, no change in LFTs, no change in hGH levels, no change in cortisol levels, and no change in testosterone levels. Another study of NCAA football players having taken creatine for 3 years showed no effect on kidney or liver function. Players had normal LFTs, normal creatinine, normal blood urea nitrogen, normal creatinine clearance, and normal urea levels after consuming creatine for 3 years. There were no reported side effects. Other retrospective studies have also found no significant adverse effects up to 5 years after ingesting creatine. However, there have been no studies of the effect of creatine longer than 5 years.

Summary

- Creatine is one of the mostly widely used supplements by athletes today. More than 30% of American professional sports teams in the NFL, MLB, NBA, and NHL actually supply creatine to their athletes. Close to 50% of NCAA Division I male athletes have used creatine. Nearly 10% of high school athletes have used creatine in the past, and 4.1% are currently using it.
- About three quarters of the high school athletes who have used creatine were informed about it from their friends—not their coaches, parents, or physicians. This highlights the importance of the medical field and, in particular, the team sports doctor being informed of the most recent sports supplements.
- The body of evidence behind creatine shows that it does increase lean muscle mass, increase maximum strength, increase short, high-intensity anaerobic endurance but lacks evidence to support longer aerobic endurance. So, it is an ergogenic aid with specific benefits.
- Besides reports of increased muscles cramping and gastrointestinal issues, creatine has no side effects. Studies have shown that it has no harmful effect on kidney function, but users should be cautioned that no study longer than 5 years has been done.
- Creatine is legal and is not banned by the IOC, the NCAA, or major professional sports.

β-Hydroxy-β-methylbutyrate

β-Hydroxy-β-methylbutyrate (HMB) is a metabolite of the essential amino acid leucine. It is metabolized to hydroxymethylglutamyl-coenzyme A. This enzyme is the rate-limiting enzyme used when cholesterol synthesis is in demand. This happens when cell membranes need to be repaired during muscle damage and to enhance recovery. HMB is found in higher quantities in catfish, citrus fruit, and breast milk. It has been marketed as an ergogenic aid that preserves LBM during fat loss and acts as an anticatabolic agent. Currently an extremely popular supplement, sales of HMB in 1998 were between $50 and $60 million.

Proven Performance Effects

Meta-analysis of supplementation with HMB compared nine studies that showed a statistically significant increase in LBM of 0.28% body mass per week and 1.40% single repetition maximal strength gain per week versus placebo groups.

As for the recuperative abilities of HMB, there is evidence that it decreases muscle breakdown, as evidenced by decreased protein breakdown and increased muscle recovery and lower levels of lactate dehydrogenase and creatine phosphokinase postexercise.

Adverse Effects

HMB supplementation has not been associated with changes in serum testosterone, cholesterol, triglyceride, urea, or glucose levels, renal function, LFTs, and lipid levels. There have been no reported side effects in any of the studies examining use of HMB.

Summary

- HMB may help aid athletes in recovering from strenuous training sessions, may increase maximal strength, and may increase fat loss while maintaining muscle mass.
- It is not banned by the IOC, the NCAA, or any other sports governing body.
- Studies examining short-term use have found no side effects or adverse effects.

Caffeine

Caffeine is the most used drug in the world and has a long history. It is estimated that 82% to 92% of the adults in North America consume caffeine on a daily basis. Nearly all American children aged 5 to 18 years drink caffeinated beverages. Caffeine is 1,3,7-trimethylxanthine, a methylated xanthine alkaloid derivative. Caffeine is metabolized in the liver into dimethylxanthines by the cytochrome P450 pathway. The three main metabolites of caffeine are the dimethylxanthines—theobromine, theophylline, and paraxanthine. Paraxanthine is the most potent caffeine breakdown product.

Actions

The structure of caffeine is similar to adenosine. In the body, caffeine binds to adenosine cell membrane receptors found in the brain, heart, smooth muscle, adipocytes, and skeletal muscle. Caffeine can simultaneously affect a wide number of tissues in the body. It stimulates the CNS and increases the release of epinephrine. Caffeine has been shown to increase heart rate, increase metabolic rate, increase respiratory center output, decrease perception of pain, decrease fatigue, and increase fat oxidation. A main benefit of caffeine's effect on performance has been linked to increased fat oxidation, causing increased serum free fatty acid levels and thereby sparing muscle glycogen. However, there is another new mechanism that shows how caffeine effects substrate utilization during exercise. Caffeine has been shown to decrease plasma potassium (K^+) levels. This is significant because during exercise, K^+ is transported out of the muscle cells. As the intracellular K^+ levels fall and extracellular levels rise, motor unit activation decreases leading to a decrease in muscular force output. Caffeine delays the outflux of K^+ from muscle cells, which delays the onset of skeletal muscle fatigue, allowing an athlete to maintain motor unit force for a longer period of time. The half-life of caffeine is 4 to 6 hours, with the mean time to reach peak plasma concentration between 30 to 60 minutes.

Proven Performance Effects

Caffeine has been studied for the past century. It is used in combination with aspirin and ephedra to form a potent fat and weight loss supplement. Because caffeine spares muscle glycogen, it has been used to increase aerobic and anaerobic endurance. As a CNS stimulant, caffeine can improve concentration. Most of the studies examining the effects of caffeine involve doses of caffeine ranging roughly from 2.0 to 9.0 mg/kg/day to 250 to 750 mg/day. For comparison, a 6-oz cup of coffee contains 100 mg, an 8-oz can of soda contains 40 mg, and a single tablet of Vivarin has 200 mg. The source of caffeine does matter in determining the efficacy. Studies have compared the effect of caffeine tablets versus coffee on performance. Caffeine from coffee causes a significantly decreased ergogenic effect. Caffeine pills release much more epinephrine and induce a greater rise in serum free fatty acids and a greater increase in time until exhaustion during exercise. Caffeine ingested from consumption of coffee is much less ergogenic. How the dosage of caffeine is divided is also important in determining its effects. Because the P450 enzymes in the liver metabolize caffeine, there is a caffeine level at which this pathway becomes saturated, and the effects of caffeine diminish at 9 mg/kg. It has been found that taking 3 to 5 mg/kg of caffeine prior to exercise and then in repeated smaller doses of 1 to 2 mg/kg during prolonged aerobic exercise is more effective.

There is clear evidence that caffeine improves performance in endurance events, with many studies supporting the use of caffeine as an ergogenic aid in swimming, cycling, skiing, running, and other sports. It has been shown to decrease race times from marathons to short sprints lasting less than 90 seconds. Caffeine has even been shown to increase maximum power generated by cyclists in 6-second sprints.

Adverse Effects

Caffeine use has been shown to cause anxiety, heart palpitations, trembling, nervousness, and facial flushing. These adverse effects are usually dose-related; more side effects were reported when subjects consumed greater than 6 to 9 mg/kg body weight. Two to three cups of coffee provide about 5 mg/kg body weight of caffeine. The lethal half-dose of caffeine is 150 to 200 mg/kg body weight, roughly 100 cups of coffee. Acute caffeine toxicity can cause hematemesis, hyperventilation, hyperglycemia, ketonuria, hypokalemia, metabolic acidosis, and cardiac arrhythmias. Tolerance to caffeine can appear after 4 to 5 days, meaning an athlete must increase his or her dose to get the same desired effect. It only takes 3 days of caffeine use for subjects to develop dependency and experience withdrawal symptoms after stopping it. The withdrawal symptoms from caffeine include mood shifts, headaches, tremors, and fatigue. Symptoms can last anywhere from 12 hours to 7 days. Even though caffeine is considered a mild diuretic, studies showed no change in serum electrolyte levels, no increased dehydration, no change in core temperature, and no change in renin concentration.

Summary

- In 1962, the IOC had classified caffeine as a banned doping agent, but in 1972, caffeine was removed from the banned list.
- Today, the IOC limits the amount of caffeine an athlete can ingest. The acceptable urine concentration for caffeine is less than 12 μg/mL, which corresponds to ingesting 9 mg/kg body weight of caffeine. This is a generous limit because a person needs to consume about six to seven cups of coffee, around 700 to 800 mg of caffeine, to exceed this limit.
- Caffeine does improve exercise performance at doses from 3 to 9 mg/kg body weight. Because of the associated health risks with higher doses, athletes are better off using lower doses, between 3 to 6 mg/kg body weight.
- Because chronic caffeine use causes tolerance and dependency, athletes are better off not consuming caffeine supplements on a daily basis, but rather small doses before specific competitions.

Ephedra

Ephedra sinica, also known as Chinese ephedra, and *Ephedra vulgaris*, also known as Ma Huang, have been around for 5,000 years. In ancient Chinese medicine, ephedra was known to relieve respiratory ailments. It was mixed into herbal teas and cold medicines. Ephedra is a stimulant that mimics the effects of norepinephrine and epinephrine. The sale of ephedra alone has been prohibited because it can be altered to make methamphetamine (also called "speed," "crystal meth," or "crank").

Actions

Ephedra is a nonselective sympathomimetic drug. It affects β_1-, β_2-, and α-adrenergic receptors. By stimulating the β_2-receptors, ephedra increases lipolysis—thereby increasing circulating levels of free fatty acids—increases heart rate, increases cardiac contractility, and increases bronchodilation. Ephedra also has a thermogenic effect; it increases resting metabolic rate, increases calorie expenditure, and decreases appetite.

Proven Performance Effects

Ephedra has been touted as a powerful weight loss supplement, with more than 50 studies of its effects on body fat loss. Ephedra causes an average of 1.0 kg of body fat loss per month compared with placebo. There were no long-term studies of the effects of ephedra because all of the weight loss studies were less than 6 months in length. Doses of ephedra ranged from 25 to 120 mg/day. There was a dose-related effect with ephedra: the higher the dose, the greater the average fat loss per month. Although ephedra is a potent fat loss agent by itself, studies have shown that, in combination with caffeine, its efficacy increases. No studies have shown that supplementation with ephedra improves strength, power, reaction time, speed, aerobic capacity, or anaerobic capacity, except for a few studies that combined ephedra and caffeine and found increased endurance.

Adverse Effects

Subjects consuming ephedra showed a wide variety of side effects, ranging from heart palpitations, hypertension, nervousness, anxiety, hyperthermia, headaches, and cardiac arrhythmias. Most of these adverse effects happen with great frequency at higher doses. Side effects of ephedra were minimized when subjects consumed less than 60 mg/day, and the adverse effects stopped after subjects discontinued ephedra use. The FDA has reported 800 adverse incidents from ephedra use, although most of these events occurred when people consumed doses in excess of the recommended daily dose. There have been 284 serious adverse events, including 5 deaths, 5 heart attacks, 11 strokes, and 4 seizures. Half of these serious adverse events occurred in people under the age of 30 years. One study showed that ephedra-containing supplements accounted for 0.82% of all supplement sales but caused 64% of supplement adverse reactions.

Summary

- As a supplement, ephedra has a positive effect on fat loss, but there is no evidence that it can improve athletic performance.
- Recommended dosages of ephedra are between 25 and 120 mg, but side effects increase when daily amounts exceed 60 mg.
- Severe adverse reactions occur at an even higher rate when athletes exceed the recognized upper limit.
- As of March 2004, ephedra-containing supplements were banned by the U.S. government. Ephedra use is also banned by the IOC, NCAA, and NFL, with many other sports soon to follow.

Glucosamine and Chondroitin Sulfate

Actions

Glucosamine is an amino monosaccharide found in human tissues, including cartilage. It is formed by adding an amino group to glucose. It is the primary building block of proteoglycans and causes increased production of hyaluronic acid. Chondroitin sulfate is a mixed group glycosaminoglycans found in articular cartilage. They are two major compounds found in healthy cartilage. Carbon-14 tagging of ingested glucosamine revealed that 4 hours after ingestion, there is increased proteoglycan synthesis and increased human chondrocyte gene expression in vitro.

Proven Performance Effects

There have been more studies examining the effects of glucosamine supplementation alone or in combination with chondroitin sulfate than chondroitin sulfate by itself. Glucosamine and chondroitin sulfate supplementation have been shown to produce symptomatic relief from osteoarthritis, decrease the progression of knee osteoarthritis, and limit joint space narrowing. Though studies have shown these results over years, glucosamine and chondroitin sulfate users show improvement even at 2 weeks, having an increase in function and a decrease in articular stiffness.

Adverse Effects

The safety of glucosamine and chondroitin sulfate is excellent. In all of the studies done on glucosamine and chondroitin sulfate, there were no serious side effects. The placebo groups had the same incidence of side effects as the treatment groups.

Summary

- There is clear evidence that glucosamine alone, glucosamine in combination with chondroitin sulfate, and chondroitin sulfate alone in doses of 1,500 mg/day provide symptomatic relief of osteoarthritis.
- Some evidence also exists showing that chondroitin sulfate and glucosamine slow the progression of osteoarthritis and improve joint function.
- Glucosamine and chondroitin sulfate are safe, effective supplements. Both are deemed legal by all of the governing bodies in sports.

Protein

Muscle mass accounts for 40% of the total amount of protein in the human body. Each gram of protein provides four calories of energy (4 g/kg). Nearly one half to one third of all protein turnover is from muscle breakdown and growth. Proteins are composed of amino acids. There are 20 amino acids, primarily classified as essential or nonessential. Nonessential amino acids are ones that the body can build on its own. Essential amino acids are ones the body needs to consume foods containing those specific amino acids. Some important amino acids that will be discussed later are glutamine (classified as a conditional essential amino acid), and the branched chain amino acids [(BCAAs); leucine, valine, and isoleucine]—all essential amino acids. Protein sources are defined as either complete or incomplete. A complete protein is one that contains all of the essential amino acids, like dairy, eggs, fish, poultry, and meat. An incomplete protein lacks at least one of the essential amino acids. Nuts, grains, fruits, and vegetables are examples of incomplete proteins. Vegetarians can often mix incomplete proteins at a meal to get all the required essential amino acids. With regard to vegetarians, a study of males in their 60s compared the effects of a meat-based protein diet with a lactovegetarian protein diet while on strength training programs. The study found that the meat-based diet group had a significantly greater increase in LBM and strength.

Requirements

The RDA is defined as the minimum amount of a particular nutritional substance—vitamin, mineral, or macronutrient—that a person must consume in order to survive. When it comes to protein, the RDA is based on the level required to maintain equilibrium in nitrogen balance. The RDA was first established in the 1970s and has not been revised since 1989, nearly 15 years ago. The RDA for protein is 0.8 g/kg body weight/day. The RDA specifically states that it does not recognize an additional protein requirement for athletes or people who exercise. According to the RDA, a sedentary, 90-year-old man who weighs 140 pounds requires more protein each day than a 130-pound female college soccer player in the middle of her sports season. This example clearly points out the shortcomings of the RDA for protein.

Protein and Exercise

One hour of aerobic exercise at 55% to 67% of Vo_{2max} leads to a 16% to 25% increase in protein oxidation. During exercise, protein is broken down at a much higher rate than when an individual is at rest. If the body's increased protein needs are not met, the body simply extracts the required protein from itself, from what it considers nonessential sources. The brain, heart, and vital organs are all deemed essential, but the body does not understand why an athlete needs additional muscle mass on his or her arms or legs, so it catabolizes it. Nitrogen balance is a way of accessing whether or not a person's body is getting enough protein. A negative nitrogen balance means an individual needs to consume more protein, whereas a positive nitrogen balance means the body is getting enough protein to build new muscle. However, there is a level at which extra dietary protein stops being useful to the body. A study examining how strength training changes dietary protein requirements showed that, only after 1 week, athletes consuming 1 g/kg body weight/day had a negative nitrogen balance. Studies have shown that athletes need at least 1.4 g/kg body weight/day and may need as much as 2.0 g/kg body weight/day.

The longer the duration of exercise and the greater the intensity, the more protein is used and the higher one's dietary needs. Resistance training increases protein synthesis in the postexercise period by 50% to 100%. There is also an increased rate of amino acid transport and increased blood flow into skeletal muscles. Skeletal muscle protein synthesis is elevated at least 50% in the 48 hours following exercise, resistance training in particular. Peak muscle growth and protein synthesis are seen primarily in the first 3 hours, where there can even be a 100% increase in protein synthesis. A study of 60- to 90-year-old men and women showed that the combination of protein supplementation and resistance training produced significantly greater increases in muscle strength and LBM than just resistance training alone. Another study found that 4 weeks of strength training while taking additional protein supplementation produced greater increases in LBM than just strength training alone.

Adverse Effects

Whenever there is a discussion about athletes consuming protein loads at levels far greater than the RDA, the topic of kidney function is raised. There is the misconception that a high-protein diet leads to or causes kidney failure. This logic comes from the fact that patients with chronic kidney disease and kidney failure are put on low-protein diets. However, no study looking at protein loads greater than the RDA has reported any side effects or health dangers. A review of the literature shows there is no evidence that high-protein diets in healthy men and women with normal kidney function leads to kidney failure.

Summary

- Athletes clearly require an increased daily amount of protein compared with sedentary individuals.
- The American College of Sports Medicine (ACSM) recommends a protein intake minimum between 1.2 to 1.4 g/kg/day for endurance athletes, between 1.6 to 1.8 g/kg/day for strength athletes, and between 1.4 to 1.8 g/kg/day for vegetarian athletes. Protein should account for <35% of daily caloric intake.
- It is recommended that athletes who participate in sports where weight reduction is required make sure that, even with a reduced caloric intake, they are getting enough protein. Such sports include crew, wrestling, gymnastics, figure skating, and cross-country running.
- Not getting enough protein leads to muscle atrophy and reduced athletic performance.
- Protein supplementation simply means adding additional protein to an athlete's diet through whole-food sources or protein shakes or powders.
- Protein supplementation in conjunction with strength training has an ergogenic effect in that it increases both lean muscle mass and strength.
- Protein ingestion in the postworkout period decreases the rate of muscle breakdown and increases muscle synthesis.
- Protein supplementation is safe and legal.

Branched-chain Amino Acids

Actions

The BCAAs are three essential amino acids—leucine, isoleucine, and valine. They make up 20% of the total amino acids found in the body. They are found in high quantities in actin and myosin, the two most abundant proteins in the body. Actin and myosin are skeletal muscle proteins, which make up 65% of all the protein in the body. BCAAs are present in most proteins (e.g., fish, chicken, red meat, eggs, and milk). For vegetarians, BCAAs are present in smaller amounts in nuts, legumes, and some vegetable and grains. The RDA has set the minimum daily allowance of BCAAs at 3 g/day. Most supplements supply between 5 to 10 g/day. During exercise, amino acids account for about 10% to 15% of the fuel used, with fats and carbohydrates providing the bulk. However, after a 90-minute strength training session, the concentration of BCAAs in muscle drops by 24%. This is because oxidation of BCAAs increases by 85% to 500% during exercise, depending on the level of intensity and the duration of the activity. This means that exercise breaks down a significant amount of BCAAs. The theory is that supplementation with BCAAs would improve postworkout recovery, limiting exercise-induced protein degradation, and create an increase in lean muscle mass. Another interesting effect of BCAAs is their relationship to the amino acid tryptophan. Many people know tryptophan as the substance in turkey that makes one tired after the Thanksgiving Day meal. An increase in the ratio of plasma tryptophan to BCAAs causes an increase in fatigue. This occurs because low levels of BCAAs enhance the uptake of tryptophan, which is used to make serotonin, and increased serotonin levels lead to increased tiredness and central fatigue.

Proven Performance Effects

In septic patients, total parenteral nutrition given with BCAAs increased mortality, showed less overnight skeletal muscle breakdown, and increased LBM during hospitalization when compared with total parenteral nutrition without BCAAs. However, other studies examining BCAA supplementation in the critically ill did not show any increased benefit. Leucine supplementation alone has been shown to stimulate greater protein synthesis than placebo. In rats, leucine administration caused a greater increase in lean muscle mass. Adding BCAAs to postworkout drinks containing a combination of carbohydrates and proteins immediately postexercise led to a reduction in serum cortisol levels, increased protein synthesis, and decreased muscle breakdown. BCAA supplementation has also been associated with an increase in LBM, a decrease in skeletal muscle degradation, and a decrease in body fat. BCAA supplementation can also aid performance and improving run times. Moreover, BCAA supplementation during aerobic endurance events—such as soccer matches, marathons, long distance cycling, and long distance swimming—can reduce fatigue and delay depletion of muscle glycogen.

Adverse Effects
BCAAs have not shown any adverse reactions or increased side effects when compared with a placebo. A review of the literature has no mention of any health risks to BCAA supplementation.

Summary
- BCAAs are safe, legal, and are not banned by the IOC, NCAA, NFL, NBA, NHL, or MLB.
- There have not been as many studies of BCAAs to produce conclusive results on its effects on athletic performance. It seems that the literature supports supplementation with BCAAs immediately postexercise, aiding in recovery and reducing muscle breakdown.
- It is not a true ergogenic aid because it does not improve field performance. However, over the course of a season or off-season, supplementation with BCAAs may be advantageous in training.

Glutamine

Glutamine is the most abundant amino acid in plasma and skeletal muscle in the human body. It accounts for nearly 60% of the free amino acids found in muscle cells. Whereas the liver has the ability to oxidize all 20 amino acids, skeletal muscle can only oxidize 6. Those six special amino acids are isoleucine, leucine, valine, aspartate, asparagines, and glutamate. The enzyme glutamine synthetase converts glutamate into glutamine. Initially, glutamine was classified as a nonessential amino acid; however, that classification has been modified. It was discovered that during times of physiological and hypercatabolic stress, the body's use of glutamine dramatically increases while synthesis of glutamine decreases. This means that during metabolic stress, the body's need for glutamine far exceeds its ability to synthesize it endogenously. Because during these periods the body is not able to produce all of the glutamine that it needs, it is now classified as a conditionally essential amino acid.

Actions
Glutamine is used by the hair follicles, the immune system, the liver, the gastrointestinal tract, the brain, and, of course, skeletal muscles. Glutamine is one of the major sources of fuel used by the gastrointestinal tract, accounting for close

to 40% of total body utilization of glutamine. In the brain, glutamine is used to build neurotransmitters. For athletes, the most important function of glutamine is on skeletal muscle. During times of high levels of physiologic stress, like the end of and after an intense training session, the body has high levels of glucocorticoids. Glucocorticoids are catabolic substances, increasing protein and muscle breakdown. Glutamine has a muscle protein-sparing effect and counteracts the actions of glucocorticoids to some degree. Glutamine increases the amount of amino acids released from skeletal muscle, reducing muscle protein degradation. It also increases the rate of muscle glycogen resynthesis. By repleting muscle glycogen stores more quickly, glutamine aids in helping the body recover from intense exercise at a faster rate. During training, glutamine helps in delaying fatigue by buffering skeletal muscle from metabolic acidosis. It does this by being converted to α-ketoglutarate and an ammonium ion (NH^{4+}). This serves to buffer the pH of the skeletal muscle, since decreasing pH leads to metabolic acidosis and reduces the body's ability to perform.

Proven Performance Effects
In times of extreme stress, the body needs additional supplementation with glucose. Burn patients, surgical patients, septic patients, and any patient who needs increased wound healing have all been shown to catabolize skeletal muscle to use the amino acids elsewhere in the body. When the body is prioritizing where it needs amino acids, preserving muscle mass is not high on the list. Administration of glutamine to these patients increases the rate of wound healing while decreasing the breakdown of skeletal muscle. This is important to athletes because overtraining and prolonged exercise create an environment of extreme stress in the body that can lead to increases in muscle breakdown and injury. By supplementing with exogenous glutamine, an athlete can aid in his or her body's healing process. Glutamine plays a role in helping the immune system function and affects lymphocyte function. In a study that examined the effect of glutamine supplementation on upper respiratory infections in athletes, significantly fewer infections developed in runners who received glutamine.

Data do not seem to support glutamine having an ergogenic effect on strength training performance. Glutamine acts as a substrate for gluconeogenesis in the liver, increasing muscle glycogen stores after prolonged exercise. This is especially useful to endurance athletes in the postworkout recovery period.

Adverse Effects
There have been no reported side effects in any of the studies examining glutamine supplementation. Also, there have been no case reports of any adverse effects from using glutamine.

Summary
- Glutamine appears to have some beneficial effects for athletes in terms of recovery and immune system function, but there is no evidence that it is a true ergogenic aid in the strict sense of improving an athlete's on-the-field performance. It can be argued, however, that, if an athlete not supplementing with glutamine is more

likely to get sick, take longer to recovery from intense workouts, and be prone to overtraining, then glutamine use does affect athletic performance.

■ The recommended dose is anywhere from 0.2 to 0.6 g/kg body weight/day, roughly 14 to 42 g/day in a 70-kg athlete.
■ Glutamine supplementation appears to be safe.
■ Glutamine is not banned by the IOC, NCAA, NFL, NHL, NBA, or MLB.

Carbohydrates

Carbohydrates are another macronutrient, like proteins, fats, and water. Carbohydrates provide the body with four calories for every gram consumed (4 cal/g). Carbohydrates are the primary fuel source used by the body during exercise, especially prolonged aerobic exercise, because it produces more ATP per unit of oxygen consumed. Glucose is the brain's primary energy substrate. Carbohydrates are classified as complex and simple. Simple carbohydrates are sugars like glucose. Examples of complex carbohydrates are breads and pastas. The definition of the RDA for carbohydrates is the minimum amount of glucose required by the brain without depending on fat or protein as alternate energy sources. However, there is no exact recommendation for how many grams of carbohydrates should be consumed in a day.

Actions

The concept behind carbohydrate supplementation in conjunction with exercise is that exercise depletes muscle glycogen and carbohydrate ingestion repletes those same stores. Decreased muscle glycogen means decreased performance, decreased isokinetic force, decreased isometric strength, and increased muscle weakness. Carbohydrate supplementation has been shown to increase the amount of work performed and to increase the duration of aerobic exercise. Taking carbohydrates in the postworkout state causes a spike in blood sugar, which begins a cascade of effects leading to increased muscle recovery and growth. The rapid rise in blood glucose releases a corresponding insulin spike. The insulin spike produces an increase in growth hormone, and this creates an anabolic environment for muscle growth and glycogen repletion.

Proven Performance Effects

Studies show that carbohydrate supplementation aids in muscle recovery and glycogen stores, but strength performance has not always been found to be increased. Other studies show that carbohydrate ingestion improves aerobic performance in those training for more than 60 minutes.

Adverse Effects

Carbohydrate consumption was not found to be associated with any negative side effects. None of the studies examined discussed any increased health risks from carbohydrates.

Summary

■ Carbohydrates are safe and legal supplements.
■ As an ergogenic aid, carbohydrates improve performance in prolonged endurance events. They also aid in the body's ability to recover better from exercise.

■ Athletes are recommended to consume between 6 to 10 g/kg body weight/day, accounting for more than 45% of daily caloric intake. During endurance events lasting longer than 60 minutes, they should consume 30 to 60 g of carbohydrates/hour. This is roughly a carbohydrate drink of a 6% glucose solution, which can be easily made by adding four tablespoons of sugar to 1 quart (32 oz) of water. Also recommended is consumption of 1.0 to 1.5 g/kg body weight in the first 30 minutes after exercise. An athlete should continue the carbohydrate dose every 2 hours for the next 4 to 6 hours.

Carbohydrate–protein Combination

Actions

The carbohydrate–protein (CHO/PRO) combination refers to a liquid concoction that provides an athlete with calories from both of these fuel sources. The idea is that there is a synergistic effect in combining the two nutrients. Carbohydrate ingestion repletes glycogen stores and creates an anabolic environment through insulin spikes. Protein increases muscle growth and decreases the rate of muscle breakdown. With the CHO/PRO combination, the rise in insulin preferentially drives glucose and amino acids into muscle cells.

Proven Performance Effects

In one study examining insulin and hGH levels after supplementation of placebo, carbohydrate, or CHO/PRO supplement, the CHO/PRO had a statistically significant greater rise in both insulin and hGH. A combination of 6 g of essential amino acids and 35 g of carbohydrates after intense resistance training created a 10-fold increase in insulin levels, a 3-fold increase in amino acid levels in skeletal muscle, and a $3\frac{1}{2}$-fold increase in protein synthesis, compared with placebo and carbohydrates only groups. The postworkout timing of when to take the CHO/PRO supplement is also important, because immediately after exercise is the time when net protein turnover is greatest. The insulin spike climbs and peaks around 90 minutes and then declines over several hours. The best time to ingest the CHO/PRO combination is immediately after exercise and then around 90 to 120 minutes postworkout.

Adverse Effects

As reported previously, carbohydrates and proteins have no serious reported side effects or health risks.

Summary

■ CHO/PRO supplements are legal and safe.
■ They may not be a true ergogenic aid, but they should have a role in an athlete's postworkout recovery.

Fats

Fats are yet another macronutrient, one that is often overlooked by athletes. Usually, athletes are looking for ways to get less fat in their diets. Fat provides more energy per gram, 9 calories worth, than carbohydrates and protein. There is no daily allowance recommendation for grams per day from the RDA. Fat is usually subdivided into saturated, polyunsaturated, and monounsaturated groups. Saturated fat comes from animal fat sources, like bacon, butter, meat, and dairy products. This is the type of fat that increases the risks of heart disease, certain cancers, and raises LDL levels. Mono- and polyunsaturated fats are healthy fats that come from vegetables, nuts, fish, olive oil, and flax seed oil. These are the fats that should be included in an athlete's diet. No more than 35% and no less than 20% of an athlete's calories should come from fat. More importantly, only one third of these fat calories should come from saturated fat. The other two thirds should come from polyunsaturated and monounsaturated sources.

Actions

Athletes need fat in their diet for hair, skin, muscle, brain, and nervous tissue development. Fat protects the body's vital internal organs. Fat can also be an important source of energy to the body during exercise, especially when muscle glycogen stores get depleted. It has been theorized that supplementation with healthy unsaturated fats might improve athletic performance. The idea is that if an athlete ingested a fat source before or during exercise, then the body might preferentially use the fats as the primary fuel source and delay using muscle glycogen. The longer the body spares muscle glycogen, the longer the athlete can train or race before fatigue begins.

Proven Performance Effects

When compared with studies looking at the effects of carbohydrate and protein supplementation in athletes, there is not nearly as much research with fats, and the studies that have been done have yielded mixed results.

Adverse Effects

Several of the studies reported that the athletes consuming the high-fat diets initially had some gastrointestinal symptoms that included primarily diarrhea, steatorrhea, and nausea. No other side effects were reported, and many of the side effects diminished as the subjects remained on the diet for a longer period of time.

Summary
- There is no conclusive evidence that high-fat diets provide an ergogenic effect to aerobic endurance exercise.
- However, athletes are hurting their training and performance if they attempt to cut out all fat from their diets. They should try to include healthy fat sources and aim for at least 20% of their calories to come from good fat sources like nuts, fish, flax seed oil, and olive oil.

Water and Fluid Replacement

With all the newest supplements on the market, many athletes forget about the beneficial and important effects of water. Water makes up 50% to 70% of the body weight of men (about 47 L), and 40% to 60% of women (about 33 L). LBM is 72% water. When our body loses water, 40% of the loss comes from muscle, and 30% comes from skin. Water is needed to help the body's metabolic pathways, cardiovascular system, thermoregulation, and neuromuscular function.

Actions

When looking at the effects of water on athletic performance, it is best to look at the effects of hypohydration. Failure to replace fluid losses leads to exhaustion ineffectiveness. For every 1% of body weight loss, there is a 0.1° to 0.2°C rise in core temperature, increasing the risk for hyperthermia. That small 1% loss of body weight due to dehydration has been shown to increase heart rate, decrease muscle strength, and decrease cardiovascular endurance.

Proven Performance Effects

Dehydration has a documented effect on strength performance and has been associated with decreased systolic blood pressures, increased heart rates, increased urine specific gravity, and increased rectal temperatures. Dehydration decreases endurance performance and has adverse effects on cognitive performance, including impaired arithmetic ability, worsened short-term memory, and decreased visuomotor tracking.

Adverse Effects

Although dehydration has negative effects on exercise performance, too much hydration can lead to serious consequences as well. Hyperhydration can lead to hyponatremia. Symptomatic hyponatremia can cause disorientation, confusion, nausea, emesis, and muscle cramps. Severe cases can lead to seizures, coma, or death. These effects can happen during an athletic event and even up to 6 hours after competition.

Summary
- Athletes need to keep themselves well hydrated, but not overhydrated.
- Recommendations are for athletes to drink about 24 oz (720 mL) of water 2 hours before exercise, 6 oz (180 mL) every 15 minutes during exercise, and then 16 oz (480 mL) for every pound of body weight lost from training.
- When exercise lasts less than 60 minutes, it is better for athletes to drink water; but, for longer than 60 minutes, a 6% glucose solution better aids performance during exercise.

RECREATIONAL DRUGS

Amphetamines

Amphetamines refer to a class of substances that are sympathicomimetic amines. Common amphetamines are dextroamphetamine (Dexedrine) and methamphetamine (Desoxyn). Methamphetamine is also called "meth" or "speed." It can be inhaled, injected, or taken in powder or tablet form. Ecstasy comes from methylenedioxymethamphetamine. Amphetamines are also called "uppers," "pep pills," and "bennies" (derived from Benzedrine). They are all CNS stimulants, acting on both β- and α-adrenergic receptors to increase the release of catecholamines. Amphetamines were given to troops during World War II to block fatigue and increase endurance. Today amphetamines are used in medicine to treat narcolepsy and attention deficit hyperactivity disorder.

Actions

As a CNS stimulant, amphetamines increase blood pressure, increase maximum heart rate, increase metabolic rate, and increase the serum concentration of free fatty acids by the endogenous releasing of catecholamines. This increase in free fatty acids spares muscle glycogen, thereby delaying the onset of fatigue.

Proven Performance Effects

Amphetamines have well-established ergogenic effects. There is a long history of amphetamines use to enhance performance of elite cyclists, including increases in quad strength, sprint acceleration, anaerobic capacity, maximum heart rate, and time until exhaustion. Increased muscle strength, increased time until fatigue, increased lactic acid levels at maximum exercise, increased heart rate, decreased appetite, and an increased baseline metabolic rate have also been reported.

Adverse Effects

Amphetamines are addictive and have high potential for abuse. Their side effects include headaches, dizziness, insomnia, anxiety, hallucinations, and mental confusion. Chronic amphetamine users are at increased risk of hypertension, stroke, arrhythmias, and ulcers. Athletes injecting amphetamines are also at increased danger of HIV, hepatitis B, and hepatitis C.

Summary

- Amphetamines are a controlled substance, and distributing them is illegal and can lead to criminal penalties. They are banned by the IOC, the NCAA, and most other sports governing bodies.
- Despite their known ergogenic effects, the health and legal risks far outweigh the benefits.

Cocaine

The plant from which cocaine is derived has been around as early as 3,000 B.C. Cocaine comes from the *Erythroxylum coca* plant, which is primarily found in South America. Cocaine is an alkaloid that is derived from the leaves of this plant. A survey showed that 1.5% of NCAA athletes used cocaine. One of the most sympathomimetic amines, cocaine indirectly stimulates α- and β-adrenergic receptors. It directly increases the release of norepinephrine, dopamine, and 5-hydroxytryptamine. Cocaine also blocks the reuptake of norepinephrine and dopamine, thereby increasing the concentration of norepinephrine at the synaptic junction. This creates that powerful stimulant effect of cocaine. Cocaine has a short half-life of 38 minutes.

There are no studies that have shown that cocaine has any ergogenic effect. It has been associated with decreased time to exhaustion, increased heart rate, increased blood pressure, and a decrease in exercise performance. Cocaine actually worsens an athlete's level of endurance. Short-term cocaine use causes peripheral ischemia, lowers seizure thresholds, causes cardiac arrhythmias, hyperthermia, stroke, and even sudden death. A single use of cocaine causes increased activity of the heart, increased heart rate, and increased blood pressure; however, at the same time, it decreases blood flow to the heart muscle. This can induce ventricular fibrillation, a life-threatening cardiac arrhythmia that can cause a myocardial infarction and death. Inhaled crack cocaine causes severe pulmonary disease. Injected cocaine carries the risk of hepatitis B, hepatitis C, and HIV. Chronic cocaine use can cause liver toxicity, mental illnesses, paranoia, severe weight loss, pulmonary disease, and physical and psychological dependence.

Summary

- Cocaine is a highly addictive drug that is banned by the IOC, NCAA, NFL, MLB, NBA, and NHL. It is classified as a schedule II substance.
- A single use can end an athlete's life.
- It has been proven to impair athletic performance, has no documented ergogenic effects, and is associated with myriad health risks.

Nicotine

Nicotine is a highly addictive compound classified as a tertiary amine. It is an alkaloid stimulant derived from the leaves of the tobacco plant. One gram of tobacco contains 10 to 20 mg of nicotine. The effects of nicotine in the body are powerful and quick, taking only 10 seconds to affect the brain after smoking a cigarette. Nearly 3.1 million teenagers smoke, with 3,000 starting every day. Thirty-five percent of all female students and 38% of all male high school students had smoked in the past month.

Nicotine is found not only in cigarettes, but also in smokeless or spit tobacco products like dip, chew, and snuff. The nicotine content in 4 to 5 dips/day is equal to a pack of 20 cigarettes. Whereas male and female athletes are less likely to smoke cigarettes than nonathletes, male and female athletes are more likely to use smokeless tobacco. The highest prevalence of spit tobacco use is in young adult males, and it is one of the only drugs that has a higher prevalence of use among athletes than nonathletes.

Nicotine crosses the blood–brain barrier rapidly. Acting as a short-term stimulant, it binds to both acetylcholine and nicotine receptors. Nicotine exerts sympathomimetic effects on the respiratory and cardiovascular systems and releases catecholamines. Studies have not shown any ergogenic effect of tobacco use. There has been no study showing any increase in strength, performance, or endurance from any nicotine product.

Nicotine is extremely habit-forming. Smoking can lead to lung cancer, chronic obstructive pulmonary disease, or other pulmonary diseases. It increases one's risks for stroke, hypertension, coronary artery disease, and a myocardial infarction. Smokeless tobacco carries some additional health dangers, such as oral leukoplakia and whitish soft-tissue lesions on the inside of the user's mouth that can develop into squamous cell carcinoma. Smokeless tobacco also increases the risk of developing oral, gingival, buccal, or pharyngeal cancers.

Summary

◼ Nicotine is not an ergogenic aid.

◼ It is not tested for by any of the sports governing bodies. It is not banned by the IOC. The NCAA has banned the use of smokeless tobacco, as has Minor League Baseball. However, MLB has not prohibited its athletes from using smokeless tobacco.

◼ Nicotine is a highly addictive drug with serious health risks.

Alcohol

Alcohol is considered by the ACSM to be the most commonly abused drug. It is the drug with the highest rate of use among high school and college athletes. In an NCAA survey, 80.5% of college athletes admitted to using alcohol in the past 12 months. Alcohol is a depressant that also has some stimulant effects. It is created by fermenting the sugars found in grains, fruits, or vegetables. Alcohol provides 7 cal/g, nearly double the calories per gram of protein and carbohydrates.

The effects of alcohol on the human body are well documented. One alcoholic beverage is enough to bring a person's blood alcohol level to 0.02. At 0.02, there is a sense of euphoria. At 0.04, there is a decline in motor skills and coordination. The legal limit for alcohol intoxication is 0.08. At this level, there is a decreased heart rate, slowed breathing, and slowed reaction time. Alcohol serves as a diuretic, causing the body to lose fluid and electrolytes. Impaired judgment, decreased coordination, and slowed reaction time are some of the neurological effects of alcohol ingestion. It was theorized that drinking a small amount of alcohol might have a beneficial effect on shooting and archery events—similar to the effects of a β-blocker—in that the alcohol would increase self-confidence and decrease anxiety and hand tremors. No actual studies have supported this claim. Race times significantly decrease with blood alcohol levels as low as 0.01. Other associations are increased systolic blood pressure, decreased hand-eye coordination, decreased pulmonary function, and increased lactic acid level. In 1982, the ACSM concluded that alcohol had a negative effect on athletic performance causing declines in strength, power, cardiovascular endurance, balance, and Vo_{2max}.

Athletes are aware that alcohol does not help them in their sport. Nonetheless, college athletes are at an increased risk for binge drinking when compared with nonathletes. This places them at an increased risk for unintended sexual behaviors, violent acts, sexually transmitted diseases, potential pregnancies, rape, and motor vehicle accidents.

Summary

◼ Athletics and alcohol are closely intertwined.

◼ Alcohol has no known ergogenic effect and is actually considered ergolytic, meaning it impairs performance.

◼ Consuming more than one drink of alcohol per day leads to long-term health risks.

◼ The IOC and other professional sports leagues do not test for alcohol, and it is not a banned substance.

Marijuana

Marijuana comes from the cannabis sativa plant. It is a psychoactive drug whose active substance is δ-9-tetrahydro-cannabinol. It is the second most widely used drug by athletes next to alcohol, being used by about 25%. Marijuana crosses the blood–brain barrier and affects the CNS.

There is no research indicating any improvement in athletic performance. Marijuana has a negative effect on coordination, short-term memory, and concentration. It impairs spacial and fine motor coordination, resulting in a decline in a variety of psychomotor skills, a decrease in complex reaction time, and a decrease in simple reaction time. Smoking marijuana causes bronchitis and asthma. One marijuana cigarette contains the same amount of tar as 5 tobacco cigarettes, and chronic marijuana use carries an increased risk of lung cancer. Marijuana affects the cardiovascular system by inducing tachycardia. In men, marijuana also leads to a decrease in testosterone production and spermatogenesis.

Summary

◼ Marijuana is classified as a schedule I drug; it is classified as having no medical use and is potentially addictive.

◼ There is some controversy to this classification, as some in the medical field would like to see it changed to a schedule II drug, meaning it has some acceptable medical use.

◼ Possession or sale of marijuana is a criminal offense. It carries clear medical risks with no ergogenic effect for athletes.

SUBSTANCES BANNED FROM USE IN COMPETITION

Throughout this chapter, it has been discussed which supplements and drugs are banned from use and which are accepted. Each of the varying professional sports has their own lists and penalties. For example, a positive drug test for marijuana or cocaine from the NCAA carries a 1-year suspension. However, the NBA does not include marijuana on its list of banned substances. Steroids have been routinely tested by the IOC, USOC, NCAA, and NFL, but 2003 was the first year that MLB ever tested baseball players.

Certain drugs are banned in one form but accepted in another. The asthma medications salbutamol, terbutaline, and salmeterol are allowed only as inhalants and require a doctor's letter and prescription. Oral consumption or injection of these substances is banned.

Athletes must pay strict attention to their sport's governing body's list. For example, the IOC allows athletes to take Seldane (terfenadine), but Seldane-D (terfenadine plus pseudoephedrine) is prohibited. Dristan nasal mist (phenylephrine HCl with pheniramine HCl) is banned, but Dristan long-lasting spray (oxymetazoline HCl) is allowed.

The NCAA has a special toll-free number for physicians to call to determine whether a drug or supplement is legal for an athlete to take. Another important resource is the *Athletic Drug Reference Book*, which is constantly updated. This book contains all the substances that comply with the NCAA and USOC rules.

One final caveat to athletes is that, because of the 1994

Dietary Supplement Health and Education Act previously discussed, the FDA cannot regulate supplements. This means that what is on the label may not always be accurate. A test on a batch of over-the-counter supplements found that many were contaminated with traces of anabolic steroids. A shipment of a pyruvate supplement manufactured by a well-known company revealed 159 μg/g DHEA, 243 μg/g testosterone, 189 μg/g 4-nor-androstenedione, and 78 μg/g 4-androstenedione. None of these ingredients were listed on the bottle, nor were they supposed to be present in the pyruvate supplement. If an athlete had taken this supplement, he or she could have been banned from competition. Athletes must realize and assume the risk involved with taking supplements, because the label may not always reflect what is inside.

INTERNATIONAL OLYMPIC COMMITTEE

The IOC is one of the biggest sports governing bodies. Its list of banned substances is broken down into prohibited classes, recreational drugs, and restricted agents. The prohibited classes are stimulants, narcotics, anabolic agents, diuretics, peptide and glycoprotein hormones, and blood doping. Recreational drugs include cocaine, amphetamines, heroin, alcohol, and marijuana. Restricted drugs are β_2-agonists, β-blockers, local anesthetics, corticosteroids, and alcohol. This list is always evolving. It is important for athletes and sports physicians to be aware of any new additions or changes.

THE FUTURE

The list of oral and injectable drugs of use and abuse is one that is constantly changing. It is an area of tremendous growth and development. Some supplements, drugs, and nutritional aids have proven ergogenic effects. Those that have been proven to be beneficial, safe, and legal may be used by athletes to enhance training and performance. However, athletes need to be aware of those that are harmful, useless, and that may result in their being suspended from competition. Team physicians must keep an open mind about the efficacy of supplements, must realize that athletes are widely using supplements, and must always keep themselves current with new research and new products entering the market to better communicate with and educate not only the athletes, but also themselves.

SUGGESTED READING

Antonio J, Uelmen J, Rodriguez R, et al. The effects of *Tribulus terrestris* on body composition and exercise performance in resistance-trained males. Int J Sports Nutr 2000;10:208–215.

Bahrke MS, Yesalis CE. Psychological and behavioral effects of endogenous testosterone and anabolic-androgenic steroids. Sports Med 1996;22:367–390.

Branch JD. Effect of creatine supplementation on body composition and performance: a meta-analysis. Int J Sport Nutr Exerc Metab 2003;13:198–207.

Brown GA, Vukovich MD, Reifenrath TA, et al. Effects of anabolic precursors on serum testosterone concentrations and adaptations to resistance training in young men. Int J Sport Nutr Exerc Metab 2000;10:340–359.

Corrigan AB. Dehydroepiandrosterone and sport. Med J Australia 1999;171:206–208.

Delbeke FT, Van Eenoo P, Van Thuyne W, et al. Prohormones and sport. J Steroid Biochem Mol Biol 2002;83:245–251.

Dempsey RL, Mazzone MF, Meurer LN. Does oral creatine supplementation improve strength? A meta-analysis. J Fam Pract 2002;51:945–951.

Fielding RA, Parkington J. What are the dietary protein requirements of physically active individuals? New evidence on the effects of exercise on protein utilization during post-exercise recovery. Nutr Clin Care 2002;5:191–196.

Graham TE. Caffeine and exercise: metabolism, endurance, and performance. Sports Med 2001;31:785–807.

Hargreaves M, Snow R. Amino acids and endurance exercise. Int J Sport Nutr Exer Metab 2001;11:133–145.

Juhn MS. Popular sports supplements and ergogenic aids. Sports Med 2003;33:921–939.

King DS, Sharp RL, Vukovich MD. Effect of oral androstenedione on serum testosterone and adaptations to resistance training in young men: a randomized controlled trial. JAMA 1999;281:2020–2028.

Knitter AE, Panton L, Rathmacher JA, et al. Effects of β-hydroxy-β-methylbutyrate on muscle damage after a prolonged run. J Appl Physiol 2000;89:1340–1344.

Koch JJ. Performance-enhancing substances and their use among adolescent athletes. Pediatr Rev 2002;23:310–317.

Kreider RB. Dietary supplements and the promotion of muscle growth with resistance exercise. Sports Med 1999;27:97–111.

Latzka WA, Montain SJ. Water and electrolyte requirements for exercise. Clin Sports Med 1999;18:513–524.

Mayhew DL, Mayhew JL, Ware JS. Effects of long-term creatine supplementation on liver and kidney functions in American college football players. Int J Sport Nutr Exerc Metab 2002;12:453–451.

Meilman PW, Crace K. Beyond performance enhancement: Polypharmacy among collegiate users of steroids. J Am College Health 1995;44:98–104.

Mero A. Leucine supplementation and intensive training. Sports Med 1999;27:347–359.

Mottram DR. Banned drugs in sport: does the International Olympic Committee (IOC) list need updating? Sports Med 1999;27:1–10.

Nissen SL, Sharp RL. Effect of dietary supplements on lean mass and strength gains with resistance exercise: a meta-analysis. J Appl Physiol 2003;94:651–659.

Olas B, Wachowicz B. Resveratrol and vitamin C as antioxidants in blood platelets. Thromb Res 2002;106:143–148.

Richy F, Bruyere O, Ethgen O, et al. Structural and symptomatic efficacy of glucosamine and chondroitin in knee osteoarthritis. Arch Intern Med 2003;163:1514–1522.

Roltsch MH, Flohr JA, Brevard PB. The effect of diet manipulations on aerobic performance. Int J Sport Nutr Exerc Metab 2002;12:480–490.

Schoffstall JE, Branch JD, Leutholtz BC, et al. Effects of dehydration and rehydration on the one-repetition maximum bench press of weight-trained males. J Strength Cond Res 2001;15:102–108.

Schwenk TL, Costley CD. When food becomes a drug: nonanabolic nutritional supplement use in athletes. Am J Sports Med 2002;30:907–916.

Shahidi NT. A review of the chemistry, biological action, and clinical applications of anabolic-androgenic steroids. Clin Ther 2001;23:1355–1390.

Shekelle PG, Hardy ML, Morton SC, et al. Efficacy and safety of ephedra and ephedrine for weight loss and athletic performance: a meta-analysis. JAMA 2003;289:1537–1545.

Taaffe DR, Pruitt L, Reim J, et al. Effect of recombinant human growth hormone on the muscle strength response to resistance exercise in elderly men. J Clin Endocrinol Metab 1994;79:1361–1366.

Yarasheski KE, Campbell JA, Smith K. Effect of growth hormone and resistance exercise on muscle growth in young men. Am J Physiol 1992;262:E261–E267.

4

FEMALE ATHLETES

JULIE GILL
SUZANNE L. MILLER

The past three decades have seen a dramatic increase in female participation in athletics. This can be partly attributed to the passage of Title IX in 1972, which prohibited sex discrimination in sports. In 1971 to 1972, there were 204,015 female high school athletic participants, compared with 2,675,874 in the 1999 to 2000 school years. At the collegiate level, there was also a dramatic increase in participation in sports by women. Excluding football, in 1999 to 2000, there were 146,618 female and 150,888 male NCAA athletes. The impact of Title IX has even had an influence at the Olympic level. Field hockey was added in 1980, and 13 new events were added in 1984. In the 2002 Olympic Games, more women than ever competed, and eight new women's events were added, including women's bobsled, skeleton, and cross-country ski sprints.

Despite the increased participation in female athletics over the past 30 years, sports medicine research focusing on female athletes is still in its early stages. The unique anatomic, physiologic, and biomechanical makeup of females deserves separate attention. Future research needs to focus on injury patterns, prevention programs, and treatment modalities. Recently, the American Orthopaedic Society for Sports Medicine published a consensus statement on female athletic issues for team physicians and other health care providers. The statement provided an overview of select musculoskeletal and medical issues important to female athletes.

This chapter provides a review of certain anatomic and physiologic differences between the sexes, the female athlete triad, common stress fractures, anterior cruciate ligament (ACL) injuries, and exercise in pregnancy.

ANATOMIC AND PHYSIOLOGIC DIFFERENCES

Although similar athletic training regimens and injury patterns are seen in both male and female athletes, there are many anatomic and physiologic variations that explain the differences in mechanics, performance, and injury rates.

- In general, females are shorter in stature and have lower body mass.
- Skeletal differences include shorter femurs (lower relative leg length with respect to total body height), narrower shoulders, a wider pelvis, and larger knee valgus angles.
- Having shorter femurs lowers the center of gravity and improves balance, an advantage in sports such as gymnastics.
- Narrower shoulders and shorter humeri alter throwing mechanics.
- A wider pelvis and greater knee valgus increases the Q-angle (the angle between a line drawn from the anterior superior iliac spine to the center of the patella and the line from the center of the patella to the tibial tubercle), predisposing females to patellofemoral problems.

51

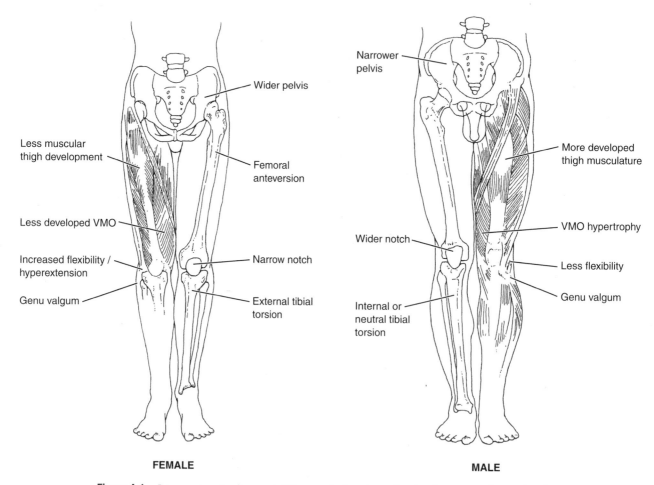

Figure 4-1   Lower-extremity alignment differences in females and males that may predispose females to increased risk of injury.

The Q-angle averages 10 ($\pm 5°$) degrees in men, compared with 15 ($\pm 5°$) degrees in women. (See Figure 4-1 for lower extremity alignment differences.)

- Females reach skeletal maturity earlier than their male counterparts at the average age of 17 to 19 years versus 21 to 22 years.
- Females can have lower bone density, which may predispose them to fractures.
- The female body composition tends to be composed of relatively more fat and less muscle mass than equally trained males.

Essential body fat, which is the normal fat that is stored in and nourishes the body's organs, is 9% to 12% in females and approximately 3% in males (the significant difference is largely the result of the fat in breasts and other gender-specific organs). In the average nonathlete, normal body fat in females is 18% to 24% and is 12% to 16% in men. Endurance athletes should maintain body fat of 12% to 18%, but this often drops dangerously to 6% to 8% in elite athletes. However, dropping below a safe level of body fat directly affects the ability to menstruate, an important component of the female triad. Greater body fat leaves females more buoyant, a potential advantage in water sports.

Greater muscle mass per pound of weight explains why males are stronger, run faster, and jump higher than equally trained females. In general, when adjusted for body mass, female strength is approximately two thirds that of males, with their upper body strength even less matched than lower body strength compared to males. Women also tend to have greater ligamentous laxity that may contribute to increased injury patterns, such as multidirectional instability of the shoulder, patellofemoral dislocations, and ankle instability.

There are several differences in physiology and aerobic capacity that are important to consider when implementing training regimens and in achieving realistic athletic goals. The major physiologic factors that contribute to aerobic differences in females include smaller body size, greater body fat, lower muscle mass, and reduced oxygen-carrying capacity. The VO_{2max} measures the body's ability to extract oxygen from the air and deliver it via the blood to muscle tissue. It is essentially a measure of aerobic capacity. The average woman has a 15% to 30% lower VO_{2max} because of several factors:

- Women have lower vital capacity, smaller tidal volumes, and faster respiratory rates due to a smaller thoracic cage.
- Cardiac output (heart rate $\times$ stroke volume) is approxi-

mately 30% less than males, secondary to their smaller heart size.

- Men have 6% higher hematocrit and 10% to 15% higher hemoglobin concentration, which results in a greater oxygen-carrying capacity of the blood.

Females also have a resting metabolic rate that is 5% to 10% lower than males, which affects the ability to lose weight with training. Because of the aforementioned physiologic differences, cardiovascular training programs and performance goals for females should be individualized on the basis of previous athletic experience and gender.

Hormonal variations throughout the menstrual cycle, as well as different stages of physiologic maturity, can have an impact on athletic performance, body composition, bone density, and injuries. Cyclic endogenous hormones, such as estrogen and progesterone, affect many physiologic systems in the body such as metabolic, thermoregulatory, cardiovascular, respiratory, and psychological. Dysregulation can certainly affect performance and may have an effect on injury. Several studies have looked at the effect of the menstrual cycle on performance and injury but the results are varied and mainly inconclusive. Although there is no definite evidence that a specific phase of the menstrual cycle increases risk of injury or decreases performance, one relatively consistent finding is that premenstrual symptoms can decrease performance and consequently increase risk of injury. Exogenous hormones, including oral contraceptives, in addition to decreasing iron deficiency anemia and protecting bone health, are known to alleviate dysmenorrhea, decrease premenstrual symptoms, and regulate menses—all of which can be beneficial to the athlete. A few studies have shown a lower incidence of musculoskeletal injuries with oral contraceptive use, likely secondary to the alleviation of premenstrual symptoms and dysmenorrhea.

FEMALE ATHLETE TRIAD

Growing concerns for women athletes led to the discussion of and need for research investigating the interrelationship between *disordered eating, athletic amenorrhea,* and *premature osteoporosis*—the three components of the female athlete triad (Fig. 4-2). The term *female athlete triad* was de-

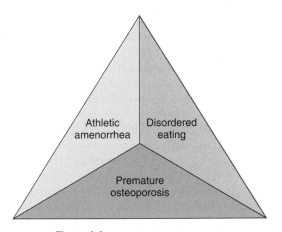

Figure 4-2 The female athlete triad.

fined at the Triad Consensus Conference in 1992, led by members of the American College of Sports Medicine. Each component of the triad occurs on a spectrum of severity and is often interrelated, which can lead to serious long-term health consequences. However, not all components of the triad need to occur simultaneously. Diagnosis of one component of the triad should alert health care providers to be suspicious about the other components.

Female athletes are often pressured to have and maintain low body weight and body fat both to enhance performance and/or for appearance. In their quest to maintain low body weight, they may succumb to disordered eating, which can cause an imbalance of energy intake versus energy expenditure. Energy depletion can lead to a dysregulation of the hypothalamic-pituitary-ovarian (HPO) axis, resulting in hypoestrogenism or athletic amenorrhea. Subsequently, a lack of exposure to the hormone estrogen can cause premature bone loss or osteopenia/osteoporosis. Thus, knowledge of the three components and how they relate is imperative when treating female athletes.

The prevalence of the female athlete triad is unknown. There are three groups of sports that have increased risk for developing the triad:

1. Sports in which subjective judging is involved—gymnastics, diving, figure skating, and dance
2. Endurance sports—long distance running and swimming
3. Sports with weight classifications—rowing, body building, and martial arts

Although elite athletes are often profiled as the classic example of being high risk for developing the triad, it can occur in any physically active female.

The first component of the triad, disordered eating, can range from simple restriction of food intake, to occasional binging and purging to laxative and/or diuretic abuse, or to frank anorexia nervosa and/or bulimia nervosa. The majority of females affected with the triad do not fit the *Diagnostic and Statistical Manual of Mental Diseases,* 4th edition (DSM IV) criteria of anorexia or bulimia, but may fit into a more broad diagnosis of eating disorder not otherwise specified (EDNOS) (Box 4-1). Studies lack consistent and valid diagnostic instruments for the assessment of disordered eating and thus prevalence studies may not be accurate. Up to 62% of female college athletes have some degree of pathologic weight control behavior. There are several instruments, such as the Eating Attitudes Tests and Eating Disorders Inventory, that attempt to document the existence and/or risk of eating disorders, but most instruments are blatant in what they are searching for and athletes may hide their signs and symptoms, thus skewing the results.

Predisposing factors for disordered eating are multifactorial and often stem from low self-esteem. The athletes often have body image disturbances. The pressures of adolescence, puberty, and competition may lead these athletes to find comfort in a false sense of control with their eating and exercise patterns. Biologic, psychologic, and social factors all contribute to predisposing risk. A history of family dysfunction, physical or sexual abuse, perfectionism, and/or long-term chronic dieting are often found in females who display signs of eating disorders. Traumatic events—

BOX 4-1 DIAGNOSTIC CRITERIA FOR EATING DISORDERS

Anorexia Nervosa
- Refusal to maintain body weight at or above 85% of normal weight for age and height.
- Intense fear of gaining weight or becoming fat, even though underweight.
- Disturbance in the way in which one's body weight or shape is experienced, undue influence of body weight or shape on self-evaluation, or denial of the seriousness of the current low body weight.
- Amenorrhea—the absence of at least three consecutive menstrual cycles.

Bulimia Nervosa
- Recurrent episodes of binge eating:
  - Eating in a discrete period of time an amount of food that is definitely larger than most people would eat during a similar period of time.
  - A sense of lack of control over eating during the episode.
- Recurrent inappropriate compensatory behavior to prevent weight gain (i.e., diuretics, enemas, self-induced vomiting, misuse of laxatives or other medications, fasting, excessive exercise).
- Binge eating and inappropriate compensatory behaviors occur, on average, at least twice a week for three months.
- Self-evaluation is unduly influenced by body shape and weight.
- The disturbance does not occur exclusively during episodes of anorexia nervosa.

Eating Disorder Not Otherwise Specified
- For females, all of the criteria for anorexia are met except that the individual has regular menses.
- All the criteria for anorexia are met except that, despite significant weight loss, the individual's current weight is in the normal range.
- All the criteria for bulimia are met except the binge eating, and inappropriate compensatory mechanisms occur at a frequency of less than twice a week or for a duration of less than 3 months.
- The regular use of inappropriate compensatory behavior by an individual of normal body weight after eating small amounts of food (i.e., self-induced vomiting after the consumption of two cookies).
- Repeatedly chewing and spitting out, but not swallowing, large amounts of food.
- Binge-eating disorder: recurrent episodes of binge eating in the absence of the regular use of inappropriate compensatory behaviors characteristic of bulimia nervosa.

such as loss of a family member, friend, or coach—change in competitive environment (i.e., high school to college and college to professional world transitions), and acute or chronic injuries can often escalate the severity of their disordered eating and lead to greater health consequences. A list of signs and symptoms of disordered eating is given in Box 4-2, and complications are given in Box 4-3. Disordered eating can severely affect athletic and academic performances. The negative energy balance created can decrease endurance, strength, speed, reaction time, and concentration—all of which increase the risk of sports-related injuries. Prolonged insufficient caloric consumption can lead to significant medical and psychological consequences such as depression and cardiovascular, endocrine, thermoregulatory, and gastrointestinal complications.

Disordered eating sets the stage for a negative energy balance. Restricting calories, along with intense training schedules, leads to a severe energy deficit that affects the HPO axis. This affects the menstrual cycle and can lead to the second component of the triad, athletic amenorrhea.

The prevalence of amenorrhea in the general population is 2% to 5%, but several studies have shown the prevalence in female athletes may be as high as 66%. The combined effect of poor nutrition and intense training regimens, leading to significant caloric deficits, disrupts the reproduction function by suppressing the HPO axis. This is currently the leading hypothesis in the mechanism of athletic amenorrhea. There is a decrease in the pulse frequency of gonadotropin-releasing hormone from the hypothalamus, which leads to dysfunction in the secretion of luteinizing hormone and follicle-stimulating hormone from the pituitary gland. Luteinizing hormone suppression leads to ovarian suppression and anovulation, resulting in amenorrhea.

Menstrual irregularity, similar to disordered eating, has a continuum of disturbances. The dysfunctions range from luteal-phase deficiency to anovulation, oligomenorrhea, and hypoestrogenemic amenorrhea. There are two forms of amenorrhea: primary and secondary. *Primary amenorrhea* is when menarche has not occurred by age 16. In this form, the reproductive axis has not yet coordinated to produce a

BOX 4-2 WARNING SIGNS AND SYMPTOMS OF EATING DISORDERS

Physical
- Dry hair
- Dull pale eyes
- Dry, flaky skin
- Lanugo
- Lack of subcutaneous fat
- Glossitis
- Cheilosis
- Gum disease
- Brittle nails
- Swollen parotid glands
- Sore throat

Psychological
- Social withdrawal
- Depression
- Secretive behavior
- Preoccupation with food or eating
- Psychosomatic complaints
- Low self-esteem
- Anxiety
- Body dissatisfaction

menstrual period. The main contributing factor to primary amenorrhea is the age at which intense training is begun. The earlier the athlete begins intense training, the greater the risk of primary amenorrhea. *Secondary amenorrhea* is when menses is halted for three or more consecutive months after the reproductive axis has previously produced at least one menstrual period.

BOX 4-3 MEDICAL COMPLICATIONS OF EATING DISORDERS

- Hypotension
- Bradycardia
- Arrhythmia
- Esophagitis, hematemesis
- Diarrhea, constipation
- Abnormal liver enzymes
- Hypokalemia
- Hyponatremia
- Hypoglycemia
- Hypothermia
- Hypercortisolism
- Lipid abnormalities
- Renal calculi
- Infertility
- Low-birth-weight infants
- Peripheral neuropathy
- Anemia
- Leukopenia
- Neutropenia
- Thrombocytopenia
- Amenorrhea
- Osteoporosis

- The primary treatment of amenorrhea is to treat the energy deficit that is likely contributing to the menstrual dysfunction.
- The goal is to optimize nutritional status and alter training intensity to maintain a positive energy balance.
- Observation with the trainer and nutritionist for 3 to 6 months is typical before pharmacologic agents should be initiated.
- Estrogen replacement therapy and oral contraceptive pills can restore menses, but low bone mineral density, a major consequence of hypoestrogenic amenorrhea, may not be restored.
- The Committee on Sports Medicine of the American Academy of Pediatrics (AAP) recommends that amenorrheic females under the age of 16 decrease their exercise intensity and increase their dietary calcium and protein. It is not recommended that they start hormone replacement therapy. The AAP does, however, recommend women over the age of 16 with hypothalamic amenorrhea and hypoestrogenism be started on a low-dose oral contraception.

Disordered eating and athletic amenorrhea are significant potential precursors to early osteoporosis or osteopenia. Osteoporosis or osteopenia is the third component of the female athlete triad. Osteoporosis is defined as bone mineral density (BMD) measured by a dual-energy x-ray absorptiometry scan (DEXA), greater than 2.5 standard deviations below that of a young, healthy, Caucasian, adult female (or a T score at or below −2.5). Osteopenia is defined as 1 to 2.5 standard deviations below a normal adult (or a T score of −1 to −2.5). Alteration of bone homeostasis (bone formation and bone resorption) leads to decreased bone mineralization and low bone density. Estrogen plays a significant role in bone homeostasis. Estrogen receptors are found in osteoblasts and osteocytes and slow the resorption of bone by decreasing osteoclastic resorption. Estrogen also alters the renal handling of and gastrointestinal absorption of calcium, which is critical for osteoblastic function and bone building. Young athletes with primary or secondary amenorrhea lack the estrogen necessary to achieve peak bone mineral density.

Ninety percent of bone mineral content is accrued by the end of adolescence. Typically, a young, adolescent, eumenorrheic female with good nutrition will gain 2% to 4% bone mass a year. A chronically estrogen-depleted state like athletic amenorrhea can cause a 2% loss of bone mass a year. Young athletes with intense training patterns and a negative caloric balance are at increased risk of skeletal fragility. This is of concern, not only for fractures and stress fractures during their current sports and training, but leaves them at tremendous risk for hip, wrist, and spine fractures later in life.

Several studies have investigated the relationship between reproductive function and bone density. Most of these studies have shown significant increased risk of fracture in those athletes with menstrual dysfunction. In fact, one study by Barrow et al. found that almost half of the college female long-distance runners with irregular menses had at one point reported a history of stress fracture.

Although return of menses can halt the process of bone resorption in adolescence, it does not reverse the damage that has already been done. The treatment of amenorrhea with estrogen replacement therapies may restore bone homeostasis at that point in time but does not make up for the prior imbalance; thus, these young athletes will never reach their potential peak BMD. Exogenous estrogen only normalizes the rate of resorption; it does not have a direct effect on bone formation.

At this time, pharmacologic treatment of osteopenia/osteoporosis in female athletes is not well studied. Bisphosphonates such as alendronate, used in postmenopausal women, are not recommended for premenopausal women of childbearing age as a result of their teratogenic effects. The selective estrogen reception modulator class of agents, such as raloxifene and tamoxifen, are also indicated for postmenopausal women but are not approved for premenopausal women. There is currently no pharmacologic treatment for osteopenia or osteoporosis that is approved by the U.S. Food and Drug Administration for premenopausal women. Treatment of the athlete with signs of osteopenia or osteoporosis consists of restoring menses, improving nutrition, having an intake of 1,500 mg of calcium/day and performing weight-bearing exercises.

The female athlete triad may potentially affect all female athletes. The three components are interrelated, and the presence of one of the components should raise suspicion for the others.

- Recognition and referral comprise the critical first step in the treatment of these athletes.
- Ultimately, effective treatment requires the communication of a multidisciplinary health care team, including physicians, athletic trainers, coaches, nutritionists, and psychologists.
- Prevention is a key objective when facing the female athlete triad. All female athletes, especially those who present with stress fractures and/or menstrual irregularities, should be screened for the triad, and preparticipation histories should include a careful and thorough menstrual and nutritional history.
- Treatment goals involve correcting the energy deficit, restoring normal menstrual function, increasing dietary calcium, maintaining and restoring bone mass density, and educating the athlete on proper nutrition and its effects on performance and health.

STRESS FRACTURES

Stress fractures are partial or complete breaks in the architecture of bone. These fractures occur as a result of the inability of bone to sufficiently remodel after exposure to repetitive overload. The diagnosis of a stress fracture can often be made on the basis of history and physical examination. Patients will often report a recent increase in training regimen (either intensity or duration) over a short period of time. Running is the most common activity that leads to stress fractures, but any sport that requires repetitive impact loading can lead to stress fractures.

- As part of the history, it is essential for the physician or treating medical personnel to obtain a detailed nutritional and menstrual history.
- Physical examination findings can include an antalgic gait, tenderness, and mild swelling over the affected area.
- If obtained early, initial radiographs (within 2 to 3 weeks) may not show evidence of callus formation, and rarely is an actual fracture line seen.
- Within the first 48 to 72 hours, a triple-phase technetium bone scan will show focal uptake at the particular site with 100% sensitivity.
  - The triple phase bone scan can also help distinguish the age of the fracture because the angiogram (phase I) and blood pool images (phase II) normalize over time.
- To help distinguish between stress injuries to bone, infections, and bone tumors, an MRI can be a useful adjunct.
- After a few weeks, plain radiographs often show evidence of callus formation (Fig. 4-3).
- A DEXA scan to determine bone mineral density may be warranted for patients who present with multiple stress fractures.

The vast majority of the literature has found that stress fractures are more common in female athletes and military recruits when compared with their male counterparts. In a

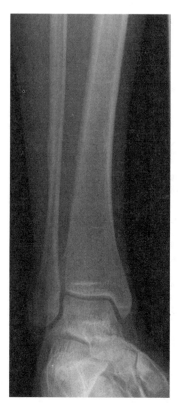

Figure 4-3 A 16-year-old female cross-country athlete presented with 4 weeks of lateral ankle pain while running. Radiograph showed a healing distal fibula stress fracture.

recent study of college athletes, stress fractures were significantly more common in women. The fractures occurred most commonly in track and cross-country athletes. Soccer was the only sport where the incidence of stress fractures was higher in males. In women, the foot was the most common anatomic region to be involved, but the tibia and the femur, respectively, were the most common bones to be involved. In men, the ankle was the most predominant anatomic site, followed by the foot and the tibia.

Many predisposing risk factors for stress fractures in the female athlete have been studied, such as age, gender, skeletal alignment, low bone density, hormonal factors, training parameters, and footwear. Risk factors for stress factors in female track-and-field athletes include significantly older age at menarche, a history of irregular menses, and restrictive eating patterns and dieting—all factors that reduce bone density. A high longitudinal arch, leg length discrepancy, and excessive forefoot varus have all been associated with increased risk of recurrent stress fractures, with the tibia being the most common location. There is an increased risk of pubic ramus fractures in integrated military training, presumably because of increased stride length set by males during marching.

- The treatment of stress fractures should not only focus on the fracture, but also identify predisposing risk factors for which intervention may be warranted.
- A multidisciplinary approach to treatment is often necessary.
  - For example, those who report disordered eating habits should be referred to a nutritionist and possibly a sports psychologist.
  - Female athletes should be educated about the inherent risks of irregular menstrual periods. Those with irregular menses should be referred to an obstetrician/gynecologist. In several studies, the use of oral contraceptive medication to help normalize menstrual irregularities seems to show a protective effect against future stress fractures. Biomechanical factors should also be addressed when appropriate.
- Treating the fracture requires a period of relative rest.
- The goal is to heal the stress fractures without allowing the athlete to become deconditioned.
  - Treatment entails avoiding the offending activity and switching to nonimpact activity, such as swimming, low-resistance cycling, or elliptical training.
  - The rate of activity progression should be determined by the athlete's symptoms. If pain occurs during an activity, stop for a few days and then gradually resume activity.
- Certain stress factors are considered to be "high-risk fractures" and warrant greater attention because of their high incidence of delayed union or complete fracture.
  - Bones commonly involved are the femoral neck, patella, anterior tibial cortex, medial malleolus, talus, tarsal navicular, fifth metatarsal, and great toe sesamoids.
  - The femoral neck stress fracture has been shown to be four times as common in female runners as in male runners.

- If the fracture is on the tensile side (superior side of the femoral neck), pinning in situ is recommended to avoid the devastating complication of a displaced femoral neck fracture. The potential complications include avascular necrosis, varus deformity, delayed union, and decreased return to play.
- If the fracture is on the compression side of the femoral neck, immediate discontinuation of the offending activity and either non-weight-bearing or partial weight-bearing should be instituted. Once pain free, a gradual return to activity should begin. If pain occurs at any point during return to activity, progression should be halted.
  - Fractures present in the proximal or distal one third of the tibia are usually on the compression or posteromedial side of the bone, and healing is generally not problematic. Casts or braces are rarely necessary unless pain persists but a quicker return to play may be possible if a brace is used.
  - Another "at-risk" fracture is on the anterior cortex of the tibia, described radiographically as the "dreaded black line." Constant tension from posterior muscle forces and the relative hypovascularity of this area predispose the site to nonunion or delayed union. Fractures at this anatomic site are common in athletes who leap or jump. Because of this fracture's unpredictable healing pattern and prolonged treatment time (average 12.5 months), intramedullary nailing has been advocated for the high-level athlete for a quicker return to sport (Fig. 4-4).
- Focus on preventive measures and recognition of stress injuries by athletes, coaches, and medical personnel should help decrease the incidence and improve treatment.

ANTERIOR CRUCIATE LIGAMENT INJURIES

ACL injuries in female athletes are 3 to 10 times more common than in males. The mechanism of injury is most commonly noncontact during deceleration, landing, or cutting. The "at-risk" position of the leg is with knee extended, hip adducted and internally rotated, and leg externaly rotated. Once a valgus moment is produced with the leg in the aforementioned position, the ACL is at significant risk. Soccer, basketball, field hockey, lacrosse, and skiing appear to be the sports with the greatest risk.

The risk factors for ACL injury have been divided into two groups:

1. Intrinsic factors—limb alignment, joint laxity, notch width, hormonal, and ligament size
2. Extrinsic factors—muscular strength and balances, neuromuscular control, body movements, shoe surface friction, and skill development

Anatomically, in females, an increased Q-angle, genu recurvatum, genu valgum, hip varus, pelvic width, and foot

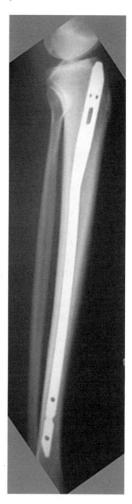

Figure 4-4   A college basketball player underwent intramedullary nailing for an anterior tibia stress fracture. This fracture was refractory to healing for 6 months prior to treatment. (Courtesy of Dr. Glen Ross.)

pronation have been implicated as contributing factors. The femoral notch size has also been implicated as a risk factor for noncontact ACL injury. Currently, anatomic factors identified in the literature include a notch width in patients with bilateral ACL tears that is less than in patients with unilateral tears. Notch width is smaller in females than males (see Fig. 4-1), and the notch width index (condylar width to notch width) in females is less than males. Some researchers have suggested that increased laxity, especially in patients with recurvatum, may contribute to the increased incidence. The increased laxity may contribute to diminished joint proprioception, causing the knee to be less sensitive to potential damaging forces.

Data on the hormonal differences between men and women as a cause of ACL injury are somewhat controversial. Some studies have suggested an increased incidence of ACL injuries during the estrogen surge at midcycle, whereas others report an increase around the time of menses. The use of oral contraceptives has also been investigated to try to understand hormonal influences but no definitive conclusions can be made at the present time.

Uhorchak et al. performed a prospective study looking at risk factors associated with noncontact ACL injuries. In women, narrow notch width, generalized joint laxity, and increased body mass index were all significant risk factors. There was a trend toward significance for knee laxity on KT-2000 testing. In these military recruits, the presence of one of these factors led to a relative risk 2.7 to 4 times those without risk factors. Using a regression model, including femoral notch width, body mass index, and generalized joint laxity, the authors were able to predict 75% of the ACL injuries.

Although it may be difficult to control potential intrinsic risk factors, changes can be made to influence potential extrinsic causes. Knee joint position during landing, landing forces, and cutting maneuvers have been implicated as potential risk factors (Fig. 4-5). Most studies report that females tend to land with the knee and hip in a more extended position. When landing with the knee in a position of extension, females tend to recruit the quadriceps eccentrically to a greater degree than the hamstrings. Research has also shown with low knee flexion angles, the maximal force generated by the quadriceps exceeds the tensile strength of the ACL. Females have also been shown to have less gluteus medius activation than in males. This is important because hip motion influences knee motion. A recent study in female athletes showed that the knee abduction angle at landing was 8 degrees greater, and the knee flexion angle at

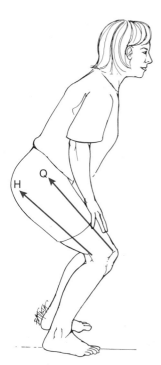

Figure 4-5   Co-contraction of the quadriceps and hamstring muscles. During co-contraction of the quadriceps and hamstrings, the pull of the hamstrings (*H*) applies a posterior shear force that protects the anterior cruciate ligament from the shear force of the quadriceps (*Q*). (From Oatis CA. Kinesiology: The Mechanics and Pathomechanics of Human Movement. Baltimore: Lippincott Williams & Wilkins, 2004.)

landing was 10 degrees lower in the ACL injured than uninjured athletes. They concluded from their study that decreased neuromuscular control (increased dynamic valgus and knee abduction moments) were risk factors for ACL injury, with 73% specificity and 78% sensitivity.

Although many athletes may possess adequate strength in the gym during isolated exercises, many cannot translate isolated muscle strength into coordinated skilled movement. As a result, there have been many neuromuscular training prevention programs developed to decrease the incidence of ACL injury and all with great success. For example, Sportsmetrics is a three-part prevention program focusing on flexibility, strengthening, and plyometrics. During phase I, proper jumping techniques are taught. Phase II concentrates on building strength and agility, and phase III focuses on achieving maximal vertical height. Data from their studies have shown a decrease incidence of ACL injuries. The program itself was found to decrease peak landing forces, decrease varus and valgus motion with landing, and increase hamstring strength, thus improving hamstring-to-quadriceps peak torque ratio. Another program is the California ACL Prevention Project: Prevent Injury and Enhance Performance PEP Program. The program has five components (avoidance, flexibility, strengthening, plyometrics,

and agilities) that are performed 2 to 3 times weekly. Randomized controlled trials using this program have shown significant decreases in ACL injuries, noncontact ACL injuries, and practice ACL injuries.

Few studies have specifically addressed outcomes for female ACL reconstructed athletes. Controversy exists in the literature regarding outcomes of ACL reconstruction when comparing men versus women. Although some studies have suggested higher clinical failure rates in women, other researchers have not found significant differences. Currently, most authors agree that gender alone should not be used as selection criteria for ACL reconstruction. In terms of graft selection, many surgeons have shown a trend in using hamstring grafts for women as a result of improved cosmesis and minimizing graft site morbidity. However, reduced peak torque of the hamstring muscles has been reported, and concern exists over a tendency toward postreconstruction residual laxity and tunnel widening. Barrett et al. performed a prospective review comparing hamstring and patellar tendon ACL reconstruction in female patients. Although not statistically significant, there was a trend toward a greater failure rate and increased laxity on physical examination and KT-1000 arthrometer differences. In the hamstring group, there was a significant increase in pain compared with the

---

BOX 4-4 AMERICAN COLLEGE OF OBSTETRICIANS AND GYNECOLOGISTS GUIDELINES FOR EXERCISE DURING PREGNANCY AND POSTPARTUM

Pregnancy and Postpartum

1. Regular exercise (at least three times per week) is preferable to intermittent activity. Competitive activities should be discouraged.
2. Vigorous exercise should not be performed in hot, humid weather or during a period of febrile illness.
3. Ballistic movements (jerky, bouncy motions) should be avoided. Exercise should be done on a wooden floor or a tightly carpeted surface to reduce shock and provide a sure footing.
4. Deep flexion or extension of joints should be avoided because of connective tissue laxity. Activities that require jumping, jarring motions, or rapid changes in direction should be avoided because of joint instability.
5. Vigorous exercise should be preceded by a 5-minute period of muscle warm-up. This can be accomplished by slow walking or stationary cycling with low resistance.
6. Vigorous exercise should be followed by a period of gradually declining activity that includes gentle stationary stretching. Because connective tissue laxity increases the risk of joint injury, stretches should not be taken to the point of maximum resistance.
7. Heart rate should be measured at times of peak activity. Target heart rates and limits established in consultation with the physician should not be exceeded.
8. Care should be taken to gradually rise from the floor to avoid orthostatic hypotension. Some form of activity involving the legs should be continued for a brief period.
9. Liquids should be taken liberally before and after exercise to prevent dehydration. If necessary, activity should be interrupted to replenish fluids.
10. Women who have led sedentary lifestyles should begin with physical activity of very low intensity and advance levels very gradually.
11. Activity should be stopped and a physician should be consulted if any unusual symptoms appear.

Pregnancy Only

1. Maternal heart rate should not exceed 140 beats per minute.
2. Strenuous activities should not exceed 15 minutes in duration.
3. No exercise should be performed in the supine position after the fourth month of gestation is completed.
4. Exercises that use Valsalva's maneuver should be avoided.
5. Caloric intake should be adequate to meet not only the extra energy needs of pregnancy, but also the exercise performed.

Maternal core temperature should not exceed 38°C.

patellar tendon group. In a case-control comparison of hamstring versus bone patellar tendon bone in female athletes, no functional differences were seen between the two groups. However, there was significantly greater kneeling avoidance, numbness/dysesthesia, and loss of passive extension in the bone-patellar tendon-bone group. The authors concluded that hamstrings were an acceptable graft alternative in the female athlete.

Because the incidence of ACL injuries is more common in women and there are increasing numbers of female athletic participants, future research needs to focus on appropriate prevention and treatment.

PREGNANCY AND EXERCISE

Most of the research on exercise during pregnancy suggests that it is beneficial, but physiological parameters must be monitored, and limitations must be applied individually. The goals throughout pregnancy should be to maintain or improve preexisting levels of fitness without risk to the mother or the developing fetus. Exercise in the supine position should be avoided because of potential risk to the great vessels from gravity acting on the uterus.

Studies have shown improvements in well-being and body image, avoidance of excessive weight gain, decreases in musculoskeletal complaints (back pain), improved labor symptoms, and facilitation of postpartum recovery. Potential risks include environmental exposure, dehydration, hypoxia, and uterine trauma. Hot and humid environments should be avoided for risk of dehydration. A meta-analysis was performed in 1992 to help determine safe exercise recommendations during pregnancy. After analyzing the 18 studies involved, the authors concluded that pregnant women can exercise safely three times a week for 43 minutes at a heart rate of 144 beats per minute. In 1994, the

American College of Obstetrics and Gynecology published revised guidelines for exercise pregnancy (Box 4-4). Thus, exercise during pregnancy can have many potential benefits, if appropriate caution is observed and certain restrictions are used.

SUGGESTED READING

Beim G, Stone DA. Issues in the female athlete. Orthop Clin North Am 1995;26:443–449.

Bennell KL, Malcolm SA, Thomas SA. Risk factors for stress fractures in female track-and-field athletes: a retrospective analysis. Clin J Sport Med 1995;5:229–235.

Hame SL, LaFemina JM, McAllister DR, et al. Fractures in the collegiate athlete. Am J Sports Med 2004;32:446–451.

Herring SA, Berfeld JA, Boyajian-O'Neil LA, et al. Female athlete issues for the team physician: a consensus statement. Med Sci Sports Exerc 2003;35:1785–1793.

Hewitt TE, Lindenfeld TN, Riccobene JV, et al. The effects of neuromuscular training on the incidence of knee injury in female athletes: a prospective study. Am J Sports Med 1999;27:699–706.

Ireland ML, Ott SM. Special concerns of the female athlete. In: Fu FH, Stone DA, eds. Sports Injuries. Philadelphia: Lippincott Williams & Wilkins, 2001:215–264.

Kazis K, Iglesias E. The female athlete triad. Adolesc Med 2003;14: 87–95.

Lephart SM, Ferris CM, Fu FU. Risk factors associated with noncontact anterior ligament injuries in female athletes. Instr Course Lect 2002;51:307–310.

Lockey EA, Tran EV, Wells CL. Effects of physical exercise on pregnancy outcomes, a meta-analytic review. Med Sci Sports Exerc 1991;23:1234–1239.

McBryde AM, Barfield WR. Stress fractures. In: Ireland ML, ed. The Female Athlete. Philadelphia: WB Saunders, 2002:299–316.

Nattiv A. The female athlete triad. In: Garrett WE, Lester GE, McGowan J, et al., eds. Women's Health in Sports and Exercise. Rosemont, IL: American Academy of Orthopaedic Surgeons, 2001: 451–465.

Uhorchak JM, Scoville CR, Williams GN. Risk factors associated with noncontact injury of the anterior cruciate ligament. Am J Sports Med 2003;31:831–842.

IMMATURE AND ADOLESCENT ATHLETES

PETER G. GERBINO

The number of immature and adolescent athletes increases yearly. Despite the oft-lamented rise in childhood obesity, sports participation by young boys and girls has continued to become an essential part of childhood for more children. Strength, speed, and sophistication have increased, raising performance levels and injury levels. As in adult sports medicine, most injuries are overuse problems that respond to rest and attention to technique. Macrotrauma injuries have also increased, as has awareness of the natural history of undertreated macrotrauma injuries. Pediatric sports medicine is the understanding and management of overuse and macrotrauma injuries by operative and nonoperative means.

All sports injuries are caused by the interplay of two or more risk factors. What would be an acceptable level of activity in one child could be excessive in another with, for example, weaker bone. Risk factors are divided into two groups: those related to the host or athlete and those arising from the athlete's environment. Surgery on athletes is for repairing damaged tissues and for modifying host risk factors. The most common host and environmental risk factors for injury in the young athlete are listed in Box 5-1.

SHOULDER

Little League Shoulder

Pathogenesis
- Little League shoulder was originally called "Little Leaguer's shoulder" and refers to a stress reaction of the proximal humeral physis.
- Risk factors include number of skilled throws per outing and open physes.
  - The disorder occurs in the throwing arm of pitchers or the racquet arm of tennis players with open physes.
- The mechanism of injury is felt to be repetitive torsion at the physis leading to physeal microfracture and widening from lateral to medial.

Diagnosis
- Diagnosis is made in an overhead throwing or racquet sport athlete with lateral shoulder pain that can sometimes radiate to the elbow.

BOX 5-1   RISK FACTORS ASSOCIATED WITH PEDIATRIC SPORTS INJURIES

Host
- Growth tissues
- Growth spurts
- Gender
- Anatomical malalignment
- Conditioning, strength, flexibility
- Preexisting medical condition
- Psychological conditions

Environmental
- Training error
- Technique error
- Coaching
- Equipment
- Playing surface
- Drugs, supplements
- Nutrition
- Weather, temperature, humidity

- There is point tenderness at the lateral physis and pain with throwing or forced shoulder rotation.
- Radiographs typically show a widened lateral physis, compared with the contralateral side (Fig. 5-1).

Treatment
- Treatment is rest from throwing or tennis until pain resolves in 6 to 8 weeks (Algorithm 5-1).
- A gradual return to throwing is begun.
- Limitations on number and types of pitches can prevent recurrence.

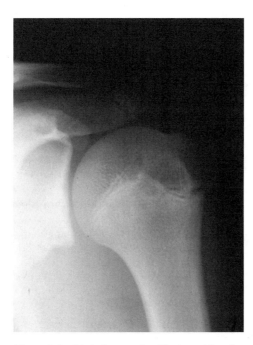

Figure 5-1   Little League shoulder is a widened lateral physis of the proximal humerus. Cause is thought to be from torsional stress.

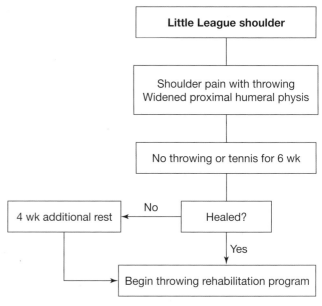

Algorithm 5-1   Management of Little League shoulder.

- Complications from untreated Little League shoulder have not been described.

Dislocation

Pathogenesis
- Shoulder dislocations are extremely rare in children younger than 12 years of age.
- In the adolescent athlete, it is similar to the adult injury, but care must be taken to rule out physeal fracture.
- Most shoulder dislocations are anterior and are caused by forced external rotation and abduction. This occurs in falls and improper tackling in football.
- The nerves of the brachial plexus can be damaged during a shoulder dislocation.

Diagnosis
- Diagnosis is made on the basis of the mechanism of injury, clinical appearance of the shoulder, and radiographs.
- An anterior dislocation will be held in abduction and external rotation.
- A standard axillary view is not usually possible, so the shoulder trauma series of anteroposterior glenoid, axillary, and scapula-Y views is modified to use a Velpeau axillary or other "protected" axillary view (Fig. 5-2).

Treatment
- Qualified personnel can reduce the dislocated shoulder immediately, but more commonly, the athlete is sent to the emergency department some time later (Algorithm 5-2).
- Several reduction techniques have been described, all of which use pain relief, muscle relaxation, and traction of the upper extremity.
- Gentle internal and external rotation may be necessary

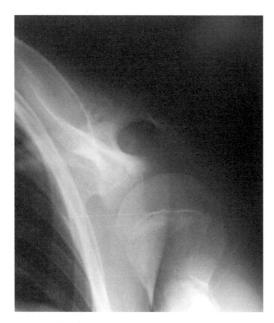

Figure 5-2   The Velpeau axillary view permits evaluation of the glenohumeral joint in the transverse plane without abduction of the shoulder.

after traction to disengage a Hill-Sachs lesion and effect final reduction.

- Postreduction management is periscapular stabilization exercises following 3 to 6 weeks of rest in a sling.
- In the competitive athlete, the case has been made for early operative repair, but this remains controversial.

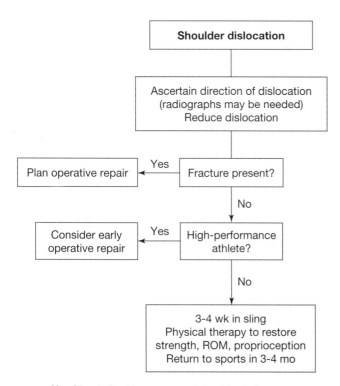

Algorithm 5-2   Management of shoulder dislocation.

- As more sports medicine orthopedists become comfortable with arthroscopic shoulder stabilization techniques, more early repairs are being recommended.
  - Despite this, the standard of care remains nonoperative treatment for first-time dislocations.
- All recurrent dislocations are stabilized by arthroscopic or open means, usually with direct repair of the Bankhart lesion.
  - Even athletes with multidirectional dislocations, traditionally not good operative candidates, are operated on if symptoms persist despite adequate nonoperative therapy.
- Untreated recurrent shoulder dislocation may lead to degenerative arthritis. Overconstraint at repair leads to rapid arthrosis and dysfunction.
- Operative repair always involves repair of a Bankhart lesion with transglenoid suture holes or suture anchors placed at or just on the articular portion of the glenoid rim.
  - If lax, the rotator interval is closed, but care is taken not to restrict external rotation so much that the athlete generates pathologic joint reaction forces in an effort to externally rotate and abduct.
  - Normally, 20 to 30 degrees of external rotation beyond neutral is considered ideal.

Microinstability

Pathogenesis

- Microinstability is a newer concept that explains the anterior shoulder pain felt by throwers, swimmers, and others with repetitive overhead shoulder use.
- The capsule and rotator cuff become attenuated and the labrum frays, tears, and/or "peels back" from the glenoid rim.
- Labral tears and peel-back can result in painful snapping, and anterior humeral head subluxation is painful at the rotator interval and coracoacromial arch.
- Damaged, painful areas result in reflex inhibition and frequently lead to muscle imbalances between the rotator cuff and major shoulder muscles causing a secondary subacromial impingement.
- Primary impingement is not believed to exist in the young athlete.
- In swimmers, posterior capsule tightness, combined with anterior capsulolabral pathology and impingement, is seen.

Diagnosis

- Microinstability with or without labral tear should be suspected in any overhead athlete with impingement symptoms.
- Positive impingement tests as described by Neer and Hawkins confirm the secondary muscle imbalance.
- Subtle anterior laxity may be detected by the shift and load test or apprehension test.
- Palpable anterior glenohumeral joint line tenderness is

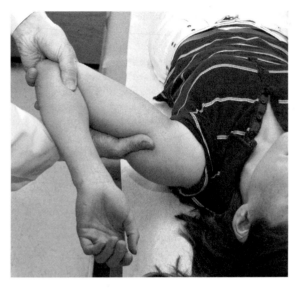

Figure 5-3   The clunk test is one of several tests useful for stressing the anterior labrum. It is performed by forcing the humeral head onto the area of suspected labral instability and then reducing the head (abduction when testing the anterior labrum) to produce a "clunk" when positive for laxity.

always present, and a labral click may be found by one of several tests for labral integrity (Fig. 5-3).
- Radiographs are normal, and magnetic resonance imaging (MRI) may miss a labral tear.
- Even a direct arthrogram MRI using intra-articular gadolinium may not identify all labral tears.

Treatment
- Initial treatment steps include rest from the causative activity and periscapular stabilization in physical therapy.
- If this fails, labral repair, closure of the rotator interval, and limited capsulorrhaphy are indicated.
- Thermal capsulorrhaphy has been used for this condition but must be used judiciously with a rehabilitation program, and prevent excessive stretching for at least 4 to 6 weeks to prevent recurrence.
- Most surgeons now use arthroscopic plication to replace or enhance thermal capsulorrhaphy.
- Overconstraint in a pitcher can result in the persistent loss of pitching ability.

ELBOW

Little League Elbow

Pathogenesis
- Originally called "Little Leaguer's elbow," this group of injuries occurs in throwers and includes medial epicondyle apophysitis from excessive traction, lateral compression–induced radiocapitellar osteochondritis dissecans, posterior ulnohumeral chondromalacia, and anterior soft-tissue tension injuries.
- Within the six phases of throwing, early and late cocking

are most responsible for the valgus stress leading to medial and lateral injuries.
- Acceleration, deceleration, and follow-through are most responsible for the anterior and posterior lesions.
- The intrinsic risk factors for injury include age-dependent tissue strength, conditioning, and muscle strength.
- Extrinsic factors include pitches thrown per outing, types of pitches, and throwing technique.

Diagnosis and Treatment
- Diagnosis and treatment are considered in Algorithm 5-3.

Medial Epicondyle Avulsion

Pathogenesis
- This can occur without warning after a single pitch or after weeks or months of medial epicondyle apophysitis.
- The medial epicondyle is avulsed by the violent valgus forces of early-to-late cocking.
- The elbow does not usually dislocate, but the ulnar collateral ligament (UCL) can be damaged by the valgus stress.
- The number of pitches (or other hard throws) is the only risk factor associated with this injury.

Diagnosis
- The athlete will have a painful swollen medial elbow.
- Ulnar neuritis can occur but is uncommon.
- There is usually a history of medial epicondyle pain and apophysitis.
- Valgus stress will be painful, and there may or may not be valgus laxity as measured by palpable gapping.
- Radiographs demonstrate a variable amount of medial epicondyle displacement (Fig. 5-4).
- A gravity stress radiograph has been advocated to assess medial integrity if there is a question.
- The MRI can be used to assess UCL integrity.

Treatment
- Nondisplaced medial epicondyle avulsions are treated closed in a cast for 4 to 6 weeks.
- Avulsions larger than 1 cm are repaired with pins or 3.5- or 4.0-mm cannulated screws and direct repair of the UCL if torn (Fig. 5-5).
- Fragments displaced between 3 and 10 mm are treated closed by some, repaired by others.
- In a throwing athlete, the trend is to treat displacement greater than 3 to 5 mm with repair, but this continues to evolve.
- Immediate repair allows early range of motion and may prevent some of the flexion contracture complications seen with closed treatment.

WRIST

Gymnast's Wrist

Pathogenesis
- Gymnasts and weightlifters place supraphysiological loads on their wrists, using them as weight-bearing

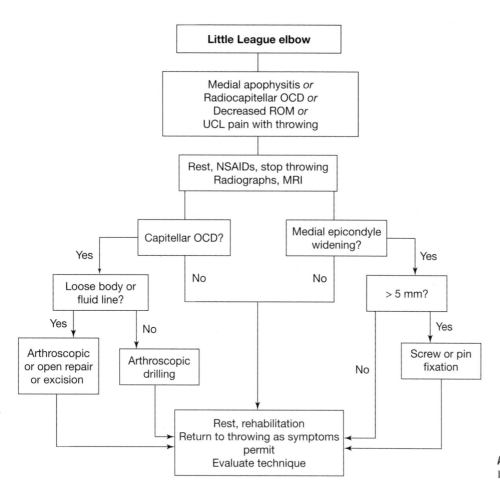

Algorithm 5-3 Management of Little League elbow.

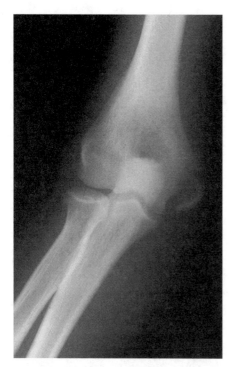

Figure 5-4 Radiograph demonstrating medial epicondyle avulsion. Comparison films may be necessary. Early repair permits immediate motion and may decrease stiffness and permit faster recovery.

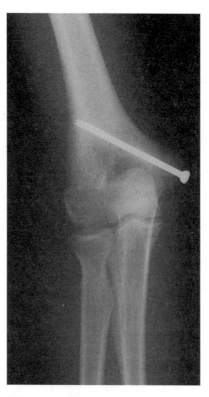

Figure 5-5 Repair of medial epicondyle avulsion with 4.0-mm cannulated screw.

joints. Over time, this can lead to physeal damage and dorsal impaction.

■ *Dorsal impaction* refers to bone bruising and synovitis at the radiocarpal joint from repetitive wrist dorsiflexion under load.

■ Both can be chronically painful, and physeal damage can lead to premature closure and a shorter or malformed distal radius (Madelung's deformity).

Diagnosis

■ Gymnasts and weightlifters with wrist pain require a thorough evaluation, but most commonly there will be dorsal tenderness at the radiocarpal joint, radial physis, or both.

■ Radiographs demonstrating positive ulnar variance, radial physeal bridging, or distal radius deformity are late findings.

■ MRI can detect paraphyseal edema, early physeal bridging or radiocarpal bone bruising.

Treatment

■ Rest will decrease pain and lead to healing of minor physeal damage or bone bruises.

■ Conservative measures include rest, technique changes, and use of wrist braces that limit dorsiflexion such as "lions-paws."

■ Physeal bridging can be resected if small, but large, physeal closures and deformity are treated with ulnar epiphysiodesis and shortening with radius osteotomy as needed.

SPINE

Spondylolysis

Pathogenesis

■ In the young athlete, 47% of all low back pain is caused by spondylolysis.

■ Repetitive spine hyperextension causes unilateral or bilateral stress fractures at the pars interarticularis, usually at L5.

■ Other levels or multiple levels may be involved.

■ Athletes in sports with spine extension (such as diving, volleyball, soccer, dance, and figure skating) are at higher risk, as are athletes with other spinal irregularities.

Diagnosis

■ The history will identify spine extension as a source of pain.

■ Physical examination confirms pain in extension, but not in flexion.

■ Radiculitis is uncommon.

■ Radiographs will show spondylolysis only when there is pars gapping or ongoing sclerosis.

■ The single-photon emission computerized tomography

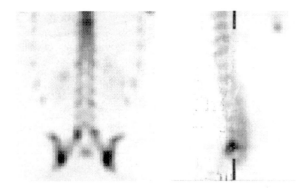

Figure 5-6 Single-photon emission computerized tomography bone scan demonstrating increased uptake at pars interarticularis. A hot bone scan indicates increased metabolic activity with or without a visible fracture. A cold bone scan does not preclude a long-standing quiescent pars fracture.

bone scan has been shown to be the best study for detecting early pars stress injury (Fig. 5-6).

■ Focal computed tomography (CT), is necessary to examine the metabolically active areas to ascertain whether fracture or stress reaction is present and to document healing after treatment (Fig. 5-7).

Treatment

■ Spondylolysis that is a partial fracture, unilateral fracture, or prefracture stress reaction will predictably heal

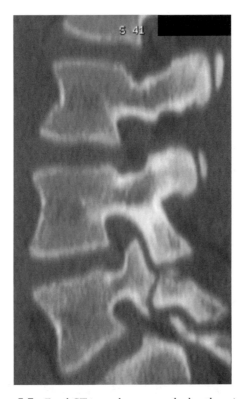

Figure 5-7 Focal CT is used to assess whether there is a visible fracture or simply prefracture stress reaction. It is also used to assess progressive healing.

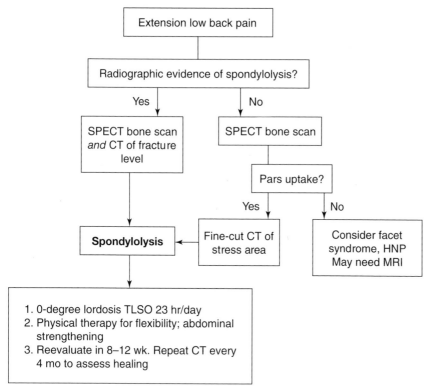

Algorithm 5-4 Management of spondylolysis.

with rest and lumbar stabilization, including therapeutic exercises and rigid bracing (Algorithm 5-4).

- It may take 6 to 9 months for complete healing.
- Bilateral fractures and those that are metabolically quiet may heal with a painless fibrous union or may remain painful.
- Persistent pain is an indication for repair or fusion.

Juvenile Disc Herniation

Pathogenesis

- A herniated nucleus pulposus (HNP) in a young athlete is caused by the same extension and twisting forces under load that cause HNP in an adult.
- There is much less collateral spine and disc degeneration in an adolescent, and the disc is as likely to herniate into an adjacent vertebral end plate (atypical Scheuermann's disease) or centrally as it is to herniate into the classic posterolateral foramen.
- HNP fragmentation is less common in this age group.

Diagnosis

- The history provided by the adolescent with HNP will typically indicate back and buttock or proximal thigh pain.
- True sciatica occurs but less commonly than in the adult.
- A negative straight-leg raising test does not rule out HNP.
- Radiographs will not show disc space narrowing or degenerative changes.
- The MRI will show the herniation, be it central, posterior lateral, or into an end plate.

Treatment

- Herniated discs in the young athlete rarely require surgery.
- They are treated with rest, supportive bracing, and physical therapy to stretch tight hamstrings and strengthen paraspinal muscles and abdominals.
- Persistent pain or sciatica sometimes responds to lumbar epidural steroid injections, and, if all else fails, surgical discectomy is warranted.

HIP

Snapping Psoas

Pathogenesis

- The iliopsoas tendon attaches to the lesser trochanter after crossing the anteromedial hip joint.
- A tight tendon, bursitis, or prominent femoral head can cause snapping with inflammatory changes and pain.
- Poor technique, such as forward pelvic rotation and lumbar lordosis, allows greater hip external rotation but shortens the psoas tendon and presents a more prominent humeral head to the tendon on external rotation.
- Painful snapping during hip external rotation is the result. The tendon snaps over the femoral head or iliopectineal eminence.
- It is believed that the rectus femoris tendon can contribute to the snapping phenomenon.

Diagnosis

- Inguinal hip pain and a palpable snap during hip external rotation are diagnostic.

- Flexing the hip, followed by external rotation and extension, brings out the snap best.
- Imaging studies rarely provide additional information.

Treatment

- Correction of technique, psoas stretching, rectus stretching, and core stabilization techniques address the cause.
- A chronic or resistant case may require fluoroscopic-guided injection of corticosteroid to the psoas and rectus femoris sheaths.
- Rarely is partial surgical release or psoas lengthening necessary.

Snapping Iliotibial Tract

Pathogenesis

- The iliotibial tract connects the gluteus maximus to Gerdy's tubercle on the anterior lateral tibia.
- Excessive use or tightness in the tract results in painful snapping at the greater trochanter.
- Bursitis ensues, eventually leading to fasciitis and fibrosis.
- Risk factors for development are controversial but are thought to include overuse of the gluteus maximus because of relative weakness in the other peripelvic muscles.
- Femoral anatomy has been theorized to be a risk factor, but no conclusive evidence has been found.

Diagnosis

- The standing patient can usually shift his or her body weight to the opposite leg by thrusting the pelvis laterally, thus causing a large "clunk" to be felt and heard.
- Many times, the clunk is painless, but chronic snapping can lead to refractory pain.
- The Ober test usually demonstrates a tight iliotibial band but often is normal.
- Hamstrings are frequently tight and quadriceps, abdominals, abductors, and paraspinals are frequently weak.

Treatment

- The mainstays of iliotibial tract treatment include avoiding the habit of making the hip snap and core muscle strengthening.
- Hamstring and quadriceps strengthening is also important, and iliotibial band stretching is needed when tight.
- Injecting the trochanteric bursa with corticosteroid can decrease pain (Algorithm 5-5).
- Resistant cases are treated with excision of the snapping section of the iliotibial tract.
- This may be a thickened window resection over the greater trochanter or a release of the posterior half of the tract.

KNEE

Meniscus Tears and Discoid Meniscus

Pathogenesis

- Meniscus tears are frequently caused by twisting injuries to the knee.

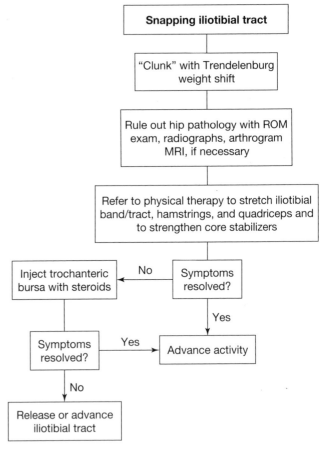

Algorithm 5-5 Management of snapping iliotibial tract.

- Compression and shear forces lead to various tear patterns.
- Peripheral meniscus avulsions can occur in tension.
- A discoid meniscus is usually lateral and congenital.
- The tear of a discoid occurs when the anterior-posterior excursion of the lateral meniscus is lost when the horns are connected because of the discoid shape.
- The meniscus can form with no posterior attachment or tear anteriorly or posteriorly to allow meniscus motion, which must occur during knee flexion-extension.
- A painless or painful clunk is usually palpable with knee flexion-extension.
- A bucket handle tear can get trapped in the notch preventing full extension.

Diagnosis

- An isolated meniscus tear is painful along the joint line in the region of the tear.
- The accompanying knee hemarthrosis occurs over several hours.
- A classic McMurray test of a painful clunk with extension after hyperflexion occurs in a small number of tears.
- Knee hyperflexion and external or internal tibial rotation stresses the posterior horns and is a very sensitive test for a tear.
- Radiographs are usually negative.

- MRI is sensitive and can rule out bone bruises that can mimic meniscus tears.

Treatment

- A locked knee needs to have the meniscus tear reduced and repaired within the first 1 to 2 weeks of injury for best results.
- Children's meniscus tears heal better than adults, but more peripheral tears still heal better than those in the avascular zone.
- Irreparable tears are excised.
- Repairs can be done using outside-in, inside-out or all-inside techniques.
    - Frequently, all-inside devices are used for the most posterior region; inside-out for the majority of the meniscus and outside-in for the anterior horn.
- Discoid meniscus tears are especially difficult and must be saucerized, as well as repaired.
- The repair is protected from full weight-bearing or range of motion (ROM) for 4 to 6 weeks.
- Sports are permitted after 3 to 4 months of physical therapy to restore ROM, strength, and proprioception.

Anterior Cruciate Ligament Tears

Pathogenesis

- Anterior cruciate ligaments (ACLs) are torn with a valgus deceleration mechanism or by hyperextension.
- The ligament fails in tension.
- Females—especially soccer, basketball, and volleyball athletes—have a 4- to 10-fold increased risk of ACL tear compared with males.
    - The reason for the discrepancy remains unknown, but hypotheses concerning landing style, muscle balance, and ligament size are most consistent with the research findings.
- The ligament can fail at the tibia, femur, or midsubstance.
- Most injuries occur close to the femoral attachment.

Diagnosis

- The athlete with an ACL tear usually describes a "pop," followed by the inability to continue with the game.
- A rapid (within 1 hour) effusion is typical.
- Early examination shows increased anterior tibial translation with the Lachman and anterior drawer test.
- Once the effusion is substantial, the athlete may not be comfortable enough to cooperate with the examination for 1 or 2 weeks.
- Other than demonstrating the soft-tissue distension from effusion, the plain radiographs are usually normal.
- The Segond or lateral capsular avulsion fracture has been described as diagnostic of ACL tear.
- MRI is diagnostic.

Treatment

- Acutely, ice is used to decrease effusion.
- Crutches allow protected weight-bearing.
- No bracing is needed acutely.
- Physical therapy can restore ROM and decrease swelling.

- Aspiration can relieve distension pain and allow earlier examination.
- Recent evidence has led to more and earlier ACL reconstruction in athletes.
- Reconstruction techniques employ patellar tendon, hamstring, quadriceps tendon, or iliotibial band autograft and allograft.
- In the immature athlete, the open physis must not be damaged.
- The adolescent with less than 2 cm of growth remaining or at Tanner stage 3 or greater is considered mature. The full spectrum of adult procedures can be used (Algorithm 5-6).
- In the postpubescent athlete with more than 2 cm growth remaining, transphyseal soft tissues (usually hamstring) grafting is used.
- In the prepubescent, every effort is first made to brace and rehabilitate the athlete nonoperatively.
- If giving way persists, an intra-articular, extraphyseal technique is used, utilizing the hamstring or iliotibial band.
    - This repair is not isometric but studies have not shown that these athletes need a second procedure after maturity.
- Rehabilitation is typically the same 6-month closed-chain adult protocol.

Tibial Spine Avulsion

Pathogenesis

- Valgus deceleration or hyperextension does not always lead to ACL tear.
- The tibial plateau bone sometimes fails before the ligament.
- This type of tibial spine avulsion has been described, depending on the degree of fragment displacement (Fig. 5-8).

Diagnosis

- Tibial spine avulsion fracture is very similar to ACL tear.
- A distinct "pop" at the time of injury is less common.
- Physical examination will show only a positive Lachman in type III, completely displaced fragments.
- Radiographs show the fracture but it can be difficult to assess a loose but anatomically positioned type III from a hinged type II.
- CT or MRI can be used to assess fragment position more accurately.

Treatment

- Type I and reducible type II fractures can be treated by 6 weeks of cast immobilization in extension (Algorithm 5-7).
- Some type II fractures have the intrameniscal ligament or anterior horn of the medial meniscus entrapped under the fragment anteriorly.
    - These may be impossible to reduce, leading to a "cyclops" lesion and loss of terminal extension.
- Some other type II fractures are completely separated from the tibia and have reduced healing potential.

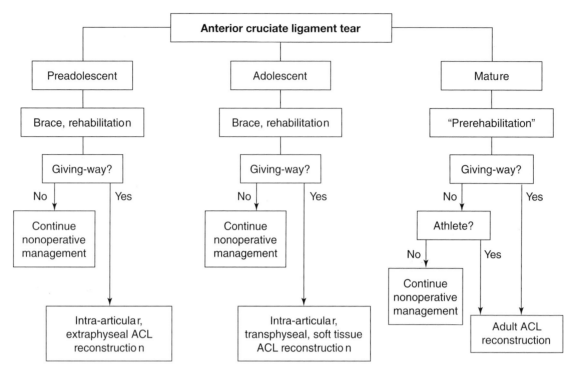

Algorithm 5-6   Management of ACL tear.

- Irreducible type II and all type III fractures are treated with operative repair.
  - This can be done open or arthroscopically with predictable healing in 6 weeks (Fig. 5-9).
- Long-term problems have not been reported for these fractures when treated properly.

Tibial Tubercle Avulsion

Pathogenesis
- A sudden supramaximal force on the tibial tubercle by the patellar tendon can avulse the apophysis.
- The highest peak forces occur with eccentric loading such as landing a jump.
- A preexisting apophyseal stress fracture (Osgood-Schlatter's syndrome) is common.

- The fracture is graded by degree of separation from minimal displacement to intra-articular extension and gross displacement (Fig. 5-10).

Diagnosis
- The athlete has pain after intensive extensor mechanism activation.
- There is swelling and a variable amount of tibial tubercle prominence.
- Straight-leg raising is painful with an extensor lag.
- The tibial tubercle is tender to palpation.
- Radiographs show minimal to complete avulsion.

Treatment
- Ice and immobilization are the first line of treatment, with casting in extension for minimally displaced fracture.

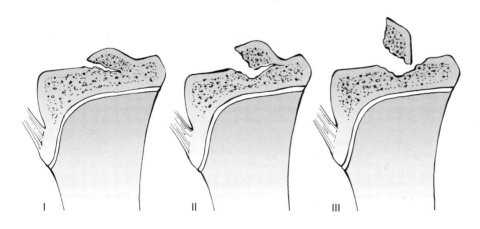

Figure 5-8   Meyers and McKeever classification of tibial spine fractures. Type I has minor displacement and is treated closed in extension. Type II is hinged posteriorly, but with plain radiographs the attachment may be difficult to assess. If reducible, type II fractures can be treated nonoperatively. Many type II fractures cannot be reduced because the medial meniscus or intrameniscal ligament is entrapped. Type III fractures always require operative repair.

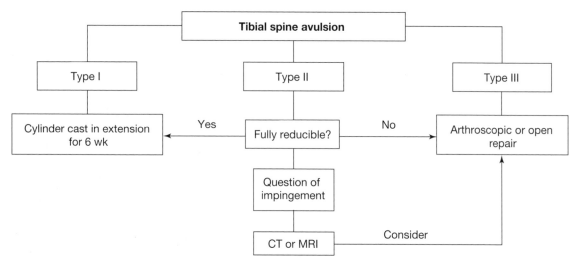

Algorithm 5-7 Management of tibial spine avulsion.

- Displacement of more than 5 mm is treated with open reduction internal fixation with two screws (Fig. 5-11, Algorithm 5-8).
- If the fracture extends into the joint, arthroscopic visualization can ensure anatomic reduction.
- With stable fixation, motion can begin immediately.
- Healing and full weight-bearing can be expected by 6 weeks.

Patellofemoral Stress Syndrome

Pathogenesis
- Patellofemoral stress syndrome represents several poorly understood injuries to the extensor mechanism.
- A major component of patellofemoral stress syndrome is joint-reactive force overload to the patella.
- Abnormal patella tracking, hamstring tightness, quadriceps weakness, patella alta, excessive foot pronation, and/or a sudden increase in activity are the usual causative factors.
- The exact pathophysiology is not known but one hypothesis for the patellar component is that patella deformation under load leads directly to patella pain.
- Synovitis, neuroma formation, and pain in the other surrounding tissues have been implicated in the genesis of this syndrome.

Diagnosis
- Anterior knee pain is very common, and it is first necessary to eliminate other sources of pain.
- If there is pain with anterior-posterior compression of the patella, the diagnosis is patellofemoral stress syndrome.
- Associated risk factors—such as quadriceps strength, hamstring tightness, patella tracking, and pes planus—are assessed.
- The prepatellar fat pad, synovium, medial plica, patella tendon, quadriceps tendon, and medial and lateral reti-

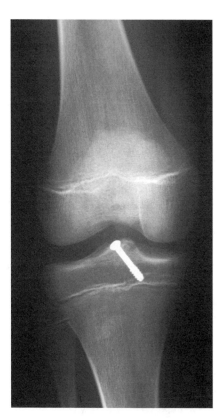

Figure 5-9 Repair of a type III tibial spine avulsion. Most surgeons are using arthroscopic means and avoiding the physis. Comminuted fractures can be repaired with suture through holes made with the ACL tibial tunnel guide.

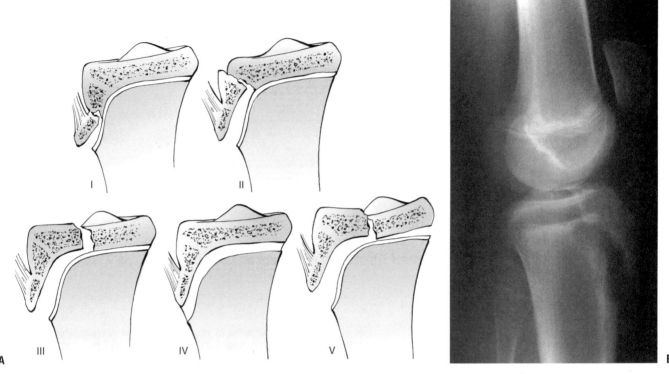

Figure 5-10   **A:** Classification of tibial tubercle fractures. Type I has minimal separation. Type II requires fixation, and type III displays intra-articular extension. Type IV is a SH-I fracture of the entire tibial physis. Type V is a combination of types III and IV. **B:** A type III fracture is shown.

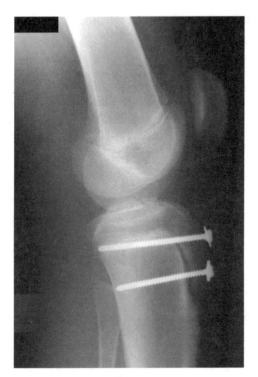

Figure 5-11   Repair of the displaced tibial tubercle fracture. The screws can cause pain with kneeling and are frequently removed. Problems with growth arrest leading to knee recurvatum have rarely been reported.

naculae should be tested separately from the patella to identify all sites of pain.

■ Radiographs demonstrating patella tilt are not necessary to make the diagnosis.

■ Other imaging studies have not been found to provide additional information.

Treatment

■ There is little evidence-based medicine to guide the treatment of patellofemoral stress.

■ Empirical studies show that quadriceps strengthening with minimal patella joint reaction forces (straight-leg raising) is effective.

■ Patella taping can improve symptoms, as can bracing to displace the patella medially.

■ Other interventions—such as orthotics for pes planus, hamstring stretching if tight, and limiting sprinting and jumping—can be helpful (Algorithm 5-9).

Patellar Instability

Pathogenesis

■ A patella can recurrently subluxate or dislocate when there is lateral patella tracking, generalized ligamentous laxity, patella alta, severe genu valgum, or medial attenuation after traumatic dislocation.

■ Virtually all patella instability leads to lateral subluxation.

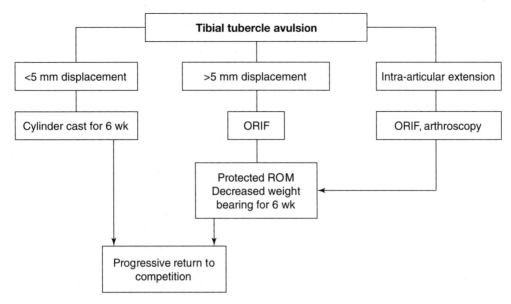

Algorithm 5-8   Management of tibial tubercle avulsion.

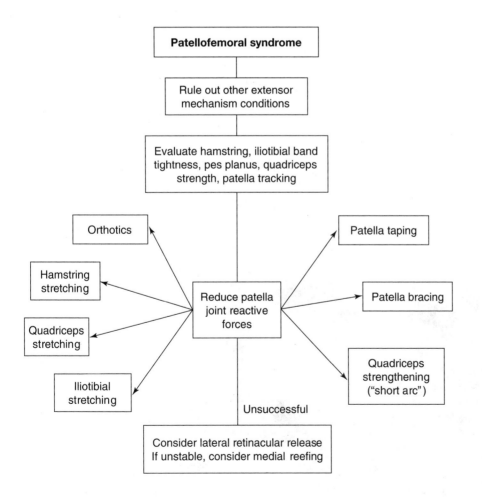

Algorithm 5-9   Management of patellofemoral syndrome.

- Medial instability can occur after surgical overcorrection.
- The medial patellofemoral ligament is the primary restraint to lateral motion.
- Genu valgum and other anatomic alignments resulting in a Q-angle greater than 20 degrees result in lateral patella displacement caused by a lateral tibial attachment.

Diagnosis

- Frequently, the athlete will be aware of the subluxation episodes. Other times, there is only a history of painful giving way.
- Physical examination will demonstrate patellofemoral pain, a positive lateral apprehension test (Fig. 5-12) and one or more risk factors, such as patella alta, lateral tracking or genu valgum.
- The J-sign (patellar tracking in a J-pattern) has been described in association with both lateral tracking and instability.
  - No studies have shown that this sign can predict pathology or effects of various treatments.
- Radiographs can demonstrate patella tilt but cannot predict instability.
- MRI can show lateral condyle bruising and medial retinacular tearing after dislocation (Fig. 5-13).

Treatment

- Acutely extending the knee and moving the patella medially will reduce a dislocated patella.
- Radiographs are obtained to ensure that no fracture or loose bodies are present.
- Most often, a 4-week course of nonoperative therapy is tried with restricted ROM and a brace to displace the patella medially.
- Straight-leg raising exercises to strengthen the quadriceps and especially the vastus medialis obliquus are begun. This is the same regimen used for chronic lateral subluxation.

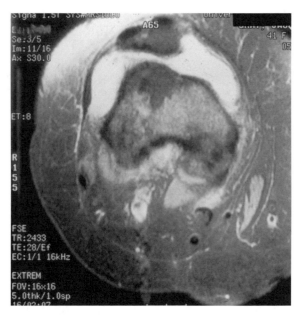

Figure 5-13   MRI of a knee after patella dislocation, lateral condyle bruising, and medial retinacular disruption are diagnostic.

- If instability persists, a medial retinacular repair, reefing, or reconstruction with or without lateral release can be done.
- Where there is gross instability, an anatomic mediofemoral patellar ligament reconstruction can be performed.
- If instability persists or recurs following proximal realignment or if there is tubercle malalignment, a medial tubercle transfer or Fulkerson procedure can be done after physeal closure (Fig. 5-14).

Osgood-Schlatter's Syndrome

Pathogenesis

- Osgood-Schlatter's syndrome is a poorly understood overuse problem at the patellar tendon's attachment to the tibia.

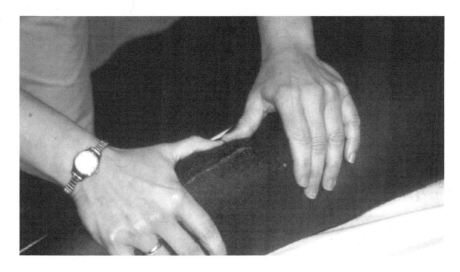

Figure 5-12   The apprehension test is performed by displacing the patella laterally. Pain or apprehension that the patella will dislocate indicates previous negative experience with lateral subluxation.

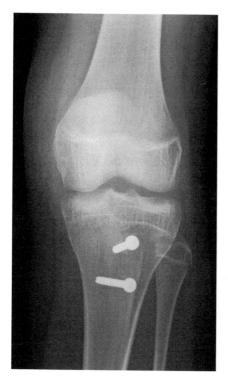
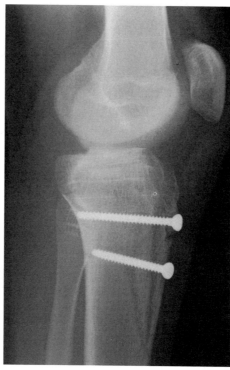

Figure 5-14   Anteriomedialization of the tibial tubercle realigns the patellofemoral mechanism distally to prevent subluxation. It elevates the tubercle to decrease joint-reactive forces.

- Variously referred to as a tendonitis, apophysitis, or enthesitis, there is no evidence that this is an inflammatory condition. Rather, it is most likely a stress fracture of apophyseal cartilage from traction forces.
- It occurs predominantly in 12- to 13-year-old boys who are running and jumping excessively.
- There seems to be relatively weak quadriceps and tight hamstrings in this population, but this has not been formally studied.

Diagnosis
- The athlete complains of pain while running and jumping.
- Symptoms may have occurred on and off in the past.
- The tibial tubercles may or may not be enlarged but will always be tender to palpation.
- The hamstrings are usually tight and the quadriceps weak for the athletic demands required.
- Radiographs and MRIs are normal early in the process.
- As the condition progresses, the more vertical portion of the tibial physis width increases, and the apophysis becomes irregular or fragmented (Fig. 5-15).

Treatment
- Osgood-Schlatter's syndrome has been treated in many ways.
- Benign neglect is advocated by some who note that, if the tubercle does not become avulsed, pain will cease when the physes close.
- Others prescribe rest from running and jumping with or without physical therapy to stretch and strengthen the thigh muscles.
- Historically, casting has been used with success.

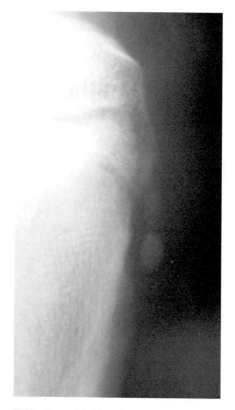

Figure 5-15   Osgood-Schlatter's syndrome with widening of the physis and fragmentation of the apophysis.

- In hyperactive boys who have failed to heal with relative rest, casting or use of an immobilizer may be the only effective treatment.
- If left untreated, complications can include chronic pain, tubercle avulsion, and painful accessory tibial tubercle ossicle as an adult.

Osteochondritis Dissecans

Pathogenesis

- Osteochondritis dissecans (OCD) is a condition occurring in the young athlete characterized by progressive injury to the subchondral weight-bearing bone.
- It has been described in most joints but is most often seen at the posterolateral aspect of the medial femoral condyle.
- One theory is that it is caused by repetitive impact with the tibial spine, but this can only explain some OCD cases. A second theory holds that these injuries result from circulation abnormalities. A third theory maintains that the subchondral bone is transiently weak during growth and susceptible to crush injury.
- Asymptomatic subchondral bone bruising and edema are the earliest signs.
- Progressive subchondral damage occurs if the stresses continue, leading to avascular necrosis, fragment separation from the underlying bone, fracture of the articular cartilage, and finally dislocation of the fragment (Fig. 5-16).

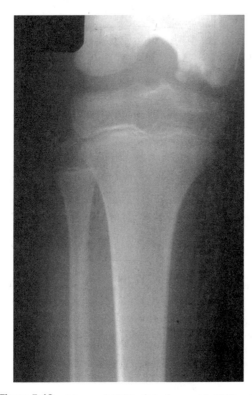

Figure 5-16   Advanced OCD of the knee with AVN and fragmentation.

Diagnosis

- When OCD becomes symptomatic, the first complaints are that of activity-related knee pain.
- The location of the pain is frequently difficult for the athlete to localize.
- Effusion will occur at more advanced stages and locking or catching only when there is a loose body.
- Palpation will frequently localize tenderness to the medial femoral condyle and the remainder of the knee examination is normal.
- Wilson's sign or an external rotation gait has not been shown to predict OCD.
- Radiographs must include a tunnel or notch view to avoid missing the typically posterior lesion (Fig. 5-17).
- Plain radiographs, bone scans, or MRIs can reveal lesion staging (Fig. 5-18).

Treatment

- MRI stage I or II lesions are treated nonoperatively by decreasing loading forces to the lesion (Algorithm 5-10).
  - Activity reduction is a part of all treatment plans.
  - Some advocate a period of cast immobilization.
  - Others will achieve the pain-free state with a combination of activity reduction, unloader bracing, and crutch gait as needed.
  - Physical therapy to optimize lower-extremity muscle balance and flexibility has been advocated.
- Surgical intervention is indicated for stage III (fragment–condyle fluid interface) or greater lesions.
- Surgery is also indicated for stage I or stage II lesions that fail to heal after 6 months of nonoperative treatment.
- For stable lesions, retrograde or transchondral drilling of the lesion stimulates the healing process.
- Intact, unstable lesions are drilled, then fixed in situ with absorbable pins or screws.
  - Headed screws must be removed prior to weight-bearing or full motion.
- Arthroscopic or open techniques can be used (Fig. 5-19).
  - Partially or fully detached lesions require removal of any soft tissue in the fragment–condyle interface prior to drilling and stabilization.
  - Fragmented lesions are debrided and the defect treated with microfracture.
  - Defects larger than 2 cm^2 or that are associated with persistent pain or locking are treated with allograft or autograft mosaicplasty or autologous chondrocyte implantation.

ANKLE

Posterior Heel Pain

Pathogenesis

- One of the most common complaints in the young athlete is posterior heel pain.
- *Achilles tendonitis, Sever's apophysitis,* and *plantar fasciitis* occur individually and in combination in this age group.

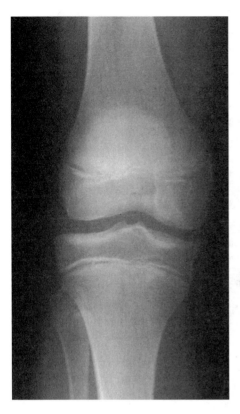
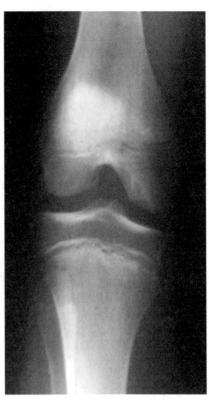

Figure 5-17 Comparison of the anteroposterior view with the tunnel view in the same knee showing the ease with which the OCD lesion can be missed.

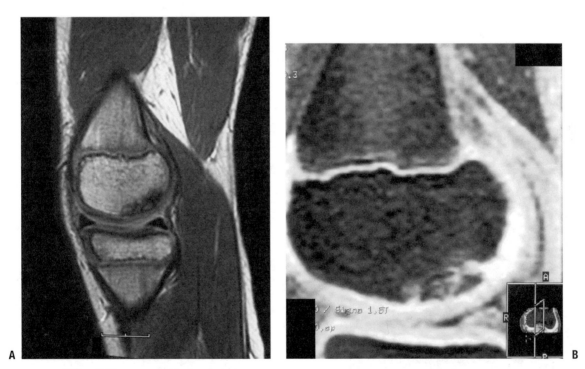

A

B

Figure 5-18 MRI staging of OCD lesions. **A:** Stage I. Homogeneous signal without fluid line or chondral breach. **B:** Stage II. Fluid line at base of lesion usually without definable chondral breach. Stages III and IV are not shown.

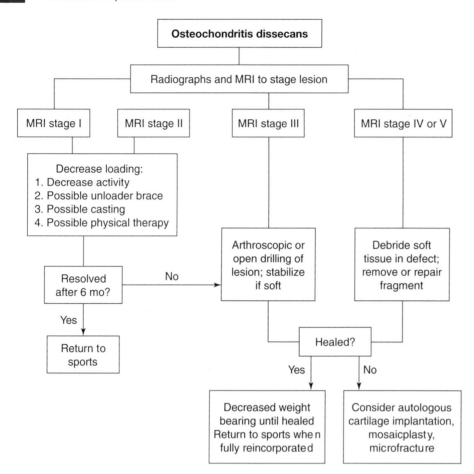

Algorithm 5-10 Management of osteochondritis dissecans.

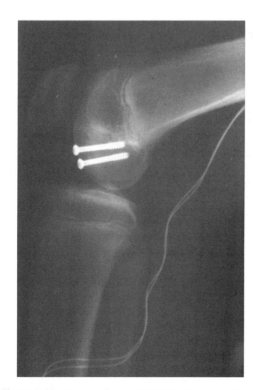

Figure 5-19 Repair of stage III OCD with screws. Good compression is achieved, but the screws must be removed before moving the knee or weight-bearing.

- Lack of adequate ankle dorsiflexion in a running or jumping athlete is always causative.
- There is a high incidence of overpronation in this population, but pronation-eversion is more likely to be compensation for lack of true dorsiflexion than to be causative.
- Athletes who wear soccer-type shoes are at greater risk because the shoes have four cleats at the heel and nine at the sole.
- This results in deeper soil penetration posteriorly, effectively, creating a "negative-heel" shoe that increases the need for ankle dorsiflexion.

Diagnosis

- The athlete complains of heel pain with activity, worsened when in soccer-style shoes.
- Physical examination shows tenderness along the Achilles tendon, at the calcaneal physis and/or at the medial plantar fascia attachment.
- Frequently, there is hypertrophy of the adductor brevis muscle. When asked to dorsiflex the ankle, the athlete will evert and pronate.
    - With the hind foot held in inversion, dorsiflexion will rarely be present beyond neutral.
- Radiographs can occasionally show advanced Sever's calcaneal apophysitis or a calcaneal spur but are not routinely obtained.
- Likewise, MRI is only obtained for chronic cases of Achilles tendonitis to look for degeneration.

Treatment

- Extensive Achilles stretching with the heel locked in mild inversion is the mainstay of treatment. Stretching several times per day is necessary to be effective.
- The knee is kept in extension as the soleus is not usually tight.
- Heel cups or lifts to allow healing can be helpful.
- Orthotics can take away compensatory pronation and exacerbate symptoms if used before adequate dorsiflexion is achieved.
- Physical therapy is prescribed to ensure proper stretching technique is followed and administer ultrasound for tendonitis or fasciitis.
- Running and jumping are permitted as symptoms resolve.

Gymnast's Ankle

Pathogenesis

- Anterior ankle pain occurring in gymnasts and cheerleaders has become increasingly common.
- Pain occurs with dorsiflexion only.
- The underlying mechanism seems to be dorsal impaction from hyperdorsiflexion, leading to bone bruising or anterior synovitis.

Diagnosis

- Anterior ankle pain on landings, dismounts, and floor exercises is the typical complaint.
- The ankle soft tissues are tender to palpation and ankle dorsiflexion increases pain.
- Forced dorsiflexion is frequently painful even without soft-tissue palpation.
- Radiographs are normal.
- MRI may show increased anterior soft-tissue volume or bone bruising at the talar neck or anterior tibial plafond but is usually normal.

Treatment

- Rest and oral anti-inflammatory medication can cure mild cases, but chronic cases can require arthroscopic soft-tissue debridement.
- Simply instructing the gymnast to avoid deep landings with forced-ankle dorsiflexion is frequently effective.
- Sometimes, the gymnast will need to strengthen the quadriceps before the technique can be corrected.
- The condition will promptly recur if the gymnast's technique is not corrected.

FOOT

Accessory Navicular

Pathogenesis

- Painful accessory navicular occurs in young athletes who have excessive tension in the posterior tibial tendon or from direct mechanical rubbing in the shoe.
- Because the function of the posterior tibial muscle and tendon is to support the arch, the typical athlete with painful accessory navicular also has pes planus.
- Whether the accessory navicular is present at birth or occurs as a result of repetitive tension on the tendon is unknown.
- Both tendonitis at the insertion and pain from the fibrocartilaginous nonunion are felt to contribute to pain.

Diagnosis

- The athlete will indicate an enlarged erythematous area on the medial midfoot as the source of pain.
- Examination will show an enlarged bony area at the insertion of the posterior tibial tendon on the navicular.
- The site may rub on the inside of the athletic shoe.
- The tendon is also tender for a variable distance from the insertion.
- Frequently, the athlete will have generalized ligamentous laxity.
- Radiographs show an enlarged navicular with an accessory ossicle medially.
- Avulsion is rare.

Treatment

- Nonoperative treatment includes rest and orthotics.
- If this fails to relieve symptoms or if the problem recurs, excision of the ossicle with navicular osteoplasty and posterior tibial tendon repair are warranted.
- The Kidner procedure is no longer advocated.

Avascular Necrosis

Pathogenesis

- There are two common sites of avascular necrosis (AVN) of the foot in young athletes: the navicular (Kohler's disease) and the second metatarsal head (Frieberg's infarction).
- The mechanism of injury is unknown, but it is thought that excessive forces lead to compression or vascular injury, thus initiating the process.
- Most cases resolve over time with rest.
- Others can progress to fragmentation and loss of joint surface congruence.

Diagnosis

- Foot pain localized to the second metatarsal head or navicular warrants radiographs.
- Radiographs show AVN at the site.
- MRI can show the extent of the lesion and whether fragmentation or instability is present.

Treatment

- Initial treatment is rest, decreasing weight-bearing until symptoms are resolved.
  - This may require casting and crutch use for several weeks.
- As pain resolves, weight-bearing is permitted.
- Healing progress is evaluated with plain radiographs and, if necessary, MRI.
- Failure of conservative therapy, loose fragments, and multiple fragments are indications for surgery.
- Stable lesions are drilled, unstable lesions are fixed, and fragmented lesions excised much the same as for OCD.

SUGGESTED READING

Borges JL, Guille JT, Bowen JR. Kohler's bone disease of the tarsal navicular. J Pediatr Orthop 1995;15:596–598.

Burkhart SS, Morgan CD, Kibler WB. The disabled throwing shoulder: spectrum of pathology. Part I: pathoanatomy and biomechanics. Arthroscopy 2003;19:404–420.

d'Hemecourt PA, Gerbino PG II, Micheli LJ. Back injuries in the young athlete. Clin Sports Med 2000;19:663–679.

DiFiori JP, Puffer JC, Aish B, et al. Wrist pain in young gymnasts: frequency and effects upon training over 1 year. Clin J Sport Med 2002;12:348–353.

Dobbs MB, Gordon JE, Luhmann SJ, et al. Surgical correction of the snapping iliopsoas tendon in adolescents. J Bone Joint Surg Am 2002;84-A:420–424.

Dorizas JA, Stanitski CL. Anterior cruciate ligament injury in the skeletally immature. Orthop Clin North Am 2003;34:355–363.

Gerbino PG. Elbow disorders in throwing athletes. Orthop Clin North Am 2003;34:417–426.

Heintjes E, Berger M, Bierma-Zeinstra S, et al. Exercise therapy for patellofemoral pain syndrome. Cochrane Database Syst Rev 2003;4:CD003472

Kartus J, Perko M. The disabled throwing shoulder: spectrum of pathology. Part II: evaluation and treatment of SLAP lesions in throwers. Arthroscopy 2004;20:336.

Katcherian DA. Treatment of Freiberg's disease. Orthop Clin North Am 1994;25:69–81.

Kocher MS, Klingele K, Rassman SO. Meniscal disorders: normal, discoid, and cysts. Orthop Clin North Am 2003;34:329–340.

Micheli LJ, Ireland ML. Prevention and management of calcaneal apophysitis in children: an overuse syndrome. J Pediatr Orthop 1987;7:34–38.

Rowe CR. Historical development of shoulder care. Clin Sports Med 1983;2:231–240.

Shea KG, Apel PJ, Pfeiffer RP. Anterior cruciate ligament injury in paediatric and adolescent patients: a review of basic science and clinical research. Sports Med 2003;33:455–471.

Tullos HS, Fain RH. Little league shoulder: rotational stress fracture of proximal epiphysis. J Sports Med 1974;2:152–153.

Wall E, Von Stein D. Juvenile osteochondritis dissecans. Orthop Clin North Am 2003;34:3413–3453.

Warme WJ, Arciero RA, Taylor DC. Anterior shoulder instability in sport: current management recommendations. Sports Med 1999;28:209–220

AGING ATHLETES

ROBERT E. LEACH

When sports medicine first started to intrude on the public consciousness, the prevailing thought was that this new specialty was largely applicable to the elite athlete group, such as professional and college athletes. The success in returning to action of such athletes as Gayle Sayers and Joe Namath convinced the public that even severe athletic injuries could be treated with a reasonable expectation of *success*. This period, roughly from 1965 to 1975, coincided with a marked growth of recreational sports and other physical activities in the general populace. Most of the populace had previously thought that many active sports were the domain of the age 40 and under group. However, certain sports—such as tennis and some others—always have had age groups for local and national tournaments, which encouraged those over 40 to continue playing at a high level. In the early 1970s, along came the fitness boom, which pushed all manner of physical activities but particularly running (jogging). It was soon evident that all age groups could participate in a variety of sporting activities, provided they followed certain rules commensurate with a particular age and physical condition.

EPIDEMIOLOGY

Now that we are ensconced in the 21st century, both the medical profession and the general public are faced with certain obvious and critical problems. Our population is aging rapidly as a variety of public health measures and other less well understood factors have come into play. At the beginning of the 21st century, the United States has

roughly 35,000,000 people who are 65 years of age or older. Although much of this group is healthy and consuming health resources at a reasonable rate, we do understand that with increasing age comes an increasing use of health care facilities, personnel, and money. Much of this commitment of personnel and money comes near the end of a person's life span. It then behooves the medical care industry and our country to encourage good health in this aging population for as long as possible.

How would this relate to sports medicine? A variety of studies done in several countries have shown that daily physical activity is one of the major keys, if not the major key, to both longevity and good health. Although there are many physical activities, which are both productive and healthful and are not sports related, many of the injuries suffered doing those same activities are similar to those occurring in sport and other recreational activities. These activity-related injuries can be well cared for by following the usual sports medicine regimens, which are based on trying to return people back to action as soon as feasible. We also realize that all population groups are becoming physically more active as they enjoy better overall health and have more time and perhaps income to enjoy the later life.

Physical activity is excellent in controlling heart disease and non-insulin-dependent diabetes mellitus, two major causes of disability and early death. Studies have shown that people who practice regular physical activity live longer, have fewer chronic conditions and illnesses, and have a much shorter period of disability, which is compressed into the last months of life, compared with those who do not stay active. Thus, the group of "potentially active senior citizens" becomes an obvious focus for sports medicine activity.

We are all aging. Thus, the concepts expressed in this chapter may be applicable to many, although when I was 40, I doubt I would have called myself an aging athlete. I believe that the primary focus of this chapter is for people over 50, with special emphasis on the large number of active people in their 60s, 70s, and 80s. My basic thought is that we, as health professionals, should pay as much attention to the aging athlete—no matter what the chronological age—as we would to their elite younger counterparts. Treatment and advice will have to be tempered for the individual person and to some extent for the age, but we must try to keep people going forward on the activity scale. On the patient's part, he/she must realize that some scaling back of certain physical activities will lead to a more healthy existence and more fun. Some body parts at age 60 are just not what they were at 25, no matter how much we wish it or work at it. All of us must have some idea of what aging does to the body as it relates to sporting and recreational activities and what simple disuse does to the same body. The latter we must advise against. The former we must be aware of and deal with.

EXPECTED PHYSIOLOGIC RESULTS OF AGING

Many of the physical components, which we associate with athletic activity, do change with age. Factors such as endurance, power, strength, agility, quickness, and flexibility all play major roles in athletic performance and all are gradually diminished by the aging process. Even an active person must accept this, but the question is, "How much diminution of our physical abilities should we accept?"

Endurance is a factor in many athletic pursuits. We know that endurance has two important aspects, the more obvious being the cardiovascular and the less obvious being the muscular response. Many people are born with the DNA potential that gives them a high Vo_{2max} and, if they train hard, they will develop excellent endurance. For others less DNA advantaged, the key will be to train harder and make the heart and the lungs respond to training. Thus, endurance is largely subject to our control. As we age, the heart and the lungs undergo certain changes. From age 25 on, there is a gradual decline in the resting stroke volume of the heart. This, with a decline in the achievable maximum heart rate, will produce a reduction in cardiac output. The return to a baseline rate after exercise slows with increasing age. The pulmonary system also undergoes changes. There is a gradual decrease in lung compliance, an increase in tidal volume, an increase in residual volume and, consequently, a gradual decrease in the Vo_{2max}. Each of these changes will reduce the ability to increase endurance. Disease of any sort for the heart and lungs may accelerate these changes.

Although these previously described changes have a negative effect on athletic performance, the good part is that, even with gradual aging, we can positively affect many of these parameters. Cardiovascular training can increase both

the cardiac output and the maximum heart rate, provided that the heart is structurally sound. This can happen even with people who are past the age of 60 and who have not previously trained. Endurance training also positively affects the Vo_{2max} significantly by decreasing the expected lowering of Vo_{2max}. A question often asked by patients is, "How much exercise must one do to effect these positive changes?" Although cardiovascular exercise at high levels is obviously most effective in producing changes, it appears that even moderate exercise done for 30 minutes a day for 4 days a week will produce positive results with regard to the heart and lungs. The point is that exercise must be done on a regular basis.

The results of aging relative to muscles and tendons can be seen even in people who are in their 30s. The problem begins with changes in the connective tissue, which include an increase in collagen crosslinks, a thickening of the basement membrane, and a decrease in the elastin of the connective tissue. Each of these changes makes the collagen stiffer and therefore weaker. Ligaments and tendons are primarily composed of collagen, and we would expect the structural integrity of these tissues to be affected. This could be very important if people expect to pursue certain stressful athletic activities throughout life. As an example, the anterior cruciate ligament (ACL) of a 50-year-old person has a markedly decreased ultimate load to failure compared with a 20-year-old person. If people age 50 continue the same activities that they did at age 20, one would expect a rash of ACL injuries, even with lesser stresses. Tendons have an even less impressive performance in the older athlete because they are subjected to some acute but more often chronic stress. A variety of tendons—including the Achilles, the wrist extensors, and the rotator cuff—might develop tendinosis as the result of repetitive use in certain sports and physical labors. Joint capsules, another tissue composed largely of collagen, are subject to the same collagen problems with resulting increased stiffness. For the patient, this can cause decreased joint motion with or without injury, and decreased joint motion may result in further injury and diminished performance.

Although the aging athlete can relatively easily positively affect cardiovascular conditioning, it may be harder to affect the collagen tissues. There are people whose genetic makeup allows them to be as loose-jointed as younger athletes, and they will always be looser than the tight-jointed individuals. However, the tighter-jointed individuals can, with regular exercise and stretching, increase capsular range of motion and musculotendinous flexibility and maintain what they have. Seeger et al. have shown that slow sustained stretching of muscle tendon units will increase flexibility to some extent. Munn, using subjects aged 65 to 88 found a significant increase in the range of motion of the subjects' wrists, shoulders, knees, ankles, etc., after a 12-week period of doing dance and flexibility exercises on a regular basis. Compared with the controls, the study group had increased flexibility.

With age, both males and females gradually lose muscle strength and power. Both of these items factor strongly in athletic performance, and muscle strength plays a major role in injury prevention, such as decreasing falls. During the middle part of the 20th century, some experts believed that endurance could be maintained by exercise but that the maintenance of strength was more difficult. Now, following some excellent studies, we know that strength cannot only be maintained but can show a gain even in an octogenarian group. Fiatarone, in 1993, published a landmark study on the effects of exercise in patients ranging in age from 89 to 92, which showed an increase of 175% in quadriceps strength over an 8-week exercise period. Many people who have remained active may have been intuitively aware that strength can be maintained, but this study showed that even those who had not been active could restore strength. Despite this knowledge, it can be difficult for even motivated and active people to stay on a program to maintain optimal muscle strength.

The medical profession and the general populace are well aware of the potential problems with bones with advancing age. Although this is a bigger concern in females than males, over the age of 80, many males will develop osteoporosis. The problem of osteoporosis may prove to be even more severe in many female athletes of the 1970s and 1980s who were running many miles. We now understand that the primary accretion of bone occurs in the 18- to 25-year-old period, and females who run a lot, keep their weight down, and have menstrual problems will have significant osteopenia as they come into their 50s. This means that some older female athletes should choose sports carefully, and those activities that have an inherent risk—such as skiing, rock climbing, and others—could pose a problem for fractures in those with osteopenia. Postmenopausal females will be more at risk than their male counterparts.

There are other tissues of the body that have changes from advancing age. The articular cartilage of joints gradually becomes thinner, loses some of its ground substance, and loses some of the water contained within. The cartilage cells become less numerous and have a decreased ability to manufacture ground substance. There is a loss of some resilience of the joint surface. The intervertebral discs gradually become thinner and less resilient as they lose some water of hydration. The knee menisci also are more subject to injury (tearing). The meniscus contains fewer cells, the ground substance undergoes changes, and there is loss of water content. The structural internal integrity of the meniscus is lessened. The junction between the meniscus and the surrounding joint capsule is weakened, and tears in this region are more likely. None of these changes can be influenced in a positive way by activity. Because of these changes, it is obvious that there are certain physical activities that may be more harmful in the older person than in the younger athlete. Meniscal tears are common in the over 50 age group, and many of the symptoms previously thought to be a result of "arthritis" are often the result of a torn meniscus.

Although there is a litany of changes that occur in the human organism, overall the news is relatively good for the over 50 athlete to remain active and to continue to play certain sports. It does not, however, mean that with exercise, your body at 50 and beyond is the same as it was at age 28. It does mean that in order to have good cardiovascular status, strength, and flexibility, one has to work at it. Lack of physical activity is the prime enemy of the aging athlete. Each single individual has to balance the known good effects of sporting activity against the possible injuries that sometimes occur.

There are certain other aspects of aging that play a huge role in those who want to continue to be active. Overall, general health and chronic diseases are usually not major factors in younger athletes but in the over 50 age group, they will be a major concern. For many people who have been active all their lives, they probably have a pretty good idea of their general health and how to deal with any concerns. The bigger concern for physical activity participants and the medical profession is that group of people who decide at a later age to take up sports. We want to encourage this latter group because it will promote good health but we must be sure that they are able to be active, to compete, etc. For active people, I would encourage them to have a general physical examination every several years even if they are doing well. For people who have not previously been very active, they must have a thorough physical, paying particular attention to the cardiovascular and pulmonary systems and to major joints. Although people may be active up to a point with a heart or lung problem or diabetes, these conditions impose certain restrictions that should be obeyed.

SPECIFIC PROBLEMS IN THE AGING ATHLETE

A major item for all older athletes is previous injury, which causes present problems. There are many sports played at a younger age with a high potential for injury (such as football, gymnastics, wrestling, skiing, and other outdoor activities) that cause many athletic people to come into their older years with significant problems. The most significant sports involve the back and knee with the shoulder and hip following.

Articular Cartilage Injuries

Osteoarthritis is not an uncommon sequela to a previous knee or hip injury. However, even without previous injury, the articular surface of the knee and the hip can be problematic for the aging athlete. With advancing age, we see an increasing number of people with osteoarthritis of the knee and hip. Looking back to instances of a previous injury, two very common scenarios play out. One concerns a meniscectomy performed on a patient during his late teens or early 20s, and the other concerns the large number of active athletes who are having ACL reconstructions and return to sports activity. We know that knees with a meniscus totally or partially removed will likely have later trouble. The articular cartilage on that side of the joint will slowly deteriorate. The evidence for this dates back to the 1940s. With regard to reconstructed ligaments, we really do not know what the final results of these knees will be when they are subjugated to long-term athletic use. However, studies from several Scandinavian countries indicate that, although the reconstructed knees remain stable, they show early degenerative changes on x-ray.

Management

■ For even a moderately active person, the treatment of osteoarthritis, no matter what the joint (but particularly in the lower extremity), will be important.

■ A careful baseline physical examination will pay particular attention to the joint range of motion, the strength of the concerned muscles, and any deformity. This physical examination plus appropriate x-rays establish the diagnosis and extent of the problem.

■ At this point, the physician has to match the physical capabilities of the patient with the activities he/she wants to perform.

　▫ In most instances, active people will want to continue the same sports activities they have always performed. Trying to change this attitude may be difficult but necessary.

■ Certainly physical therapy has a major role to play in patients who have arthritic joints.

　▫ Increasing the range of motion of an afflicted joint helps performance and may decrease pain.

　▫ Strength gain in the muscles around that joint will help stabilize it, and increased muscle strength can help to absorb the energy of foot strike.

　▫ The key is always trying to find ways of increasing strength without causing pain to the joint.

■ Judicious nonsteroidal anti-inflammatory drug (NSAID) use is helpful in the aging athlete.

　▫ In most instances, pain will be decreased and make it possible to play, and might also be helpful in the rehabilitation process.

　▫ A major decision for the doctor is how much NSAID use is reasonable.

　▫ If the use is gradually increasing or if there is increased pain following activity after NSAID use, this might be the time to re-examine the use of medications.

　▫ Patients often mistakenly believe that NSAIDs are curative, and they must be made to understand the difference between decreasing pain and curing the disease.

■ During the past decade, it seems there has been a gradual increasing patient and doctor acceptance of various braces.

　▫ This is particularly true with regard to the knee where we see common usage of either a knee stabilizer or a knee unloader brace.

　▫ It is important to approach the question of using a brace by giving the patient sufficient information to help him/her make a decision, which may be obvious to you.

　▫ In dealing with aging athletes, extra time spent explaining the situation seems to pay off with happy patients and less-frequent visits.

　▫ Paramount to the successful use of bracing for both doctor and patient is having a sound brace person available.

　▫ A careful fit makes a huge difference to the patient, and detailed instructions as to how best apply and use the brace are vital.

■ Intra-articular steroid injections will quiet down a synovitis and make the pain substantially better for a while.

　▫ This is a short-term solution and if the person becomes much more active using the joint, the synovitis will return in full force.

　▫ There is evidence to show that intra-articular steroids may increase the rate of cartilage degeneration, and so this is a short-term, somewhat limited solution, particularly if the person tries to stay active.

■ Viscosupplementation is another method of helping to decrease joint pain.

　▫ It is quite expensive and must be done in a series of shots.

　▫ Infection remains a possibility but is not common.

　▫ The bigger problem is how long pain relief will last and whether it is logical to repeat the series of shots several times.

Muscle Strains

One of the most common problems for any athletic population is a muscle strain. Although this may occur in the younger age group as the result of abnormal muscle endeavor (often eccentric exercise) in the trained athlete, in the older age group it is much more common. In this second group, muscle strains often occur after what appears to be even moderate exercise. This can be very discouraging to that person trying to remain active. Over time, it can test the patience of the aging athlete, the doctor, the therapist, and even family members.

One basic problem is that we active people all remember or think we remember what was for us, at one point in time, normal physical activity. We then go out and replicate that activity, failing to realize that we are no longer in the physical shape that we once were and that there have been some tissue changes. Absolutely, the person who has remained in muscular shape can go out and perform at a higher level than the person who has not. However, even the trained older athlete at some point in time has to make some concessions as to the amount of time he/she can spend doing an activity and the absolute amount of muscle stress he/she wants to exert. People who have continued to do the same athletic activity over time do gradually adjust to the aging process, and they are keeping the active muscles in shape for that sport. That is why we often see problems in people who take up certain activities later in life. However, there is no reason to not take up new activities. Just be sure to get the musculoskeletal system ready for that sport. Usually, this means doing some resistance exercises to increase strength and endurance of the muscle groups that will be used. Stretching the muscle-tendon groups and the involved joints is also a requisite.

Management

■ Treatment of muscle strains in the older athlete may be roughly the same as for the younger group, except that it may take longer to reach complete resolution.

■ Distinguishing between muscle soreness, usually as a result of an increased period of time using a certain muscle group, and muscle strain—which is a microscopic injury to the muscle fibers—may take a bit of history taking and a good physical examination.

　▫ Soreness tends to be associated with stiffness and

to involve a whole muscle group. After several days, it has receded and mild analgesics or NSAIDs have sufficed.

- Muscle strains usually involve a particular area of the muscle, have local tenderness, occasionally an ecchymosis, and are painful with use not just sore.

- The usual treatment of compression, ice, medications, possibly protection, and gentle stretching after pain has receded must then include a well-ordered program of regaining muscle strength of the involved muscle.
- Many times, the aging athlete has gradually lost muscle strength and with even a small strain may fall prey to further weakness and subsequent repetitive injury.
- Most younger athletes will gradually regain strength after injury, but even in that group, many do not work hard enough to protect themselves from another strain.
  - In the aging athlete, the problem is magnified and many are less likely to think of going beyond just stretching the injured area.

REHABILITATION

We all recognize the importance of aggressive and prolonged rehabilitation in the treatment of sports injuries. We usually think of this in terms of the elite or competitive athlete wanting to lose as little time as possible from competition. However, aggressive and long-term rehabilitation may be even more important in the aging athlete than it is the younger one. The time away from sports in the older person and the subsequent loss of conditioning, both cardiovascular and muscular, may make it difficult to return to previous activity levels—not just athletic activities but those of daily living. The older athlete is starting from a lower baseline level of overall conditioning. It is unlikely that either his muscle strength or cardiovascular condition is at the level of the younger person. This makes it imperative that the sports medicine doctor, who must be a believer in aggressive therapy even in the older age groups, be the overseer of the physical therapy program. It is also important to set up a program taking into account that the older athlete may not be able to rehabilitate in precisely the same way that the younger athlete does.

- Regaining muscle strength, improving joint motion, and aiding in the return of proprioception are the important parameters for this rehabilitation program.
- Gaining strength in various muscle groups will often be a primary focus.
  - The aging athlete may not be able to use some of the more traditional progressive resistance exercise programs. Instead of using free weights or even machines, we may use something such as rubber tubing to initially provide resistance.
  - Most of the time, we will start with light resistance and gradually increase repetitions before going on to heavier resistance.
  - The fallacious concept of "no pain, no gain" is even less applicable in the older athlete.
- Ancillary muscles for a particular area or injury may need substantial work.

- For instance, in a knee injury, we often think of the quadriceps as the primary focus with a less emphasis on the hamstrings. In the older person, we may need to focus on the hip musculature, too, as it falls prey to the disuse resulting from the knee problem.
- We must always be aware of the effect of our prescribed exercises on neighboring joints and muscles.
  - Many elders have some loss of back mobility, and an exercise program for the knee may put stress on the back that interferes with the overall rehabilitation.
- The basic concept must be that there is always a way to carry out the program but it will take some thought on the part of the therapist with input from the physician to solve the problem.
- Regaining full joint motion will be difficult or impossible in many cases, and there is always the problem of figuring out exactly what that particular person's joint motion norm was prior to the present injury.
  - Patients are not good at remembering how well they were doing. They gradually become used to loss of motion or strength and are surprised to find the extent of the loss when they are measured.
  - Regaining joint motion can result in decreased pain and increased function athletically. It makes many activities of living easier.
- Short periods of stretching several times a day are far more effective than one longer episode.
- Working with a therapist for a period is very helpful in teaching the patient what to do and may result in some gains by using a bit of active assistive activity, which is difficult to achieve alone.
  - It is the extended work done by the patient at home or alone at a facility, however, that will determine the final physical capabilities.
- The use of heat and cold as adjuncts to help with exercises must be carefully monitored, because some aging athletes will have circulatory problems, diabetes, etc.
  - The application of either heat or cold directly to the skin is contraindicated.
- The upper age group requires more time and thought to start the rehabilitation process, but the flip side is that these athletes can usually follow instructions well and will do so.
- With the cost of physical therapy and the restrictions often put on Medicare payment for patients, you may find yourself recommending health club facilities for extended therapy.
  - Knowledge of local facilities and particularly some of the so-called personal trainers who work within certain clubs is useful. Although some may have had competent training and be excellent, others are simply not suitable for your patients.
  - The overly aggressive personal trainer may cause the patient injury, and you may lose them forever.
- One final positive sign for older athletes is that they are often intelligent, very motivated to return to their activities and, after age 60 or so, often have the time available to rehabilitate.

SURGERY

Although many aspects of surgery are the same in the aging athlete as in his/her younger counterpart, in other instances, there are significant differences. In each instance, our stated aim should be to return the afflicted patient to previous athletic and daily activity levels. Yet, in the older athlete, we realize that this may not prove entirely feasible. We may have to have both the surgeon and the patient take a realistic view of what can be expected. Overall, the less complicated the surgery and the shorter the expected rehabilitation period, the better, but sometimes major procedures are all that will accomplish the job.

As in the young athlete, the meniscus in the aging athlete is prone to tears, which with activity are even more likely to occur in the older group than in the 20- to 40-year-old age group. In the older group, there is going to be no chance to repair the meniscus, and most tears will be posterior horn degenerative tears. The remaining meniscus will not have the internal structure of the 20-year-old, and surgeons must refrain from trying to resect meniscal tissue back to "normal" tissue because it will be a total removal by then. The state of the joint articular surface may be very different than that of the younger patient, and the surgeon may have to make decisions regarding the surface. If the articular cartilage is down to bone in certain areas, the possibility of cartilage cell transplants or multiple drill holes must be considered. However, this is not going to be a spur of the moment decision and is a likely follow-up to meniscal surgery. Minimal articular cartilage debridement is often done in association with meniscal resection. Various procedures to "smooth" the articular cartilage have been advocated but, as yet, long-term results have not proven the effectiveness over minimal debridement.

The previous state of the articular surface and what you do to it will have a great effect on how well the patient will do after a meniscal procedure and may slow up the return to activity. Patients have to be aware of this possibility before surgery to avoid later disappointment and friction with the surgeon. The older athlete may compare himself/herself to a younger person having the "same" procedure or what he/she remembers from previous years. The athlete has to understand the potential for degeneration of the joint surface.

Another anatomical area commonly involved in the older athlete is the rotator cuff. Tendinosis and/or tears, major or minor, are frequently seen. Several aspects of this deserve special mention. The tissue to be repaired may not be very good, and some surgical accommodation may have to be made to obtain a good closure of the cuff and thus a potential for return to good shoulder function. With this in mind, the surgeon will have to consider which procedure, open repair, arthroscopic repair, or arthroscopic debridement would be best for that particular patient. Another aspect to consider is that many of the aging athletes who have had shoulder problems have had trouble for quite a while. As a consequence of this, there is a major loss of shoulder strength. This means that the return of strength is going to be hard to achieve and will necessitate a long rehabilitation period, even 1 to 2 years to gain a final hoped-for result.

Arthroplasty

Many of the active people in the older age group with a lower-extremity joint problem may need either a knee or hip replacement. During the initial phases of joint replacement, the prevailing thought was that this surgery was not to allow people to return to such activities as skiing, tennis, and other similar sports. However, with better prosthetic devices, stronger methods of bone anchoring, and an understanding of wear and tear characteristics, it is apparent that many people can and will return to active lives. One would think that such activities would probably induce more severe wear on the prosthetic devices, and this is likely true. The question for many somewhat younger and active people is whether the risk of another needed surgery is worth the pleasure of a certain number of years of continued activity in a favored sport. This brings up the first and perhaps the most important of decisions that physician and patient have to make. Both must understand what the expectations of the patient are. Then, the patient must understand what can reasonably be expected from a total hip or knee. The patient has to realize that if another replacement is needed, it is not as easy to perform and that the remaining bone stock has been jeopardized. With the success that we often hear about, it seems as if patients believe that if one hip wears out, it is easy to just replace it with another, with no expected loss of function or durability.

The patient who wants to return to certain physical activities must be well aware of the potential for wearing down the replacement and the possibility of loosening as a result of various causes.

Having warned any patient of what can or cannot be expected, it seems clear to me that both hip and knee replacements have, in many instances, allowed people to return to many activities, and that 5 years, 10 years, and longer periods have elapsed for many patients to enjoy their lives. Maintenance of muscle strength must be one of the major considerations for such patients, and long-term muscle therapy seems warranted and, indeed, mandated. The older patient will not put as much stress on the device as a 35-year-old but also may not have the protective muscle power that the younger person might have. Patients often get their knowledge from other patients who have been operated on and who have done well. Although this can be a source of information, it may not always be applicable to another's status. Patients tend to hear what they really want to hear and, in the active person facing a joint replacement, they are very likely to hear all the positives of the new joint and very little of the negatives, with respect to wear and tear as a result of physical activity.

SUMMARY

An aging population is going to put tremendous strains on our health care system. Anything that the medical profession can do to improve the health of the over 50 population will affect the system both significantly and positively. Active people have fewer major illnesses and demand less health care resources than those who are inactive. Events of the past 25 years have demonstrated that people can continue to be very active and athletic into their 60s, 70s, and 80s. Although there may be a physical price to pay for this activity at times, sports medicine practitioners are well suited to care for such problems and to encourage the general populace to maintain sports activities. Many of the effects on the body previously thought to be a result of aging are actually because of disuse. Sports medicine is in a unique position to increase the well-being of many aging people by keeping them active and thus healthy.

SUGGESTED READING

Cooper KH, Pollack, ML Martin RP, et al. Physical fitness levels vs. selected coronary risk factors: a cross-sectional study. JAMA 1976; 236:166–169.

Fiatarone MA, Marks EC, Ryan ND, et al. High intensity strength training in nonagenarians. JAMA 1990;263:3029–3034.

Huang Y, Macera CA, Blair SN, et al. Physical fitness, physical activity, and functional information in adults aged 40 and older. Med Sci Sports Exerc 1998;30:1430–1435.

Kirkendall DT, Garrett WE. The effects of aging and training on skeletal muscle. Am J Sports Med 1998;26:598–602.

Kohn WM, Malley MT, Coggan AR, et al. Effect of gender, age, and fitness level on response of VO_{2max} to training in 60 to 70 year olds. J Appl Physiol 1991;71:2004–2011.

Kujala UM, Sarna S, Kaprio J, et al. Hospital care in later life and former world-class Finnish athletes. JAMA 1996;276:216–220.

Munns K. Effects of exercise on the range of joint motion in elderly subjects. In: Smith EL, Serfass RC, eds. Exercise and Aging: The Scientific Basis. Hillside, NJ: Enslow Publishers, 1981:167–178.

Paffenbarger RS, Hyde RT, Wing AL, et al. The association of changes in physical activity level and other lifestyle characteristics with mortality among men. N Engl J Med 1993;328:538–545.

Sarno S, Kaprio J, Kujala UM, et al. Health status of former elite athletes. The Finnish experience. Aging 1997;9:35–41.

Smith EL, Serfass RC. Exercise and Aging: The Scientific Basis. Hillside, NJ: Enslow Publishers, 1981.

Taylor DC, Dalton JD, Seaber AV, et al. Viscoelastic properties of muscle-tendon units. The biomechanical effects of stretching. Am J Sports Med 1990;18:300–309.

Thompson LV. Effects of age and training on skeletal muscle physiology and performance. Phys Ther 1994;74:71–81.

Vita AJ, Terry RB, Hubert HB, et al. Aging, health risks, and cumulative disability. N Engl J Med 1998;338:1035–1041.

Woo SL, Hollis JM, Adama DJ, et al. Tensile properties of the human femur-anterior cruciate ligament–tibia complex: the effect of specimen age and orientation. Am J Sports Med 1991;19:217–225.

HEAD INJURIES

ROBERT V. CANTU
ROBERT C. CANTU

Over the past decade, sport-induced head injuries have received increasing attention. This is the result of the early retirement of well-known professional athletes, such as Steve Young, Troy Aikman, Pat Lafontaine, Merrill Hodge, and others who have sustained multiple concussions. There is an increasing awareness of the frequency and effects of head injury in sports. This chapter will provide information to help physicians, coaches, and trainers to diagnose, treat and, hopefully, prevent head injuries in athletes.

PATHOGENESIS

Etiology

The most common head injury sustained by an athlete is a concussion. Multiple definitions of concussion exist. The word itself is derived from the Latin verb *concussus*, which means "to shake violently." The Committee on Head Injury Nomenclature of the Congress of Neurological Surgeons defines concussion as "a clinical syndrome characterized by immediate and transient posttraumatic impairment of neural function, such as alteration of consciousness, disturbance of vision, equilibrium, etc., as a result of brainstem involvement." As Kelly has stated, a concussion is a "trauma-induced alteration in mental status that may or may not involve loss of consciousness." The American Orthopaedic Society for Sports Medicine defines concussion as "any alteration in cerebral function caused by a direct or indirect (rotation) force transmitted to the head resulting in one or more of the following acute signs and symptoms: a brief loss of consciousness, light-headedness, vertigo, cognitive and memory dysfunction, tinnitus, blurred vision, difficulty concentrating, amnesia, headache, nausea, vomit-

ing, photophobia, or balance disturbance. Delayed signs and symptoms may also include sleep irregularities, fatigue, personality changes, inability to perform usual daily activities, depression, or lethargy."

Although some have suggested that a concussion is a physiologic disturbance without structural damage, animal and human data have shown that neurochemical and structural changes with loss of brain cells can occur. A neurochemical cascade begins within minutes after a concussion and can continue for days. It is during this period that neurons remain in a vulnerable state, susceptible to minor changes in cerebral blood flow, increases in intracranial pressure, and anoxia. Animal studies have shown that, during this susceptible period, a decrease in cerebral blood flow that normally would have little consequence can produce extensive neuronal cell death.

A term first defined by Schneider is *second impact syndrome*. This syndrome occurs in an athlete who has sustained an initial head injury, most often a concussion, and returns to play while still symptomatic and sustains a second head injury. The second impact to the symptomatic brain can result in a loss of cerebral autoregulation, leading to rapid cerebral vascular congestion, increased intracranial pressure, and brain herniation. The condition typically occurs in adolescents aged 14 to 16 and is uncommon in adults. It appears to have a common pathophysiology with "diffuse cerebral swelling" or "malignant brain edema" syndrome in children.

Epidemiology

Sporting activities account for an estimated 20% of the 1.54 million head injuries each year in the United States. High school football alone accounts for about 250,000 brain injuries each year. Approximately 1 in 20 high school football players sustain a concussion in a given season. Head injury accounts for 75% of all fatalities in high school football. Of these fatalities, the majority (74.4%) are the result of subdural hematomas. Between 1980 and 1993, 35 football players succumbed to the second impact syndrome.

Although the overall number of head injuries is highest is football, many other sports pose a risk for head injury (Table 7-1). During a single season of Canadian intercollegiate ice hockey, the incidence of concussion was 1.55 per 1,000 athletic exposures. Concussion rates among college soccer players are estimated to be about 1 per 3,000 athletic exposures. Concussions occur in many other sports, including wrestling, lacrosse, motor sports, bicycling, diving, basketball, baseball, field hockey, gymnastics, rugby, volleyball, track and field, and softball. One study sampling students from a boarding school with mandatory sports participation reported that 97% of athletes aged 14 to 19 years had sustained at least one sports-related concussion.

Concussion is a common injury at the professional level. In the National Football League, it is estimated that 100 to 120 concussions occur per year, or about one every two to three games. In professional soccer, 52% of players have reported at least one concussion in their career. The National Hockey League (NHL) has seen an increase in the number of concussions, with the rate from 1997 to 2002 more than triple that of the preceding decade. Multiple theories have been proposed for the increase, such as bigger, faster players, new equipment, and harder boards and glass. Fortunately, the rate has reached a plateau since 1997, which was the year the NHL instituted its concussion program.

There is some evidence to suggest that younger athletes may be at higher risk for concussion. For example, the concussion rate for collegiate soccer players is estimated at

1 per 3,000 athletic exposures, whereas the rate for high school players has been reported at 1 per 2,000 exposures. Among Canadian amateur hockey players aged 15 to 20, 60% have reported sustaining a concussion during either a practice or a game. Authors have expressed concern that injury during adolescence may impair the plasticity of the developing brain.

The National Athletic Trainers' Association study found gender differences in regard to concussion rates. In high school sports, females were found to be at higher risk for sustaining a concussion than males competing in the same sport. The rate in soccer was 1.14 concussions per 100 player-seasons in females and 0.92 per 100 player-seasons in males. In basketball, females had a rate of 1.04 concussions per 100 player-seasons, whereas males had a rate of 0.75 per 100 player-seasons. In softball, the rate was 0.46 for females and 0.23 for males. This trend does not remain at all levels. At the collegiate level, the concussion rate for soccer and basketball players appears to be nearly identical. At the Olympic level, 89% of male and 43% of female soccer players have reported a prior history of concussion.

Pathophysiology

The pathophysiology of traumatic brain injury can be divided into several categories: primary injury, secondary injury, inflammatory response, and repair/regeneration process. The primary injury generally occurs after an external impact to the head. Contact forces can cause a focal injury, such as a skull fracture, epidural hematoma, subdural hematoma, or coup or contra coup injury (Fig. 7-1). Inertial or accelerative forces to the head can cause these focal injuries, as well as more diffuse injury such as diffuse axonal shear.

Secondary injury develops over hours to days after a brain injury and is associated with the production and release of neurochemicals that alter cerebral blood flow, ion homeostasis, and metabolism. After a concussion or minor traumatic brain injury, disruption of the neuronal cell membrane, stretching of axons, and opening of potassium channels lead to an efflux of potassium out of affected neurons. Depolarization of neurons leads to release of glutamate, which further induces an efflux of potassium. The extracellular potassium leads to a release of excitatory amino acids and further depolarization, both serving to further increase extracellular potassium. Increased adenosine triphosphate (ATP) is required to restore the imbalance in potassium and membrane potential. Glucose utilization increases, leading to a state of hyperglycolysis that in rat studies lasts several hours but in humans may last significantly longer. Lactate levels increase, which can cause neuronal damage and lead to increased vulnerability to cell damage.

After a concussive injury to the brain, there is an influx of calcium into neuronal cells. Elevated intracellular calcium may activate proteases and cause cell damage or death. Oxidative phosphorylation slows, which results in decreased ATP availability and a further increase in glycolysis. Cerebral blood flow has been seen to decrease 50% after concussion. This drop may further impair the neurons' ability to maintain a normal electrolyte balance.

Injured cells also see a decrease in intracellular magnesium, which may not return to normal for four days.

TABLE 7-1 1989–1998 NCAA INJURY SURVEILLANCE SYSTEM CONCUSSION DATA

Sport	Concussion as a Percentage of All Game Injuries
With head protection	
Ice hockey	7.5
Men's lacrosse	5.2
Football	4.5
Softball	3.6
Baseball	2.7
Without head protection	
Field hockey	13.0
Women's soccer	11.0
Men's soccer	9.0
Women's lacrosse	8.5
Women's basketball	8.0
Wrestling	4.3
Men's basketball	3.1

Data from the National Collegiate Athletic Association (NCAA) official web site.

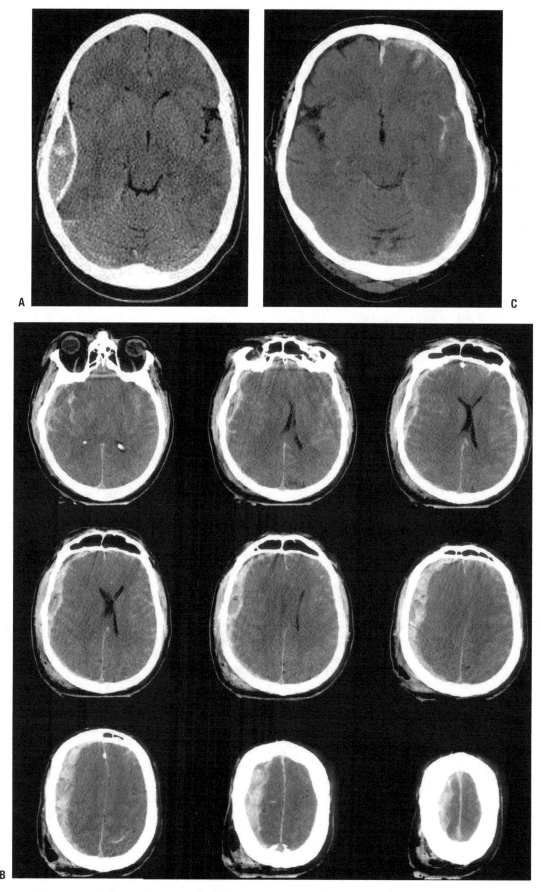

Figure 7-1 **A:** Computed tomography (CT) scan appearance of epidural hematoma. **B:** CT scan appearance of subdural hematoma. **C:** CT scan appearance of subarachnoid hematoma.

TABLE 7-2 EVIDENCE-BASED CLASSIFICATION SCHEMES FOR CONCUSSION

Classification System	Mild: Grade 1	Moderate: Grade 2	Severe: Grade 3
Cantu	No LOC, PTA/PCCS <30 min	LOC <1 min, PTA >30 min but <24 hr, PCCS >30 min but <7 days	LOC >1 min PTA >24 hr PCCS >7 days
American Academy of Neurology	Transient confusion; no LOC; symptoms or abnormalities resolve in <15 min	Transient confusion; no LOC; symptoms or abnormalities last >15 min	Any LOC

LOC, loss of consciousness; PCCS, postconcussion signs and symptoms other than amnesia; PTA, posttraumatic amnesia (anterograde/retrograde).

Decreased magnesium can cause a further influx of calcium. It is also associated with impairment of glycolysis, oxidative phosphorylation, and protein synthesis.

Electrolyte imbalance usually returns to normal four days after the concussion. In the hours to weeks after injury, damage may be seen in both the microtubule and neurofilament structure. Structural changes may occur, such as focal axonal swelling and axonal bulbs. This swelling is also referred to as a "retraction bulb" because the axonal ending appears severed from its distal segment and is characteristic of diffuse axonal injury.

In severe traumatic brain injury, ischemia can lead to a release of oxygen free radicals. Stimulation of cyclooxygenase, monoamine oxidase, and nitric oxide synthase can result in the production of these oxygen free radicals, which can cause cell membrane damage through lipid peroxidation and result in release of arachidonic acid. Production of leukotrienes and thromboxane B_2 from the arachidonic acid cascade has been shown to cause neurodegeneration and result in poor outcomes in experimental models. Animal studies have used ibuprofen and indomethacin, inhibitors of cyclooxygenase, to limit the arachidonic acid cascade. These compounds have been shown to improve cerebral metabolism and reduce neurologic dysfunction in mice after brain injury.

Classification

The most common head injury sustained in sports is a concussion, also referred to as minor traumatic brain injury. Several attempts have been made to classify concussions based on their severity, with guidelines for return to play. The most commonly used classifications have three grades, with a type 1 described as mild, type 2 as moderate, and type 3 as severe. The classification schemes vary somewhat, but are all based on clinical presentation of the athlete and duration of symptoms. Table 7-2 provides a comparison of two commonly used classifications.

DIAGNOSIS

History and Physical Examination

Clinical Features

- The athlete who has sustained a severe head injury is usually easy to identify. Typically, there has been a significant impact or acceleration/deceleration to the head, and the athlete may be rendered unconscious.

- The challenge lies in identifying the athletes who have sustained less severe head injuries, such as a grade 1 concussion.
  - The impact to the head may not seem out of the ordinary or may not have been seen at all by the team physician or trainer.
  - Athletes often minimize symptoms in an effort to remain in play but may use terms such as "having my bell rung" or feeling "in a fog" (Box 7-1).
  - Classic acute symptoms include headache, dizziness, nausea, and difficulty concentrating.
  - Athletes may seem to have a vacant stare or ask repetitive questions and express emotional lability.
  - It is not unusual for the athlete to develop a sense of euphoria after such an injury.

BOX 7-1 POSTCONCUSSION SIGNS AND SYMPTOMS

"Bell rung"
Depression
Dinged
Dizziness
Excess sleep
Fatigue
Feeling "in a fog"
Feeling "slowed down"
Headache
Inappropriate emotions or personality changes
Loss of consciousness
Loss of orientation
Memory problems
Nausea
Nervousness
Numbness/tingling
Poor balance/coordination
Poor concentration, easily distracted
Ringing in the ears
Sadness
Seeing stars
Sensitivity to light
Sensitivity to noise
Sleep disturbance
Vacant stare/glassy eyed
Vomiting

On-field Evaluation

- The initial approach to an unconscious athlete is similar to that for any traumatized patient, and the "ABCs" (Airway, Breathing, and Circulation) should be followed.
- It is important to assume the athlete also sustained a neck injury until proven otherwise, and spine precautions should be followed.
- The facemask on football helmets can be removed, but usually the rest of the helmet is left on and used to help stabilize the neck.
- For less-severe injuries, a detailed sideline examination can be performed.
  - A neurologic examination should include an assessment of level of consciousness, speech, balance, memory (antegrade and retrograde and to event), and orientation to person, place, and time.
- Athletes should not return to play until symptoms have resolved both at rest and with exertion, such as running a sideline sprint.
  - One recent study found that some high school athletes, whose symptoms were thought to have cleared quickly postconcussion, scored below their baseline on neuropsychologic testing at 48 hours, suggesting that perhaps no athlete with a documented concussion should return to play the same day.
- The use of neuropsychologic testing has received increasing attention.
  - Given the wide variation among individuals on these tests, it is necessary to have a preseason baseline evaluation for comparison after a traumatic brain injury.
  - A decline in neuropsychologic test results has been shown to correlate with severity of postconcussive symptoms at 1-week postinjury.

Diagnostic Workup Algorithm

- Athletes who have sustained a prolonged loss of consciousness, or exhibit neurologic deficits, should be triaged to a medical center for further evaluation.
- Abbreviated neurologic examinations, such as the Glasgow Coma Scale, are useful in predicting outcome after a severe head injury (Table 7-3).
- On arrival at a medical center, a full neurologic examination should be performed, including assessment of mental status, speech, memory, motor and sensory function, cranial nerve function, and reflexes (normal and abnormal).
- A computerized tomography scan is helpful in the evaluation of potential intracranial hemorrhage and skull fracture.
- Magnetic resonance imaging will identify more diffuse injury, such as diffuse axonal shear.

TREATMENT

Return-to-play Decision

- Because the subject may not lend him/herself to prospective, randomized studies, the guidelines for return to play after a traumatic brain injury are based largely on retrospective analysis and judgment.

TABLE 7-3 GLASGOW COMA SCALE

Sign	Evaluation	Score[a]
Eye opening (E)	Spontaneous	4
	To speech	3
	To pain	2
	None	1
Best motor response (M)	Obeys	6
	Localizes	5
	Withdraws	4
	Decorticate	3
	Decerebrate	2
	None	1
Verbal response (V)	Oriented	5
	Confused conversation	4
	Inappropriate words	3
	Incomprehensible sounds	2
	None	1

[a] Total EMV score by adding best response in each category. Range from 3 to 15.

- A primary goal is to avoid secondary injury, such as a more severe concussion, or worse yet a second impact syndrome. It is for this reason that athletes who remain symptomatic after even a grade 1 concussion should not return to play.
- Another goal is prevent the long-term effects of multiple minor traumatic brain injuries that can lead to permanent changes, such as the classic description of "dementia pugilistica" seen in boxers. It is with these aims in mind that the guidelines in Table 7-4 were developed.
- Factors other than the concussion severity must be weighed in the return-to-play decision.
  - The athlete's concussion history: the total number, time between injuries, and severity of the blow causing the concussion are all important factors.
  - When making the return-to-play decision, one should consider all pieces of the concussion puzzle and, when in doubt, err on the side of caution: "If in doubt, sit them out."
- A relatively recent finding is that athletes who possess the apolipoprotein E4 allele may be at increased risk after minor traumatic brain injuries.
  - This allele is already well known to correlate with the incidence of Alzheimer's disease. There is increasing evidence that patients who have the apolipoprotein E4 allele have a worse outcome after head injury and may be predisposed to earlier-onset of dementia after repetitive concussions.
  - Knowing an athlete has this allele may factor into the retirement decision after head injury.

Medical Treatment

- The first step in medical treatment is making an accurate diagnosis.
  - What at first may appear to be a relatively minor head injury may actually be a developing subdural

TABLE 7-4 GUIDELINES FOR RETURN TO PLAY AFTER CONCUSSION

Concussion	Grade 1	Grade 2	Grade 3
First	Athlete may return to play that day in select situations if clinical examination results are normal at rest and with exertion, otherwise return to play in 1 week	Athlete may return to play in 2 weeks if asymptomatic at rest and with exertion for 7 days	Athlete may return to play in 1 month if asymptomatic at rest and exertion for 7 days
Second	Return to play in 2 weeks if asymptomatic for 1 week	Minimum of 1 month; may return to play then if asymptomatic for 1 week; consider terminating season	Terminate season; may return to play next season if asymptomatic
Third	Terminate season; may return to play next season if asymptomatic	Terminate season; may return to play next season if asymptomatic	

or epidural hematoma. If an athlete is suspected to have sustained such an injury, he should be triaged to the closest medical center that provides neurosurgical services.

- Intracranial hematomas may require prompt craniotomy and removal, but their treatment is beyond the scope of this chapter.

- On the field, treatment of athletic head injuries begins with preparation, including having appropriate personnel and equipment available.

- For the unconscious athlete, full spine precautions should be followed, including use of a spine board and cervical collar.
- Maintaining an adequate airway is of primary concern.
- The facemask should be removed and, if there is respiratory compromise, on-the-field intubation may be required.
- Continuous blood pressure monitoring is performed, and cardiopulmonary resuscitative equipment should be available if needed.
- The shoulder pads should be loosened in the front to allow for chest compressions and defibrillation.
- For patients in whom a spine injury is suspected, the Inter-Association Task Force for Appropriate Care of the Spine-Injured Athlete has outlined four instances in which the athletic helmet and chin strap should be removed (Box 7-2).

- The awake athlete for whom cervical spine injury has been ruled out can be helped to a sitting position.
- If stable in the sitting position, the athlete may be helped off the field for more detailed examination.

- The primary focus is preventing a second impact that could have more severe consequences. For this reason, the athlete should not return to competition until asymptomatic, both at rest and with exertion.

Surgical Treatment

Indications and Contraindications

Surgical treatment is typically performed for large or expanding intracranial hematomas. Although subdural is the most common intracranial hematoma resulting in death after athletic head injury, the epidural hematoma can be a rapidly fatal lesion without immediate surgical treatment. Epidural hematoma classically results from injury to the middle meningeal artery (Fig. 7-2), whereas a subdural hematoma occurs after disruption of the venous connections between the dura and the brain. The patient with an epidural hematoma may sustain an initial loss of consciousness, followed by an awake and more lucent period, and then quickly develop loss of mental status and lapse into coma.

Results and Outcome

Guidelines for return to play after concussion are developed in part to protect the injured brain from further insult, as

BOX 7-2 INSTANCES IN WHICH AN ATHLETIC HELMET SHOULD BE REMOVED IN HEAD-INJURED PATIENTS

- If the helmet and chin strap do not hold the head securely, such that immobilization of the helmet fails to immobilize the head
- If the design of the helmet prevents adequate airway management even after removal of the facemask
- If the facemask cannot be removed in a reasonable amount of time
- If the helmet prevents immobilization for transportation in an appropriate position

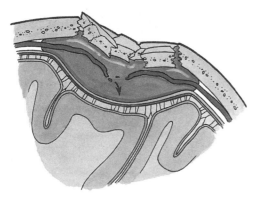

Figure 7-2 Extradural or epidural hemorrhage between the endosteal layer of the dura and the calvaria may follow a blow to the head. Typically, a brief concussion results, followed by a lucid interval of some hours. This is followed by drowsiness and coma. Most bleeding from the torn meningeal arteries results in an extradural or epidural hematoma—a slow, localized accumulation of blood. As the blood mass increases, compression of the brain occurs, necessitating evacuation of the blood and occlusion of the bleeding vessels. (From Moore KL, Agur A. Essential Clinical Anatomy, 2nd ed. Philadelphia: Lippincott Williams & Wilkins, 2002.)

well as to try to minimize the cumulative effects that multiple concussions can cause. Boxing is perhaps most recognized for this, with fighters having been described as permanently "punch drunk" or suffering from "dementia pugilistica." The cumulative effects of minor traumatic head injuries are becoming better understood in many other sports as well. Athletes who have sustained prior concussions appear more prone to future head injury, often with less force required to cause impairment. In one prospective study of high school football players, those players who had sustained three prior concussions were 9.3 times more likely to demonstrate on-field signs (such as loss of consciousness, anterograde amnesia, and confusion) with a concussion, compared with players sustaining their first concussion.

Age may play a role in the outcome of a concussion, even between high school and college age athletes. In one prospective study, high school athletes with concussion showed prolonged memory dysfunction, compared with college athletes with concussion. By three days postconcussion, the college athletes scored similar to aged-matched controls on neuropsychological testing. At seven days postconcussion, the high school athletes still scored below age-matched controls. The exact cause for this age difference is not fully understood. Children have shown a more diffuse and prolonged cerebral swelling after traumatic brain injury, compared with adults. It is hypothesized that the immature brain is more sensitive to excitotoxic brain injury and may show prolonged metabolic dysautoregulation.

The grading of concussions serves as a guideline for return to play but is clearly open to individual variation and clinical judgment. Duration of posttraumatic amnesia is one factor in the Cantu scale of concussions. In one study, the athletes who self-reported memory problems at 24 hours postconcussion were an indicator of the severity of the con-

cussion. Athletes who reported memory problems on follow-up examination in general had longer duration of symptoms, scored worse on neurocognitive tests, and had more overall symptoms. All postconcussion signs and symptoms are important, as is their duration. Thus, grading of a concussion should ideally await resolution of symptoms.

The ultimate goal when discussing athletic head injuries is prevention. The increased attention on head injuries in sports has made athletes, trainers, physicians, and fans more aware of the potential dangers of brain injury in sports. Football was one of the first sports to focus on prevention of head and neck injury, as evidenced by the rule change in 1976 prohibiting initial contact with the head ("spear tackling"). The number of fatalities as a result of head injuries in football has declined from a high of 162 during the 10-year span from 1965 through 1974 to a low of 32 during the 10 years from 1985 through 1994.

Other sports are attempting to decrease head injuries by means of rule changes, improved protective equipment, and better data collection to analyze outcomes. The NHL began data collection on head injury when it instituted its concussion program in 1997. Improved equipment, such as the Bull Tough helmet (Bull Tough, San Antonio, TX), seems to help decrease the incidence of head injury in professional and amateur bull riders (Fig. 7-3). Equally important is the increasing realization by athletes that returning to competition while symptomatic from a concussion could lead to significant worsening of their symptoms and even second impact syndrome.

In conclusion, head injury is prevalent in many sports, with football resulting in the highest overall number per year in the United States. What may seem to be a minor injury, such as a grade 1 concussion, can cause metabolic and potentially structural changes in the brain, thus making it more susceptible to further insult. Appropriate identification and on-the-field management of head-injured athletes can limit further injury. There appears to be age- and gender-related differences in the rate and severity of head injury in athletics. Through increased data collection and analysis,

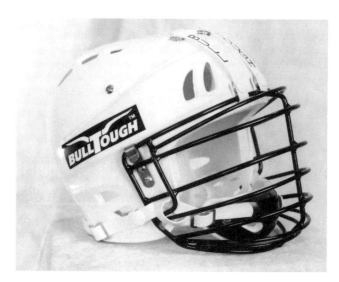

Figure 7-3 Bull Tough headgear. (Courtesy of www.bulltough.com.)

rule changes, education, and equipment development, hopefully, the incidence of head injury in athletics will decline.

SUGGESTED READING

Brandenburg MA, Archer P. Survey analysis to assess the effectiveness of the Bull Tough helmet in preventing head injuries in bull riders: a pilot study. Clin J Sports Med 2002;12:360–366.

Cantu RC. Guidelines for return to contact sports after a cerebral concussion. Phys Sports Med 1986;14:76–79.

Cantu RC. Recurrent athletic head injury: risks and when to retire. Clin Sports Med 2003;22:593–603.

Cantu RC, Mueller FO. Brain injury-related fatalities in American football, 1945–1999. Neurosurgery 2003;52:846–853.

Collins MW, Lovell MR, Iverson GL, et al. Cumulative effects of concussion in high school athletes. Neurosurgery 2003;51:1175–1179.

Cooper MT, McGee KM, Anderson DG. Epidemiology of athletic head and neck injuries. Clin Sports Med 2003;22:427–443.

Echemendia RJ, Cantu RC. Return to play following sports-related mild traumatic brain injury: the role of neuropsychology. Appl Neuropsychol 2003;10:48–55.

Erlanger D, Kaushik T, Cantu RC, et al. Symptom-based assessment of the severity of a concussion. J Neurosurg 2003;98:477–484.

Field M, Collins MW, Lovell MR, et al. Does age play a role in recovery from sports-related concussion? A comparison of high school and collegiate athletes. J Pediatr 2003;142:546–553.

Ghiselli G, Schaadt G, McAllister DR. On-the-field evaluation of an athlete with a head or neck injury. Clin Sports Med 2003;22:445–465.

Grindel SH. Epidemiology and pathophysiology of minor traumatic brain injury. Curr Sports Med Rep 2003;2:18–23.

Lovell MR, Collins MW, Iverson GL, et al. Grade 1 or "ding" concussions in high school athletes. Am J Sports Med 2003;32:1–8.

McKeever CK, Schatz P. Current issues in the identification, assessment, and management of concussions in sports-related injuries. Appl Neuropsychol 2003;10:4–11.

Okonkwo DO, Stone JR. Basic science of closed head injuries and spinal cord injuries. Clin Sports Med 2003;22:467–481.

Schneider RC. Head and neck injuries in football: mechanisms, treatment, and prevention. Baltimore: Williams & Wilkins, 1973.

Webbe FM, Barth JT. Short-term and long-term outcome of athletic closed head injuries. Clin Sports Med 2003;22:577–592.

Wennberg RA, Tator CH. National Hockey League reported concussions, 1986–87 to 2001–2. Can J Neurol Sci 2003;30:206–209.

SPINAL INJURIES

CHRISTOPHER M. BONO
MARC A. AGULNICK
MARK G. GROSSMAN

The spine is commonly involved in sports injuries. Although not the usual focus of a sports medicine practitioner, its importance should not be overlooked. Spinal conditions can have substantial effects on an athlete's performance, as well as important implications of the propensity for neurological injuries. It is the goal of this chapter to review the essentials of spinal examination, specific injuries of the cervical and lumbar spine, and the current recommendations for return to sport after athletic head injuries.

SPINAL EXAMINATION

On-field Examination

- Among the most crucial tasks of the on-field physician is to decide when a potential spine injury is benign or requires immediate stabilization and further workup.
- The following features are indications for immediate stabilization and immobilization and transfer to an emergency department for evaluation:
  - The athlete is down on the field.
  - No voluntary or spontaneous movement is noted.
  - Loss of consciousness has occurred.
  - There are objective neurological or cognitive deficits.
  - A palpable step-off is appreciated.
  - Localized tenderness and pain with a high index of suspicion.

- In such cases, imaging studies—such as x-rays, computerized tomography (CT), or magnetic resonance imaging (MRI)—are indicated.
- The athlete needs to be immobilized carefully and securely for transfer.
- The on-field examination of an injured athlete starts with evaluation of the "ABCs" (Airway, Breathing, Circulation).
  - The Glasgow Coma Scale is a useful method of assessing quickly the neurocognitive status (see Table 7-3 in Chapter 7).
  - The pupils should be examined for reactivity and the gaze noted for signs of ocular deviation.
- A detailed neurological examination should be performed.
  - The athlete should not be moved from a supine position.
  - Motor strength of individual muscles or motions can be tested and graded (in the fully contracted or shortened position) in the upper and lower extremities to assess function of individual nerve root levels (Table 8-1 and Table 8-2).
- Sensation to light touch should be graded as normal, diminished, or absent in each dermatome.
- Importantly, rectal tone should be assessed, particularly in the unconscious patient, as it may be the only possible site of motor strength assessment. In the awake patient, perianal sensation is a reflection of the most distal sacral nerve root function (S2-5).

TABLE 8-1 GRADING OF MUSCLE STRENGTH[a]

Grade	Description
5	Full strength
4	Can overcome gravity with some but not full resistance
3	Can overcome gravity without resistance
2	Can move extremity with gravity eliminated
1	Visible muscle contraction without limb movement
0	No muscle contraction

[a] Test in the fully contracted (or shortened) position.

- Deep tendon reflexes should also be tested. These include the biceps (C5), brachioradialis (C6), triceps (C7), patella tendon (L4), and Achilles tendon (S1) reflexes.
  - The bulbocavernosus reflex (assessed by squeezing the glans of the penis or clitoris or gently tugging a Foley catheter) results in involuntary contraction of the anal sphincter.
  - Hyperreflexia (3+) is an indication of upper motor neuron dysfunction, such as spinal cord compression.
  - Hyporeflexia (0 or 1+) is an indication of lower motor neuron dysfunction (such as compression of the cauda equina or peripheral nerves).
  - Clonus is elicited by jerking the ankle into dorsiflexion. More than four beats are considered pathologic.
  - An upgoing Babinski response is also an indication of upper motor neuron disease.
- The spinous processes and paraspinal muscles should be palpated.
  - This can be performed by carefully logrolling the patient from side to side, although a supine examination can often suffice.
  - Importantly, a helmet should be *left in place*. Removing a helmet can cause harmful motion of an injured cervical spine.
    - The facemask and chin strap can, and should,

TABLE 8-2 MUSCLE NERVE ROOT LEVELS

Muscle/Test	Nerve Root Level
Deltoid	C5
Biceps/wrist extension	C6
Triceps/wrist flexion	C7
Finger flexors	C8
Finger abduction	T1
Hip flexion	L1–L2
Knee extension	L2–L3
Ankle dorsiflexion	L4
Toe dorsiflexion	L5
Ankle plantarflexion	S1

be removed to allow assessment of the airway and eyes.
- If a spinal injury is suspected, the athlete is then immobilized.
  - A transfer board is usually used.
  - The athlete is logrolled from side to side to place him/her on the board.
  - Taping or strapping the head and body to the board is the most effective method of immobilizing the spine. A cervical collar can also be used.
  - Once again, the helmet should stay in place.

Ambulatory (Office) Examination

- Although many components are the same, the in-office spinal assessment includes more detailed history and neurological and palpatory examinations.
- A history of movements (e.g., extension versus flexion) that aggravate pain should be sought.
- Tenderness of the spinous processes, facet joints, sacroiliac joints, ribs, and paraspinal muscles can be differentiated.
- Though it should never be performed in the acute traumatic setting, neck and back range of motion should be quantified.
- In addition to the motor, sensory, and reflex examination, the ambulatory neurologic examination should include assessment for pathologic reflexes, such as Hoffmann's and inverted radial reflexes and root tension signs such as the straight-leg raise and femoral stretch test.
- Imaging studies are indicated for patients with:
  - Worsening symptoms
  - A progressive neurological deficit
  - Symptoms that continue beyond 4 to 6 weeks
- Following a general imaging protocol may be helpful.

LUMBAR SPINE INJURIES

- Low back pain usually affects athletes at some point in their career. It can be from an "overuse syndrome" or acute trauma. Complaints may range from mild pain to severe pain after a game or practice.
- Some injuries are characteristic of certain sports: lumbar herniated disks in weight lifters, sacral stress fractures in runners, and spondylolysis in football players and gymnasts.
- Predominantly, axial low back pain suggests internal disc disruption from degenerative disc disease.
- Predominantly, leg symptoms suggest radiculopathy from a herniated disc.
- Infections, tumors, or inflammatory arthritis are more typically suggested by nonmechanical back pain. Other red flags are night pain, pain at rest, fever, or weight loss.
- The differential diagnosis of lumbar spine injuries in athletes can be divided into two categories: serious acute injuries and benign and chronic injuries (Box 8-1).

BOX 8-1 DIFFERENTIAL DIAGNOSIS OF LUMBAR SPINE INJURIES IN ATHLETES

Serious Acute Injuries
■ Acute fracture or dislocation
■ Large herniated disc/cauda equina syndrome
■ Epidural hematoma
■ Spinal cord injury

Benign and Chronic Injuries
■ Lumbar strain/sprain
■ Degenerative disc disease
■ Spondylolysis/spondylolisthesis
■ Facet syndrome

Fractures

■ Lumbar fractures are not uncommon with sports injuries.
■ The most benign of these are compression fractures, noted by mild anterior wedging of the anterior vertebral body. By definition, they do not involve the posterior vertebral body and are stable fractures.
■ Importantly, flexion-distraction (seatbelt type) injury should be ruled out, because this is inherently unstable and most often surgically stabilized.
■ *Simple compression fractures* are typically treated non-operatively with a brace for 6 to 12 weeks. An athlete can return to play after negative flexion-extension films, resolution of pain, and full restoration of range of motion.
■ *Burst fractures* are higher-energy injuries that can present with or without a neurological deficit and may be stable or unstable.
   ■ The fracture involves the posterior vertebral body and typically has canal compromise from retropulsed bone fragments.
   ■ Nonoperative treatment can include a custom-molded thoracolumbar orthosis or extension cast for 12 weeks. Our criteria for nonoperative treatment include:
      ■ No neurological deficit.
      ■ Intact posterior ligaments (suggested by <25 degrees kyphosis, no interspinous process widening, no facet joint gapping, and confirmed by MRI inspection of the ligaments).
   ■ Patients with evidence of posterior ligament injury but no neurological deficit can usually be treated by posterior fixation alone (e.g., pedicle screw stabilization).
      ■ We prefer to perform an anterior decompression and reconstruction for those patients with a neural deficit associated with retropulsed bone. Supplemental posterior stabilization may also be considered.
   ■ Returning to play after treatment for a burst fracture is controversial. There are little to no data of any established criteria.
      ■ In our practice, return to play criteria after non-

operative treatment is similar to those described for compression fractures.
   ■ After surgical treatment of a burst fracture, most physicians would probably not recommend return to contact sports.

Disc Herniations and Cauda Equina Syndrome

■ Cauda equina syndrome (CES) is most commonly associated with a large lumbar disc herniation.
■ The clinical signs and symptoms of CES are:
   ■ Saddle anesthesia (inner thighs and perineum)
   ■ Bowel/bladder incontinence
   ■ Variable lower extremity sensory and/or motor deficit
■ The treatment of CES is surgical discectomy and is best performed within 48 hours from the onset of symptoms.

Sprains and Strains

■ The most common cause for low back pain in athletes is a lumbar strain (muscular) or sprain (ligamentous).
■ They are caused by a subcatastrophic stretch of the muscle or ligament fibers and usually result in self-limited pain. In some cases, pain can become chronic.
■ A strain is associated with paraspinal muscle tenderness and sometimes a "trigger point" spasm, whereas a sprain demonstrates tenderness localized to the interspinous process region.
■ Treatment of both sprains and strains includes a short (1 to 2 days) period of rest, ice, and then a stretching program directed by a trainer or physical therapist.
■ Return to play after a strain or sprain is allowed once the pain has subsided and range of motion and endurance have been restored.

Degenerative Disc Disease

■ The link between degenerative disc disease (DDD) and low back pain is still unclear, although it is commonly believed that inflammatory factors within the nucleus leak out through annular tears (Fig. 8-1) to stimulate nociceptive nerve endings within the annulus and dorsal root ganglion. This is because radiographic studies have detected high rates of DDD and other degenerative abnormalities in asymptomatic patients.
■ Compared with nonathletes, competitive athletes have a higher rate of degenerative changes in their lumbar spines.
   ■ Gymnasts, weight lifters, and football players are among the most at-risk athletes.
   ■ While competing, athletes appear to have a higher rate of low back pain than nonathletes; however, once retired, past participation in sports does not seem to be a substantial risk factor.
■ DDD is irreversible. Treatment is directed toward decreasing the intensity and frequency of symptoms, thus improving lumbar mechanics and muscle physiology.
   ■ In most cases, a carefully planned and executed physical therapy program is effective.

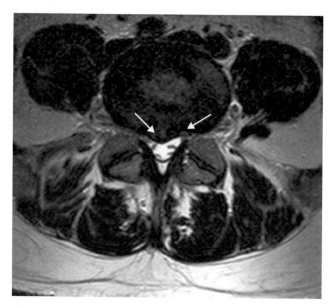

Figure 8-1 Axial T_2-weighted MRI image of an athlete with severe low back pain and no radicular symptoms. Note the annular fissuring *(white arrows)*, which are thought to allow inflammatory factors from the degenerated nucleus pulposus to "leak out" and stimulate nociceptive nerve endings in the posterior annulus.

- After treatment, the authors' return-to-play criteria are:
  - Full painless range of motion
  - Ability to maintain a neutral posture during sports-specific exercises
  - Full muscle strength, endurance, and control
- In the rare cases that nonoperative treatment fails, an interbody fusion with or without stabilization can be performed.
  - Return to play after lumbar fusion is controversial because clear criteria have not been established. We have a minimum requirement of solid radiographic fusion, in addition to those criteria outlined previously for nonoperative treatment.

Spondylolysis

- Stress fractures are common in athletes. The most common region of the spine to be affected is the pars interarticularis of the L5 (and less commonly L4) vertebra.
- This is termed *spondylolysis* and can be a frank, non-healed fracture or a stress "reaction" that can only be noted on an MRI or bone scan.
- Importantly, an adolescent athlete with substantial back pain longer than 3 weeks should be evaluated with plain lumbar radiographs and a bone scan, or a single-photon emission computed tomography scan.
  - A retrospective study comparing 100 adolescent athletes and 100 adults with acute low back pain showed that 47% of the adolescent athletes had spondylolysis, compared with only 5% in the adult subjects.
  - The presence and grade of spondylolysis/spondylolisthesis can influence the decision to allow return to play.

- The prevalence of spondylolysis varies from sport to sport and is highest in sports that require frequent or sustained lumbar hyperextension maneuvers, such as diving (43%), wrestling (30%), weight lifting (23%), throwing sports (27%), and gymnastics (17%).
- Symptoms are localized to the low back, although referred pain to the buttocks or upper thighs is not uncommon.
  - Pain is exacerbated by hyperextension and relieved by flexing or squatting down.
  - A single-leg hyperextension test can be useful in determining whether one or both sides have symptoms.
  - Eighty-five percent of defects are detectable on a lateral lumbar film.
  - CT is the most sensitive modality for detecting an established defect. Single-photon emission computed tomography scan is the most sensitive method of detecting an occult stress reaction.
- Nonsurgical treatment of spondylolysis includes rest, brace immobilization, and pain control.
- Medications include nonsteroidal anti-inflammatory drugs.
- An antilordotic (Boston) brace (worn for up to 6 months) leads to resolution of symptoms in about 80% of cases.
- Unilateral defects heal better than bilateral defects, though healing is not necessary for return to play.
- Athletes can return to sports after nonoperative treatment of a pars defect if:
  - There is no pain with extension on examination.
  - The athlete remains pain-free after the brace is removed.
  - Functional restoration of endurance and range of motion has been achieved.
- In recalcitrant cases, surgery might be considered. Although a single-level fusion remains the current gold standard, a pars defect repair may be considered in some cases (Fig. 8-2).

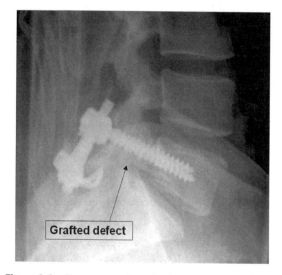

Grafted defect

Figure 8-2 Postoperative lateral radiograph of an athlete who underwent a pars repair instead of a lumbar fusion for recalcitrant pain from a spondylolytic defect of the L5 vertebra.

CERVICAL SPINE INJURIES

Fractures and Spinal Cord Injuries

- Cervical spine injuries continue to make up a large percentage of spinal injuries in sports.
- Injuries range from cervical sprains to catastrophic complete spinal cord injuries (SCIs).
- An estimated 10% to 15% of football players experience an injury to the cervical spine.
  - The overall incidence of SCI in the high school and college populations is around 1 in 100,000. Most are incomplete with preservation of varying degrees of neurologic function.
  - In an analysis of football players from 1977 to 1989, catastrophic SCIs were secondary to fracture dislocations or anterior compression (burst) fractures in 33% and 22% of cases, respectively.
- Preexisting spinal stenosis predisposes to SCI; in such cases, athletes can sustain cord injury without bony or ligamentous disruption.
- The mechanism of injury is often direct axial load.
  - Particularly in football players, the cervical spine is flexed (which straightens it from its usual lordotic posture) on impact. This decreases its ability to dissipate the load. With increasing loads, the spine fails in flexion, thus resulting in vertebral body comminution (subluxation) of facet joint dislocation.
  - Experimentally, Maiman et al. found the average axial load to failure to be less with a straightened versus normolordotic posture. The greatest force applied to the spine was found when the load was applied to the vertex of the skull. This decreased as the load was moved forward on the skull.
  - Torg et al. described the "spear tackler's spine." It occurs in athletes who use improper tackling technique, using the top of their football helmet to hit an opposing player head-on.
    - This is associated with an increased risk for permanent neurologic damage.
    - Affected athletes demonstrate narrowing of the cervical spinal canal, persistent straightening or reversal of the normal lordotic curve, and concomitant preexisting posttraumatic roentgenographic abnormalities of the cervical spine.
    - Although axial loads combined with flexion cause the majority of fracture dislocations of the cervical spine, other mechanisms can cause injuries as well.
  - Rotation, extension, and shear forces alone or in combination have been implicated in various fracture patterns observed in the cervical spine.
  - Although the multiple fractures experienced by athletes participating in contact sports such as football are beyond the scope of this chapter, they have led to the National Collegiate Athletic Association (NCAA) Football Rule Committee outlawing the use of one's helmet to tackle an opponent.
- Contact sports such as football, rugby, and wrestling place patients at high risk for injury.
  - Most cervical spine injuries in football players result

from hyperflexion, but other mechanisms—including hyperextension, rotation, and lateral bending—have been reported.
  - Wrestlers commonly exhibit neck hyperflexion but also may endure rotational and horizontal shearing forces that place great stresses on the intervertebral disks, facet joints, and spinal ligaments.
- SCI has also been documented in noncontact sports, such as diving, surfing, and gymnastics.
  - These events usually result from the individual striking his/her head at the bottom of the pool or body of water, thus causing neck hyperflexion.
  - Gymnasts may sustain injuries after "missed" maneuvers that result in an uncontrolled fall.
- A player may be permitted to return to play after treatment of a cervical fracture in the following situations:
  - The fracture is fully healed, and there is normal alignment.
  - A single-level fusion has been performed below the level of C2.
  - There is no residual canal compromise.
  - There is no pain or neural deficit.
  - There is no instability or olisthesis on flexion-extension films.
- A player may *not* be permitted to return to play in the following cases:
  - The fracture is healed in a kyphotic posture.
  - A multilevel (2 or more) fusion has been performed.
  - C1–C2 fusion has been performed.
  - Rotatory instability is present.
  - There is residual canal compromise.
  - A residual neural deficit exists.
  - Pain persists.
  - There is evidence of instability on flexion-extension films.

Sports-specific Conditions

Transient Quadriplegia

- *Neurapraxia* of the cervical cord, otherwise known as transient quadriplegia, is fairly common in contact sports participants.
- It is characterized by bilateral burning pain, tingling, and loss of sensation in the upper and/or lower extremities.
  - Burning dysesthesias and paresthesias usually occur in a glove-like distribution.
  - Motor deficits can vary from mild weakness to total paralysis, depending on the extent of insult to the spinal cord.
- By definition, symptoms are transient, and complete recovery usually occurs within 10 to 15 minutes but may take up to 48 hours.
- Axial load with hyperextension or flexion of the cervical spine is often the inciting event. A pincer mechanism that theoretically causes a brief compression of the cord is thought to play a role in the transient nature of the symptoms.
- Standard radiographic evaluation of the cervical spine is usually negative for fractures or dislocations but incidental findings—such as congenital stenosis, spon-

dylosis, Klippel-Feil syndrome, or evidence of intervertebral disk disease—may be present.

- Preexisting cervical stenosis may be a predisposing factor.

■ Reversible MRI spinal cord signal abnormalities have been documented.

■ The decision to allow an athlete to return to play after an episode of transient quadriplegia is controversial.

- Torg et al. have held that an athlete may play after one or two episodes, provided there is full neurologic recovery.
- Others are more reluctant, recommending no play after just one episode, particularly if there is any underlying spinal canal stenosis.
- From this, the term *functional stenosis* has arisen, which denotes loss of the cerebrospinal fluid space anterior and posterior to the spinal cord on a midsagittal MRI (Fig. 8-3), has been used as a contraindication to return to play.

Stingers and Burners

■ Burner syndrome is one of the most common injuries in contact sports. The "burner" or "stinger" was named after the pain, tingling, and burning experienced in the upper extremity of the athlete after contact.

■ These injuries usually occur after the athlete strikes his head against another player, a wall, or a mat.

- The athlete experiences sudden pain, burning, and sometimes tingling that begins in the neck, radiates into the shoulder, and continues down the arm and into the hand.

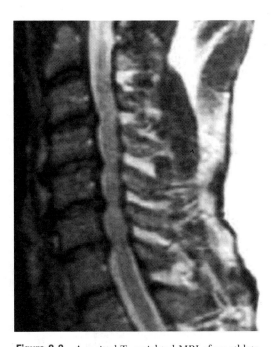

Figure 8-3 A sagittal T$_2$-weighted MRI of an athlete with functional stenosis, noted by complete effacement (or loss) of cerebrospinal fluid anterior and posterior to the spinal cord. This is thought to increase the risk for SCI with athletic trauma to the neck.

- Symptoms do not follow a dermatomal pattern. Weakness of the supraspinatus, infraspinatus, deltoid, and biceps muscle are often noted, which usually presents hours to days after the injury.

■ Burners are a type of brachial plexus injury, usually resulting from traction to the brachial plexus or compression of the cervical root at the intervertebral foramen. Direct impact to the plexus within the supraclavicular region has also been reported.

- Traction injuries can occur with tackling. This causes sudden lateral deviation of the head away from the affected side and simultaneous depression of the ipsilateral shoulder.
  - These injuries are more frequent in high school athletes, possibly because of less developed supportive neck musculature.
- Cervical root compression occurs at the level of the intervertebral foramen. The foramen is dynamically narrowed during activities that cause cervical spinal extension, compression, and rotation toward the symptomatic side.
  - These injuries are more commonly seen in collegiate or professional athletes and present with more neck pain and diminished range of motion than the patients with traction injuries.
- Direct trauma to the supraclavicular region at Erb's point can produce Burner syndrome with upper trunk deficits predominating.
- Spurling's test (lateral flexion and rotation of the head toward the symptomatic side) is used to evaluate compression-type injuries, whereas the brachial plexus stretch test (lateral flexion away from the symptomatic side) can be used to evaluate traction-type injuries.

■ Central cervical canal and foraminal stenosis are reported as risk factors for recurrent burners. Logically, this association has been described for compression and extension-type injuries but not traction mechanisms.

- Athletes with a history of recurrent burners, associated DDD, or congenital stenosis should abstain from participation in contact sports.

■ The physician must determine whether symptoms are from cervical cord or root pathology. This important distinction is often made on the playing field.

- By definition, burners present with unilateral arm symptoms.
- Athletes who present with bilateral upper or any lower extremity symptoms are more likely to have had a more serious SCI.
- Focal neck tenderness or severe pain with motion should raise suspicion of a fracture or ligamentous injury to the cervical spine.
  - In these cases, the spine should be immobilized using a collar and backboard, and the patient transported to a hospital for immediate imaging.
  - Burners are self-limited syndromes that usually do not cause permanent sequelae. Even with this favorable natural history, certain restrictions should be placed on athletes after sustaining these injuries to prevent more severe problems in the future.
- Patients who are experiencing significant muscle

weakness should rest the involved extremity until symptoms improve. At that time, physical therapy can begin and advanced as tolerated.

- Athletes should also be started on year-round trapezial strengthening programs. Theoretically, strengthening the neck musculature may increase the shock-absorbing capacity of the cervical spine.
- Athletes must fulfill particular criteria before they can return to play:
  - Complete resolution of paresthesias
  - Full range of motion of the neck
  - No pain
  - Negative Lhermitte's test (axial compression of head results in electric-like sensation down to the lower back)
  - Normal strength
- Athletes who are prone to burners can use special equipment to help prevent injuries.
  - Commonly used devices are thicker shoulder pads, neck rolls, springs, and the "cowboy collar." They must fit correctly and be used with properly fitting shoulder pads to be effective.
- Educating participants about proper athletic technique is also important. Proper tackling and blocking techniques, with avoidance of spearing, should be taught to young football players as they are first learning the sport.

Sprain and Strain

- Neck pain, or the so-called "jammed neck," is one of the most common complaints among athletes, especially football players.
- Patients can sustain an injury to the musculotendinous unit (sprain) or paraspinal muscle itself (strain). Therefore, one sprains a tendon but strains a muscle.
- Typically, the athlete will present with localized neck pain without radiation to the arms or back.
  - Athletes may have decreased cervical range of motion secondary to pain.
  - Sometimes the pain may be localized to one specific cervical level.
  - There are no neurologic deficits.
- Treatment is based on severity and etiology.
  - Generally, the use of a cervical collar and analgesic medications is continued until pain and spasm subsides.
  - After the collar is removed, range-of-motion exercises can begin.
  - Return to athletic participation is delayed until painless full range of motion is achieved.
  - Instability may necessitate surgical stabilization to prevent future neurologic injury.

Degenerative Conditions

Disc Herniations

- Acute disc herniations in contact sports are rare.
- Head-on collisions or other events leading to axial loading can result in increased intradiscal pressure. If large enough, cord compression can manifest as either transient or permanent quadriplegia or quadriparesis. Patients may present with acute paralysis of all four extremities, as well as loss of pain and temperature sensation.
  - Patients may also present with anterior cord syndrome. However, acute radicular symptoms can occur alone.
- MRI is the study of choice to detect a herniated disc.
- Patients with persistent clinical and radiological evidence of spinal cord compression should be offered surgery, which may include anterior cervical diskectomy and interbody fusion.
- Radiographic evaluation of the cervical spine of football players can reveal asymptomatic cervical spondylosis.
  - In one study, 7% of freshman college football players demonstrated abnormally narrowed disk spaces.
  - Early degenerative changes have been attributed to years of repetitive loading from tackling.
  - Severe degenerative changes—including foraminal stenosis, central canal stenosis resulting from posterior osteophytes, and the loss of normal cervical lordosis—can result in the classic "spear tacklers spine."
- Contraindications to returning to play after a cervical disc herniation are:
  - Presence of pain (axial neck or radicular)
  - Neural deficit
  - Limitation of range of motion
  - *Any* evidence of myelopathy (walking imbalance, hyperreflexia, pathological reflexes) (e.g., Hoffmann's or inverted radial reflex)

Stenosis and Myelopathy

- Narrowing or stenosis of the cervical spinal canal can predispose athletes to SCI.
- Two forms of cervical stenosis have been described in athletes: developmental and acquired.
  - *Developmental stenosis*, otherwise known as congenital stenosis, is present at birth and is characterized by shortened pedicles causing an abnormally narrow canal, sometimes described as funnel-shaped.
  - *Acquired stenosis* is the result of reactive bony thickening and ligamentous hypertrophy that can result from repeated collisions in sports over time. Other pathoanatomic features include disc bulges, spondylolysis, and osteophytes.
- Methods for diagnosing and quantifying cervical stenosis have been suggested.
  - Sagittal canal diameter is measured on a standard lateral cervical spine radiograph. The measurement is recorded as the anteroposterior distance between the posterior aspect of the vertebral body and the nearest point along on the spinolaminar junction.
    - Wolfe et al. established normal parameters for this dimension.
    - The average diameters at C1, C2, and C3–C7 were 22 mm, 20 mm, and 17 mm, respectively. Sagittal canal diameters of more than 15 mm were established as normal, and diameters of less than 13 mm were defined as stenotic.
    - Evaluation of the sagittal canal diameter on a lateral cervical spine radiograph is limited by er-

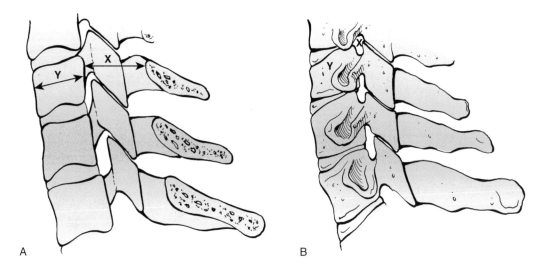

Figure 8-4   The Torg ratio is calculated by dividing the sagittal diameter of the vertebral canal (*X*) by the diameter of the vertebral body (*Y*).

rors related to magnification, roentgenographic technique, and measurement variability.

■ Taking different vertebral sizes into account, Torg et al. derived a ratio of the anteroposterior canal diameter to the anteroposterior vertebral body diameter. A value below 0.8 was defined as spinal stenosis (Fig. 8-4).

　■ Herzog et al. have questioned the reliability of the Torg ratio, finding it to have a high sensitivity but a poor positive predictive value for detecting clinically significant cervical narrowing.

　■ Studies that have evaluated the cervical spines of clinically asymptomatic professional football players showed abnormal Torg ratios in 33% to 49%.

　■ The high incidence of these abnormally low ratios is the result of the large vertebral body size in this population, with absolute dimensions of the spinal canal being adequately capacious for the spinal cord.

　■ MRI evaluation of these players revealed adequate space available for the cord in these athletes and thus no true stenosis.

　■ Currently, evaluation for functional spinal stenosis, with either MRI or CT myelogram, is becoming the new standard.

■ Functional spinal stenosis is defined as obliteration of the cerebrospinal fluid cushion surrounding the cervical spinal cord.

■ This method of evaluation is being used by many team physicians for decision making regarding athletes' return to play, as well as treatment and activity modifications.

Congenital Anomalies and Participation in Sports

■ Congenital anomalies of the cervical spine can predispose an athlete to spinal injuries by changing the me-

chanics and load dissipating properties of the cervical spine.

■ Congenital anomalies can occur by failure of formation or segmentation.

■ Klippel-Feil syndrome is secondary to failure of segmentation that may involve one or more motion segments.

　■ Torg and Glasgow classified Klippel-Feil syndrome into two types:

　　■ *Type I* involves a long congenital fusion (more than two segments).

　　■ *Type II* has one or two fused segments.

　■ As the number of fused segments increases, the ability of the cervical spine to dissipate loads decreases. More force is concentrated on the unfused motion segments, increasing the chance for injury in these regions with contact sports.

■ Failure of formation can present as odontoid agenesis, hypoplasia, or os odontoideum.

　■ These can result in atlantoaxial instability, which places athletes participating in contact sports at great risk for SCI.

■ In some instances, an athlete can have failure of formation of the atlanto-occipital junction.

　■ These individuals are prone to experience compression of the posterior columns of the spinal cord at the posterior margin of the foramen magnum and should be restricted from contact sports.

■ Spina bifida occulta is another congenital anomaly. It is usually an incidental finding and is asymptomatic.

　■ It should not usually hinder participation in athletics.

HEAD INJURIES AND CONCUSSIONS

■ On-field examination of a suspected head injury should include pupillary examination and an assessment of the level of consciousness.

　■ The Glasgow Coma Scale is a useful measurement.

- In cases of athletic head injuries, treatment should include immediate immobilization (as described previously for cervical spine injuries) and removal of the facemask, leaving the helmet in place.
  - Trendelenburg (head lower than body/heart) hypotonic intravenous fluids are *contraindicated* because they can cause further increases in intracerebral pressure.
- Among all sports, teenage football is associated with the highest risk of head injury. Between 75% and 85% are concussions.
  - A concussion is caused by temporary diminished cerebral blood flow after an impact.
  - In 90% of cases, there is no loss of consciousness, thus making diagnosis difficult.
  - After having one concussion, an athlete is at four times the risk for another one.
  - Tables 7-2 and 7-4 in Chapter 7 cover grading and management of concussions.
- The concept of the *second impact syndrome* is important to understand. This refers to a minor second injury after an incomplete recovery from a previous head injury.
  - This can lead to massive intracerebral hypertension.
  - Mortality has been reported in about 50% of cases because patients can die without any prodromal loss of consciousness.
  - Second impact syndrome is associated with a 100% rate of permanent neurological sequelae. This highlights the importance of understanding the criteria for return to play after athletic concussions.

SUGGESTED READING

Bono CM. Low back pain in athletes. J Bone Joint Surg Am 2004; 86–A;382–396.

Cantu RC, Mueller FO. Catastrophic spine injuries in football (1977–1989). J Spinal Disorders 1990;3:227–231.

d'Hemecourt P, Zurakowski D, Kriemler S, et al. Spondylolysis: returning the athlete to sports participation with brace treatment. Orthopedics 2002;25;653–657.

Durand P, Adamson GJ. On-the-field management of athletic head injuries. J Am Acad Orthop Surg 2004;12:191–195.

Epstein JA, Carras R, Hyman RA, et al. Cervical myelopathy caused by developmental stenosis of the spinal canal. J Neurosurg 1979; 51:362–367.

Giovanni MA, Day AL. Spinal injuries in athletes with cervical stenosis. Tech Neurosurg 1999;5:185–193.

Herzog RJ, Wiens JJ, Dillingham MF, et al. Normal cervical spine morphometry and cervical spinal stenosis in asymptomatic professional football players: plain film radiography, multiplanar computed tomography, and magnetic resonance imaging. Spine 1991; 16(suppl):S178–S186.

Kiwerski J. Cervical spine injuries caused by diving into water. Paraplegia 1980;18:101–106.

Maiman DJ, Sances A Jr, Myklebust JB, et al. Compression injuries of the cervical spine: a biomechanical analysis. Neurosurgery 1983; 13:254–260.

Maroon JC. "Burning hands" in football spinal cord injuries. JAMA 1977;238:2049–2051.

Meyer SA, Schulte KR, Callaghan JJ, et al. Cervical spinal stenosis and stingers in collegiate footfall players. Am J Sports Med 1994; 22:158–166.

Penning L. Some aspects of plain radiography of the cervical spine in chronic myelopathy. Neurology 1962;12:513–519.

Thomas BE, McCullen GM, Yuan HA. Cervical spine injuries in football players. J Am Acad Orthop Surg 1999;7:338–347.

Torg JS. Cervical spinal stenosis with cord neurapraxia and transient quadriplegia. Sports Med 1995;20:429–434.

Torg JS, Glasgow SG. Criteria for return to contact activities following cervical spine injury. Clin J Sports Med 1991;1:12–26.

Torg JS, Pavlov H, Genuario SE, et al. Neurapraxia of the cervical spinal cord with transient quadriplegia. J Bone Joint Surg Am 1986; 68:1354–1370.

Torg JS, Truex RC Jr, Marshall J, et al. Spinal injury at the level of the third and fourth cervical vertebrae from football. J Bone Joint Surg Am 1977;59–A:1015–1019.

Torg JS, Truex R Jr, Quedenfeld TC, et al. The National Football Head and Neck Registry: report and conclusions 1978. JAMA 1979;241: 1477–1479.

Torg JS, Vegso JJ, O'Neill MJ, et al. The epidemiologic, pathologic, biomechanical, and cinematographic analysis of football induced cervical spine trauma. Am J Sports Med 1990;18:50–57.

Wilberger J, Abla A, Maroon JC. Burning hands syndrome revisited. Neurosurgery 1986;19:1038–1040.

Wolfe BS, Khilnani M, Malis L. The sagittal diameter of the bony cervical spinal canal and its significance in cervical spondylosis. J Mt Sinai Hosp 1956;23:283–292.

Wu WQ, Lewis RC. Injuries of the cervical spine in high school wrestling. Surg Neurol 1985;23:143–147.

STRESS FRACTURES

LEE A. MANCINI
BRIAN D. BUSCONI

Stress fractures are one of the most common forms of overuse injuries seen in athletes. Stress fractures account for 10% of the visits made to a sports medicine specialist. They were first described by the Prussian military physician Breithaupt in 1885. He called stress fractures of the metatarsal shaft, "march fractures." Stress fractures develop when excessive, repetitive loads are placed on the bone without adequate periods of rest. This causes an increase in osteoclast activity, which creates an imbalance between bone resorption and bone formation. The osteoclasts resorb bone, and the osteoblasts form new bone. This metabolic imbalance with greater osteoclast than osteoblast activity is called a fatigue fracture. Stress fractures are more common in weight-bearing activities, especially running and jumping activities. More than 90% of stress fractures occur in the lower extremities. In nature, only three types of animals get stress fractures: race horses, racing greyhounds, and humans.

BONE REMODELING

Bone has a remodeling response to applied mechanical stress. Wolf's law states that bone develops the structure and form that is most suited to resist the forces acting on it. Thus, the mechanical strain and forces on the affected bone influence bone remodeling. Both cancellous and cortical bone remodel throughout their life cycle. A bone's response to stress is a function of multiple factors: number of loading cycles, cycle frequency, amount of strain, strain rate, and strain duration/cycle. How effectively bone responds to stress depends on the subject's metabolic state, nutritional status, age, sex, ethnicity, and level of fitness. Tensile forces create a positive electrical charge and stimulate osteoclasts and bone resorption. Compressive forces create a negative electrical charge and stimulate osteoblasts and new bone formation.

EPIDEMIOLOGY

Who gets stress fractures? There is some debate in the literature as to whether or not women sustain a higher number of stress fractures than men. Military studies show that male recruits sustain a stress fracture rate of 0.9% to 4.7%. Female recruits sustain stress fracture rates between 1.1% and 13.9%. However, studies comparing stress fracture rates between male and female athletes do not support any gender difference. These studies showed male athletes with a rate of 0.54 stress fractures per 1,000 training hours, and females at 0.86 per 1,000 training hours. There was no significant statistical difference between these rates.

RISK FACTORS

There are two classes of risk factors: extrinsic and intrinsic. An intrinsic risk factor is any variable that is based on a person's body type or characteristics, whereas an extrinsic risk factor is any outside environmental variable. Some extrinsic risk factors are training regimen, footwear, and training surface. Athletes who maintain a high training volume are at increased risk for stress fractures. Also, athletes who have abrupt increases in the duration, frequency, or intensity of training are at greater risk of developing a stress fracture. Sports medicine physicians often see this when athletes make the jump from junior varsity to varsity or from high school to college-level sports participation. Improper program design and training errors are the most frequently encountered cause of stress fractures. One study showed that training errors were responsible for 22.4% of all stress fractures. Another extrinsic risk factor is poor footwear. Athletic shoes older than 6 months increase the risk of an athlete developing a stress fracture; however, the more shock-absorbing ability a pair of running shoes has, the greater the decrease in an athlete's risk of getting a stress fracture (Fig. 9-1). Often, the higher the price of the shoe, the more powerful is the shoe's ability as a shock reducer on the user. Just as more cushioning in the footwear can reduce the force on the runner, so can the type of training surface. Harder, less compliant surfaces—like cement, pavement, and asphalt—increase the risk of stress fracture when compared with rubberized tracks, grass, and sand. Uneven terrain also increases one's risk for developing a stress fracture.

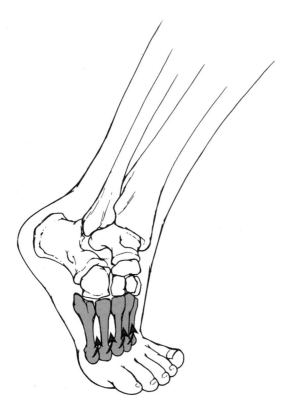

Figure 9-1 The loads on the metatarsal heads during gait produce bending moments in the metatarsal bones that may contribute to stress fractures. (From Oatis CA. Kinesiology: The Mechanics and Pathomechanics of Human Movement. Baltimore: Lippincott Williams & Wilkins, 2004.)

Although there are many extrinsic factors that affect one's risk for developing a stress fracture, there are even more intrinsic factors. Some examples of intrinsic risk factors are gender, age, race, foot structure, nutrition status, and many more. Women are at greater risk than men for developing femoral, metatarsal, or pelvic stress fractures. Data from the military show that white individuals are at greater risk than black individuals for stress fractures. Athlete data are more limited, but the results suggest the same conclusion. One study showed two times increased risk of stress fractures in whites. There has been conflicting evidence about the role the age of an athlete plays with regard to stress fractures. One retrospective study looked at 20,422 military recruits and found a positive association between increasing age (17 to 34 years) and the incidence of stress fractures in both men and women. This meant that as the age of a military recruit rises, so does the risk that he or she will develop a stress fracture. However, a later study showed that for each year of age increase between ages 17 and 26, the risk for all stress fractures decreased by 28% per year.

There are several biomechanical intrinsic factors that affect an athlete's risk for stress fractures: bone mineral density (BMD), bone geometry, and foot structure. BMD relates to the quality of the bone present in an athlete. Low BMD has been clearly shown to be associated with an increased risk of stress fracture. Studies have found that lower BMD in the lumber spine, femoral neck, total hip, and foot were significant predictors of stress fracture development in both male and female track and field athletes. Bone geometry refers to the amount of force a bone can withstand based on its cross-sectional area and cross-sectional moment of inertia. The wider a bone's cross-sectional area and cross-sectional moment of inertia, the more force the bone can handle. One study of military recruits revealed that 31% of recruits with femoral, tibial, or foot stress fractures had narrower medial to lateral tibial widths than the recruits who did not sustain a stress fracture under identical training conditions. Tibial moment of inertia as measured on x-rays correctly predicted 92% of stress fractures during the first year of military training in male recruits. This concept is presently being studied in the athletic population. No clear relationship has been found between an individual's specific foot structure and his or her risk for developing stress fractures. Foot type does have an effect on what type of stress fracture an individual is at greater risk for developing. A pes cavus, or high-arched, foot absorbs less stress and transmits greater force to the tibia and femur. A pes planus, or low-arched, foot absorbs more stress in the foot itself, placing those bones at greater risk for a stress fracture. This is a correlation between pronated feet and tibial stress fractures and cavus feet with metatarsal and femoral stress fractures.

Nutrition

It has been shown that athletes with stress fractures had a lower intake of calcium compared with those without stress fractures. The Recommended Daily Allowance for calcium is 1,000 mg/day; but, for athletes, there is much debate about whether or not this amount is too low. Athletes should aim for 1,200 to 1,500 mg of calcium/day, as well as for 400 to 800 IU of vitamin D/day. Vitamin D increases calcium transport, stimulates osteoblasts, and decreases parathyroid hormone.

Female Athlete Triad

The female athlete triad consists of amenorrhea, eating disorders, and stress fractures. Female runners with a history of stress fractures are more likely to have a history of oligomenorrhea or amenorrhea. Menarche is the age at which a female first begins menstruating. The long-term effects of delayed menarche are unknown. One study of female college distance runners revealed that 50% had irregular menstrual cycles. Some of the potential complications are osteopenia, stress fractures, and scoliosis. Estrogen deficiency at any age lowers bone mass. Lower fat intake per kilogram of body weight was more likely to sustain a stress fracture. There is still a lack of large prospective longitudinal studies on the effect of hormone replacement or birth control therapy pills on BMD in young female athletes.

Exercise and Resistance Training

Weight-bearing exercise provides a mechanical stimulus that is important for the maintenance and/or improvement of bone health. Physical inactivity is associated with bone loss, osteopenia, and osteoporosis. Resistance training has a more profound site-specific effect than aerobic exercise. Cross-sectional studies performed on female athletes show that resistance training is positively correlated with bone density. Females who combined aerobic and strength training had a higher lumbar spine BMD when compared with control subjects who participated in aerobics without resistance training. One study showed that children who engage in modest physical activity had a higher BMD than their sedentary peers.

DIAGNOSIS

History

- Taking a proper history and physical examination is vital for early diagnosis of a stress fracture.
- No matter the site of the stress fracture, there are some common threads that are found in both the history and the physical examination.
- There is usually an insidious onset of pain over a 2- to 3-week period or even longer.
  - At first, the athlete recalls the pain only appearing at the end of a contest or practice, and the pain quickly resolves with rest.
  - As time passes, the onset of pain is earlier and earlier in the practice or game, and it needs more and more rest before it goes away.
  - The pain finally becomes so severe that the athlete needs to modify his or her activity or else he or she will be unable to compete.
  - Eventually, minimal activity causes pain even with the athlete having stopped sports participation.

- Often, the onset of pain correlates with a recent change in training habits or equipment.
  - An athlete may have dramatically increased his or her mileage, may have changed his or her running shoes, or may have started running on asphalt instead of the school track.
- The pain is localized to the area of the body receiving the repetitive stress.
- There is no history of an acute or traumatic event.
- Careful nutrition and menstrual history should be obtained for all female athletes.

Physical Examination

- The hallmark of the physical examination is tenderness over the affected bone.
- There may or may not be localized edema around the stress fracture site, but rarely is a deformity seen at the site.
  - One study of stress fractures showed that 66% of the patients had localized tenderness over the fracture site, whereas only 25% had soft-tissue swelling.
- Percussion of the bone at a site away from the actual stress fracture may produce pain.
- Functional testing, such as hopping on one foot, may elicit pain.

Radiologic Examination

- Three of the most common imaging studies to use in the diagnosis of a possible stress fracture are plain films, triple-phase bone scan, and magnetic resonance imaging (MRI).

Plain Radiographs

- Plain radiographs are normal during the initial 2 or 3 weeks that an athlete develops symptoms. In fact, they may not reveal any abnormal findings for several months.
- Seventy percent of plain films are normal in patients who are ultimately diagnosed with a stress fracture.
- Abnormal findings on a plain film are usually a thin incomplete radiolucent fracture line, a fluffy periosteal reaction, or a thin linear area of sclerosis that is perpendicular to the major trabecular lines.
- A positive plain radiographic finding is usually cortical bone, periosteal reaction, cortical lucency, or a fracture line.
- In cancellous bone, the findings are more subtle and consist of a bandlike area of focal sclerosis without periosteal reaction.

Triple-phase Bone Scans

- Triple-phase bone scans are highly sensitive but lack specificity. They can detect increased uptake in a bone as soon as 2 or 3 days after the onset of clinical symptoms.
- Increased uptake in a stress fracture is seen in all three phases of the bone scan: the blood flow or angiographic

phase, the blood pool or soft-tissue phase, and the delayed phase.

- In contrast to stress fractures, shin splints are positive only in the delayed phase.
- Acute stress fractures reveal clear, localized areas of increased uptake on all three phases.
- As healing occurs, the flow phase returns to normal first, and then the pool phase reverts to normal.
- Lagging behind clinical resolution, activity on the delayed phase decreases over 3 to 18 months as the bone remodels. For this reason, bone scans should not be used to monitor healing and return to activity.

Magnetic Resonance Imaging

- MRI has several advantages over the other imaging methods:
  - It has a sensitivity on par with bone scans but a much greater specificity.
  - It does not expose the patient to any ionizing radiation.
  - It takes a shorter imaging time than a triple-phase bone scan.
  - It gives a more precise anatomic location to the stress fracture site.
  - It allows for the determination of both the extent and the orientation of the stress fracture.
- There are two stress fracture patterns seen on MRI—a bandlike fracture line and no clearcut fracture line.
  - The bandlike fracture line, which is more common, is a low signal on all imaging sequences and is surrounded by a larger, more poorly defined area of bony edema. The fracture line is continuous with the cortex and extends into the medullary space.
    - The high signal intensity of the surrounding edema decreases the longer an athlete has the symptoms.
  - The fracture pattern without the fracture line is called a *stress response* and represents an earlier stage in the evolution of the stress injury.
- The MRI is a sensitive test for early detection of periosteal and marrow edema along a fracture line.
  - A stress reaction reveals only grade I or II marrow edema and periosteal reaction, whereas a grade III or IV means a stress fracture is present.

SPECIFIC SITES

Femur

Stress fractures of the femur occur most commonly in distance runners. Femoral neck stress fractures account for 5% to 10% of all stress fractures. Femoral shaft stress fractures account for slightly less than 5%. There are two distinct types of femoral neck stress fractures: tension and compression. Compression stress fractures occur on the inferior and medial cortex of the femoral neck. Compression stress fractures are low-risk fractures and rarely displace. Young, healthy patients are more likely to develop compression fractures. As muscles tire, they lose their ability to absorb stress, increasing the forces across the femoral neck and,

over time, creating the stress fracture. Tension stress fractures occur on the superior cortex of the femoral neck. Tension stress fractures are high-risk fractures because they have a tendency to displace.

- Early diagnosis is extremely important in treating tension stress fractures because of this risk.
- Patients with a femoral stress fracture usually present with an insidious onset of pain in the groin, which gets worse with impact loading.
- Athletes also have a painful hip range of motion on the affected side.
- Femoral shaft stress fractures cause athletes to complain of mild deep thigh pain with weight-bearing.
- Both the "hop" test and the "fulcrum" test are helpful in making the diagnosis of a femoral shaft stress fracture.
- The most common site for a femoral shaft stress fracture is the medial compression side of the femur at the junction of the proximal and middle thirds of the shaft.
- The differential diagnosis for femoral stress fractures should include muscle strains, bursitis, synovitis, infection, neoplasm, slipped capital femoral epiphysis (SCFE), Perthes disease, development dysplasia of the hip (DDH), and osteoid osteoma.

Patella

- Patellar stress fractures are extremely rare.
- The differential diagnosis should include patellofemoral pain syndrome and patellar tendonitis.

Tibia

The major sports associated with tibial stress fractures are distance running, soccer, and basketball. The athlete usually presents with a pain that progressively worsens in both intensity and frequency. The pain is also aggravated by impact loading. Often, the sports medicine physician may elicit a history of the athlete changing his or her footwear, running surface, or increasing the training intensity, mileage, or frequency. The most common location for a tibial stress fracture is at the junction of the middle and distal thirds of the tibia in the posteromedial cortex, the compression side of the tibia (Fig. 9-2). Less common, but more concerning, areas for stress fractures of the tibia are the anterior cortex of the midtibia and the medial malleolus.

- The sports medicine physician should evaluate the athlete's gait for pronated feet.
- The differential diagnosis for tibial stress fractures should include nerve entrapment, muscle strains, popliteal artery compression syndrome, shin splints (medial tibial stress syndrome), and exertional compartment syndrome.

Fibula

Fibular stress fractures are found predominantly in distance runners. In particular, distance runners who train on hard surfaces are at increased risk. The most common site on the fibula is the distal third just proximal to the inferior

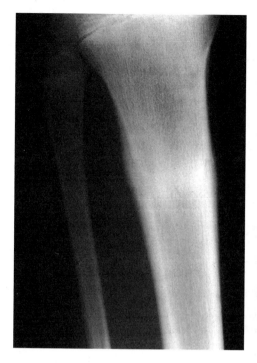 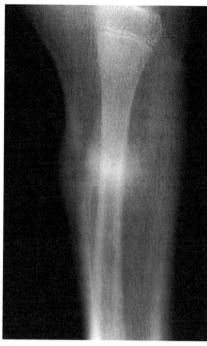

Figure 9-2 A stress fracture in a young male athlete. Note the sclerosis and widened cortices associated with bone healing. (From Bucholz RW, Heckman JD. Rockwood and Green's Fractures in Adults, 5th ed. Lippincott Williams & Wilkins, 2002.)

tibiofibular ligaments at the junction of cortical and cancellous bone.

The two major groups who often present with fibular stress fractures are young men and middle-aged women. The young men develop a stress fracture that is 5 to 6 cm proximal to the distal tip of the lateral malleolus. In middle-aged women, the common site is 3 to 4 cm proximal to the malleolar tip. Fibular stress fractures that develop in middle-aged women are usually because of metabolic problems such as osteoporosis or osteopenia. Athletes who have a valgus hindfoot have an increased risk of developing distal fibular stress fractures.

■ Surgery is seldom needed to treat a fibular stress fracture.
■ In most cases, immobilization in a short leg cast or boot for 6 to 8 weeks is sufficient.

Calcaneus

There are few cases of calcaneal stress fractures. The majority of athletes who present with heel pain have a soft-tissue injury and not a stress fracture. Calcaneal stress fractures are most common in long-distance runners, military recruits, and older, osteoporotic patients.

■ Patients present with tenderness and pain at the postero-superior calcaneus just anterior to the apophyseal plate.
■ On physical examination, an athlete has pain both dorsal and anterior on the calcaneal tubercle, as well as on the medial and lateral sides of the heel anterior to the Achilles tendon.
■ Calcaneal stress fractures are usually incomplete and show up as a vertical condensation within the cancellous bone of the calcaneal tubercle.

■ Radiographs taken 2 weeks or more after the onset of symptoms usually reveal a sclerotic line perpendicular to the trabecular stress lines in the posterosuperior aspect of the calcaneus.
   ■ This is the most common site for a calcaneal stress fracture.
   ■ A less common location is adjacent to the medial tuberosity on the calcaneus.
■ A sports medicine physician must have a high index of suspicion for a calcaneal stress fracture to avoid misdiagnosis.
■ Because plain films are usually negative, MRI is the diagnostic tool of choice.
■ The differential diagnosis for calcaneal stress fractures should include plantar fasciitis, Achilles tendonitis, and retrocalcaneal bursitis.
■ Treatment is immobilization with a short leg cast or boot for 8 to 12 weeks.

Talus

Talar stress fractures are uncommon. They are found primarily in runners, military recruits, dancers, and jumping athletes. The classic location is at the talar neck, but they can also be found at the lateral, posteromedial, and postero-lateral parts of the talus. In ballet dancers, the number one type of stress fracture is a posterolateral talar fracture. There is a disruption of the synchondrosis between the os trigonum and the posterior body of the talus. The posterior impingement of the os trigonum against the posterior tibia causes pain. This posterior impingement often occurs in ballet dancers when they go into the en pointe position, which involves dancing on one's toes in hyperplantar flexion on the tibiotalar joint.

- Plain radiographs are usually negative, and MRI is needed for definitive diagnosis.
- The healing time for these stress fractures is usually 3 to 4 months.

Navicular

Navicular stress fractures are seen most commonly in basketball players, football players, soccer players, and runners. Athletes usually describe an insidious onset of vague midfoot pain, tenderness over the dorsum of the foot medially, tenderness on the medial aspect of the longitudinal arch, foot pain that is worse with activity, and pain that is reproduced by standing on one's toes. The most common site for a navicular stress fracture is at the junction of the medial two-thirds and the lateral one-third of the bone. Navicular stress fractures are the most difficult stress fracture of the foot and ankle to treat. This is because the location of the stress fracture corresponds to the zone of avascularity of the bone. The blood supply to the navicular bone is an interosseous blood supply, which enters the medial and lateral poles of the bone but diminishes in the zone where the stress fracture usually occurs.

- Athletes with a navicular stress fracture tend to present much later than with other lower-extremity stress fractures.
- Plain radiographs rarely show navicular stress fractures.
- The telltale sign is sclerosis in the subchondral bone adjacent to the talonavicular joint.
- A computed tomography (CT) scan (or MRI) is the imaging test of choice, since it can show the vertical fracture line in the sagittal plane.

Cuboid and Cuneiform

Cuboid and cuneiform stress fractures are rare. They occur most often in distance runners. The predisposing factor for developing a cuboid fracture is an overload on the lateral column of the foot, such as subtalar ankylosis or a varus hindfoot position. The middle and lateral cuneiforms are most likely to develop a stress fracture instead of the medial cuneiform because of the forces on the foot transmitted through the second and third metatarsals. Both of these types of stress fractures heal well because they involve cancellous bone.

- Treatment of both of these stress fractures is conservative.
- A soft-soled, supportive shoe that is custom-molded and cushioned to correct for any stiffness or varus deformities in the patient should be worn.

Metatarsals

Metatarsal stress fractures, the original "march fracture," is more common in military recruits than in athletes. Athletes participating in ballet, football, gymnastics, and basketball are most at risk. Metatarsal stress fractures are the most common lower-extremity stress fractures. The most common site is usually the shaft (diaphysis or neck) of the second or third metatarsals (Fig. 9-3). Both pes cavus and pes planus feet are associated with an increased incidence of metatarsal stress fractures.

A Morton's foot is one in which the individual possesses a short first metatarsal, a long second metatarsal, and a hypermobile first metatarsal ray. This condition predisposes

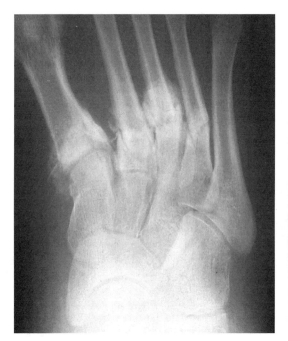
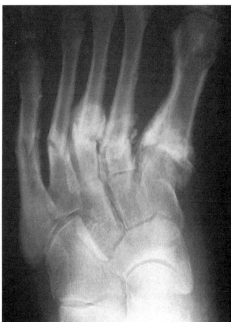

Figure 9-3   Stress fractures of the metatarsal bones. These two radiographs show the progression of fractures from medial to lateral along the metatarsals in an insensate individual. (From Bucholz RW, Heckman JD. Rockwood and Green's Fractures in Adults, 5th ed. Lippincott Williams & Wilkins, 2002.)

an athlete to a second metatarsal stress fracture. One study showed that six of eight ballet dancers with stress fractures of the second metatarsal had a Morton's foot. Forefoot pain may be exacerbated by running, jumping, or dancing; a callus is often felt.

There are two types of stress fractures to the fifth metatarsal: a Jones-type fracture and a "dancer's fracture." A "dancer's fracture" is an acute fracture at the base of the fifth metatarsal. This fracture at the proximal metaphysis is not a stress fracture. However, a Jones fracture, named after Sir Robert Jones, is a stress fracture at the metaphyseal–diaphyseal junction of the fifth metatarsal. Jones stress fractures are more common in basketball and football players.

- Special care must be taken with the proximal diaphyseal fifth metatarsal stress fractures because there is a high incidence of nonunion due to poor blood supply.
- Plain radiographic films are usually negative so treat symptomatic patients conservatively.
- Immobilize the patient to strict non-weight-bearing in a short leg cast for a minimum of 6 weeks.
- If patient has persistent, unresolved pain, is an elite-level athlete, develops an established pseudarthrosis, or fails conservative treatment, then operative intervention is indicated.
- Differential diagnosis for metatarsal stress fractures should include Morton's neuroma, Freiberg's infraction, and metatarsal phalangeal joint instability.

Sesamoid

Sesamoid stress fractures are not uncommon in athletes. They are seen in all active populations. In particular runners, football players, golfers, and gymnasts are at increased risk. The mechanism for injury is during weight transfer onto the medial column of the forefoot. There is very little soft-tissue padding in this area. The medial sesamoid bone is more likely to develop a stress fracture because it is the larger of the two sesamoid bones.

- An athlete usually presents with a story of insidious onset of medial forefoot pain, which gets worse with jumping, running, and toe-off activities.
- Usually, the patient presents with pain on palpation of the sesamoid bones, as well as pain with dorsiflexion of the metatarsophalangeal joint of the great toe.
- Plain radiographs using a metallic marker over the area of pain using anteroposterior and sesamoid views may be helpful in visualizing the stress fracture. Otherwise, an MRI is the imaging method of choice.
- Conservative treatment is the primary method of choice.
- The athlete uses off-loading orthoses, a protected weight-bearing cast, or a boot.
- Surgery is needed only if conservative management fails.
- Surgery consists of the excision of the offending sesamoid bone and reconstruction of the flexor hallucis brevis and intersesamoid ligaments.

Pubic Ramus

Pubic rami stress fractures are relatively rare. They occur more often in women than in men. The primary stress fracture site is in the inferior pubic ramus adjacent to the symphysis pubis.

- The athlete presents with groin pain that is exacerbated by activity.

Sacrum

Sacral stress fractures are also rare. They happen most often in runners and weight lifters.

- The symptoms of a sacral stress fracture may mimic that of a herniated disc.
- An athlete may complain of low back and sacral pain that radiates into the buttocks.

Pars Interarticularis

A defect in the posterior neural arch of the pars interarticularis is called a spondylolysis. Stress fractures of the pars interarticularis are seen primarily in adolescents involved in gymnastics or dancing. This is a fatigue-type injury that occurs secondary to repetitive microtrauma. The mechanism is chronic and repetitive loading of the lumbar facet joints due to hyperextension.

- Athletes often present with low back pain made worse with hyperextension.
- To confirm the diagnosis, an MRI or single-photon emission computed tomography (SPECT) scan is usually needed.

Rib

Rib stress fractures are most commonly seen in rowers; however, golfers and baseball players have also been found to be at increased risk for rib stress fractures. In rowers, the ribs that are usually affected are the fourth through the ninth. Rowing stress fractures are usually associated with long-distance training. The mechanism for a rib stress fracture is from the repetitive bending forces on the ribs, especially in exhalation caused by the pull of the serratus anterior and the external oblique muscles. During rowing, the harmful position is believed to occur at the end of the drive phase, with shoulder extension and scapular retraction. In golfers, it is the posterolateral part of the rib in the leading side of the trunk that is the most common site. As in rowers, the lower ribs are more at risk. Electromyographic analysis of a golfer's swing shows that the serratus anterior is the primary force on the ribs during the swing. Golfers at increased risk for developing a rib stress fracture are those with a poor technique, those that take more strokes, and those who create larger divots. First rib stress fractures have been reported in baseball players.

- Treatment of rib stress fractures is largely symptomatic.
- Physical therapy focusing on strengthening and stretching of the serratus anterior is critical.
- Also, addressing an athlete's mechanics of either his or her rowing form, golf swing, or baseball throwing or hitting motion is vital.

Sternum

Stress fractures of the sternum are rare. They are most often seen in wrestlers and golfers.

- Athletes report pain in the center of their chest.
- Symptomatic treatment is all that is needed.
- Treat athletes with rest, ice, anti-inflammatories, and avoid contact sports until pain-free.
- Usually, it takes 6 to 12 weeks for an athlete to return to play.

Humerus

Stress fractures of the humerus are usually seen in throwing athletes. They may occur in the shaft of the humerus in adult baseball players, especially pitchers. In skeletally immature throwing athletes, stress fractures of the humerus may develop through the proximal growth plate. The mechanism of injury is the creation of opposing muscular contractions during throwing, which cause torsional and tension forces on the growth plate. The muscles of the rotator cuff are attached proximally to the physis, and the deltoid, pectoralis major, and triceps all are attached distally to the growth plate.

- Athletes complain of pain made worse by hard throwing.
- On examination, there is usually focal tenderness and discomfort to manual resistance to shoulder abduction and internal rotation.
- In younger throwers, widening of the lateral portion of the physis (growth plate) may be present on external rotation anteroposterior radiographs.
- The radiographs may also show lateral fragmentation, sclerosis, or cystic changes of the humerus.

Olecranon

This is another upper extremity stress fracture that is common in throwing athletes. Usually, this type of stress fracture is more common in adolescents and kids. Olecranon stress fractures are due to repetitive extension overload.

- Patients complain of pain on the lateral border of the ulna.
- On examination, the athlete experiences pain over the olecranon with resisted extension.
- If this stress fracture is not recognized early, displacement can occur.
- Plain radiographs show fractures only occasionally. A CT scan or MRI is the best imaging study for viewing an olecranon stress fracture.
- Conservative treatment is preferred.
- Once point tenderness over the olecranon ceases, athletes can begin light strength training on their triceps and biceps, as well as rotator cuff exercises.
- If symptoms persist and conservative treatment has failed, then surgical intervention is needed.
- A single axial large cannulated screw is inserted through the distal triceps tendon.

Radius

Radial stress fractures are most often seen in gymnasts, in which their upper extremity serves in weight-bearing. In about one-third of cases, a gymnast has bilateral stress fractures.

The most common site is at the distal radial physis.

- On examination, the athlete has pain along the distal radial physis, with extremes of wrist dorsiflexion and axial loading.

MANAGEMENT

General Principles

- Once the initial diagnosis of a stress fracture is made, a treatment plan must be implemented as soon as possible.
- The first goal of treatment is to control the athlete's pain using nonsteroidal anti-inflammatory drugs, ice, and stretching.
- The two basic principles are rest and immobilization of the stress fracture site.
  - It is important to break the athlete's cycle of destructive, repetitive trauma through rest.
    - Rest allows the reparative phase to dominate over the resorption phase helping the fracture to heal.
    - In general, at least 6 to 8 weeks are needed for most stress fractures to heal, although some may take longer.
  - For immobilization of the stress fracture, we use prefabricated braces, orthoses, and walking boots.
    - The advantage of these over casts it that they can be removed, enabling the athlete to perform active range-of-motion exercises to try and maintain muscle tone and bulk and to reduce joint stiffness.
- Surgery should be considered for bones in which a complete fracture can lead to long-term disability.
  - These troublesome bones include stress fractures of the tibia, the navicular, the fifth metatarsal, and the femoral neck.
- A close look must be taken at the athlete's nutritional status.
  - The sports medicine physician should evaluate the athlete's intake of calcium and vitamin D and determine whether or not an eating disorder exists.
    - If an eating disorder is uncovered, a multidisciplinary approach should be used.
  - In a female athlete, if abnormal menstrual patterns are identified, estrogen supplementation should be considered.
  - The treating physician must make sure there are no medical conditions present that may affect bone integrity.

Return to Play

- For athletes looking to return to play, there is a definite progression to the activities to which they are allowed to participate.

- The first conditioning allowed should be swimming, which is a non-weight-bearing activity.
- Nonimpact exercise such as biking comes next, followed by weight-bearing nonimpact activities like the elliptical machine, cross country skier machine, and stair climber.
- The final activities allowed should be weight-bearing impact exercises such as walking, progressing to jogging and finally running.

- At each specific activity, the duration should progress from short to long, and the intensity level from low to high.
- For each impact activity, an athlete should have a pain-free progression from low intensity–short duration to low intensity–long duration to high intensity–short duration to high intensity–long duration before advancing to the next impact activity level.
- Only after this complete, pain-free progression over at least 6 to 8 weeks can an athlete return to his or her sport.

Femoral Stress Fracture

- In compression-type stress fractures of the femoral neck, the patient should be made non-weight-bearing with crutches until the patient is pain-free and has full range of motion.
  - Usually, this is at least 4 to 6 weeks.
- Athletes are allowed to return to sports only when they are pain-free, have a full range of motion, and radiographs show evidence of a healed fracture.
- If the fracture becomes complete or does not heal with non-weight-bearing and conservative management, pinning is recommended.
- For tension-type stress fractures of the femoral neck, athletes should have surgical intervention.
  - Tension-type stress fractures have a high likelihood of becoming displaced fractures.
  - Displaced fractures require open reduction and internal fixation.
  - Postoperative management consists of 6 weeks of non-weight-bearing, followed by gradual progression of weight-bearing over the next 6 weeks.
- The initial treatment for femoral shaft stress fractures is for the athlete to rest for 2 to 4 weeks.
  - During this period, the athlete progresses from toe-touch weight-bearing to full weight-bearing.
- If, after these initial 4 weeks, the athlete is able to weight-bear pain-free, he or she is allowed to begin low-impact activity.
- If low-impact activity is tolerated pain-free, the athlete is progressed slowly to higher-impact activities.
  - This process takes place over a course of 6 to 8 weeks.
- If the stress fracture has delayed union, nonunion, or progresses to a complete fracture, intermedullary nailing is performed.

Tibial Stress Fracture

- For athletes with a tibial stress fracture, the first 6 weeks of treatment consist of complete rest while using either crutches, a short leg cast, or a boot.

- Posteromedial cortex stress fractures respond well to rest.
- After the pain has subsided, the athlete may begin some low-intensity, nonimpact aerobic activities such as swimming or biking.
- Re-evaluate the athlete after 6 weeks.
  - If the athlete is pain-free, he or she may begin a gradual progression back in play.
  - Do not increase the athlete's volume or intensity by more than 10% each week.
- If at the 6-week mark the athlete still has pain, radiographs should be repeated.
  - If the radiographs have positive findings, complete rest should be continued for another 6 weeks.
  - If the radiographs are negative, the athlete can begin a slow return to activity.
- If after 12 weeks the athlete still has pain, a CT scan or MRI should be obtained.
- Surgical excision and bone grafting may be required if the fracture does not heal with rest and immobilization.

Navicular Stress Fracture

- Navicular stress fractures are a difficult problem to treat.
- Incomplete fractures are treated with immobilization in a cast or boot, and athletes are made non-weight-bearing for 6 to 8 weeks.
- A return to weight-bearing and activity is based on the clinical picture and evidence of radiographic healing.
- For complete, nondisplaced fractures, attempt nonoperative treatment with cast and non-weight-bearing for 6 to 8 weeks.

Metatarsal Stress Fracture

- The definitive initial treatment for metatarsal stress fractures is rest, putting the patient in a boot or on crutches for 6 weeks.
- The one exception is Jones-type stress fractures of the fifth metatarsal, which require the athlete to be in a short-leg cast or a boot for 12 weeks of non-weight-bearing.
- With these specific types of fractures, many athletes choose operative management with an intramedullary cancellous or cannulated screw and return to sports slowly after 6 weeks.

PREVENTION

In this chapter, we have examined the risk factors for developing stress fractures, specific stress fractures, and the diagnosing and treatment of stress fractures. In this final section, we will discuss steps athletes, coaches, and team physicians can take to prevent stress fractures. Nutrition plays a key role. The athlete must be sure to take in enough calcium and vitamin D in his or her diet, as well as to take in enough calories. The sports medicine staff should be looking for red flags pointing to possible eating disorders in their athletes. Athletes (especially distance runners) should also use proper footwear and try to train on softer, impact-absorbing surfaces. An athlete's training program should contain a cyclical progression in terms of intensity and distance. Cross-training should be encouraged. Training should place an emphasis on quality over quantity. Most importantly, sports medicine physicians should educate parents, coaches, and athletes about stress fractures.

SUGGESTED READING

Barbaix E. Stress fracture of the sternum in a golf player. Int J Sports Med 1996;17:304–305.

Barrow GW, Saha H. Menstrual irregularity and stress fractures in collegiate female distance runners. Am J Sports Med 1988;16: 209–216.

Bennell KL, Malcolm SA, Thomas SA. The incidence and distribution of stress fractures in competitive track and field athletes. Am J Sports Med 1996;24:211–217.

Brudvig TJS, Grudger TD, Obermeyer L. Stress fractures in 295 trainees: a one-year study on incidence as related to age, sex, and race. Mil Med 1983;148:666–667.

Brukner PD, Bradshaw C, Khan KM. Stress fractures: a review of 180 cases. Clin J Sports Med 1996;6:85–89.

Giladi M, Milgrom C, Simkin A. Stress fractures and tibial bone width. A risk factor. J Bone Joint Surg Br 1987;69:326–329.

Gilaldi M, Milgrom C, Stein M, et al. Stress fractures, identifiable risk factors. Am J Sports Med 1991;19:647–652.

Green NE, Rodgers RA, Lipscomb AB. Nonunion stress fractures of the tibia. Am J Sports Medicine 1985;13:171–176.

Gurtler R, Pavlov H, Torg J. Stress fracture of the ipsilateral first rib in a pitcher. Am J Sports Med 1985;13:277–279.

Karlson KA. Rib stress fractures in elite rowers. Am J Sports Med 1998; 26:516–519.

Khan K, Brown J, Way S, et al. Overuse injuries in classical ballet. Sports Med 1995;19:341–357.

Khan KM, Fuller PJ, Brukner PD, et al. Outcome of conservative and surgical management of navicular stress fracture in athletes. Am J Sports Med 1992;20:657–666.

Knapp TP, Garrett WE. Stress fractures: general concepts. Clin Sports Med 1997;16:339–356.

Matheson GO, Clement DB, McKenzie DC. Stress fractures in athletes: a study of 320 cases. Am J Sports Med 1987;15:46–58.

Nuber G, Diment M. Olecranon stress fracture in throwers. Clin Orthop 1992;278:58–61.

Roy S, Caine D, Singer KM. Stress changes of the distal radial epiphysis in young gymnasts. A report of twenty-one cases and a review of the literature. Am J Sports Med 1985;13:301–308.

Umans HR, Kaye JJ. Longitudinal stress fractures of the tibia: diagnosis by magnetic resonance imaging. Skel Radiol 1996;25:319–324.

Van Hal ME, Keene JS, Lange TA. Stress fractures of the great toe sesamoids. Am J Sports Med 1982;10:122–128.

Voss LA, Fadale PD, Hulston MJ. Exercise-induced loss of bone density in athletes. J Am Acad Orthop Surg 1998;6:349–357.

10

SOFT-TISSUE ALLOGRAFTS

JOSHUA S. HORNSTEIN

Soft-tissue allografts have been used in orthopaedics for more than a century. More recently, implantation of these tissues has become more common as their safety and efficacy have been established. The procurement and sterilization process for allografts has improved with the addition of newer testing methods. Allografts can and have been used as a substitute for nascent tissues and autogenous grafts. The safety and clinical outcome of procedures using allografts has improved, as we have gained a better understanding of the basic science behind the biologic incorporation of these tissues. We present a historical review of allograft utilization, current procurement and testing techniques, and case presentations to exemplify their clinical applications.

Allograft tissue has been used in orthopaedics since early in the 20th century. The first documented use of a musculoskeletal soft-tissue allograft was by MacEwen in 1880. More recently, Noyes and Shino reported on their use of allografts in ligament reconstruction in 1981. Over the past decade, soft-tissue allografts have been used more commonly to decrease patient morbidity and substitute for tissue that is deficient or not available for implantation. The screening and preparation of allogeneic tissues have changed and improved as well. In this review, the different sterilization and screening techniques of allografts will be covered. The clinical applications of these tissues will be presented. Today, quality soft-tissue allografts are available as a viable substitute for harvesting the patient's own tissues.

ADVANTAGES AND DISADVANTAGES

Six different tissue banks process more than 85% of all soft-tissue allografts. Some procedures mandate the use of allograft (e.g., multiple ligamentous injuries of the knee). Allografts have both advantages and disadvantages (Box 10-1). Donor-site morbidity is eliminated with the use of allografts. Graft size is not an issue as a result of the ability to preselect based on the donor. Operative times are decreased because autograft procurement is unnecessary. Studies comparing matched autograft and allograft bone-patellar tendon-bone anterior cruciate ligament (ACL) reconstructions have found less loss of motion in the allograft group, no difference in hop strength, side-to-side KT-1000 measurements and International Knee Documentation Committee (IKDC) ratings.

Allografts are not without their shortcomings. Disease transmission is the greatest concern on the part of both the physician and patient. The risk of disease transmission of any kind is currently estimated at 1:1.67 million. Currently, newer tests are being implemented to discover human immunodeficiency virus (HIV) during the early infection "window period," which goes undetected by current testing methods. A host-versus-graft T cell–mediated immune response may occur, causing graft rejection. Also, antibody-mediated rejection can occur.

Delayed graft incorporation is a theoretical concern related to soft-tissue allografts. In a study comparing patellar tendon autografts to fresh-frozen allografts using a goat

115

BOX 10-1 ADVANTAGES AND DISADVANTAGES OF ALLOGRAFTS

Advantages
No donor site morbidity
Cosmetically better outcome
No size limitation, therefore useful in revisionary situations
Shorter operating time (autograft harvesting is eliminated)
Decreased incidence of postoperative knee stiffness

Disadvantages
Possibility of disease transmission, the biggest fear of
    recipients
Host immune response
Delayed incorporation
Local bone resorption
Cost

model, Jackson found that allografts lose a great proportion of their time-zero strength during the remodeling phase. The speed of remodeling is not as rapid in allogeneic tissues as it is in autografts. They found that, although both grafts proceeded through the same biologic process, allografts went at a slower rate when compared at 6 months postreconstruction. In contrast, Shino compared fresh patellar tendon autografts with frozen patellar tendon allografts in replacing the canine ACL. The authors found a more rapid conversion of graft collagen to host collagen in the allograft model. Similar degrees of vascular and histologic incorporation were found.

The final disadvantage of allografts is the cost of the implant. Soft-tissue allografts range in price from $795 each for fresh-frozen tibialis tendon, $1,590 for semitendinosus and gracilis, and $2,800 for a cryopreserved graft.

PROCUREMENT, DISEASE TRANSMISSION, AND SCREENING

Tissue handling and screening are the key elements in the prevention of disease transmission. The American Association of Tissue Banks (AATB) requires their member organizations to follow a strict protocol for the preparation and storage of soft-tissue allografts. Procurement standards have been established by the AATB and were most recently updated in April 2001. Potential donors are examined via an exhaustive medical, social, and sexual history completed by the donor's family. A physical examination is also performed for any signs of infectious disease. Any positive finding that raises suspicion of communicable or metabolic disease disqualifies the individual as a donor.

Tissue harvesting often occurs within a few hours of death, usually after procurement teams have removed the donor's solid organs. Musculoskeletal tissues can be removed by means of an aseptic, completely sterile, or clean technique, where absolute sterile technique is not used. Secondary sterilization with gamma irradiation is required after a clean harvest but not necessarily after a sterile technique is used. If radiation is used, the source and dosage must be clearly documented in the allograft processing record. Once they are harvested, the tissues are cooled, cleaned of body fluids, and transported to the local tissue bank. Final determination of tissue acceptance is made by the medical director of the tissue bank after all the medical and serologic data are considered.

Both the U.S. Food and Drug Administration and AATB require multiple laboratory tests to be performed on the donor's serum. These include antibodies to HIV 1 and 2, hepatitis B surface antigen, hepatitis C antibodies, syphilis antibodies, human T cell lymphotrophic virus antibodies, and aerobic and anaerobic cultures, as well as tissue cultures from the individual allografts.

A window period exists when a donor can be infected with HIV yet not produce serum antibodies. This period can range from 25 days to 6 months. Most tissue banks utilize polymerase chain reaction (PCR) testing to identify small amounts of viral DNA. With the addition of PCR to the battery of testing, the window period can be reduced to 19 days with an added processing cost of $120 to $150. Seven-hundred fifty thousand allografts have been tested with PCR and implanted without a single HIV seroconversion. Buck calculated that the risk of contracting HIV from an implanted bone allograft was estimated at 1 in 1,667,000. Meticulous screening of donors is the primary reason for this extremely small risk. Theoretically, if this screening were not followed, testing only for HIV antibodies, the risk would increase to an unacceptable 1 in 161. The risk assessment of Buck, which was proposed in 1989, is likely higher than the risk under current screening techniques.

GRAFT PREPARATION AND STORAGE

A number of processing techniques have been used since the inception of allografts. Freeze-dried allografts have been in use since 1951. Once the allograft is procured, it is frozen pending the results of the donor's serology. The tissue is then thawed and soaked in an antibiotic solution, refrozen, and lyophilized to a moisture content of less than 6% by weight. Allowable storage time after this technique is from 3 to 5 years. Before implantation, the graft is rehydrated for 30 minutes. This graft has been shown to provide adequate initial strength.

The most commonly used graft preparation technique is fresh-frozen. The allograft is procured and frozen, pending the results of the donor's serology. The tissue is then thawed, soaked in an antibiotic solution, packaged dry, and refrozen from $-70°C$ to $-80°C$. When the tissue is ready for implantation, it is rapidly thawed in warm water and implanted. This graft can be stored up to 3 to 5 years. Cellular survival is essentially zero with this preservation process. This process is inadequate for meniscal and osteochondral allografts because of the need for cell survival in these tissues. Ultimate failure strength has been shown to be adequate when tissue warming lasts for 2 hours.

The technique of cryopreservation is a method of deep-freezing, which allows for fibroblast survival. In this process, grafts are initially cooled to 0°C and processed within 24

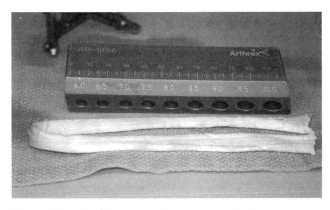

Figure 10-1   Typical example of a cryopreserved soft-tissue allograft—in this case a tibialis tendon.

hours of death. Second, they are stored and processed through an antibiotic "cocktail" at 37°C for 24 hours and then undergo a time-controlled freezing to a final temperature of −150°C. This technique is ideal for allografts that depend on the survival of its cellular elements (i.e., menisci). Cryopreservation has been shown to protect up to 80% of cells in meniscal allografts and up to 70% in a tibialis anterior tendon graft (Fig. 10-1).

Because freezing does not kill the HIV virus, secondary sterilization techniques have been developed. Ethylene oxide, commonly used to sterilize surgical instruments, was initially used to sterilize allografts prior to implantation. Jackson et al. showed that the ethylene oxide byproducts—ethylene glycol and ethylene chlorohydrin—cause graft failure and sterile persistent effusions after allograft ACL reconstruction. The AATB requires a measurement of residual levels of these byproducts to be documented in the processing record of the allograft. Ethylene oxide weakens the mechanical strength of the allograft and potentially causes synovitis postoperatively. Newer techniques that inactivate pathogens via chemical and antibiotic treatment add significant expense to the overall cost of the allograft.

Gamma irradiation is currently the more commonly used secondary sterilization technique for soft tissue grafts. Gamma irradiation can inhibit HIV uptake by T lymphocytes. Bone allografts have been looked at more closely in regard to the effect of radiation. Many authors have concluded that deep-freezing, in conjunction with 1.5 to 2.5 mrad of radiation, adequately eliminated HIV while causing minimal damage to the collagenous substrate of the allograft. Although gamma irradiation kills graft cells, it is a necessary step to ensure sterilization of the allograft.

BIOLOGICAL INCORPORATION OF ALLOGRAFTS

All implanted biologic tissues, whether allograft or autograft, undergo a sequence of graft necrosis, host cellular repopulation, revascularization, and remodeling. Jackson et al. eloquently outlined the biologic incorporation of soft-tissue allografts in a goat ACL model. His group looked at freeze-dried allograft ACL reconstructions and compared them with a control group of intact ACLs. One year after implantation, these two groups were compared on both histologic and microvascular bases. They found a similar vascular pattern surrounding both the nascent and allograft ACL. In a follow-up study, the histological and mechanical properties of patellar tendon autografts and allografts were compared. The allograft induced greater vascular and inflammatory responses at 6 weeks, compared with the autografts. Both groups were similar histologically at 2 months, with all the cellular elements being from the host. The allografts had a 27% average load to failure (compared with the nascent ACL), compared with 62% for the autograft. Other authors have found that at 26 weeks, allograft ACLs have a maximum of 43% load to failure and were histologically similar to the nascent ACL.

SURGICAL TECHNIQUES

Upper Extremity

Acromioclavicular Joint

More than 100 different procedures for the repair or reconstruction of the acromioclavicular joint have been described. The procedure depicted is a derivation of that described by Lemos and Morrison in which a GORE-TEX® loop was placed through both the coracoid and distal clavicles. Weaver and Dunn resected 1 cm of distal clavicle and transferred the coracoacromial ligament into the medullary canal with fixation through drill holes. We performed a technique using a semitendinosus allograft for the reconstruction of the coracoclavicular ligaments. No long-term, prospective, randomized study of this technique has been performed comparing allograft reconstruction to methods involving augmentation or internal fixation. Currently, this is the technique of choice in our institution.

- The AC joint is debrided of fibrous scar tissue and organized hematoma, and 1 cm of distal clavicle is removed.
- A 4.5-mm drill hole is made in the distal clavicle 1 cm medial to the previous resection.
- This drill hole is enlarged using sequentially larger curettes to an approximate size of 8 mm.
- On a separate table, a semitendinosus-gracilis allograft of 255 mm in length is prepared in the following manner.
  - A running no. 5 nonabsorbable "baseball" stitch is placed in either end of both the semitendinosus and gracilis allografts.
  - This graft is tensioned at 20 ft-lb to remove any creep.
  - A "safety strand" composed of three no. 5 nonabsorbable sutures is then braided together.
  - A 90-degree Mixter clamp is passed around the inferior border of the coracoid, and the allograft and suture braid are brought around the coracoid.
  - The lateral tail of the graft and suture braid is passed over the clavicle and through the 8-mm drill hole.
  - The clavicle is overreduced 5 mm, and the allograft is sewn to itself using a no. 5 nonabsorbable suture.
  - The "safety stitch" is tied to itself as well (Fig. 10-2).

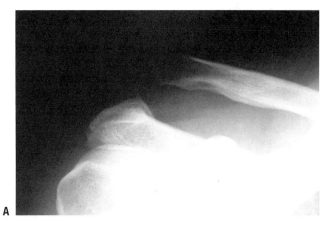

A

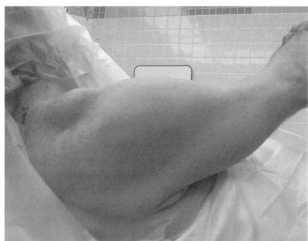

B

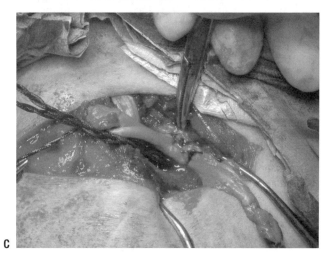

C

Figure 10-2   **A:** Radiograph of type V acromioclavicular joint separation. **B:** Clinical appearance of type V acromioclavicular joint separation. **C:** Semitendinosus allograft woven through distal clavicle and around coracoid in acromioclavicular joint reconstruction.

■ The patient is immobilized for 7 days and then begins on a progressive motion and strengthening program.

Scapular Winging

The technique of pectoralis major transfer for serratus anterior palsy has yielded good results. In our institution, we have modified this technique by using a soft-tissue allograft to lengthen the normally stout pectoralis tendon.

■ The procedure is performed using the two-incision technique as described by Warner, substituting a hamstring allograft for the fascia lata autograft.
■ The patient is placed in the lateral decubitus position, allowing access to both the patient's chest and inferomedial scapula.
■ Through a limited deltopectoral approach, the sternocostal head of the pectoralis major is identified and detached from its humeral insertion.
■ On a back table, a semitendinosus allograft is prepared in a similar fashion as described previously.
■ The graft is not tensioned prior to use.
■ The single graft is then woven into the pectoralis tendon with a no. 5 suture (Fig. 10-3).
■ Attention is then directed to the inferomedial angle of the scapula, which is displaced medially and superiorly.
■ An 8-cm oblique incision in the direction of Langer's lines is made in between the current and reduced positions of the patient's scapula.
■ The latissimus dorsi is retracted laterally, and the rhomboid major, infraspinatus, and subscapularis are subperiosteally dissected off the inferomedial angle of the scapula.
■ While protecting the underlying chest wall, an 8-mm drill hole is made from posterior to anterior in the inferomedial angle of the scapula.

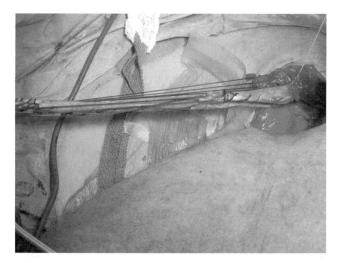

Figure 10-3   Semitendinosus tendon "leader" for pectoralis tendon transfer for scapular winging.

- Using blunt dissection, a tunnel is made from the anterior to the posterior wound along the chest wall.
- A large Kelly clamp is then passed from posterior to anterior and opened, serving to dilate the tunnel.
- The clamp is then repassed, transferring the tendon/allograft to the posterior incision.
- The scapula is reduced, and the composite is brought through the scapula and sutured to itself with a no. 5 suture.
- For additional fixation, the graft is secured via drill holes and a no. 2 suture to the medial scapula.
- The patient is placed in a "gunslinger" brace in 30 degrees of abduction, neutral rotation, and flexion.
- This position is held for 6 weeks, at which point gentle range of motion in scaption is begun.

Ulnar (Medial) Collateral Ligament

Several authors have looked at the strength of the nascent medial collateral ligament (MCL), palmaris longus, and gracilis tendons. Hamner found that a fresh-frozen, single gracilis tendon had a strength of 837 ± 138 Newtons. Fresh-frozen gracilis tendon exhibits adequate strength characteristics for replacement of the anterior band of the MCL. Morgan and Schepsis (personal communication, 2005) have established a series of MCL reconstructions utilizing gracilis allograft and a docking technique. All 16 athletes have returned to sports, and no complications were reported. Of note, approximately 15% of patients do not have a palmaris tendon and, if an allograft is not utilized, graft sources include the less desirable extensor indicis pollicis, toe flexors, or plantaris.

The docking technique described by Altchek may be used, although a split instead of an elevation of the flexor-pronator mass can be performed.

- An 8-mm longitudinal incision is made, slightly anterior to the cubital.
- The ulnar nerve is dissected from its cubital tunnel and released proximally at the intermuscular septum, as well as distally at the split of the flexor carpi ulnaris.
- After identification of the flexor-pronator mass, it is split longitudinally from the medial epicondyle to the sublime tubercle of the proximal ulna.
- The attenuated MCL is directly deep to the flexor-pronator mass.
- This ligament should be split longitudinally for later imbrication over the graft.
- A gracilis allograft is pared down to approximately 50% of its original size. The graft is prepared on a back table by placing a no. 2 nonabsorbable suture baseball stitch into one end.
- The graft is not tensioned prior to implantation.
- Using a 3.2-mm drill bit, two drill holes are made 45 degrees to each other in the sublime tubercle.
- These drill holes are then connected using medium-sized curettes to form a tunnel.
- Attention is then directed toward the inferior and distal aspects of the medial epicondyle.
- Two 3.2-mm drill holes are placed retrograde at 45 degrees to each other, aiming proximally.

- These tunnels are not connected.
- Then, using a 2.5-mm drill bit, two "docking" tunnels are made from the superior aspect of the epicondyle into the respective tunnel.
- Using a suture passer, the graft is passed through the ulnar tunnel.
- Then, the graft end, with the suture attached, is "docked" retrograde into its ulnar tunnel.
- The remaining graft end is then shortened so that it will be the proper length to "dock" into its drill hole.
- A no. 5 nonabsorbable suture is then placed into this graft end and docked in an identical fashion.
- The two no. 5 sutures are then tied to each other with a varus force placed on the elbow.
- The nascent MCL is then imbricated over the allograft.
- The ulnar nerve is subcutaneously transposed, the skin is closed with interrupted suture, and the extremity is placed in a compressive dressing and in a locked, hinged, unilateral elbow brace.
- The standard rehabilitation protocol as per Wilk et al. was followed.
- Complications associated with this procedure are ulnar nerve injury, which can be decreased with the muscle splitting technique, medial antebrachial cutaneous nerve injury, and ulnar tunnel fracture.

Distal Biceps Tendon

Distal biceps disruptions usually occur in the dominant extremity of men in the fourth through sixth decades of life. No cases have been reported in women. The mechanism of injury is a single traumatic event in which an unexpected extension moment is placed across the elbow while the arm is flexed 90 degrees. The tendon typically avulses from the radial tuberosity. The bicipital aponeurosis may rupture or remain intact.

Distal biceps ruptures can be classified as partial or complete. Partial tears can often be difficult to diagnose, with magnetic resonance imaging (MRI) possibly being of assistance in delineating the percentage of tendon remaining intact. Partial tears can be treated with protection, followed by range of motion and progressive strengthening. If the patient is still symptomatic, the tendon can be released completely, debrided, or repaired back to the radial tuberosity. Complete tears can be classified as acute (<4 weeks) and chronic (>4 weeks). Acute tears can be repaired using a one- or two-incision technique. Chronic tears present a difficult problem with regard to direct repair. The biceps tendon usually retracts proximally into the distal arm and fibroses to the underlying brachialis. The bicipital aponeurosis will often limit this retraction. The goal of treatment is anatomic repair of the tendon into the radial tuberosity. Loss of tendinous tissue and tendon length should be expected preoperatively. Autogenous grafts have been described in the literature by a number of authors. We have taken the results from these studies and expanded them with the use of allografts to bridge the gap in chronic biceps tendon disruptions. Our technique for repair of a chronic distal biceps tears is described.

- A 6-cm gap between the mobilized distal biceps muscle and the scarred tendon in the radial tuberosity is identified.
- A cryopreserved semitendinosus allograft is used for reconstruction.
- The graft is woven through the distal bicipital musculotendinous junction, brought distally and sutured to itself using a no. 2 Ethibond suture.
- The doubled tendon unit is fixed to the radial tuberosity with double fixation, using a trough and drill holes, as well as a suture anchor.

Lateral Ulnar Collateral Ligament

There have been no reported cases of allograft reconstruction of the lateral ulnar collateral ligament. In the classic article by O'Driscoll et al., 3 of 5 patients had reconstruction of the lateral ulnar collateral ligament, 2 with palmaris longus and 1 with triceps fascia autografts. Instability symptoms resolved in all patients in this series. There have been no studies looking at the use of allograft hamstrings in the treatment of posterolateral instability of the elbow. We present the following example of lateral ulnar collateral ligament reconstruction.

The patient was brought to the operating room where examination under anesthesia revealed a positive pivot shift for posterolateral rotatory instability of the elbow. Elbow arthroscopy revealed no intra-articular pathology. Lateral ulnar collateral ligament reconstruction was then performed using cryopreserved gracilis tendon. Utilizing the technique described by O'Driscoll for autogenous palmaris longus reconstruction, an allograft gracilis tendon was used to reconstruct the attenuated lateral ulnar collateral ligament.

At final follow-up, approximately 8 months after surgery, the patient subjectively noted excellent function of the shoulder and no longer had the subjective complaints that she had preoperatively. On examination, she had a stable elbow with full range of motion.

Lower Extremity

Anterior Cruciate Ligament

There has been little written on the use of soft-tissue allografts in ACL reconstruction. We recently performed a 2-year prospective study comparing autograft to allograft hamstring ACL reconstruction. Both clinical and functional data were assessed. This prospective investigation involved 70 patients, 41 of whom had soft tissue allograft and 29 with autograft double-stranded semitendinosus gracilis ACL reconstructions. Concomitant injuries were similar between the two cohorts. There was no statistical difference in Tegner and Lysholm functional scores. The number of normal and near-normal IKDC scores was equal as well. Side-to-side KT-1000 differences were 1.08 mm for the autografts and 0.68 mm for the allografts. This is the only study to compare soft tissue autografts and allografts for ACL reconstruction.

Posterolateral Corner Reconstruction

Reconstruction of chronic posterolateral corner injuries has been addressed by a number of authors. Multiple techniques have been proposed, ranging from tissue transfers to autograft and allograft reconstructions. All of these different techniques have displayed good results.

Posterior Cruciate Ligament Reconstruction

Reconstruction of the posterior cruciate ligament (PCL) is usually indicated in two different scenarios. First, an isolated grade III tear of the PCL (>1 cm of posterior translation) with patient complaints of instability is an indication for reconstruction of the PCL. Second, PCL reconstruction should be considered in the face of a multiple-ligament injured knee, when the central hinge of the knee (ACL/PCL) has been injured. We present a surgical case to exemplify both our indications for surgery and surgical technique.

A 16-year-old high school football player presented 3 days after being injured in the first game of his junior season. The patient recalled that three different players struck his right knee. He heard a loud "pop," then felt extreme pain in his knee, and was carried off the field. He was taken to an emergency department and had radiographs, which revealed an avulsion fracture of the lateral epicondyle. On examination, the patient had a large effusion and an active range of motion of 5 to 30 degrees. He had a 3+ Lachman, 3+ opening without end point with varus stress and normal valgus stability. Posterior drawer and dial testing could not be performed as a result of pain. Distal pulses were normal, and peroneal nerve function was 4−/5. A diagnosis of acute ACL, lateral collateral ligament (LCL), and posterior ligament complex (PLC) disruption was made, with suspicion of a PCL injury. The patient was placed in a straight-leg brace, instructed to keep the extremity iced and elevated, and scheduled for an MRI. The MRI revealed the suspected ACL, LCL, PLC, and PCL disruptions, as well as bimeniscal capsular disruptions (Fig. 10-4). At follow-up, the effusion had decreased to allow testing of the injured structures. A 3+ posterior drawer and, at 30 degrees of knee flexion, a 15-degree side-to-side difference in dial testing were observed (Fig. 10-5).

The patient was scheduled for acute operative repair of the PLC, ACL, and PCL tibialis allograft reconstruction, and meniscal repair or meniscectomy. Medial and lateral meniscal repairs were performed using the Fast-Fix (Smith and Nephew, Mansfield, MA) meniscal repair system. Standard endoscopic ACL reconstruction was completed using a continuous loop endobutton (Acufex, Smith and Nephew, Mansfield, MA) for femoral fixation. A single-bundle PCL was performed endoscopically using a posteromedial portal and a 70-degree scope. A biointerference screw was used for femoral fixation. Neither graft was secured in its tibial tunnel. Attention was then directed to the PLC. The extremity was exsanguinated and the tourniquet inflated to 300 mm Hg. A 10-cm longitudinal incision was made along the lateral knee, traveling just anterior to the biceps femoris and extending to Gerdy's tubercle distally. A large hematoma was evacuated, and the peroneal nerve was present in the center of the wound (Fig. 10-6). The iliotibial band and biceps femoris had been avulsed from their distal attachments. The peroneal nerve was dissected distally to the fibu-

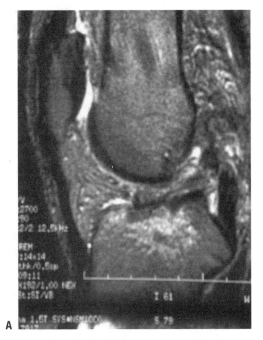
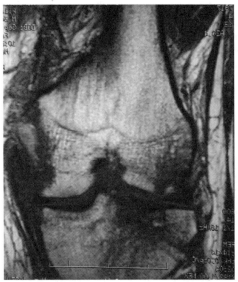

Figure 10-4   Sagittal **(A)** and coronal **(B)** MRIs of an ACL/PCL/PLC injured knee.

lar head and protected. The LCL had been avulsed from its fibular attachment. Posterior retraction of the lateral gastrocnemius revealed a musculotendinous disruption of the popliteus and avulsion of the popliteofibular ligament and joint capsule. Using suture anchors, the capsule was reattached to its tibial insertion, the popliteofibular ligament was reapproximated to the fibular head, and the popliteus was sutured with a no. 2 nonabsorbable suture. The LCL and biceps femoris were replaced into the fibula using suture anchors as well. The iliotibial band was repaired to

itself. An Intrafix (Mitek, Norwood, MA) device was used for the ACL tibial fixation and a screw-in-screw and washer were used for the PCL fixation. Postoperatively, the patient was placed in a locked hinged brace, made strictly non-weight-bearing, and started on CPM 0-40 up to 90 degrees for 8 weeks.

Medial Collateral Ligament Reconstruction

Although rarely necessary, reconstruction of the MCL of the knee can be performed with an allograft. Numerous studies have shown the excellent integration potential of allografts in an extra-articular setting. We present the following case of the reconstruction of a chronic grade III MCL injury with instability.

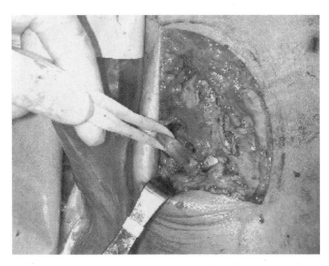

Figure 10-5   Positive, right-sided dial test indicating likely posterolateral corner injury.

Figure 10-6   Peroneal nerve in subcutaneous tissue associated with posterolateral corner injury.

A 19-year-old male presented with complaints of 2 years of left knee instability. He initially injured his knee while playing football and opted to continue participation in both football and as a hockey goaltender with a functional brace. Now in college, the patient was experiencing daily instability that limited him in his normal activities.

Upon his initial presentation, the patient had an antalgic gait with varus thrust and knee alignment. He had 3 + opening with valgus stress at both 0 and 30 degrees of flexion. He also had a 3 + Lachman test with no end point. The dial test, varus stress test in extension, and recurvatum test were normal. The patient's MRI revealed a complete tear of the ACL, a grade III tear of the MCL, and a capsular disruption of the medial meniscus. Full-length standing radiographs showed 12 degrees of knee varus.

The patient's condition indicated a staged procedure. First, an arthroscopic medial meniscal repair, an opening wedge tibial osteotomy (Arthrex, Naples, FL), and an Achilles allograft MCL reconstruction would be performed. The technique of Caborn et al. would be used for reconstructing both the MCL and the posterior oblique ligament (POL). A capsular avulsion red-red medial meniscal tear was repaired with three Fast-Fix (Smith and Nephew). The leg was then exsanguinated, and a direct medial 6-cm incision was over the distal insertion of the MCL. The pes anserinus tendons and MCL were retracted posteriorly, and an opening wedge tibial osteotomy with a 12-degree correction was completed. The Achilles allograft was prepared on a back table. A 10 × 30 mm bone plug was prepared. The tendinous portion of the graft was split and a whip stitch of a no. 2 Fiberwire (Arthrex) was placed in each limb. A 2-cm incision was made over the medial epicondyle, and the MCL origin was split longitudinally. A transepicondylar pin was placed across the femur and a 10 × 35 mm tunnel was drilled. The Allograft bone plug was press fit into the tunnel and fixed with a 10 × 28 mm biointerference screw. A Kelly clamp was then used to tunnel under the superficial MCL, and the tendinous limbs were brought antegrade to the level of the proximal tibia. Two 9 × 30 mm tunnels were drilled

into the proximal tibia at the relative isometric points for the MCL and POL. The graft limbs were then passed into these tunnels and the anterior limb was fixed with a 9 × 25 mm biointerference screw with the knee in 30 degrees of flexion, varus, and internal rotation. The posterior limb was fixed in a similar manner with the knee at 60 degrees of flexion (Fig. 10-7).

The patient began immediate protected weight-bearing and range of motion exercises. A tibialis ACL reconstruction was planned once his osteotomy was fully healed and the MCL integrated.

Medial Patellofemoral Ligament Reconstruction

In several cases, we have employed the use of a cryopreserved semitendinosus allograft for reconstruction of the medial patellofemoral ligament for patients with chronic recurrent patellar dislocation secondary to traumatic chronic insufficiency of the medial patellofemoral ligament. The method used is similar to that described by Drez, utilizing a free tendon graft that is secured by suture anchors to the adductor tubercle origin of the medial patellofemoral ligament and then secured to the proximal medial third of the patella. The following is an illustrative case.

A 19-year-old male presented 1 year after an acute patellar dislocation during a football game. This was reduced on the field by the trainer, and radiographs in the emergency room were negative for any type of osteochondral fracture. The patient was treated elsewhere with 4 weeks of immobilization in a straight-leg knee immobilizer, followed by physical therapy. Subsequent to this, the patient had 5 to 6 further lateral patellar dislocations over the following year. At the time of initial presentation, he was noted to have a normal Q-angle with markedly abnormal lateral excursion of the patella. The patient was brought to the operating room for arthroscopy and proximal realignment of the extensor mechanism. At the time of arthroscopy, it was noted that he had a grade II lesion of the medial patellar facet for which an arthroscopic chondroplasty was performed. An open proximal realignment was performed in combination

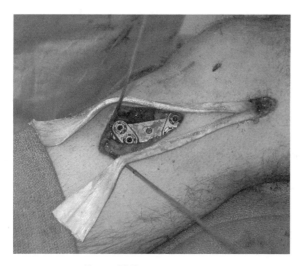 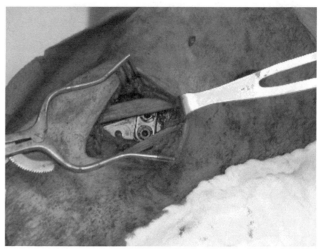

Figure 10-7   Reconstruction of the MCL with a split Achilles tendon allograft. An opening wedge tibial osteotomy was performed concomitantly.

with a lateral retinacular release. At the time of reconstruction, it was noted that the medial retinaculum and the medial patellofemoral ligament were markedly thin and attenuated. Imbrication of this tissue, as well as advancement of the vastus medialis obliquus (VMO), would have been insufficient to reconstruct the medial patellar restraints. A cryopreserved semitendinosus allograft was used to reconstruct the medial patellofemoral ligament. This was secured to the origin of the medial patellofemoral ligament through a transverse incision in the retinaculum, thus exposing the adductor tubercle. After creating a bleeding bone bed in this area, two bioabsorbable suture anchors were placed into the adductor tubercle, and two additional anchors were placed at the proximal medial border of the patella at the junction of the proximal third and the middle one third of the patella. The patella was reduced to recreate the normal lateral patellar excursion, and both sets of anchor sutures were passed through the semitendinosus allograft. The graft was then folded back on itself and sutured to itself using a no. 2 nonabsorbable suture. Postoperatively, the patient was immobilized in extension for approximately 3 weeks, at which time range-of-motion exercises were begun. No active quadriceps exercises were allowed until 6 weeks postoperatively. At 1-year follow-up, the patient had returned to football with no further episodes of instability.

Patellar Tendon Reconstruction

Allograft reconstruction of the extensor mechanism is commonly associated with chronic attenuation after total knee arthroplasty. Also, allografts have been used in revision or in chronic and undiagnosed patellar tendon rupture. Primary, acute patellar tendon ruptures are universally manageable through primary repair. Chronic, neglected tears and retears often require augmentation and, in extreme cases,

complete reconstruction of the patellar tendon unit. We present an illustrative case below.

A 27-year-old male presented with complaints of 7 weeks of left knee pain. He initially injured his knee during a pickup basketball game. He heard a "pop" and was unable to return to play. On examination, the patient was found to have a complete patellar tendon rupture and was indicated for operative repair, which was performed 8 weeks postinjury. Three weeks later, the patient presented for follow-up and had an obvious disruption of his repair. On returning to the operating room, the patient was found to have a deep wound infection. Irrigation and debridement were performed, and broad-spectrum antibiotics were started. *Pseudomonas* and *Enterobacter* were cultured from the wound. After 6 weeks of antibiotics and the presence of a sterile surgical wound, the patient was returned to the operating room for an Achilles tendon allograft reconstruction of the patellar tendon (Fig. 10-8A). The patient began range of motion at 6 weeks and at 4 months obtained a range of motion of 0 to 90 degrees with integration of the Achilles graft (Fig. 10-8B).

Achilles Tendon Reconstruction

Little has been written regarding allograft hamstring reconstruction of the Achilles tendon. For treatment of chronic Achilles tendon ruptures, reruptures, or tendinosis, most authors recommend either the advancement of local tissues or transfer of the plantaris or flexor hallucis longus (FHL) muscle-tendon unit. Tendinosis and chronic unrepaired disruptions of the Achilles tendon need to be reconstructed rather than repaired. Numerous procedures have been described that involve the transfer of the FHL, flexor digitorum longus (FDL), or plantaris musculotendinous unit into the deficient Achilles tendon. These transfers are indi-

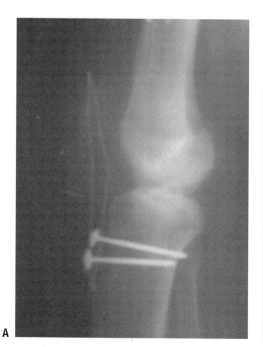
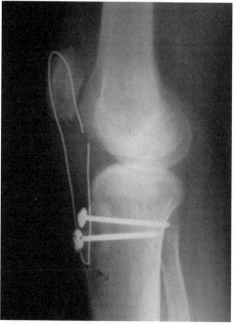

A   **B**

Figure 10-8   Initial **(A)** and final **(B)** radiographs of an Achilles tendon allograft reconstruction of a failed, infected patellar tendon repair.

cated when a gap in the Achilles is present when the foot is put in neutral or if greater than 50% of the tendon has been removed as a result of degeneration or poor tissue quality. These transferred tendons are meant to provide additional vascularity, as well as structural support. Soft-tissue allografts provide immediate structural support, as well as a scaffold for ingrowth of new, vascular fibrous tissue.

A 42-year-old male truck driver presented with complaints of many years of intermittent left Achilles pain and swelling. He has tried stretching, nonsteroidal anti-inflammatory drugs, and heel lifts without improvement. His MRI revealed fusiform enlargement of his Achilles tendon with extensive degenerative tendinosis. As a result of his conservative measures failure for more than 1 year, the patient's condition indicated Achilles tendon debridement and reconstruction. The preoperative plan was to reconstruct the Achilles tendon if greater than 50% of the tendon had degenerated. The patient's left lower extremity was exsanguinated. A 10-cm incision was made just medial to the Achilles tendon through skin and subcutaneous tissue only. The peritenon was identified, split longitudinally, and elevated off the tendon. The Achilles was firm and rubbery, with little resemblance to a normal tendon for the large majority of its length and width. The central 75% of the tendon was excised, leaving only the normal periphery remaining. On a back table, an 8 mm × 255 mm tibialis anterior allograft was prepared with a no. 5 nonabsorbable "baseball" stitch in either end of the graft. The allograft was then woven through the remaining Achilles tendon and, with the foot in gravity plantarflexion, sutured to the remaing tendon and itself. The paratenon is closed separatel and the skin secured with interrupted nylon sutures. The patient was then placed in a gravity plantarflexion below-knee cast and remained non-weight-bearing for 6 weeks with weekly cast changes. The patient did well postoperatively and returned to work as a truck driver at 6 months.

Proximal Hamstring Avulsion

Proximal hamstring avulsions are relatively uncommon when compared with the more common midsubstance musculotendinous hamstring tears that are seen in the orthopaedic surgeon's office. Most of these have been described as a result of water skiing. Proximal hamstring avulsions are one of the rare indications for surgery after hamstring tears. We present the use of a semitendinosus allograft for surgical reconstruction after a chronic proximal hamstring rupture.

A 42-year-old male presented with a proximal hamstring rupture after he slipped down some stairs and noted some acute pain and a tearing sensation in the area of the proximal hamstring and buttocks. His condition indicated nonoperative treatment. After several months of physical therapy, however, he noted persistent fatigue, weakness, and deformity. Despite continuing a rigorous stretching and strengthening program, he was unable to return to his normal activities of tennis and golf without symptoms. Approximately 9 months after his injury, he presented to our office with an obvious proximal hamstring avulsion with distal retraction of all three hamstring muscles. Another course of physical therapy and isokinetic strengthening was pre-

scribed; however, the patient returned 3 months later with the same symptoms and was not happy with his abilities.

Approximately 1 year after injury, the patient was brought to the operating room for attempted repair/reconstruction of the proximal hamstrings. At the time of surgery, the conjoined tendon of the semitendinosus and biceps was mobilized and reattached directly to the ischial tuberosity through drill holes. The semimembranosus, however, had retracted distally and there was a large gap of approximately 10 cm after mobilization between the proximal end of the semimembranosus and the ischial tuberosity. A semitendinosus allograft was used to bridge the gap. The allograft was weaved through the proximal end of the semimembranosus and then attached to the ischial tuberosity via suture anchors and drill holes. Postoperatively, the patient was maintained in a brace, keeping his knee at 90 degrees of flexion and his hip extended for approximately 6 weeks, and the patient was started on a gradual rehabilitation program. After a lengthy rehabilitation program, the patient was able to return to all his activities and was very satisfied with his outcome, being able to return to golf and tennis approximately 6 months after surgery.

SUGGESTED READING

Altchek DW, Hyman J, Williams R, et al. Management of MCL injuries of the elbow in throwers. Tech Shoulder Elbow Surg 2000;1:73–81.

American Association of Tissue Banks. Standards for tissue banking: 2001 update. Hollywood, FL: American Association of Tissue Banks, 2001.

Arnoczky SP, Warren RF, Ashlock MA. Replacement of the anterior cruciate ligament using patellar tendon allograft: an experimental study in the dog. J Bone Joint Surg 1986;68A:376–385.

Borden PS, Kantaras AT, Caborn DN. Medial collateral ligament reconstruction with allograft using a double bundle technique. Arthroscopy 2002;18(4):E19.

Bowen MK, Warren RF, Cooper DE. In Insall J (ed): Surgery of the Knee. New York: Churchill Livingstone, 1993:505–554.

Buck BE, Malinin TI, Brown MD. Bone transplantation and human immunodeficiency virus: an estimate of risk of acquired immunodeficiency virus (AIDS). Clin Orthop 1989;240:129–136.

Chrisman OD, Snook GA. Reconstruction of lateral ligament tears of the ankle. An experimental study and clinical evaluation of seven patients treated by a new modification of the Elmslie procedure. J Bone Joint Surg 1969;51:904–912.

Coughlin MJ, Matt V, Schenck RC Jr. Augmented lateral ankle reconstruction using a free gracilis graft. Orthopedics 2002;25:31–35.

Emerson RH Jr, Head WC, Malinin TI. Extensor mechanism reconstruction with allograft after total knee arthroplasty. Clin Orthop 1994;303:79–85.

Harner CD, Olson, E, Irrgang JJ, et al. Allograft versus autograft anterior cruciate ligament reconstruction. Clin Orthop 1996;324:134–144.

Horibe S, Shino K, Nagano J, et al. Replacing the medial collateral ligament with an allogeneic tendon graft. An experimental canine study. J Bone Joint Surg 1990;72B:1044–1049.

Jackson DW, Corsetti J, Simon TM. Biologic incorporation of allograft anterior cruciate ligament replacement. Clin Orthop 1996;324:126–133.

Jackson DW, Grood ES, Wilcox P, et al. The effects of processing techniques on the mechanical properties of bone-anterior cruciate ligament-bone allografts: an experimental study in goats. Am J Sports Med 1988;6:101–105.

Jones HP, Lemos MJ, Schepsis AA. Salvage of failed acromioclavicular joint reconstruction using autogenous semitendinosus tendon from the knee. Am J Sports Med 2001;29:234–237.

Larson RV, Simonian PT. Semitendinosus augmentation of acute patellar tendon repair with immediate mobilization. Am J Sports Med 1995;23:82–86.

Mandelbaum BR, Bartolozzi A, Carney B. A systematic approach to reconstruction of neglected tears of the patellar tendon. A case report. Clin Orthop 1988;235:268–271.

Noyes FR, Barber SD, Mangine RE. Bone-patellar ligament-bone and fascia lata allografts for reconstruction of the anterior cruciate ligament. J Bone Joint Surg 1990;72A:1125–1136.

Noyes FR, Barber-Westin SD. Reconstruction of the anterior cruciate ligament with human allograft. Comparison of early and later results. J Bone Joint Surg 1996;78A:524–537.

O'Driscoll SW, Bell DF, Morrey BF. Posterolateral rotatory instability of the elbow. J Bone Joint Surg 1991;73:440–446.

Peterson RK, Shelton WR, Bomboy AL. Allograft versus autograft patellar tendon anterior cruciate ligament reconstruction: a 5-year follow-up. Arthroscopy 2001;17:9–13.

Prokopis PM, Schepsis AA. Allograft use in ACL reconstruction. Knee 1999;6:75–85.

Schepsis AA, Jones H, Haas AL. Achilles tendon disorders in athletes. Am J Sports Med 2002;30:287–305.

Shelton WR, Treacy SH, Dukes AD, et al. Use of allografts in knee reconstruction: I. Basic science aspects and current status. J Am Acad Orthop Surg 1998;6:165–168.

Shino K, Nakata K, Horibe S, et al. Quantitative evaluation after arthroscopic anterior cruciate ligament reconstruction. Allograft versus autograft. Am J Sports Med 1993;21:609–616.

Shino K, Inoue M, Horibe S, et al. Maturation of allograft tendons transplanted into the knee. An arthroscopic and histologic study. J Bone Joint Surg 1988;70-B:556–560.

Wascher DC, Summa CD. Reconstruction of chronic rupture of the extensor mechanism after patellectomy. Clin Orthop 1998;357:135–140.

Wilk KE, Arrigo C, Andrews JR. Rehabilitation of the elbow in the throwing athlete. J Orthop Sports Phys Ther 1993;17:305–317.

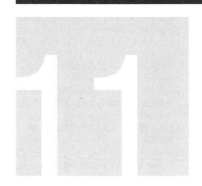

PRINCIPLES OF ARTHROSCOPIC SURGERY

MARK H. GETELMAN
MARK J. ALBRITTON

The practice of arthroscopic surgery continues to advance at a rapid pace. Arthroscopic techniques have significantly changed the approach to the diagnosis and treatment of orthopaedic joint pathologies. A high degree of clinical accuracy, combined with low morbidity, has encouraged the use of arthroscopy to assist in diagnosis, to determine prognosis, and often to provide treatment. Two critical aspects of arthroscopic surgery are the correct placement of arthroscopic portals and the avoidance of complications. During arthroscopy of any joint, accurate placement of the portals is essential to adequately accomplish the intended goal of the procedure without complications. Fortunately, complications during or after arthroscopy are infrequent and are usually minor. Most complications can be prevented with careful and thorough preoperative and intraoperative planning and attention to the details of arthroscopic techniques.

KNEE ARTHROSCOPY

Portals

Critical components of knee arthroscopy are appropriate illumination and distention of the joint, as well as accurate placement of the portals. With improper portal position, it may be difficult to obtain adequate visualization of the intra-articular anatomy and to maneuver the instruments to all locations within the joint. Improperly placed portals can cause the surgeon to force the arthroscope or instrument into position and can result in articular injury, instrument damage or breakage, and/or other problems. Accurate portal placement can be obtained by a thorough understanding of the anatomy. Specifically, the surgeon must know where the medial and lateral joint lines are, the border of the patella and patella tendon, and the posterior contours of the medial and lateral femoral condyles. These areas can be marked with a skin-marking pen before joint distention.

The standard portals for diagnostic knee arthroscopy are anterolateral, anteromedial, posteromedial, and superolateral.

Anterolateral and Anteromedial Portals

- The anterolateral and anteromedial portals are made with the knee in flexion.
- Vertical or horizontal incisions are placed adjacent to the patella tendon and approximately 1 cm above the joint line, typically just below the inferior pole of the patella (Fig. 11-1).
- The scalpel is used to incise the skin only, and the joint capsule is penetrated with a blunt-tipped obturator, and aimed toward the notch to avoid articular cartilage injury.
- If the portal is placed too close to the joint line, the anterior horn of the meniscus can be damaged.

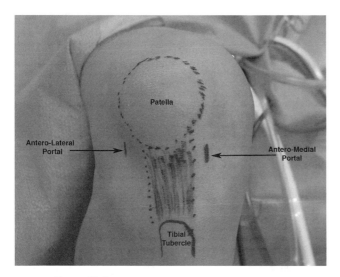

Figure 11-1 Knee landmarks and portal locations.

- Also, the arthroscope can pass either through or beneath the anterior horn of the meniscus, resulting in damage to the anterior horn or difficulty in maneuvering the arthroscope within the joint.
- If the portal is placed too superior to the joint line, it prevents the view of the posterior horns of the menisci and other posterior structure.
  - An arthroscope placed immediately adjacent to the edge of the patellar tendon can go through the fat pad, causing difficulty in viewing and maneuvering the arthroscope in the joint.
- With the use of a 4-mm diameter, 30-degree oblique arthroscope through an appropriately placed anterolateral portal, the structures within the knee joint can be visualized.

Posteromedial Portal

- The posteromedial portal is positioned in a soft spot formed by the posteromedial edge of the femoral condyle and the posteromedial edge of the tibia.
  - This location can be palpated with the knee flexed to 90 degrees.
  - With the knee fully distended and flexed to 90 degrees, this portion of the compartment will balloon out.
- The location of this portal is approximately 1 cm above the posteromedial joint line and approximately 1 cm posterior to the posteromedial margin of the femoral condyle.
- To aid with precise location of this portal, the arthroscope can be inserted through the notch along the lateral portion of the medial femoral condyle (modified Gillquist view) and into the posterior aspect of the knee to visualize the placement of a spinal needle in the posteromedial portal (Fig. 11-2).
- The arthroscope's light illuminates the area around the portal, allowing visualization of the saphenous vein, which should be avoided when making this portal.
- This portal is always established with a blunt-tipped obturator.

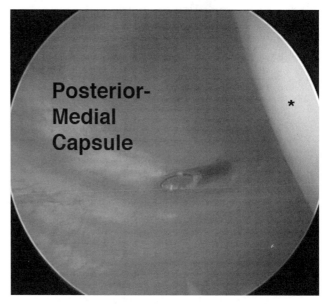

Figure 11-2 Arthroscopic view from the anterolateral portal showing insertion of a spinal needle, localizing the best position for establishing the posteromedial portal. Asterisk indicates the posterior medial femoral condyle.

Superolateral Portal

- The superolateral portal is typically used for inflow or outflow.
- It can also be useful for viewing and accessing the dynamics of the patellofemoral articulation and can be helpful for excising a medial plica.
- This portal is located just lateral to the quadriceps tendon and about 2 to 3 cm superior to the superolateral corner of the patella.
- Viewing the patellofemoral joint from this portal using a 70-degree arthroscope allows evaluation of patellar tracking, patellar congruity, and lateral overhang of the patella as the knee is inspected through a range of motion.

Posterolateral Portal

- The posterolateral portal is made with the knee flexed about 90 degrees and the joint maximally distended.
- The posterolateral portal is about 2 cm above the posterolateral joint line at the posterior edge of the iliotibial band and the anterior edge of the biceps femoris tendon.
- Care must be taken not to place the portal too far posterior because the common peroneal nerve can be injured.
- A small skin incision is made, and the posterior edge of the lateral femoral condyle is palpated with a blunt trocar.
- By slipping off the posterior condyle, directing it slightly inferiorly, the sheath will be directed into the posterolateral compartment.
- Be cautious not to damage the articular surface of the posterior femoral condyle with the trocar.
- Care must be taken not to plunge in, because the popliteal space could be inadvertently entered.

- The arthroscope may be positioned into the posterolateral joint via the anteromedial portal (similar to the Gillquist view), and a spinal needle can again be used to localize the appropriate position.

Midpatellar Portal

- The optional midpatellar portal is used to improve the viewing of the anterior compartment structures, the lateral meniscocapsular structures, and the popliteus tunnel.
- This portal is also used to minimize crowding with the arthroscope during procedures requiring several accessory instruments.
- These portals are located just off the medial and lateral edges of the midpatella at the broadest portion of the patella.

Far Medial and Lateral Portals

- The accessory far medial and lateral portals can be used for bringing accessory instruments into the knee.
- They are located 2 to 3 cm medial or lateral to the standard anteromedial and anterolateral portals.
- Medially, these portals are near the anterior edge of the tibial collateral ligament; laterally, they should be well anterior to the fibular collateral ligament and popliteus tendon.
- One technique is to insert a spinal needle through the skin and capsule and into the compartment under direct vision with the arthroscope.
- The needle can be adjusted and directed to its desired location to help ensure the instrument will be able to reach this location easily.
- There can be increased risk of damage to the meniscus, collateral ligaments, and the articular surface of the femoral condyle with these portals, and extreme care should be exercised when making them.

Transpatellar Tendon Portal

- The transpatellar tendon portal is located approximately 1 cm inferior to the inferior pole of the patella through the patellar tendon and is angulated to pass above the fat pad.
- This portal incision is made through the skin and subcutaneous tissue with the knee flexed 90 degrees.
- The tendon is then split with the sharp trocar.
- The knee is then extended to 45 degrees, and the sheath and obturator are aimed toward the superomedial compartment.
  - This helps prevent passing the arthroscope into the fat pad.
- This portal can be used for central viewing or grasping.
- This portal is not recommended secondary to the risk of injuring the patella tendon and potential for anterior knee pain.

Complications

In 1986, Small presented a report on 395,566 arthroscopies—375,069 of which were knee arthroscopies—from the Committee on Complications of the Arthroscopy Association of North America. The overall complication rate was 0.56%. In the knee, there were 239 infections, 12 vascular injuries, 683 cases of thrombophlebitis, and 190 cases of reflex sympathetic dystrophy. The complication rate in meniscal repair was 2.4%, including 30 saphenous nerve injuries, 6 peroneal nerve injuries, 22 infections, 3 vascular injuries, and 4 cases of thrombophlebitis. With anterior cruciate ligament procedures, the complication rate was 1.8%, including 7 stiff knees, 1 infection, 2 neurological injuries, and 12 loose or poorly placed staples.

In 1988, Small published a prospective study of complications from the Arthroscopy Association of North America. In this series of 8,741 knee arthroscopies, the overall complication rate was 1.8%. Sixty-five percent of the complications were hemarthrosis. The complication rate for meniscal repair had decreased to 1.29%. The complication rate for medial meniscectomy was 1.78%. Only one neurological injury was recorded, a saphenous nerve injury during a medial meniscal repair. The complication rate for anterior cruciate ligament surgery was only 2%, and no neurological or vascular injuries were reported.

At present, complications associated with knee arthroscopy occur at a rate similar to that reported by Small. Complications may increase with the difficulty and length of the case. Saphenous and peroneal nerve injuries are still being reported with arthroscopic meniscal repairs. However, with all inside meniscal repair techniques, the incidence may decrease. The incidence of arthrofibrosis associated with anterior cruciate ligament reconstruction is increased when meniscal repair is performed concurrently. Likewise, the incidence of infection associated with anterior cruciate ligament reconstructions is slightly increased when the reconstruction is performed in conjunction with meniscal repair. The reasons can probably be attributed to the additional exposure, surgical time, and potential for joint contamination during the passing and retrieving of needles.

Careful attention to detail during surgery—including proper sterilization techniques, handling of the graft, and appropriate preparation and draping—can help to prevent postoperative infections. When a postoperative knee infection occurs, urgent and thorough arthroscopic irrigation and debridement are indicated with repeat irrigation and debridement at 48 to 72 hours if the patient is still symptomatic. Anterior cruciate ligament grafts can be salvaged if no extensive deterioration of the graft is present. The appropriate intravenous antibiotics generally are prescribed for 2 to 3 weeks, followed by oral antibiotics to complete a 6-week course of antibiotic treatment.

Early surgical intervention for ligamentous injuries and meniscal repairs before regaining muscular tone and motion is associated with arthrofibrosis. Allowing the patient to regain motion before surgery greatly decreases the incidence of postoperative stiffness and arthrofibrosis.

Reflex sympathetic dystrophy is a poorly understood condition that possibly could be decreased by better patient selection, decreased operating time, and early physical therapy. The best way to help minimize any complication is proper patient selection, through preoperative evaluation and operative plan, meticulous and skilled surgical technique, and close patient follow-up.

SHOULDER ARTHROSCOPY

Shoulder arthroscopy has become extremely useful as both a diagnostic and therapeutic tool. The advantages of arthroscopic versus open procedures include less invasive surgery, muscle preservation, smaller incisions, improved visualization and access, and quicker rehabilitation.

Portals

- Routine diagnostic arthroscopy is usually carried out through an anterior and a posterior portal (Fig. 11-3).
- Additional portals are used for special applications.

Posterior Portal

- The posterior portal insertion point is chosen after palpating the posterior shoulder anatomy and balloting the humeral head.
- The exact position is dependent on the thickness of the soft tissue and bony anatomy.
- In the average-sized individual, the portal is approximately 2 cm inferior and 1 cm medial to the posterior lateral acromion.
  - For larger patients, the portal is more inferior and medial.
- Make a small incision through the skin without piercing the muscle or capsule.
- Insert the arthroscope with a tapered-tip obturator through the muscle until the posterior head is palpated, while the opposite hand palpates the anterior shoulder joint.
- Balloting the head back and forth helps establish the position of the joint line.

- Direct the cannula medial to slide off the humeral head to feel the step-off between the head and the glenoid.
- Finally, insert the cannula through the posterior capsule into the joint (usually feeling a definitive pop).
  - A common error is inserting the cannula too lateral or proximal.

Anterior Portal

- The anterior portal should be created before performing the diagnostic examination.
  - It is necessary for outflow and to palpate the anatomy.
- The ideal location can only be determined after visualizing the anterior anatomy.
- Note the condition of the superior labrum and anterior ligaments before determining which anterior portal to make.

Anterior-superior Portal

- If anterior reconstruction or superior labrum, anterior to posterior (SLAP) lesion require repair, a high anterior-superior portal should be made.
  - This helps improve visualization of the anterior labral anatomy and allows adequate room for an anterior mid-glenoid portal.
- The anterior-superior portal can be made with an outside in technique.
- Insert a spinal needle into the skin 1 cm off the anterior lateral corner of the acromion into the joint through the rotator interval, just anterior to the biceps tendon.
- Angle the needle to approach the anterior anchor point of the biceps tendon.
- Make an incision at the needle puncture sight and insert a cannula with a tapered tip obturator.

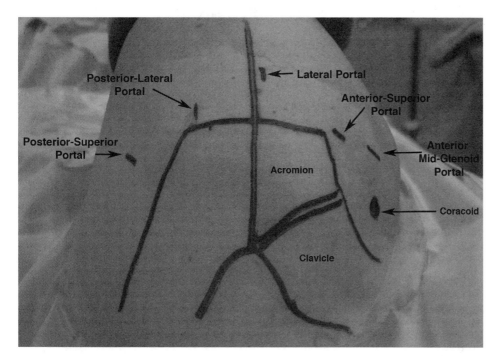

Figure 11-3 Shoulder landmarks and portal locations.

Midglenoid Portal

- When doing diagnostic arthroscopy and no SLAP repair or anterior reconstruction is planned, a standard anterior midglenoid portal can be established.
- To create this portal, an inside-out technique may be used.
- Pass the tip of the arthroscope into the anterior triangle between the biceps and subscapularis tendons.
- Then angle the scope a few degrees superiorly and laterally, and hold it against the anterior capsule.
- Remove the scope, insert a taper-tipped guide rod (Wissinger rod) into the cannula, puncture the anterior capsule, and tent the skin.
- Make a small incision adjacent to the guide rod tip (it should be approximately 2 cm inferior and 1 cm medial to the anterior lateral edge of the acromion).
- Pass the guide rod out of the incision and pass a cannula over the rod and insert it into the joint.
- Outflow can be connected to the cannula, the scope can be inserted into the posterior-superior portal, and the diagnostic arthroscopy can be performed.

Subacromial Access

- The subacromial bursa diagnostic examination is performed through the already established posterior-superior portal and the anterior-superior portal.
- Using the posterior portal incision, a cannula with a tapered tip obturator can be directed into the bursal space.
  - This can be achieved by sliding the cannula between the acromion and rotator cuff.
  - It can then be positioned under the anterior-lateral portion of the acromion.
- Next, a Wissinger rod can be placed through the cannula and passed underneath the coracoacromial ligament and continued out the anterior-superior portal incision.
- A cannula can then be placed over the rod and slid into the bursa.
- In addition, a third bursal portal, the lateral acromial portal, is helpful when working in the subacromial space.
- The portal is made approximately 3 cm off of the lateral border of the acromion.
- The anterior-posterior position of this portal is critical when performing an arthroscopic rotator cuff repair.
- To ensure correct position of your portal, a spinal needle should first be inserted into the bursa to help locate the correct position.
- An incision is made where the needle was removed and a cannula is inserted into the bursa.
- A standard reference point is a line drawn perpendicular to the lateral margin of the acromion in line with the posterior aspect of the acromioclavicular joint.

Supraspinatus Portal

- An additional portal, preferred by some surgeons, is the supraspinatus (Neviaser) portal that is used for inflow or for visualization of the anterior glenoid.

- This portal is placed in the corner of the supraspinatus fossa and oriented slightly anterior and lateral.
- It should also be placed with the arm adducted and the trocar angled posteriorly to avoid injury to the tendinous portion of the rotator cuff.

Complications

Complications associated with shoulder arthroscopy performed by experienced arthroscopic shoulder surgeons are uncommon. Portal placement and maneuvering in the shoulder can be more difficult than the knee as a result of the thickness of the muscles surrounding the shoulder. There are greater chances for complications as the procedures become more complex.

Neurovascular injury is a concern with any arthroscopy, and the shoulder is no different. Excessive traction on the shoulder or improper positioning can lead to transient or permanent nerve injury. Reports have indicated transient paresthesia rates as high as 30% when performing shoulder arthroscopy with traction. Anterior portal placement risks neurovascular injury if the portal is placed too medial or inferior. Posterior portal placement risks injury to the axillary nerve if placed too inferior or lateral and risks injury to the suprascapular nerve if placed too medial.

Although infection is a concern with any surgical procedure, the incidence with shoulder arthroscopy is extremely low. Limited exposure, the rich blood supply, and the irrigation solution minimize the chances for infection. Sterile technique is critical in infection prevention, and this can be accomplished through careful preparation, appropriate draping, and meticulous surgical technique.

Infection should be an infrequent complication because of the limited incisions, the rich vascularity about the joint, and the dilutional effect of the irrigating solution. However, infection can occur with violations of sterile technique.

ANKLE ARTHROSCOPY

Portals

Proper portal placement is critical to perform successful diagnostic and therapeutic ankle arthroscopy. Improperly placed portals can make diagnosis and treatment extremely difficult. A thorough understanding of ankle anatomy is critical to avoid complications.

Anterior Portals

- The anteromedial and anterolateral portals are the primary anterior portals used in ankle arthroscopy.
- The placement of the anteromedial portal is just medial to the anterior tibialis tendon at the joint line.
  - At this location, there is a premalleolar depression that often bulges in the presence of an effusion.
  - The appropriate position can be determined by first placing a 22-gauge needle at the anticipated position.
- When confirmed, the portal is established by making a skin incision superficially and then bluntly spreading through the soft tissue with a mosquito clamp.

- A blunt-tipped obturator with a small diameter cannula is then advanced into the joint.
- Care must be taken to avoid injuring the saphenous vein and nerve as they cross the ankle joint on the anterior aspect of the medial malleolus.
  - The anterolateral portal is placed just lateral to the peroneus tertius tendon at or slightly proximal to the joint line.
  - A branch of the superficial peroneal nerve, the intermediate dorsal cutaneous nerve, passes over the inferior extensor retinaculum, crosses the common extensor tendons of the fourth and fifth digits, and runs toward the third metatarsal space before dividing into the dorsal digital branches.
  - The other branch of the superficial peroneal nerve, the medial dorsal cutaneous nerve, passes over the common extensor tendons.
  - It parallels the extensor hallucis longus and then divides into three dorsal digital branches distal to the inferior extensor retinaculum.
  - These nerve branches need to be avoided during portal placement.
- An additional anterior portal is the anterocentral portal.
  - It may be developed between the tendons of the extensor digitorum communis at the joint line.
  - The portal is placed between the tendons to help decrease risk of injuring the dorsalis pedis artery, branches of the deep peroneal nerve, and medial branches of the superficial peroneal nerve.
  - The dorsalis pedis artery and the deep peroneal nerve run deep in the interval between the extensor hallucis longus and the extensor digitorum communis tendons.
  - In the past, this portal has been used to allow easier passage of instruments and the arthroscope from the anterior and posterior compartments.
- However, the use of this portal is strongly discouraged because of the high potential for complications.

Accessory Anterior Portals

- Anterior accessory portals can be useful while excising soft tissue or bony lesions in the medial and lateral gutters.
- The anterolateral and anteromedial accessory portals are commonly used.
- The accessory anteromedial portal is established 0.5 to 1 cm inferior and 1 cm anterior to the anterior border of the medial malleolus.
  - This portal is particularly helpful for removing ossicles inherent to the deep deltoid ligament while viewing from the standard anteromedial portal.
- The accessory anterolateral portal is established 1 cm anterior to and just distal to the tip of the anterior border of the lateral malleolus, near the anterior talofibular ligament.
  - This portal is useful for removing ossicles and probing the anterior and posterior talofibular ligaments.

Posterior Portals

- Posterior portals may be established posteromedial, posterolateral, or trans-Achilles.

- The posterolateral portal, the most commonly used and the safest, is placed just lateral to the Achilles tendon and 1.0 to 1.5 cm proximal to the tip of the fibula.
  - There are branches of the sural nerve and the small saphenous vein that must be avoided when establishing this portal.
- The trans-Achilles portal is made at the same level as the posterolateral, but through the central portion of the Achilles tendon.
  - The portal was originally designed to allow a posterior two-portal technique, while avoiding injury to the neurovascular structures medial to the tendon.
  - This portal has been discouraged because it does not allow easy mobility of the arthroscope and instruments and may lead to increased morbidity of the Achilles tendon.
- The posteromedial portal is established just medial to the Achilles tendon at the level of the joint.
  - The posterior tibial artery, tibial nerve, flexor hallucis longus tendon, and flexor digitorum longus tendon must be avoided.
  - Also, the calcaneal nerve and its branches divide from the tibial nerve proximal to the ankle joint and run in an interval between the tibial nerve and the Achilles tendon.
  - This portal is also discouraged because of the high potential for serious complications.

Accessory Posterior Portals

- The accessory posterolateral portal is established 1 to 1.5 cm lateral to the standard posterolateral portal and at the same level or slightly higher.
- Extreme caution must be used to avoid injury to the peroneal artery, small saphenous vein, and sural nerve.
- This portal is useful for removing posterior loose bodies and for debridement and drilling of very posterior osteochondral lesions of the talus.

Transmalleolar and Transtalar Portals

- Transmalleolar portals are used to establish better access to the osteochondral lesions of the talar dome.
  - These portals are particularly useful for drilling Kirschner wires through the tibia or fibula into the talar dome under arthroscopic visualization.
  - It can also be helpful for bone grafting certain osteochondral lesions of the talus.
- Transtalar portals can be used to drill or bone graft osteochondral lesions of the talus.

Complications

Ankle arthroscopy is rapidly progressing as technology advances. Newer techniques continue to develop as equipment and instruments improve. As the number of arthroscopic procedures has increased and more demanding procedures have been developed, the opportunity for potential complications has also increased. The reported rates are significant and emphasize that extreme caution must be taken when performing ankle arthroscopy.

The most frequently reported complications are nerve injuries and infections. Other reported complications include synovial fistulae, adhesions, fractures, instrument breakage, and reflex sympathetic dystrophy. Most complications associated with ankle arthroscopy are neurologic. Neurovascular injuries can be caused by incorrect portal placement, prolonged or inappropriate distraction, or excessive tourniquet time. This usually involves a temporary paresthesia of the superficial nerves but can be associated with permanent paresthesia or paresis. Painful neuromas can also occur from nerves injured during surgery. The anteromedial portal is associated with injury to the greater saphenous vein or saphenous nerve. The anterocentral portal is not recommended because of the high risk of injuring the dorsalis pedis artery and deep peroneal nerve. The anterolateral portal is associated with significant risk to the superficial peroneal nerve. This is the most common nerve injured. Preoperatively, it is critical to mark out the path of the nerve and its branches to help avoid injury. Unfortunately, in some patients, particularly those who are obese, the nerve may not be seen directly or through transillumination. To help minimize potential for nerve damage, incisions should be made vertically and only through the skin, followed by careful blunt spreading of the subcutaneous tissue before penetrating the capsule. The posterolateral portal places the lesser saphenous vein and sural nerve at risk. The posteromedial portal should not be used due to the high risk of injury to the neurovascular bundle. If paresthesias or pain develop postoperatively, this should be carefully examined and documented. The patient should be informed of the findings and followed carefully. A positive Tinel's sign over a portal site may indicate a neurapraxia or neuroma formation.

The use of a tourniquet is helpful for ankle arthroscopy to improve visualization with a bloodless field. The complications associated with tourniquet use include paresthesias, paresis, thigh pain, and perhaps thrombophlebitis. Proper application, adequate padding, low pressures, and keeping tourniquet times as low as possible can minimize problems related to tourniquet use.

Many of these complications can be avoided by careful patient selection, a clear understanding of ankle anatomy, and meticulous surgical technique (especially with regard to portal placement and the use of blunt dissection down to the capsule). Assurance of clear vision by maintaining good fluid flow without overdistention, noninvasive traction, and the use of a small-joint (2.7-mm) scope and instruments help prevent intra-articular surgical damage.

ELBOW ARTHROSCOPY

Elbow arthroscopy has experienced remarkable growth and advancement in the treatment of elbow disorders. Although useful both for diagnosis and treatment, elbow arthroscopy can be demanding. With the proximity to the major neurovascular structures about the elbow, there is potential for injury, and a thorough understanding of anatomy is required.

Portals

■ The anterolateral portal, usually the standard diagnostic portal, typically is the first established after elbow distention (Fig. 11-4).

    ■ Anterolateral portals may include the distal anterolateral portal approximately 2 to 3 cm distal and 1

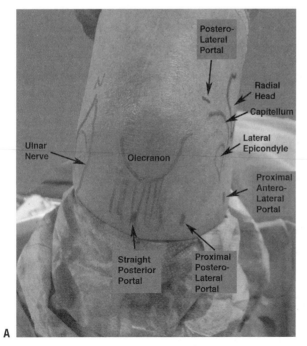
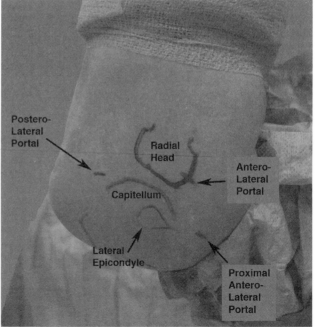

Figure 11-4 Elbow landmarks and portal locations. **A:** Lateral. **B:** Posterior.

cm anterior to the lateral epicondyle, the midantero-lateral portal just proximal and approximately 1 cm anterior to the palpable radiocapitellar joint, and the proximal anterolateral portal 2 cm proximal and 1 cm anterior to the lateral epicondyle.

- The proximal portal is significantly farther from the radial nerve than other anterolateral portal sites.
  - This portal allows for an excellent view of the anterior radiohumeral and ulnohumeral joints, as well as the anterior capsular margin.
  - The elbow is kept flexed during trocar insertion because extension brings the radial nerve closer to the joint, placing it more at risk.
  - A superficial skin incision should be made carefully, avoiding deep penetration to protect the lateral and posterior antebrachial cutaneous nerves.
  - Next, a hemostat is used to spread down to the capsule before entering the joint with a blunt trocar.
- The anteromedial portal is placed approximately 2 cm anterior and 2 cm distal to the medial epicondyle.
  - This portal can be established using an outside in technique with a spinal needle for localization.
  - The elbow should be flexed to 90 degrees as the portal is established.
  - The median nerve is approximately 1 to 2 cm anterior and lateral to this portal.
- The proximal anteromedial portal is located approximately 2 cm proximal to the medial epicondyle and immediately anterior to the intermuscular septum.
  - When making this portal, ensure the position of the intermuscular septum is clearly demarcated, then make a small portal incision, followed by blunt dissection.
  - The trocar is inserted over the anterior surface of the humerus aiming for the radial head.
  - Contact should be maintained with the anterior humerus at all times to reduce risk to the neurovascular structures.
  - This portal allows visualization of the anterior elbow, including the anterior joint capsule, medial condyle, coronoid process, trochlea, capitellum, and the radial head.
  - The radial head is best visualized from the proximal anteromedial portal.
  - The nerves at risk with this portal include the ulnar nerve, medial brachial cutaneous, medial antebrachial cutaneous, median nerve, and brachial artery.
- The posterolateral portal is located in the center of the anconeus triangle bordered by the radial head, lateral epicondyle, and the tip of the olecranon.
  - This portal can be used to visualize the posterior elbow structures, including the olecranon fossa.
  - The use of a 2.7-mm, 70-degree scope facilitates visualization of the radiocapitellar joint.
  - This portal allows debridement of the capitellum.
- The straight posterior portal is placed 3 cm posterior to the olecranon tip and approximately 2 cm medial to the posterolateral portal.
  - It can be used as a second posterior portal if needed.

- If the portal is placed too far medial, the ulnar nerve is at risk.
- The portal can be established under direct vision; appropriate position of the portal can be confirmed by placement of a spinal needle.
- In stiff elbows, the direct posterior portal can sometimes be more easily established than the posterolateral portal, and the use of a 2.7-mm arthroscope can make visualization of the posterior compartment easier.

Complications

Elbow arthroscopy is a technically demanding procedure in which high attention to detail is critical to help prevent complications. Temporary or minor complications following elbow arthroscopy are not rare. In a review of 473 consecutive elbow arthroscopies by Kelly et al., complications occurred in 11%. The reported prevalence of neurologic complications after elbow arthroscopy has ranged from 0% to 14%. In this study, there were no permanent neurologic injuries, whereas 10 of the 473 (2.5%) patients did suffer transient nerve palsies. The nerve-to-portal distances increase with joint distension although the nerve does not move further away from the capsule. Also, capsular distension is often difficult in elbows with contractures.

Nerve injuries associated with elbow arthroscopy can result from compression, local anesthetic, direct trauma, prolonged tourniquet compression, and/or forearm compression from wrapping too tight. When making incisions, cutting only through the skin and dragging the skin rather than making a stab, can help protect the superficial nerves.

Permanent nerve injuries from transections of all three major nerves have been reported. The anterolateral and the anteromedial portals are the most likely to be associated with nerve injury due to the closeness of the radial, posterior interosseous, ulnar, and median nerves. The distances between the nerves and the portals can be increased substantially by flexing the elbow to 90 degrees and distending the joint with fluid. With distention of the joint using 15 to 25 mL of fluid, the nerves can be displaced away from the portals, but the average intracapsular capacity of a stiff elbow is only about 6 mL. Therefore, in stiff elbows, the capsule cannot be distended away from the instruments.

To prevent serious complications of elbow arthroscopy, one must have a thorough understanding of the anatomy of the elbow and surrounding neurovascular structures, the effects of joint distention, and correct portal placement. In addition, recognition of the procedures that place specific nerves at risk, and excellent arthroscopic skills are also crucial. In conclusion, two critical aspects of arthroscopic surgery are: the correct placement of arthroscopic portals and the avoidance of complications. During arthroscopy of any joint, accurate placement of the portals is essential to adequately accomplish the intended goal of the procedure, and to do so without complications.

Fortunately, most can be prevented with careful and thorough preoperative and intraoperative planning and exquisite attention to detail.

SUGGESTED READING

Ferkel RD. Arthroscopic Surgery: The Foot and Ankle. Philadelphia: Lippincott-Raven, 1996.

Guhl JF. Foot and Ankle Arthroscopy, 2nd ed. Thorofare, NJ: Slack, 1993.

Kelly EW, Morrey BF, O'Driscoll SW. Complications of elbow arthroscopy. J Bone Joint Surg Am 2001;83:25.

Small NC. Complications in arthroscopy: the knee and other joints. Committee on Complications of the Arthroscopy Association of North America. Arthroscopy 1986;2:253–258.

Small NC. Complications in arthroscopic surgery performed by experienced arthroscopists. Arthroscopy 1988;4:215.

Snyder SJ. Shoulder Arthroscopy, 2nd ed. Philadelphia: Lippincott Williams & Wilkins, 2003.

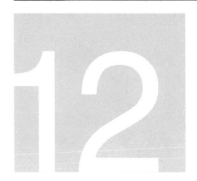

MEDICAL CONCERNS OF THE TEAM PHYSICIAN

JOSEPH BERNARD
PHILIP CRUZ
J. HERBERT STEVENSON
BRIAN D. BUSCONI

The team physician is faced with a variety of medical issues in athletes that can range from dermatologic conditions to cardiac anomalies. It is important for the team physician to be aware of common medical conditions that affect athletes, as well as their impact on safe participation. A sound understanding of these conditions allows for an accurate assessment and initiation of an effective treatment program. Common medical conditions that affect athletes are listed below with a focused overview, and pearls to diagnosis and effective treatment options are outlined. Keys to return to play and clearance are addressed for relevant conditions.

PULMONARY CONCERNS

EXERCISE-INDUCED BROCHOSPASM

Background

Exercise-induced asthma, more appropriately termed exercise-induced bronchospasm (EIB), describes the transient airway narrowing after exercise or physical activity that occurs in some individuals. Asthma (Fig. 12-1) is a common respiratory disease in many children and young adults, and exercise is one of the most common precipitating factors of an acute attack. EIB is caused by the loss of heat, water, or both from the lungs during exercise, as the ventilated air during exercise is drier and cooler than that in the respiratory tree. Between 80% and 90% of patients with asthma may also have EIB. However, there are many patients who only have bronchospasm associated with exercise. Stimuli thought to be associated with triggering EIB include environmental pollutants (such as found in indoor ice arenas, including a high level of nitrogen dioxide and carbon monoxide) and sulfur dioxide. Although swimmers have generally been described to be at lower risk secondary to their warm, humid environment, chlorine compounds in swimming pools have been described as a possible trigger in swimmers who do develop symptoms of EIB. A high prevalence has also been found in elite ski racers who race in cold/dry ambient conditions and distance runners associated with respiratory allergies. Other stimuli may include viral illness or cigarette smoking.

Diagnosis

History and Physical Examination
- Athletes complain of shortness of breath, chest tightness, coughing, or wheezing associated with participation in their sport or with exercise.

A

Cross section

B

Mucus plugs

Swelling

Constriction

Cross section

Close-up of a bronchiole, showing spasm, edema

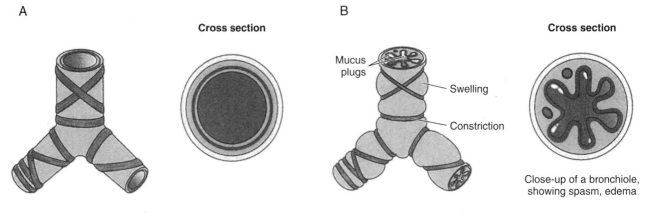

Figure 12-1   Asthma. **(A)** Normal bronchiole and **(B)** bronchiole under asthma attack. (From Willis MC. Medical Terminology: The Language of Health Care. Baltimore, MD: Williams & Wilkins, 1996: 233.)

- They may notice a decrease in their exercise endurance as well.
- Symptoms typically occur during or shortly after onset of exercise, peak 8 to 15 minutes after exercise, and spontaneously resolve within 30 to 60 minutes.
  - A refractory period of up to 3 hours after recovery is often seen, during which time there is less bronchospasm seen with exercise.
- When initially evaluating an athlete for EIB, it is important to distinguish between exacerbation of chronic asthma and EIB.
- Types and levels of exercise that precipitate the problem and the exact symptoms that develop should be addressed.
- Common physical examination findings observed include cough and expiratory wheezing after exercise.

Testing

- Confirmation of the diagnosis of EIB is accomplished by recording a fall in the forced expiratory volume in 1 second of 15% or more after an exercise challenge test with spirometry.
- A level of exercise must generate 85% of an athlete's maximum heart rate and should last for 4 to 8 minutes to maintain an appropriate ventilatory rate.
  - This can be accomplished by having the athlete run on a treadmill or pedal on an exercise bike to try to evoke symptoms.
  - This may be more difficult in elite athletes or in those individuals who have an environmental stimulus (i.e., who may require testing in their sport-specific environment to elicit their symptoms).
- Spirometry is performed at 3- to 5-minute intervals up to 30 minutes after this level of exertion is reached.
- If the ability to do exercise challenge testing is logistically difficult because of access to spirometry or space, consider use of peak flows recorded before and during their sports participation.
- Differential diagnosis includes exacerbation of chronic asthma and vocal cord dysfunction.

- In chronic asthma, there may be night symptoms or symptoms seen at times other than with exercise and may necessitate more intensive treatment.
- With vocal cord dysfunction, inspiratory rather than expiratory wheezing (as well as stridor) may be seen.
- If the diagnosis is in question, consider referral to an ear, nose, and throat specialist for evaluation.

Treatment

- The main treatment goal of EIB is focused on prevention and/or modifying the severity. This can be accomplished through a variety of nonpharmacologic and pharmacologic approaches.
- Some nonpharmacologic suggestions include modifying the environment in which the exercise occurs, such as avoiding cold, dry air by exercising in warmer and more humid conditions.
- Type of exercise should also be considered, as more severe symptoms usually are related to greater intensity and duration.
  - High-minute ventilation activities (long distance running and cycling) and activities taking place in a cool, dry climate (ice hockey, figure skating, speed skating) are more likely to induce EIB.
- Warming up before exercise may allow competitive participation to occur during the refractory period where less bronchospasm is present and may decrease development of EIB.
- Pharmacologic treatment should be considered if there is no improvement with exercise modifications or if the athlete's particular sport does not allow for this type of modification.
- The most common first-line therapy for EIB is inhaled β_2-adrenergic agonists.
  - These are short-acting bronchodilators that can be used 5 to 30 minutes before exercise for prophylactic use, as well as during exercise for symptomatic relief if needed.

- Other treatment alternatives include a long acting β_2-agonist, which can be used 30 to 60 minutes before exercise and can last for up to 12 hours, as well as leukotriene inhibitors.
- Other medications used include cromolyn sodium and theophylline.
- If common EIB therapies are not causing improvement in symptoms, re-evaluation for possible exacerbation of chronic asthma should be considered.
- It is important to consider that some of these drugs may be banned by the National Collegiate Athletic Association (NCAA) or the International Olympic Committee (IOC), and therefore the medication used may vary, depending on the athlete's level of participation and the sport involved.

Clearance

- An athlete who has been appropriately diagnosed and is under adequate treatment is cleared to participate as tolerated.
- If pharmacologic treatment is used, athletes should carry the medication with them at all times if they are involved in any form of exercise.
- Review of NCAA, IOC, or relevant governing body guidelines should be taken before allowing a specific treatment to be used while in competition.

EXERCISE-INDUCED ANAPHYLAXIS

Background

Exercise-induced anaphylaxis, although rare, is generally characterized by a spectrum of symptoms that occur with physical activity, ranging from milder cutaneous manifestations to more severe findings of hypotension, syncope, and death. Ingestion of certain foods (seafood, celery, wheat, and cheese) or medications (aspirin or nonsteroidal anti-inflammatory drugs) before exercise has been considered as possible predisposing factors. Although the severe symptoms are rare, urticaria is much more common and may affect 10% to 20% of the population at some time.

Diagnosis

History

- With exercise-induced urticaria, athletes report symptoms of cutaneous warmth, erythema, and pruritus during or after exercise.
- If symptoms progress to wheezing, dyspnea, or syncope, exercise-induced anaphylaxis should be considered.
- A personal history of atopy may help support the diagnosis.

Testing

- The exercise challenge test can help diagnose an athlete with suspected exercise-induced anaphylaxis.
  - This can be done by using a treadmill or exercise bicycle under controlled conditions with emergency equipment available.

- A positive test, with reproduction of the signs and symptoms, helps confirm the diagnosis; however, a negative test is nondiagnostic, as the athlete may still have exercise-induced anaphylaxis that was not triggered.

Treatment

- Similar to EIB, modification of activities that may precipitate the event is an important first-line consideration.
- Athletes should have an EpiPen or anaphylaxis kit in their possession or near by while exercising.
- Acute reactions may also be treated with antihistamines and steroids in addition to the epinephrine.

Clearance

- If an athlete has a history of life-threatening anaphylaxis, this is generally a contraindication to participation.
- There are, however, no firm guidelines, and switching to a less strenuous sport may be considered if risks and benefits are thoroughly reviewed.
- In less serious situations, participation can be allowed as long as precautions are undertaken, including EpiPen and resuscitation equipment.

CARDIOVASCULAR CONCERNS

HYPERTROPHIC CARDIOMYOPATHY

Background

Hypertrophic cardiomyopathy (HCM) is a genetic cardiac disease that is the most common cause of sudden cardiac death in young athletes. It is relatively common in the general population, affecting approximately 1 in 500 people. It is inherited as an autosomal dominant trait. It is caused by the mutation of a gene that encodes proteins of the cardiac sarcomere. Currently, there are three mutant sarcomeric genes that predominate: β-myosin heavy chain, cardiac troponin T, and myosin-binding protein C.

The clinical course can be variable, ranging from asymptomatic to sudden death. Its pathologic feature is left ventricular wall hypertrophy without dilatation (Fig. 12-2). In the absence of other causes, this can be diagnostic of HCM. On histologic evaluation of the cardiac muscle at autopsy, cardiac muscle cell disorganization is seen. Screening during the preparticipation examination has become a focus as to a way to prevent many of the sudden cardiac deaths that result from HCM.

Diagnosis

History

- The wide range of presentations seen in HCM makes diagnosis a challenge.

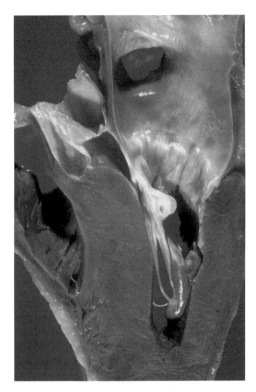

Figure 12-2 Hypertrophic cardiomyopathy. The heart has been opened to show striking asymmetric left ventricular hypertrophy. The interventricular septum is thicker than the free wall of the left ventricle and impinges on the outflow tract. (From Rubin E, Farber JL. Pathology, 3rd ed. Philadelphia: Lippincott Williams & Wilkins, 1999.)

- Athletes may present with symptoms such as dyspnea, chest pain, syncope, or arrhythmia. Any of these symptoms should heighten consideration for a cardiac cause, such as HCM.
- The presentation may be sudden death in a young athlete after strenuous exertion.
    - Sudden death is most common in children and young adults ages 10 to 30.
- The preparticipation screening examination may be the opportunity to detect an athlete who is at high risk for HCM before the unfortunate event of sudden death occurs.
    - Screening questions should include a family history of cardiac disease; specifically, early cardiac death before the age of 50.
    - The athlete should be asked about history of chest pain, dyspnea, syncope, or near-syncopal episodes in relation to exercise.

Physical Examination

- Any positive history findings during the screening examination should cause increased awareness during the physical examination; but, because many athletes are asymptomatic, the cardiac examination may be your one opportunity for early detection of HCM.
- Clinical findings include a systolic ejection murmur at the left sternal border that increase with provocative

maneuvers that decrease venous return, such as Valsalva maneuver or going from a squatting to a standing position.
- Any murmur grade III/IV or greater should be further investigated.
- Most patients with HCM do not have obstruction to flow under resting conditions; therefore, physical examination is not reliable on its own as a screening tool.

Radiologic Examination

- The diagnosis can be reinforced by diagnostic tests such as an electrocardiogram (ECG) or a two-dimensional echocardiogram.
- Findings on ECG include criteria for left ventricular hypertrophy.
- An echocardiogram shows left ventricular wall thickening (LVWT) with a nondilated left ventricular chamber.
    - Findings of LVWT >15 mm are highly suggestive of HCM.
    - HCM should be strongly considered in any male athlete with LVWT >12 mm and in any female athlete with LVWT >11 mm with a nondilated left ventricle.
    - LVWT between 13 and 15 mm is a diagnostic gray zone.
- Stress echocardiography may also help distinguish between athlete's heart and HCM.
    - Some athletes who have undergone intense physical training may have a physiologic increase of LVWT >15 mm, but they will demonstrate an absence of left ventricular outflow tract gradient on exercise echocardiography.
    - If there is diagnostic uncertainty, genetic testing can be definitive.
        - It is not routinely available because of its complexity, cost, and time consumption.

Treatment

- Pharmacologic options for treatment of symptomatic patients include β-adrenergic blocking drugs and verapamil.
    - β-Blockers have a negative inotropic effect, therefore prolonging diastole and allowing increased ventricular filling. This helps to improve symptoms such as chest pain and dyspnea and allows improvement in exercise tolerance.
    - Verapamil also helps with symptoms by improving ventricular filling.
    - In asymptomatic patients, there is no evidence that either β-blockers or verapamil protect against sudden cardiac death.
    - Exceptions that may be treated are asymptomatic patients with significant outflow tract obstructions.
- Atrial fibrillation is a common arrhythmia to develop in patients with HCM and is often treated with amiodarone.
- Nonpharmacologic therapy for unresponsive HCM includes myomectomy and alcohol septal ablation.
- Dual-chamber pacing and implantable cardiac defibrillators have also been used.

Clearance

- The 36th Bethesda Conference recommended that all persons with HCM, even those with no symptoms or who have received treatment, be excluded from competitive sports, with the possible exception of low-intensity athletics (IA).
- They found no good evidence that exceptions should be made to this policy.

CONGENITAL ANOMALIES OF THE CORONARY ARTERIES

Background

Congenital coronary anomalies are another common and often unrecognized cause of sudden cardiac death, accounting for up to 20% of cases in young athletes. A congenital coronary anomaly is the ectopic origin of a coronary artery. It is classified based on the artery involved and its origin and path. Many of these types produce few or no symptoms, but others can be more serious and even cause sudden death. Some of the types described include the left coronary artery arising from the right sinus of Valsalva, the right coronary artery arising from the left sinus of Valsalva, or the absence of the left coronary artery/single coronary artery (attributed to the death of "Pistol Pete" Maravich, a previous hall-of-fame basketball star).

Diagnosis

History and Physical Examination

- There is frequently the absence of any symptoms, therefore making it difficult to diagnose. If there are symptoms present, they may include chest pain or syncope.
- Often, there is no associated physical examination findings associated with a congenital coronary anomaly, once again explaining the difficulty in diagnosis. Occasionally, a murmur may be present.
- Congenital coronary anomalies often are not diagnosed until autopsy.

Radiologic Examination

- If the patient has symptoms, workup may include an electrocardiogram (usually normal) or a two-dimensional echocardiography with color Doppler imaging (which may reveal the coronary artery anomalies).
- If the echocardiogram is nondiagnostic, coronary angiography, ultra-fast computed tomography (CT) and/or a magnetic resonance imaging (MRI) may be necessary to delineate.

Treatment

- The patient should be referred to a cardiothoracic surgeon for potential surgery to reduce the risk of cardiac death.
- Possible options include coronary artery bypass grafting or coronary artery reimplantation.

Clearance

- The 36th Bethesda Conference recommended that participation in competitive sports should be prohibited once congenital anomalies are detected.
- Three months after successful surgical treatment, participation could resume, assuming the athlete has no ischemia, ventricular or tachyarrhythmia, or dysfunction during maximal exercise testing.

LONG QT SYDROME

Background

The most common cause of sudden cardiac death in the general population is considered to be arrhythmias. In young persons without any identifiable structural heart defect, long QT syndromes (LQTS) are common causes. There are multiple genes identified that encode cardiac ion channels (mostly potassium and sodium) that cause LQTS. It occurs as an inherited disorder or can be acquired. One cause of acquired LQTS is the use of certain medications, such as antiarrhythmics, antihistamines, psychotropic drugs, antifungal drugs, and macrolide antibiotics. It can also be acquired through electrolyte disturbances such as hypokalemia. The result is prolongation of ventricular repolarization, which can lead to fatal arrhythmias, most commonly from polymorphic ventricular tachycardia or ventricular fibrillation.

Diagnosis

History

- Patients may complain of palpitations or a syncopal episode.
- Potentially, the presentation could be cardiac arrest or sudden death.
- Review of the athlete's family history during preparticipation screening is important.
- If a patient presents with symptoms, a review of their current and recent medications should take place.

Physical Examination

- In the symptomatic patient, a cardiac arrhythmia will be detected, possibly ventricular tachycardia.

Testing

- LQTS is usually diagnosed with an ECG.
- There is a prolonged QT interval with correction for heart rate QT_c of >460 to 480 msec.
- There is also often a relative bradycardia, T-wave abnormalities, and episodic ventricular tachyarrhythmias.
- Genetic testing can also be done to determine the genotypic type.

Treatment

- Current treatment usually involves initiation of a β-blocker at the time of diagnosis.

- When there is failure with medical therapy, sympathectomy or implantation of an automatic cardioverter defibrillator have been tried.
- Genetic-based therapy has also been described.

Clearance

- The 36th Bethesda Conference recommended excluding from all competitive sports (except class IA category) anyone who has had cardiac arrest outside of a hospital or who has had a suspected syncopal episode precipitated by LQTS.
- Asymptomatic patients with QT prolongation may participate in IA sports.
- Patients identified with QT prolongation by genetic testing who are genotype-positive/phenotype-negative LQTS may participate in competitive sports, with the exception of swimming.
- Patients with LQTS/pacemaker should not participate in collision or contact sports as a result of risk of damage to the pacemaker. The presence of an implantable cardiac defibrillator (ICD) should restrict individuals to class IA activities.

HYPERTENSION

Background

Systemic hypertension is the most common cardiovascular condition observed in competitive athletes. A blood pressure reading in adults over the age of 18 should be below 120/80. A reading above that is considered hypertensive. When dealing with patients under 18, hypertension is defined as average systolic or diastolic levels greater than or equal to the 95th percentile for gender, age, and height. Blood pressure measurement should be a standard part of any examination to clear competitive athletes for competition.

The most recent report by the Joint National Committee VII classifies blood pressure into normal (<120/80), prehypertension (120 to 139/80 to 89), stage 1 hypertension (140 to 159/90 to 99), and stage 2 hypertension (≥160/100).

Diagnosis

History

- When evaluating an athlete with hypertension, the history should include questions about diet, salt intake, caffeine use, excessive alcohol consumption, stimulants, decongestants, herbs, dietary supplements, and illicit drugs.
- Other things that may need to be considered are stress levels, gender (male >female), race (blacks >whites), and family history of hypertension.

Physical Examination

- When measuring blood pressure, proper cuff size and technique should be used to ensure accuracy.

- Diagnosis should not be made on an isolated reading in the office, because many patients will exhibit "white coat" hypertension.
- At least three separate readings on separate days should be documented before labeling someone as hypertensive.

Testing

- Laboratory tests to exclude secondary causes of hypertension or to identify end-organ damage include a complete blood count, sodium, potassium, blood urea nitrogen, creatinine, glucose, cholesterol levels, urinalysis, and ECG.

Treatment

- Nonpharmacologic treatments include dietary and lifestyle changes.
  - Some specific recommendations may include a decrease in sodium intake and an increase in potassium intake, avoiding stimulants and caffeine use, regular aerobic exercise, and weight loss.
  - If stress is a concern, relaxation techniques may be tried.
  - Regular cardiovascular exercise can also assist in lower blood pressure.
- Hypertension not controlled with lifestyle changes often requires use of pharmacologic treatment.
- There are multiple pharmacologic choices available but some may have an adverse affect on exercise tolerance, and some are banned for use by the IOC or the NCAA.
- Possible classes of drugs include thiazide diuretics, β-blockers, angiotensin-converting enzyme inhibitors, angiotensin receptor blockers, calcium channel blockers, and α-blockers.
- Choices may be driven by their side effects and their effect on heart rate and exercise tolerance.
  - Athletes tend to tolerate thiazide diuretics and ace inhibitors best.
  - β-Blockers tend to cause exercise intolerance and therefore are not tolerated as well.

Clearance

- Before individuals begin a competitive training program, they should have undergone an evaluation of their blood pressure.
- The 36th Bethesda Conference defines multiple different recommendations with regard to participation based on the level of the blood pressure and the presence of end-organ dysfunction.
- Mild-to-moderate hypertension is usually not a contraindication to athletic participation in the absence of end-organ damage.
- Certain high-intensity sports may need to be restricted until hypertension is controlled.
- It is important to make sure any pharmacologic treatment is not classified as a banned substance with the appropriate governing board.

OTHER CARDIOVASCULAR CONCERNS

Congenital Anomalies

- Multiple cardiac congenital anomalies can exist in athletes that require individual evaluation and consideration with regard to athletic participation.
- Some examples include atrial septal defect, ventricular septal defect, patent ductus arteriosus, coarctation of the aorta, tetralogy of Fallot, transposition of the great vessels, and Ebstein's anomaly.
- Many of these may have been present at birth and were surgically corrected.
- Specific recommendations are made with regard to active or corrected congenital cardiac anomalies before athletic clearance.
- It is important to ask about history of any cardiac problems, and the Bethesda recommendations should be reviewed before clearance for participation in athletics.

Valvular Heart Disease

- Valvular heart disease may be detected by the presence of a cardiac murmur or characteristic physical examination findings.
- Some examples include mitral stenosis, mitral regurgitation, aortic stenosis, aortic regurgitation, tricuspid regurgitation, tricuspid stenosis, mitral valve prolapse, and prosthetic heart valves.
- Athletes should be referred to the appropriate physician who is comfortable in managing these diseases before clearance to play should be allowed.
- The Bethesda recommendations offer guidelines to consider in asymptomatic individuals, and symptomatic individuals will often need referral for consideration of valvular replacement or repair.

Arrhythmogenic Right Ventricular Dysplasia (ARVD)

- ARVD is a disorder that is characterized by ventricular arrhythmias and structural abnormalities of the right ventricle.
- It is caused by progressive replacement of the myocardium with fibrofatty tissue.
- Symptoms may include palpitations, syncope, or sudden cardiac death, although the patient may be asymptomatic.
- Treatment usually consists of antiarrhythmic drugs or use of an ICD.
- Recommendations from the 36th Bethesda Conference state that athletes with ARVD should be excluded from most competitive sports, with the possible exception of those of low-intensity (class IA).

Coronary Artery Disease (CAD)

- It is thought that regular cardiovascular activity reduces the risk of CAD.

- In those individuals with known CAD though, risk stratification should be undergone before clearance for intense physical activity.
- Evaluation may consist of a maximal treadmill or exercise test to assess their exercise capacity.
- ECG stress testing before participation in athletics should be included for those at moderate to high risk for CAD.
- More specifically, this includes men >40 to 45 years old or women >50 to 55 years old with 1 or more independent coronary risk factors.
- A risk factor would be hypercholesterolemia (total cholesterol >200 mg/dL, low-density lipoprotein >130 mg/dL, high-density lipoprotein <35 mg/dL in men, or < 45 mg/dL in women), systemic hypertension (>140/90), cigarette smoking, diabetes mellitus, a history of myocardial infarction, or sudden cardiac death in a family member <60 years of age, any symptoms of cardiac disease, or anyone ≥65 years of age in the absence of risk factors.
- The 36th Bethesda Conference has made recommendations for intensity of sports activities that should be allowed based on the patient's risk stratification level.
- Athletes with mildly increased risk can usually participate in low-to-moderate intensity sports, but should be re-evaluated annually for risk stratification.
- If an athlete is in the increased risk group, he or she is generally restricted to low-intensity sports.
- Athletes with a recent myocardial infarction should avoid training until cleared by the cardiologist.

Marfan Syndrome

- Marfan syndrome is an autosomal dominant connective tissue disorder that consists of a variety of clinical manifestations of the skeletal system (tall stature, arachnodactyly, increased arm span to height ratio, ligamentous laxity, and chest wall deformities) and ocular injuries (lens dislocation).
- The cardiovascular system may also be affected by aortic dilatation and possible dissection (Fig. 12-3).
- In athletes with suspected Marfan syndrome, they should undergo further evaluation with an echocardiogram to evaluate the aortic root.
- Certain restrictions in activities are recommended based on the history, symptoms, and aortic root size.
- Referral to a cardiologist or a specialist in evaluation of Marfan syndrome should be considered if there is any question about diagnosis or decisions on recommended activity levels.

VASCULAR CONCERNS

RAYNAUD'S PHENOMENON

Background

Raynaud's phenomenon is characterized by episodic vasospasms of the extremities that is precipitated by cold or

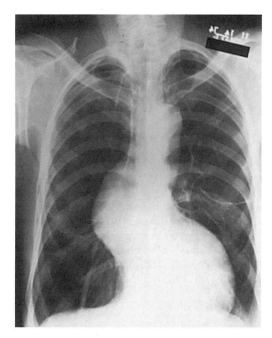

Figure 12-3 Marfan syndrome with hyperinflation, bullous changes, dilated tortuous aorta, and "tall" lungs. (From Crapo JD, Glassroth JL, Karlinky JB, et al. Baum's Textbook of Pulmonary Diseases, 7th ed. Philadelphia: Lippincott Williams & Wilkins, 2004.)

stress and causes ischemia of the fingers and toes. It was first described in 1862 by Maurice Raynaud as a phenomenon of cold-induced digital pallor followed by cyanosis and erythema. Fingers are the most commonly affected (Fig. 12-4), followed by the toes. Other potential sites include the tongue, nose, ears, and nipples. It can be seen worldwide but has a higher prevalence in cold weather climates. Females have a higher risk for development of the disorder than do males. Having a family history of the disorder or

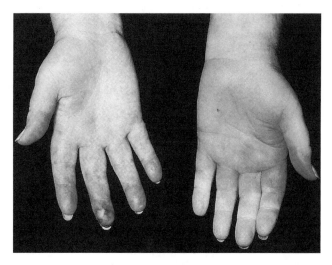

Figure 12-4 Hallmarks of Raynaud's disease are color changes. (From Effeney DJ, Stoney RJ. Wylie's Atlas of Vascular Surgery: Disorders of the Extremities. Philadelphia: Lippincott Williams & Wilkins, 1993.)

having a personal history of related connective tissue disorders are also risk factors.

Raynaud's phenomenon can be divided into primary (there is no known underlying illness) or secondary (a related disorder is detected). A frequent association is seen between scleroderma and Raynaud's phenomenon. Other secondary causes include occupational exposure to mechanical vibration, medications (chemotherapeutic agents), and more widespread vasospastic processes. Typically, primary disease is seen in the second or third decade of life, and secondary disease is usually after the age of 40.

Diagnosis

History

- When obtaining a history from the athlete, details should be obtained regarding occupation, sports participation, medical history, and medications.
- The description of the digits may consist of initial pallor caused by digital artery vasoconstriction, followed by cyanosis from slow blood flow, and then a reactive hyperemia as the vessels reopen in response to warmth.
- Some athletes may notice only cyanosis or may observe the entire spectrum of findings.
  - Typically, it will initially involve only one or two fingers and may then progress to all of them.
- Sometimes the symptoms will resolve spontaneously, and others will only respond to warming.

Physical Examination

- Often, the clinician does not witness the event, as it has resolved by the time of presentation.
- As team physicians may be on the sidelines during cold-weather sports, it is possible that the athlete may present with the initial pallor or cyanosis for advice.
- Physical examination should consist of careful inspection of all of the digits on the hands and feet and peripheral pulses.
- Further workup should ensue in an athlete with the above history and examination findings to look for potential primary causes.

Testing

- Diagnostic tests should include a complete blood count, erythrocyte sedimentation rate, chemistry profile, autoantibody screen, urinalysis, and radiographs of the hands and chest.
- Other rheumatologic testing may be necessary to rule out related disorders.
- Differential diagnosis should include peripheral vascular disease, Buerger's disease (thromboangiitis obliterans), polycythemia, scleroderma, systemic lupus, CREST syndrome (calcinosis cutis, Raynaud's phenomenon, esophageal dysmotility, sclerodactyly, and telangiectasia), thoracic outlet syndrome, carpal tunnel syndrome, occupational injury, and drugs (chemotherapeutic agents).

Treatment

- Differentiation between primary and secondary diseases should be determined, as treatment options differ.

- Primary disease often responds to more conservative measures.
  - Some modalities include layered clothing, woolen gloves and sheepskin mittens (i.e., two layers rather than one), gloves made from specially insulating fabric, and electrically heated gloves.
- If there is an occupational exposure suspected, then it should be avoided if possible.
- For moderate symptoms, in addition to the preventive measures, the athlete may try a topical vasodilator.
- With more severe symptoms, if conservative measures are not effective, calcium channel blockers can be tried, such as nifedipine or diltiazem.
- Recent studies have also shown that selective serotonin reuptake inhibitors, such as fluoxetine, may be effective in reducing the severity and frequency of attacks.

Clearance

- There are no specific contraindications to participation in sports but, depending on the severity, athletes may need to modify the environment in which they are participating.
- Uncontrolled symptoms despite modifications and medical treatment may necessitate discontinuation of sport.

GASTROINTESTINAL CONCERNS

TRAVELER'S DIARRHEA

Background

Athletes and teams who are involved in foreign travel or competition may expose themselves to traveler's diarrhea. Traveler's diarrhea was first described in travelers to Mexico and is now endemic in many parts of the world. The etiology of most traveler's diarrhea is bacterial, but viral and parasitic infections have been implicated. Potential bacterial pathogens that have been isolated include enterotoxigenic *E. coli* (most common), *Shigella* species, *Campylobacter* species, *Salmonella* species, *Aeromonas* species, *Plesiomonas shigelloides*, and noncholera *Vibrios*. Viral etiologies include Norwalk virus, rotavirus, and enteric adenoviruses. Parasitic causes include *Giardia lamblia*, *Entamoeba histolytica*, *Cryptosporidium parvum*, and *Cyclospora cayetanensis*. Most cases of traveler's diarrhea come from contaminated food and water.

Diagnosis

- Traveler's diarrhea is often associated with travel to developing and tropical areas.
- It is defined as the passage of at least three unformed stools in a 24-hour period, with associated nausea, vomiting, abdominal pain or cramps, fecal urgency, tenesmus, or the passage of bloody or mucoid stools in a person who normally resides in an industrialized region and travels to a developing tropical or semitropical country.
- This includes illness that develops within the first 7 to 10 days after returning home.
- A typical course consists of 3 to 10 unformed stools daily for 3 to 5 days.
- In the presence of the above symptoms, the diagnosis can be confirmed with examination of the stool.
  - If fecal leukocytes are present, a bacterial pathogen is likely.
  - If fecal leukocytes are absent, it does not rule out that a bacterial pathogen may still be present.
- Other diagnostic tests include stool cultures looking for the specific pathogen.

Prevention and Treatment

- Prevention strategies are essential to avoid acquiring traveler's diarrhea in at-risk regions.
- Consuming bottled water and carbonated beverages—while avoiding tap water, ice cubes, and fresh vegetables—are simple measures that can help prevent an infection.
- Initial treatment should focus on replacement of fluids and electrolytes to prevent dehydration from diarrhea.
- Most traveler's diarrhea will respond to antibiotic treatment.
  - As a result of resistance to trimethoprim/sulfamethoxazole (TMP/SMX), most travelers will respond to treatment with the fluoroquinolones.
  - First-line therapy can be ciprofloxacin 500 mg twice a day for 5 to 7 days.
  - In areas where resistance has been seen, azithromycin has been used effectively in all bacterial pathogens.
- A nonantibiotic treatment includes bismuth subsalicylate, which can reduce the number of unformed stools and decrease symptoms.
- Loperamide, an antimotility agent, can also help symptoms by decreasing intestinal motility and enhance the intestinal absorption of fluids and electrolytes.
  - Loperamide should be avoided though in the presence of dysentery, with symptoms such as high fever, chills, and bloody diarrhea.
- Prophylactic treatment should be considered when traveling to high-risk areas.
  - Bismuth subsalicylate in the form of two 262-mg tablets four times a day has been effective in decreasing attacks.
- Self-treatment with loperamide and oral hydration can be used for onset of mild symptoms and an antibiotic, such as a fluoroquinolone, can be added when more severe symptoms are present.

Clearance

- In an athlete diagnosed with traveler's diarrhea, there are no formal guidelines for participation.

- If the athlete is dehydrated, has systemic symptoms, is actively vomiting, or is febrile, strong consideration should be given to not participating in a competition until status improves.

HEMATOLOGIC CONCERNS

ANEMIA

Background

Anemia is a state in which a person has a level of hemoglobin that is lower than the expected range for someone their gender and age. The correlation between exercise and anemia has sparked more investigation about this subject. The mean hemoglobin concentration of the exercising versus the nonexercising population is lower. The difference is even more notable in the more elite endurance athletes. Anemia is often misconceived as a disease, opposed to the result of a physiologic response or aberrancy.

Dilutional pseudoanemia secondary to plasma volume expansion is the most common cause of anemia in the athlete. Dilutional pseudoanemia should not affect other parameters in a complete blood cell count (CBC) (mean red cell volume, ferritin) or haptoglobin. It should not be associated with symptoms. When training ceases, the hemoglobin should normalize in 3 to 5 days.

Foot strike hemolysis (intravascular hemolysis) has also been seen in endurance athletes. It is primarily the result of mechanical trauma but is also linked to exercise intensity.

Iron deficiency with or without frank anemia is also seen in athletes. In one study, 80% of young female athletes and 30% of elite male athletes were found to be iron deficient. The causes of iron deficiency anemia are many. Some of the etiologies include poor nutrition, exercise-induced hemoglobinuria or hematuria, gastritis, and hemorrhoids.

Diagnosis

- The diagnosis is made by laboratory evaluation, which should include CBC, haptoglobin, urinalysis, and iron studies (iron, ferritin, and total iron-binding capacity).
- If more suspicious and searching for another possibility, one may also choose to get other studies, including reticulocyte count, hemoglobin electrophoresis, fecal occult blood tests, and coagulation profile.

Treatment

- Treatment is inevitably to address underlying cause if a true anemia is detected.
- The treatment may be as simple as diet manipulation or supplementation.

Clearance

- Usually, athletes self-preclude if their symptoms do not allow expected performance.
- There are no guidelines for individual events.

THALASSEMIA AND SICKLE CELL ANEMIA

Background

Numerous blood disorders are encountered in athletes. Sickle cell anemia, thalassemias, and clotting disorders are a few of the important ones to review. These disorders are genetically inherited, and a complete family history is important in these situations.

The people who are afflicted with sickle cell anemia can possess the sickle cell gene in either a homozygous (disease-HbS) or heterozygous state (carrier-HbS). The carriers usually do not have crises. Homozygous individuals can experience acute chest syndrome and aplastic crises among other complications.

Thalassemia presents with numerous genetic variants. These are multifactorial anemias characterized by defects in the α- and/or β-subunit of the hemoglobin tetramer. Hemolysis occurs chronically in people with thalassemias.

People with clotting disorders (hemophilia, various factor deficiencies) have aberrancies in their clotting cascade, rendering them unable to clot in an organized way. Hemostasis normally occurs via a series of well-choreographed steps (coagulation cascade). A vascular response initially helps to form a platelet plug. This process is followed by the activation of coagulation factors leading to the stabilization of the platelet plug by fibrin.

Diagnosis

- Blood samples should be ascertained for the above disorders if there is clinical suspicion.
- Sickle cell and thalassemias need CBC, peripheral smear, hemoglobin electrophoresis (in some instances), and reticulocyte count (especially in crisis).
- A haptoglobin level and liver function tests (bilirubin direct and indirect) can also be done if there is an acute hemolytic event. Clotting disorders need laboratory evaluation as well.
- In clotting disorders, PT, PTT, and INR are important, as are CBC and a peripheral smear.

Treatment

- Treatment involves addressing the underlying cause.
- In many instances, careful observation is the only intervention that can be pursued.
- Hydration is the key preventive measure, especially with heat or outdoor activities.

Clearance

- It is recommended that those who are afflicted with HbS (disease), as well as other coagulopathies, not be involved in contact sports.

- Most providers recommend against heavy exertion because this could increase oxygen debt and cause crisis.
- High-altitude participation, including flying in unpressurized cabins, is also not favorable for those afflicted.
- One must use clinical judgment because no specific "exclusion" criteria exist.
- Participants with thalassemia and HbS (carriers) should not have restrictions but should be monitored.

BLOOD DOPING

Background

Doping is the use of any substance to enhance athletic performance. Blood doping is a scientifically proven illegal means of enhancing athletic performance. In the past, athletes would donate blood a few weeks before a competition and then replace this blood before competition. This process would in turn increase this athlete's hemoglobin concentration, hence causing their oxygen-carrying capacity to increase. This "autologous" type of transfusion is virtually obsolete after the advent of rHuEpo. Erythropoietin is a genetically engineered copycat kidney hormone that stimulates the bone marrow to produce red blood cells. Numerous side effects are known to occur from blood doping. Some of these documented side effects are pulmonary embolism, myocardial infarct, and stroke, just to name a few. There were a few documented deaths in the early 1990s in Dutch cyclists before erythropoietin was banned.

Diagnosis and Prevention

- There are very sensitive tests to test urine via liquid chromatography to detect exogenous erythropoietin and also other subtle peptides.
- Prevention involves education about possible side effects and avoidance.

Clearance

- If detected, the participant is disqualified because erythropoietin and blood doping are banned in most competitive endurance sports.
- The IOC banning occurred in 1996, and testing occurred at the Olympic Games in Atlanta 1996.

HEAD AND NECK AREA CONCERNS

EYE TRAUMA

Background

More than 42,000 sports and recreational eye injuries were reported in the year 2000. Of those injuries, more than 70% occurred in people under 25 years of age, and two thirds of the injuries occurred in persons between the ages of 5 and 25. The cause of these injuries is multifactorial. Some of the factors may include the number of people involved in athletic activities, the aggressive nature of play, and at times the lack of supervision. The most common eye injuries in sports affect the anterior globe. Corneal abrasions account for 83% of nonperforating anterior globe injuries. Subconjunctival hemorrhage, foreign bodies, hyphema, retinal detachment, and globe rupture are a few injuries that can also occur. Subconjunctival hemorrhage occurs from blunt trauma, as does hyphema and often retinal detachment.

Diagnosis

- Diagnosis of most of the aforementioned ocular injuries is made by physical diagnosis.
- An important part to precede the physical examination is the history.
  - Ask about the person's vision and examine the pupils.
  - If the patient is unable to open the eye, do not force the lid open, because a globe rupture may be present.
- The main complaint with detached retina is visual disturbance.
- Corneal abrasions can be seen after application of fluorescein stain (Fig. 12-5).
- If a foreign body is seen during this examination, one may take this opportunity to remove it if it is superficial.
- In a subconjunctival hemorrhage, the conjunctiva becomes erythematous and has a bloodshot appearance (Fig. 12-6).
- Extensive hemorrhage should make one worry about a ruptured globe.
- A hyphema is when there is blood in the anterior chamber (see Fig. 12-6).

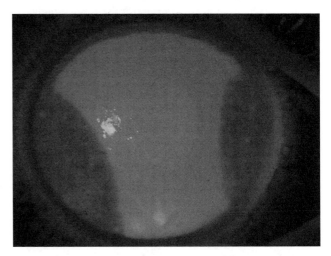

Figure 12-5   A large, traumatic corneal abrasion stains brightly after topical fluorescein instillation. (From Tasman W, Jaeger E. The Wills Eye Hospital Atlas of Clinical Ophthalmology, 2nd ed. Lippincott Williams & Wilkins, 2001.)

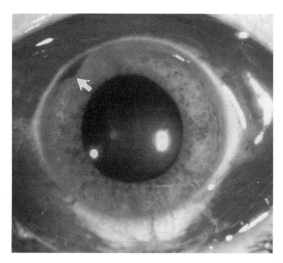

Figure 12-6   Subconjunctival hemorrhage extending for 360 degrees. Note the small hyphema (*arrow*). (From Fleisher GR, Ludwig W, Baskin MN. Atlas of Pediatric Emergency Medicine. Philadelphia: Lippincott Williams & Wilkins, 2004.)

Treatment

- Corneal abrasions
  - Apply topical anesthetic, then apply fluorescein strips to the conjunctival sac.
  - Identify the abraded epithelium, which is the area that is fluorescent green when viewed with a cobalt blue light.
  - Antibiotic should be applied.
  - Mandatory 24-hour follow-up is necessary.
  - Pain and blepharospasm may make it difficult to open the eye.
  - The athlete may not return to play.
- Superficial corneal foreign body
  - Apply topical anesthetic.
  - Remove the foreign body with sterile irrigation solution or a moistened sterile cotton swab.
  - Never use a needle to remove the foreign body.
  - Apply topical antibiotic.
  - Mandatory 24-hour follow-up.
  - If unable to remove the foreign body, do not allow return to play.
- Concealed foreign body
  - Usually located under the eyelid or lower fornix, as frequently suggested by vertical linear corneal abrasions that show after fluorescein strip staining.
  - Evert upper eyelid and irrigate with sterile irrigation solution or moistened swab.
  - Follow corneal abrasion guidelines if present.
  - If there is no corneal abrasion, the athlete may return to play.
  - Patching is not recommended.
- Hyphema
  - Blood is present in the anterior chamber.
  - Intraocular pressure may increase.
  - The eye should be shielded and immediate referral should be made.
  - No return to play is acceptable.

- Patients with visual complaints (such as floating bodies and/or papillary defect) and any of the other diagnoses should be referred to an ophthalmologist for possible retinal issues or optic neuropathy.

Clearance

- Participation should be withheld until proper treatment is implemented and vision returned to baseline.
- Information about proper eyewear in various sports arenas should be discussed, because up to 90% of eye injuries may be avoidable.
- Improper eyewear and protective eyewear are often overlooked.

NASAL INJURIES

Background

Nasal injuries, specifically fractures, account for a large percentage (40%) of bony injuries in facial trauma. In children, play and sports account for a majority of nasal fractures. In a nasal injury, there are other problems besides fractures that should be evaluated. A septal hematoma or deformity, as well as epistaxis, can also occur. A septal hematoma is a blood-filled cavity between the nasal cartilage and the perichondrium. This area can become infected, and necrosis can ensue. Epistaxis at times can impair the ability to perform a thorough examination. The vascular anatomy of the nose renders it susceptible to bleeds. There is a dense vascular network that supplies the nose called "Kisselbach's area." This plexus is responsible for most simple nosebleeds. The bleeding that occurs secondary to a fracture is usually from the sphenopalatine artery (posterior) or the anterior ethmoid artery (anterior). Septal hematomas often occur with nasal trauma and can result in septal deformities.

Diagnosis

- Diagnosing nasal injuries is performed via history and physical examination.
  - An idea of the type of force involved will either broaden or narrow the differential diagnosis.
  - Epistaxis may be the only finding in some nasal fractures.
  - Palpation may uncover crepitus or step-off deformities during the examination.
  - Ecchymosis and edema will usually occur within minutes to an hour after the injury.
- With a nasal speculum and good light, one should examine the nasal septum, mucosa, floor, and turbinates. Also check for airway patency.
  - Internal examination of the nares will often be obscured by blood or clots.
  - Saline irrigation or removal with cotton-tipped applicators may aid in the examination.
  - One should be able to visualize if a septal hematoma is present.
  - One should also check for clear rhinorrhea.

- The surrounding structures of the nose should be examined as well.
  - Disconjugate extraocular movements give concern for orbital fractures.
  - Tenderness over other facial areas gives concerns for other fractures, including the zygomatic arch, malar eminences, and mandible fractures.
- X-rays are often obtained for simple fractures but may be of limited value for occult or complex fractures as a result of poor sensitivity and specificity.
- If there are other concerning signs (such as clear rhinorrhea or disconjugate gaze), CT imaging is indicated.

Treatment

- Epistaxis should initially be treated with direct pressure for stasis.
  - If stasis becomes an issue, packing can be performed.
- With nasal fractures, if reduction of a gross deformity is required, it should be performed within 5 to 10 days of the injury.
  - If there is no mucosal injury, septal hematoma, or deformity, splinting may be used.
- If there is an open fracture or mucosal injury, the injured participant's tetanus status should be ascertained; infection may possibly occur.
  - Appropriate referral should be made.
- Septal hematomas need to be drained because a saddle deformity may result.
  - Immediate needle aspiration under local anesthetic should be done.
  - Referral once again would be optimal.

Clearance

- Because reinjury (including the possibility of airway compromise) exists, as well as an increased chance of rebleeding, one should err on the side of caution and use good judgment for return to play.
- Generally, return is allowed if homeostasis is obtained and the area can be protected with a facial shield or mask.
- No set guidelines exist.

OTITIS EXTERNA (SWIMMER'S EAR)

Background

Otitis externa (OE) is inflammation or infection of the external auditory canal (Fig. 12-7). It is caused by a breakdown in the normal skin barrier in the ear canal, often related to elevated humidity and warmer temperatures. It is commonly associated with water sports such as swimming or water polo. Other risk factors are local trauma to the external ear or maceration of the skin. The common bacteria that normally populate the healthy external auditory canal are *Staphylococcus auricularis*, *Staphylococcus epidermidis*, and diphtheroids. When the skin barrier breaks down, infection develops, with the predominate pathogens being *Pseudomonas aeruginosa* and *Staphylococcus aureus*.

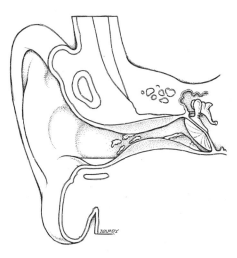

Figure 12-7   Illustration of otitis externa (swimmer's ear). (Courtesy of Neil O. Hardy, Westpoint, CT.)

Diagnosis

- Diagnosis is clinical, based on the clinical history and physical examination findings.
  - The most common complaint with OE is pain, often severe, with itching preceding the pain.
  - Patients may also complain of purulent secretions or a feeling of fullness secondary to edema.
  - A history of recent water exposure is usually present.
- On physical examination, the physician should evaluate the external auditory canal for signs of inflammation or infection.
  - Erythema or thick drainage may be seen.
  - There is usually pain on manipulation of the external ear.
- Evaluation of periauricular lymph nodes should also be performed, as enlargement of these nodes may signify an infection.
- Differential diagnosis needs to include acute otitis media and necrotizing OE.
- The tympanic membrane needs to be evaluated, and if it is erythematous and bulging, treatment for acute otitis media should be considered.
- Necrotizing externa is a malignant rare variant of OE that is caused by *Pseudomonas aeruginosa* and is associated with systemic invasion.
  - It has primarily been described in elderly adults who have diabetes mellitus.
  - They note severe pain, especially at night, as well as discharge, hearing loss, and a sensation of fullness.
  - They may develop facial nerve palsy.
  - Examination reveals inflammation and granulation tissue at the bony–cartilaginous junction.

Treatment

- First-line treatment for OE is topical.
- Choices include 2% acetic acid or a topical antibiotic containing aminoglycoside, polymyxin, or fluoroquinolone.

- Topical corticosteroids are also effective in combination with a topical antibiotic.
- Topical or oral analgesics are used for the treatment of pain.

Clearance

- There are no specific contraindications to sports participation with OE.
- Treatment should be initiated to decrease symptoms.
- Preventative measures may include the use of earplugs while swimming or prophylactic use of 2% acetic acid to decrease the amount of moisture in the ear.

OTITIS MEDIA

Background

Acute otitis media (AOM) is an infection of the middle ear that represents the most frequent diagnosis when children present to a physician with a complaint. The most frequent bacterial pathogens in AOM are *Streptococcus pneumoniae*, *Haemophilus influenzae*, and *Moraxella catarrhalis*. Other, less common bacterial causes are *Staphylococcus aureus*, *Streptococcus pyogenes*, enterococcus, group B *streptococcus*, and *Pseudomonas aeruginosa*. Viral pathogens include respiratory syncytial virus, parainfluenza, influenza, cytomegalovirus, enterovirus, rhinovirus, adenovirus, herpes simplex virus, and coronavirus.

Diagnosis

- AOM is often preceded by a recent upper respiratory tract infection.
- The eustachian tube fails to drain the middle ear effectively and provides a culture medium for bacteria.
- Once the middle ear becomes infected, patients may complain of ear pain or fever.
- A history of sick contacts or recent upper respiratory infection symptoms must be addressed.
- Physical examination should include evaluation of vital signs, including evaluation for the presence of a fever.
  - Characteristic findings on examination include a bulging tympanic membrane with purulent fluid visible in the middle ear (Fig. 12-8).
- Pneumatic otoscopy can also be used to demonstrate decreased mobility of the tympanic membrane, suggestive of middle ear fluid.
- Diagnosis of AOM can be difficult because there are no good diagnostic tests.
- Diagnosis relies on the presence of an acute illness and middle purulent ear fluid.

Treatment

- Most cases of AOM will resolve spontaneously without use of antibiotic therapy. Therefore, watchful waiting is an acceptable approach in managing AOM in the age group of most athletes.

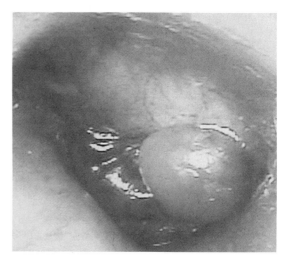

Figure 12-8   Acute otitis media with bullae formation and fluid visible behind the tympanic membrane. (Courtesy of Alejandro Hoberman, Children's Hospital of Pittsburgh, University of Pittsburgh.)

- Symptomatic treatment with oral fluids to prevent dehydration and analgesics for pain can be used.
- Despite the high frequency of spontaneous resolution, antibiotics are still frequently prescribed by physicians.
- Common antibiotics used include amoxicillin, erythromycin-containing preparations such as azithromycin, and amoxicillin/clavulanate (for nonresponsive infections).
  - Judicious use of antibiotics should be used to prevent creation of resistant organisms.

Clearance

- In athletes who develop an AOM, there are no specific return-to-play restrictions.
- Symptoms should guide the athlete's decision.
- Participation with a fever ≥38°C should restrict the athlete from participating as a result of the risk of developing heat illness.

AURICULAR HEMATOMA

Background

Auricular hematoma is a condition of the pinna of the ear where there is a collection of blood beneath the perichondrial layer. If untreated, this will progress to become "cauliflower ear." It is a common condition seen in wrestlers, boxers, and martial artists but can also occur in the helmeted athlete and other activities. It occurs with blunt trauma or repetitive shearing forces to the ear's pinna.

Diagnosis

- An auricular hematoma is diagnosed by history and PE.
- On physical examination, an edematous region at the pinna is palpable and easily seen (Fig. 12-9).

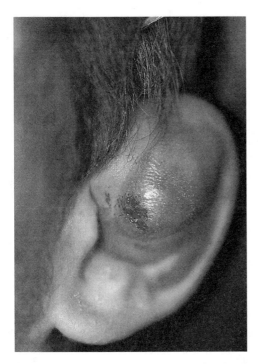

Figure 12-9 Auricular hematoma. The smooth, discolored mass obscuring the normal contour of the pinna is a hematoma. (From Fleisher GR, Ludwig S, Baskin MN. Atlas of Pediatric Emergency Medicine. Philadelphia: Lippincott Williams & Wilkins, 2004.)

Treatment

- No single method has proved better than another for long-term outcomes.
- One wants to drain the hematoma and place a compression dressing on it to avoid reaccumulation of blood.
  - This can be done with a needle under sterile conditions or via incision.
  - If incised, the sutures should remain in place for up to 14 days.
  - This intervention for long-term outcome is even controversial.
- Silicone splinting has been recommended for a quicker return to play and decreased reoccurrence.

Clearance

One should abstain from possible contact to the area for a minimum of 24 hours. On return, they should wear proper protective gear (i.e., wrestler's headgear). Some recommend continued compression dressing for the remainder of the season.

BAROTRAUMA

Background

Barotrauma refers to tissue damage to an air-filled body cavity or space when there is failure to equalize a change in barometric ambient pressure. It often occurs in water sports either with rapid descent/ascent in self-contained underwater breathing apparatus (SCUBA). Barotrauma can occur at the middle ear or the inner ear. Contact at the air–water interface in diving, water-skiing, and other water activities can cause rupture of the tympanic membrane.

Diagnosis

- Diagnosis is made by history more than physical examination, with the exception of ruptured tympanic membrane.
- Neurologic symptoms include change in hearing, vertigo, pain and, at times, Bell's palsy.
- In inner ear barotrauma, the symptoms may also include emesis, nystagmus, and tinnitus.

Treatment

- Antihistamines and analgesia in many cases will suffice.
- If there in a tympanic rupture, one should consider antibiotics.
- In a more severe case (as in inner ear barotraumas, bed rest with head elevation, and stool softeners), one may also highly consider ENT referral if symptoms are prolonged.

Clearance

- Participation is dependent on symptoms.
- Usually, participants will self-preclude.
- Athletes with perforated tympanic membrane need to avoid water immersion and swimming until perforation resolves.

DENTAL MANDIBLE AND SKULL INJURIES

Background

Although not as common as dentoalveolar; ear, nose, and throat; and head injuries, skull and mandible fractures do occur. High velocity or impact is needed for these types of injuries to occur.

Dentoalveolar injuries can also occur in conjunction with these types of injuries, although they can also occur as an isolated injury. It is estimated that 35% of all dental injuries are the result of sports injury. Fifty-six percent of dentoalveolar injury occurred with other associated injuries. Mandible fracture etiology has changed over the past two decades. In the past, these types of injuries were mostly secondary to motor vehicle accidents, violence, and assaults. Sports injuries have now been steadily rising as an etiology as per some studies. Cycling, skiing, and hockey—among other sports—have an increased incidence of mandible fractures.

Skull fractures, if nondisplaced and without any type of concurrent bleeding, have good outcomes. There are times that a depressed fracture may occur. Appropriate field management will be discussed.

Diagnosis

- History and clinical findings are important in the diagnosis.
- Gross deformities such as a palpable depressed skull fracture or a mandibular deformity are more easily diagnosed.
- The subtle findings of malocclusion or cerebrospinal fluid oto/rhinorrhea are also clinical clues pointing toward fractures.
- Radiologic studies are helpful in these cases.
  - Plain x-rays in suspected mandible fractures are often diagnostic, whereas findings on plain x-ray are less useful in suspected skull fractures.
  - CT scan is the diagnostic standard if a skull fracture is likely.
- Some dental fractures are difficult to assess where frank avulsions and luxations are not.
- Skull fractures, if a palpable deformity is evident, need immediate follow-up.
  - If no deformity is evident but suspicion is high, clinical hospital referral is appropriate.
- There are some specific bruising patterns that correlate with certain fractures of the skull.
  - Raccoon eyes and battle signs are two of these patterns that happen a few hours after the trauma.
- Plain radiography is of little use, whereas CT is more sensitive and specific, especially in determining concurrent intracerebral injury.

Treatment

- Dentoalveolar injuries have a specific protocol for specific injury.
  - Complete avulsion ("knocked out of socket") treatment includes rinsing the tooth with saline (do not scrub), replacing it in the socket, and following up immediately with a dentist.
    - If unable to replant, place tooth in milk or in the buccal vestibule of the athlete with emergent dental follow-up.
  - Tooth fracture, where there is no sensitivity to air, generally allows for return to play that game with dental follow-up within 24 to 48 hours.
  - Severe pain may be associated with a more significant tooth fracture or occult fracture.
    - These athletes should be withheld from playing and have emergent dental follow-up.
  - Tooth luxations (partial dislocation) have other protocol depending on if the tooth is extruded, intruded, or laterally luxated.
  - Overall, if there is a possible underlying alveolar fracture, do not try to reduce the tooth.
  - Dental referral is recommended in most situations.
- Many mandible fractures are managed by closed maxillomandibular fixation or occlusal splinting.
- Skull fractures need appropriate referral and intervention.

SPECIAL SITUATIONS

There are numerous situations that require extra evaluation prior to participation. A physician's responsibility changes as an on-site medical provider at an athletic event. Providers should be aware of special situations, especially single organ or structure, that may be encountered on the playing field.

- Single- or one-eye blind may be encountered.
  - Acuity of 20/40 is considered to provide good vision.
  - Athletes with less than this level of visual acuity with correction should be considered functionally one-eyed.
  - Because there are numerous protective devices for the eyes, many athletes can participate in various sports with knowledge of their inherent dangers.
  - Sports have been rated in an eye injury risk classification.
- Players with a single testicle or undescended testicle should wear protective cups.
  - They should also be warned of the increased incidence of testicular cancer in an undescended testicle.
  - No restrictions are given to these participants.
- Athletes with a single kidney, single functioning kidney, or a pelvic kidney have restrictions in sports.
  - Though the incidence is rare, the ability of the participant to injure his or her only functioning kidney would render the individual in need of a transplant or lifelong dialysis.
  - The recommendation from most health care providers would be to not indulge in contact or collision sports.
  - There are no formal restrictions.
  - If the player decides to play, special recommendations for protective gear, such as a flack jacket, should be encouraged.
- People with diabetes may participate in any sport, although there is a recommendation against endurance activity involvement (marathon, triathlon).
  - The most important factor is of course glycemic control.
  - If the player has a finger-stick blood glucose level >250 with ketosis or a finger-stick blood glucose level >300, then the player should be held out.
  - If the glucose level is <100, the athlete should ingest a substance with carbohydrates.
  - The player should also stay ahead of their fluids.
  - Sports classified as high risk for people with diabetes because of their ability to become hypoglycemic include SCUBA, rock climbing, and skydiving.

SUGGESTED READING

Adams BB. New strategies for the diagnosis, treatment, and prevention of herpes simplex in contact sports. Curr Sports Med Rep 2004;3: 277–283.

American Academy of Pediatrics, Committee on Sports Medicine and Fitness and the American Academy of Ophthalmology, EYE. Health and Public Information Task Force. Protective eye wear for young athletes [joint policy statement]. Ophthalmology 2004;111: 600–603.

Bowling JCR, Dowd PM. Raynaud's disease. Lancet 2003;361: 2078–2080.

Dienst WL Jr, Dightman L, Dworkin MS, et al. Pinning down skin infections: diagnosis, treatment, and prevention in wrestlers. Physician Sportsmed 1997;25.

Kucik, CJ, Clenney T, Phelan J. Management of acute nasal fractures. Am Fam Physician 2004;70:1315–1320.

Maron BJ. Hypertrophic cardiomyopathy: a systemic review. JAMA 2002;287:1308–1320.

McFadden ER, Gilbert IA. Exercise-induced asthma. N Engl J Med 1994;330:1362–1367.

Methicillin-resistant *Staphylococcus aureus* infections among competitive sports participants—Colorado, Indiana, Pennsylvania, and Los Angeles County, 2000–2003. MMWR 2003;52:793–795.

Mitten MJ, Maron BJ, Zipes DP. 36th Bethesda Conference: eligibility recommendation for competitive athletes with cardiovascular abnormalities. J Am Coll Cardiol 2005;45:1318–1373.

National Collegiate Athletic Association: 2003–2004 Wrestling Rules, Appendix D. Skin Infections. Indianapolis, 2004.

Promoting oral health: interventions for preventing dental caries, oral and pharyngeal cancers, and sports-related craniofacial injuries. MMWR 2001;50(RR 21):1–13.

Seventh Report of the Joint National Committee on Prevention, Detection, Evaluation, and Treatment of High Blood Pressure. The National Heart, Lung, and Blood Institute National Institute of Health. May 2003;3:5233.

Shaskey DJ, Green GA. Sports haematology. Sports Med 2000;29;1.

Shlim DR. Update on traveler's diarrhea. Infect Dis Clin North Am 2005;19:137–149.

Whitman JH. Upper respiratory tract infections. Clin Family Pract 2004;6:35–74.

13

DERMATOLOGIC AND INFECTIOUS DISEASES

MATTHEW A. PECCI
SHAWN M. FERULLO
PHILIP CRUZ
J. HERBERT STEVENSON

Infectious skin rashes and upper respiratory infections are very common in athletes. The close quarters of locker rooms, shared equipment, and skin-to-skin contact with other athletes aids in transmission of these infections. In addition, warm, moist skin is an ideal environment for many types of skin infections to flourish. It is essential for sports medicine physicians to be able to recognize the signs and symptoms of common infections. It is also important to understand what conditions may call for temporary disqualification of an athlete from competition.

In this chapter, we will outline and discuss some of the most common infectious skin rashes and respiratory infections encountered. We will discuss the course and treatment of these illnesses. Finally, we will discuss special considerations in athletes.

DERMATOLOGIC CONDITIONS

HERPES SIMPLEX

Pathology

Herpes simplex is a DNA virus that has two distinct types: herpes simplex 1 (HSV1) and herpes simplex 2 (HSV2). These two types produce identical lesions and are treated the same. Therefore, it is not essential to make the distinction between the two types at diagnosis. Generally, HSV1 produces oral lesions such as the common "cold sore" and is more common in infections obtained from athletic events. HSV2 tends to be more common in genital infections. Herpes is spread by direct contact with herpes lesions or by contact with fluid that contains the virus, such as saliva or cervical secretions. The herpes virus does not live long outside of the body, so skin-to-surface spread is uncommon. After exposure, there is a variable incubation period of 2 to 14 days before lesions first appear. The first time someone is infected with herpes is considered the primary infection. The primary infection differs from the secondary infection because the lesions generally last longer and are preceded by prodromal symptoms—such as body aches, fever, generalized fatigue, headaches, and tender lymph nodes—all of which may occur a few days before the appearance of herpes lesions. Typically, the lesions of herpes in a primary infection last 2 to 6 weeks. After the lesions heal, the virus then enters peripheral nerves at the site of inoculation and ascends to the dorsal root ganglia, where it remains until reactivated in a secondary infection. Herpes is a chronic infection and can never be completely cleared from the body.

The secondary infection of herpes occurs when the latent virus in the dorsal root ganglia is reactivated. The virus then travels back through the peripheral nerve and causes lesions in the same area as the previous primary infection. The herpes virus is opportunistic and generally reactivates at times of stress or skin compromise. The stress that may cause reactivation is variable. Common causes are upper respiratory infections, fatigue, menstruation, or (in athletes) stress as a result of an upcoming event or match. Also, any skin trauma, such as a cut or scrape or even a sunburn in the area of prior infection, may cause reactivation. The secondary infection is not preceded by prodromal symptoms, and lesions generally last 10 to 14 days.

Diagnosis

- The appearance of skin lesions in a herpes infection is typically preceded by some localized symptoms in the area of the lesion, including pain, burning, and tingling—all of which can occur 1 to 2 days before the lesion appearance.
- The classic description of the lesions of herpes is grouped vesicles on an erythematous base (Fig. 13-1).
  - The vesicles contain clear to serosanguineous fluid and may coalesce with adjacent vesicles to form larger lesions.
  - The virus is contained within the fluid of the vesicle, and therefore these vesicles are considered contagious.
  - The skin under the vesicles tends to be erythematous but this does not extend far beyond the lesions.
  - The vesicles rupture in a few days forming shallow erosions covered by a yellowish crust.
  - These erosions will then heal in 8 to 14 days.
  - The lesions of herpes are in the outermost layer of the skin or the epidermis, and therefore should generally heal without scarring.
- The diagnosis of herpes can often be made from the appearance of the lesions; but when in doubt, laboratory evaluation can be performed.
  - A herpes culture is most definitive for diagnosis.

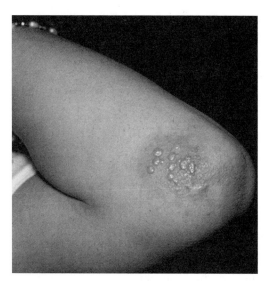

Figure 13-1 Herpes simplex : grouped vesicles on an erythematous base. (From Goodheart HP. Goodheart's Photoguide of Common Skin Disorders, 2nd ed. Philadelphia: Lippincott Williams & Wilkins, 2003.)

- Culture specimens can be taken from the fluid contained in the vesicles or swabbed from the base of a moist ulcer.
- Culture yield is low once the lesions begin to dry.
- Results of a herpes culture may take up to 1 week but can be available as soon as 1 to 2 days.
- The other testing method is called a Tzanck smear, which attempts to visualize multinucleated giant cells (cells infected with the herpes virus).
  - The specimen for a Tzanck smear is collected by scraping the base or edges of an ulcer with a scalpel.
  - The collected specimen is then placed on a slide, fixed, and stained.
  - The benefit to this method is that a diagnosis can be made within minutes.

Treatment

- Herpes is a chronic, incurable disease.
- Treatment is aimed at decreasing the time course of an outbreak, rather than curing the disease.
- It is most effective if it is begun early in the course of an outbreak when the virus is rapidly replicating.
  - In primary infections, this is usually when the lesions first appear and are diagnosed.
  - In secondary infections, this can be before the lesions even appear, especially if a patient has localized symptoms before the outbreak.
- At the first indication that a patient may be developing a secondary outbreak such as localized burning or tingling in the area of a prior outbreak, medication should be started.
- There are three antiviral medications available for the treatment of herpes: acyclovir, famciclovir, and valacyclovir.

- In a primary infection, begin acyclovir 400 mg three times per day (TID) for 10 days, famciclovir 250 mg TID for 10 days, or valacyclovir 1,000 mg two times per day (BID) for 10 days.
  - Topical acyclovir may also be effective in primary infections and can be applied every 4 hours for 10 days.
- In secondary infections, begin acyclovir 400 mg TID for 5 days, famciclovir 125 mg BID for 5 days, or valacyclovir 500 mg BID for 3 days.
  - Again, treatment is not curative but lessens the time to lesion healing.
- Patients may also try a variety of drying agents in an attempt to hasten resolution of lesions, such as alcohol, bleach, or Betadine—none of which are medically recommended.
- A patient with frequent outbreaks of herpes, or herpes that reoccurs predictably at times of stress, may be prescribed prophylactic treatment.
  - The prophylactic doses of the medications are acyclovir 400 mg BID, famciclovir 250 mg BID, or valacyclovir 500 mg QD.

Athletic Considerations

- Herpes in the athlete is typically caused by HSV1.
- It is called herpes gladiatorum because of its frequency in wrestlers but it can occur in athletes in any contact sport.
- It is seen most commonly in areas of contact such as the face, neck, upper trunk, and upper extremities.
- Because of the contagiousness of this disease and its incurable nature, athletes are disqualified from competition in any contact sport or swimming if he or she has active herpes lesions, even if the lesions encompass a very small area that can be covered with a dressing or clothing.
  - Athletes may return to competition only when the lesions are completely dry.
- Many sports governing organizations, including the National Collegiate Athletic Association (NCAA), require that an athlete has had no new lesions for a 72-hour period before competition is allowed.
  - Furthermore, the NCAA also requires that an athlete be treated with systemic antiviral medication for at least 5 days before the event and be taking the medication at the time of competition.
- As stated previously, athletes may use a variety of topical agents in an attempt to dry the lesions as quickly as possible.
  - Athletes may also use these agents in an attempt to make the diagnosis difficult for the untrained clinician and thereby avoid disqualification.
  - If there is any question of herpes, however, an athlete should be disqualified from contact sports until further evaluation can be undertaken.
- Because secondary herpes can occur at times of stress, it is very common for athletes to suffer outbreaks during times of important meets.
  - If this is known to occur in a given athlete, it may be appropriate to consider prophylactic treatment with antiviral medications at these times.

MOLLUSCUM CONTAGIOSUM

Pathology

Molluscum contagiosum is a pox virus that infects the epidermis of the skin. Similar to herpes, there are two types of molluscum viruses: MCV-1 and MCV-2. Again, it is not important to make the distinction between the two types because they cause similar lesions and are treated the same.

Molluscum lesions are spread by direct skin-to-skin contact, so lesions are typically seen in areas of exposed skin such as the face, neck, and arms. The lesions can be spread from person to person but can also be spread to different areas of a given individual by autoinoculation. Although not truly considered a sexually transmitted disease, lesions can also be present in the genital area and therefore can be spread through sexual activity.

Diagnosis

- The lesions caused by molluscum contagiosum are papules 1 to 2 mm in size (Fig. 13-2).
  - They are typically white to skin-colored and are generally grouped in clusters.
- One of the most characteristic traits of a molluscum contagiosum lesion is a central dimple or umbilication.
  - The umbilication is most easily seen on large lesions and is caused by a keratotic plug.
  - If this umbilication is not readily apparent on first inspection, it can sometimes be observed after treatment with liquid nitrogen.
- Typically, the skin surrounding the lesions appears normal; however, individual lesions may have a surrounding erythematous halo.
  - This erythema may be caused by an immune reaction to the lesion and indicates it may soon clear spontaneously.

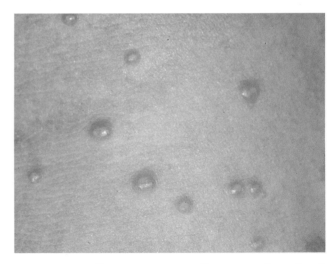

Figure 13-2   Molluscum contagiosum. Characteristic dome-shaped papules, some with central umbilication. (From Goodheart HP. Goodheart's Photoguide of Common Skin Disorders, 2nd ed. Philadelphia: Lippincott Williams & Wilkins, 2003.)

- The diagnosis of molluscum is typically made by examination.
- If the diagnosis is unclear, however, a Giemsa stain of the keratotic plug may reveal cells containing inclusion bodies that are typical of molluscum.
- These intracytoplasmic inclusion bodies may also be seen on biopsy specimens.

Treatment

- Molluscum lesions may undergo spontaneous resolution, but this may take up to 6 months to occur.
- For quicker resolution, lesions can be destroyed by a variety of different methods.
- If only a few small lesions are present, they can be removed with a curette.
- More diffuse lesions may be treated with liquid nitrogen, electrodesiccation, or laser.
- If the lesions are too numerous to treat completely, treating at least some of the lesions may stimulate the body to mount an immune response against the remaining lesions and cause spontaneous resolution.
- It is important to remember that any of the previously described treatments may leave a scar or area of hypopigmentation, especially in dark-skinned individuals.
  - A patient should be counseled and consented as to this possibility before treatment is attempted.

Athletic Consideration

- Because molluscum contagiosum is highly treatable, and does not spread systemically, athletes with lesions may engage in contact sports, provided the lesions can be adequately covered.

IMPETIGO

Pathology

Impetigo is an infection of the epidermis caused by the bacteria *Staphylococcus aureus* or *Streptococcus pyogenes*. This infection typically occurs in areas of minor superficial breaks in the skin. The bacteria are most prevalent in skin areas with warm, ambient temperatures, and humidity. Therefore, outbreaks are frequent around the nose and mouth. Also, dryness and cracking of the skin around the lips, and trauma from shaving in this area may provide an entrance point for the bacteria. There has also been some association of outbreaks with poor hygiene, which may lead to a prevalence of the bacteria on the skin. Between 20% to 40% of normal adults may have nasal colonization of S. *aureus*, and about 20% may have colonization of the axilla or perineum.

Although impetigo is considered an epidermal infection, if left untreated it can progress to a deeper skin infection such as a cellulitis, or may even cause a systemic bacteremia. The exotoxin produced from S. *aureus* may produce detachment of the superficial layers of the epidermis causing bullous lesions, or in certain cases widespread desquamation called *staphylococcal scalded skin syndrome*. Exoto-

xins produced from either bacteria may cause scarlet fever. More clinically concerning complications from systemic bacteremia such as rheumatic fever and acute glomerulonephritis, although not common, have also been associated with untreated impetigo.

Diagnosis

- The classic impetigo lesion is described as an erythematous, moist-appearing macule with a honey-colored crust (Fig. 13-3).
- This appearance, together with a common location around the lips or nose, is generally enough to make the diagnosis.
- There may be small lesions or larger lesions formed from confluence of these smaller ones.
- In addition to this classic appearance, impetigo may appear bullous with small blister-like lesions or may appear dry and scaly as it is starting to heal.
- If the diagnosis is in doubt based on appearance, the lesions can be swabbed for Gram stain and culture to confirm the presence of *Staphylococcus* or *Streptococcus*.

Treatment

- Although the lesions of impetigo may resolve spontaneously, it is recommended that treatment with either oral or topical antibiotics be initiated at the time of diagnosis because of the risk of localized spread and systemic complications.
- Very localized infections with few lesions may be treated with topical agents.
- Mupirocin is the topical treatment of choice for impetigo because it is effective against even resistant strains of both staphylococci and streptococci.
  - Two-percent mupirocin ointment is applied to the lesions three or four times per day until the lesions have completely cleared.

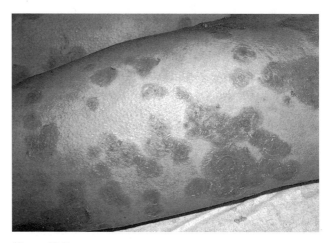

Figure 13-3 Streptococcal impetigo. Erythematous macules with moist crust. (From Rubin E, Farber JL. Pathology, 3rd ed. Philadelphia: Lippincott Williams & Wilkins, 1999.)

It may also be beneficial for the infected individual to wash with an antibacterial soap such as Betadine or pHisoHex once per day.

For more widespread outbreaks, oral antibiotics are recommended.

- Penicillin is generally not adequate for treatment because of known staphylococcal resistance.
- Erythromycin may be inadequate because of increasing staphylococcal resistance.

The preferred treatment is with an antistaphylococcal penicillin such as cloxacillin or dicloxacillin, or a first-generation cephalosporin such as cephalexin.

- The course of treatment depends on the extent of the infection, generally from 5 to 10 days.

For those individuals who are allergic to penicillin, azithromycin, or clarithromycin may be used.

For those infections that do not seem to be improving with oral antibiotics, it is recommended that a culture be performed.

A culture can identify the bacteria involved and its specific antibiotic sensitivities and can therefore guide treatment.

In addition to antibiotics, infected individuals should take measures to prevent further localized spread (such as minimizing friction or skin trauma in the infected area), avoid shaving the infected area, and cover lesions if possible, especially if the lesions are moist.

Athletic Considerations

Impetigo is commonly seen in the athlete.

It is typically spread from skin-to-skin contact and is frequently seen in sports such as wrestling.

The infection can also be spread from surface-to-skin contact.

- Therefore, wrestling mats, locker rooms, or other common-use equipment may be the source of some infections.
- It is essential that wrestling mats and other common-use equipment be cleaned regularly with antiseptic cleaners to prevent widespread outbreaks.

Because of the highly infectious nature of impetigo and the possibility of systemic complications, infected athletes are disqualified from contact sports until the lesions of impetigo are completely dried and clear of any crusting, even if the area can be adequately covered.

- In most cases, this degree of clearing occurs after about 5 days of appropriate antibiotic treatment.

The NCAA requires an athlete have had no new lesions for 48 hours before the event before competition is allowed.

In widespread outbreaks among teams, careful consideration as to possible sources of the infection should be explored.

- As previously described, common-use equipment that is not adequately cleaned may be a source.
- Another potential source is nasal colonization of team members.
- If this is suspected, cultures can be performed, or team members may be empirically treated with 2%

mupirocin ointment applied in the nares 3 times per day for 1 week.

FOLLICULITIS

Pathology

Folliculitis is inflammation of hair follicles that can be caused by physical irritation or, more commonly, by a bacterial infection. Infectious folliculitis is typically caused by *Staphylococcus aureus*, but there is a variant of infectious folliculitis associated with the use of hot tubs called *hot tub folliculitis*. In hot tub folliculitis, the offending agent is often *Pseudomonas aeruginosa*. Similar to impetigo, the bacteria tend to proliferate and cause infection in warm, moist environments; thus, folliculitis is commonly seen in areas of occlusion such as under tight clothes or in skin folds. The lesions in hot tub folliculitis frequently develop on areas that were covered with a bathing suit. Shaving also predisposes to hair follicle infections, because this activity can spread bacteria and provide breaks on the skin where bacteria may enter and cause infection.

Diagnosis

The typical infection of folliculitis is confined to the ostium, or superficial, portion of the hair follicle.

The characteristic lesions are pustules associated with hair follicles (Fig. 13-4)

- Often, hair from the follicle can be seen extruding from the center of the pustule.
- These infected follicles are generally grouped closely and surrounded by erythematous halos.
- When theses pustules rupture, they appear as superficial, moist erosions, which form a crust before they heal.

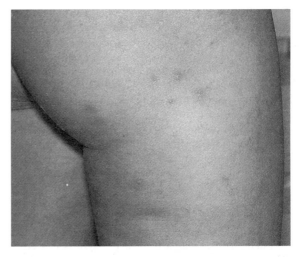

Figure 13-4 Folliculitis. Pustules associated with hair follicles. (From Goodheart HP. Goodheart's Photoguide of Common Skin Disorders, 2nd ed. Philadelphia: Lippincott Williams & Wilkins, 2003.)

- Because the infection is superficial, the lesions often heal without scarring, but may cause postinflammatory pigment changes, particularly in dark-skinned individuals.
- Even though the infection of impetigo and folliculitis both may be caused by *Staphylococcus,* in folliculitis the bacteria seem to be confined to the hair follicle, making risk of person-to-person transmission much less with folliculitis.
- Although the infection is typically limited to the hair follicles, if left untreated it may progress to a deeper dermal infection called a "furuncle."
    - A furuncle appears as a larger erythematous nodule, which can become an abscess filled with pus and necrotic debris. Multiple furuncles can coalesce to form a carbuncle.
    - A carbuncle is characterized by a larger area of erythema and multiple skin openings draining pus.
    - When these deeper infections occur, there is greater risk of systemic bacteremia.
- Pustules can be unroofed with a scalpel or needle and cultured, which can aid in guiding treatment. This is especially recommended in cases that do not respond to common antibiotic treatment.

Treatment

- Treatment is through the use of antibiotics to eradicate the infecting bacteria.
- In localized infections, 2% mupirocin ointment can be applied 3 times per day until the lesions have cleared.
    - Washing with an antibacterial soap daily may hasten clearance and prevent spread.
- For more widespread infections, systemic antibiotics should be used.
    - The choice of these medications is the same as with impetigo.
    - The course again varies with the severity of the infection from 5 to 10 days.
- Infections that have spread and become a furuncle or abscess may need to be incised and drained, in addition to the use of topical antibiotics.
- Measures to prevent spread should be discussed, such as avoiding shaving (until the infection has cleared) and avoiding the use of occlusive clothing or dressings.
    - If *Pseudomonas* is suspected, topical treatment with silver sulfadiazine cream may be effective.
    - More widespread infections should be treated with an oral antibiotic with antipseudomonal activity such as ciprofloxacin.

Athletic Considerations

- Like impetigo, folliculitis is very common in the athlete due to warm, moist skin, and use of occlusive clothing.
- Since the risk of spread is low, and systemic complications are rare, athletes with folliculitis may participate if the area can be adequately covered.
- If the lesions have progressed to a draining furuncle or carbuncle, however, an athlete engaging in a contact sport should not be allowed to participate until the lesion is no longer draining.

TINEA

Pathology

Tinea refers to infection with a fungus or dermatophyte often of the *Trichophyton* genus. It is classically named based on the area of the body infected. Tinea capitis refers to an infection on the head, tinea cruris the groin, tinea pedis the feet, and tinea corporis the body. Like many of the bacterial infections discussed, tinea favors warm, moist environments, so infections are commonly seen in the web space of the toes, between the legs, and in skin fold areas. The degree of infection seems to depend on the infected individuals cellular-based immune response. So many individuals may carry spores on their skin but never develop a rash, whereas others are very prone to recurrent outbreaks. The dermatophytes infect the superficial or keratin layer of the skin, but may infect hair and nails as well. The fungus may also live for a variable period of time on surfaces such as shower room floors, so surface-to-skin transmission is common.

Diagnosis

- The skin lesions of tinea can take on different appearances but are classically described as well-demarcated patches that may have a slightly raised border.
    - These patches are often erythematous and have some superficial scaling.
    - Over time, the central erythema may clear forming an erythematous ring, hence the term *ringworm* is often used to describe this classic tinea rash (Fig. 13-5).
    - The lesions of tinea are generally very itchy.
- Tinea pedis commonly infects the toe web spaces, and can cause cracked, macerated, moist appearing lesions (Fig. 13-6).

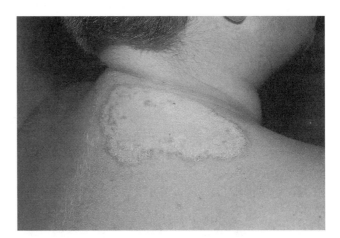

Figure 13-5 Tinea corporis. Erythematous, scaly macule, with central clearing ("ringworm"). (From Goodheart HP. Goodheart's Photoguide of Common Skin Disorders, 2nd ed. Philadelphia: Lippincott Williams & Wilkins, 2003.)

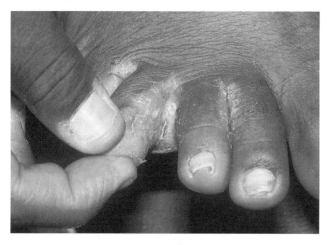

Figure 13-6 Tinea pedis ("athlete's foot"). (From Goodheart HP. Goodheart's Photoguide of Common Skin Disorders, 2nd ed. Philadelphia: Lippincott Williams & Wilkins, 2003.)

- Because bacteria are prevalent on the feet, this cracked skin may provide a site for bacteria entrance and superinfection.
- This should be considered in web space infections that are very erythematous and moist.
- Tinea capitis can cause the classic skin lesions but may also cause some overlying alopecia or hair loss.
- Tinea cruris is very common in males and typically begins in the crural folds and extends onto the inner thigh.
  - Over time, the lesion may change from erythematous to a more red-brown color (Fig. 13-7).
  - It is uncommon for tinea cruris to infect the scrotum; therefore, if the scrotum is involved, one should consider the possibility of another type of infection such as *Candida*.
  - Bacteria and even repetitive friction can cause a similar-appearing groin rash; thus, these diagnoses should be considered when examining a groin rash.
- Tinea is often diagnosed based on the location and appearance of the lesions.

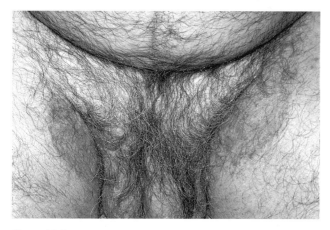

Figure 13-7 Tinea cruris ("jock itch"). (From Goodheart HP. Goodheart's Photoguide of Common Skin Disorders, 2nd ed. Philadelphia: Lippincott Williams & Wilkins, 2003.)

- When there is doubt, skin scrapings can be examined for the presence of the fungal organisms or hyphae.
  - The lesions are gently scraped with the edge of a glass slide or a scalpel, and these skin fragments are collected onto a slide.
  - A 10% potassium hydroxide solution is then applied to these fragments and a coverslip applied. The potassium hydroxide serves to lyse skin cells, thereby making the hyphae easier to visualize.
  - The slide can then be examined under low power on a microscope for the presence of hyphae.
  - Hyphae appear as branching, translucent filaments that appear to be separated into uniform segments by traversing septa.

Treatment

- There are many different types of topical preparations for the treatment of a tinea infection, and all are available without a prescription.
- These medications function by disrupting synthesis of a substance in the fungal cell membrane, leading to cell lysis and death.
- Two of the major classes of topical medications are imidazoles and allylamines.
  - The imidazole class contains medications such as miconazole, clotrimazole, and ketoconazole.
  - Allylamines contain the medication terbinafine or Lamisil.
- Both classes are effective against dermatophyte infections of the skin.
  - Some studies have shown that terbinafine may have a higher cure rate and more rapid response than the medications in the imidazole class.
- These medications are available as creams, lotions, aerosols, or powders.
  - Generally, cream or lotion is applied to the infected area twice per day until the rash clears.
- Tinea infections of the nails or more widespread infections that cannot be adequately treated with topical medication may need a course of oral antifungal medication.
- There are many different oral agents available, of which the more common ones will be reviewed here.
  - Griseofulvin has been around for more than 20 years and is effective only against dermatophyte infections.
    - The typical adult dose for tinea infection of the skin is 500 mg/day, for anywhere from 2 to 6 weeks, depending on the severity of symptoms.
    - The main reported side effects are gastrointestinal upset and headaches.
  - Ketoconazole is effective against both dermatophytes and yeast.
    - The typical adult dose for tinea infection of the skin is 200 to 400 mg/day for 2 to 4 weeks.
    - One of the most concerning side effects of ketoconazole is hepatitis, which has proved fatal in several cases.

- Liver enzymes should be monitored before starting oral treatment with ketoconazole and intermittently throughout the course of treatment.
- Another oral imidazole is itraconazole, which is less hepatotoxic than ketoconazole.
  - The typical adult dose for tinea infection of the skin is 200 to 400 mg/day for 2 to 4 weeks.
- Finally, there is an oral form of terbinafine.
  - The typical dose for tinea infections of the skin is 250 mg/day for 2 to 6 weeks.
- In addition to using medication, it is essential to correct factors that may predispose one to developing the infection.
  - The skin should be washed daily and thoroughly dried before dressing, with special attention to drying skin fold and web space areas.
  - Talcum powder can be applied in the socks or underwear to absorb any excess moisture.
  - If clothes do get wet or sweaty, it is essential to change these as soon as possible.
  - Dermatophytes do survive on surfaces other than skin; therefore, in an infected individual, all clothes should be washed in hot (>60°C) water.
  - Any old shoes or sneakers should be discarded.
  - Shower or bathroom floors should be cleaned thoroughly with bleach.

Athletic Considerations

- Tinea is so common in athletes that it has taken on common athletic names. Tinea pedis is commonly referred to as *athlete's foot*, and tinea cruris is commonly referred to as *jock itch*.
- The obvious reason for its frequency in athletes is that an athlete often has hot sweaty skin that favors the growth of dermatophytes. Also, athletes frequent areas such as locker rooms and common shower rooms that can harbor dermatophytes.
- Some control measures in athletes include not sharing equipment, or towels; avoiding occlusive clothing; wearing shower shoes when showering or walking in common-use areas; and making sure locker rooms and shower room areas are cleaned thoroughly between usages.
- Because tinea is very treatable, infected athletes are allowed to participate in contact sports as long as the rash can be adequately covered.
  - There is debate over how long an individual must be receiving treatment before being considered noninfectious, but 5 days is used as the general rule.
  - Therefore, an athlete with a more widespread infection, which cannot be adequately covered, should not be allowed to participate until he or she has been treated for at least 5 days.
- The NCAA requirements are slightly more lax, requiring only a minimum of 72 hours of topical treatment of an uncovered skin lesion, but 2 weeks of systemic treatment for a scalp lesion before competition can be allowed.
  - However, the NCAA does allow for decisions about competition to be made on a case-by-case basis, by physicians or certified athletic trainers.
- Table 13-1 is a summary of dermatologic conditions and their treatment.

CELLULITIS, ABSCESS, AND METHICILLIN-RESISTANT STAPHYLOCOCCUS AUREUS

Pathology

Cellulitis is a diffuse, painful inflammation of the skin, often secondary to a local insult. The border of erythema advances in cellulites. There are numerous etiologic bacteria that cause this illness, including *Streptococcus pyogenes*, group A β-hemolytic *Streptococcus*, and methicillin-resistant *Staphylococcus aureus* (MRSA). Cellulitis often occurs on the lower extremities or the hands, but can occur anywhere on the dermis. An abscess is a fluctuant soft tissue mass with overlying erythema. Abscesses are deep tissue infections with a pocket of pus that makes the area fluctuant.

Diagnosis

- Diagnosis is made clinically.
- Skin temperature and color are important clinical findings.
- It is important to monitor the infection closely.
- Occasionally, cellulitis may progress to or indicate an underlying abscess.
- With the new emergence of MRSA, cultures of an abscess must be considered.
- Monitoring the infection for clinical response remains very important.

Treatment

- The mainstay treatment of cellulitis is oral antibiotics based on underlying bacterial infection.
- First-line antibiotics include dicloxacillin, cephalexin, and erythromycin.
- If the infection is not responding well to oral treatment, parenteral may be necessary.
- An abscess is treated with antibiotics, as is cellulitis.
  - It must first be incised and drained for maximal antibiotic benefits.
- Infections secondary to community-acquired MRSA are usually sensitive to Bactrim among other antibiotics (vancomycin, clindamycin, tetracycline, and quinolones [some resistance already documented with quinolones]).

Athletic Considerations

- Community-acquired MRSA has recently become a more prevalent pathogen responsible for abscesses, especially in high school and college athletes.

TABLE 13-1 SUMMARY OF DERMATOLOGIC CONDITIONS COMMONLY EXPERIENCED BY ATHLETES

Condition	Appearance	Location	Diagnosis	Treatment	Contact Sports Participation
Herpes	Grouped vesicles on an erythematous skin base	Anywhere, but most common in areas of skin-to-skin contact (i.e., face, neck, upper trunk)	By classic appearance, Tzanck smear, or culture	Incurable. Antiviral medication may decrease time of outbreak	When lesions are completely dry
Molluscum	Grouped papules, may have central umbilication	Anywhere, common on trunk and extremities	By classic appearance, or Giemsa-stain of keratotic plug	Destruction by curettage, liquid nitrogen, electrodessication, or laser	If area can be adequately covered, or after treatment
Impetigo	Erythematous macule, with moist "honey-colored" crust	Common around nose and lips	By location and appearance, or Gram stain and culture	Dicloxacillin, cephalexin, azithromycin	When lesions are completely dry
Folliculitis	Pustules associated with hair follicles	Common on extremities	By appearance, or Gram stain and culture	Dicloxacillin, cephalexin, azithromycin	If area can be adequately covered
Tinea	Well-demarcated erythematous, scaly macule. May exhibit central clearing	Anywhere, but common in warm moist environments such as the groin and toe web spaces	By appearance, or scraping, application of potassium hydroxide and visualization of hyphae under the microscope	Topical imidazoles, allylamines. Consider oral antifungal medication in widespread cases	If area can be adequately covered, or after 3 to 5 days of treatment

- MRSA was first reported on sports teams in 1998. Other incidences on sports teams have now been more recently reported by the Centers for Disease Control and Prevention.
- Guidelines for clearance do not exist.
- If the lesions can be covered adequately and the athlete is afebrile, exclusion should not be the only option.
- Many people are using similar criteria as is being used for herpes and impetigo in wrestling.

ACNE

Pathology

Acne is a common disorder of the skin that affects 79% to 95% of American adolescents in the United States. Although this problem often commences at puberty, it may persist into adulthood. Up to 12% of females and 3% of males have persistent acne through middle age. The increased activity of the pilosebaceous glands occur secondary to a change in androgen levels. Acne also develops as a result of increased sebum production, pore clogging, rapid *Propionibacterium acne* production, and inflammation. This disease of the skin gives rise to eruptions of papules and/or pustules. A papule is a small, elevated circumscribed lesion. A pustule is a pus-filled papule. Other types of le-

sions that present in acne are comedones, macules, cysts, and nodules.

Acne mechanica usually occurs secondary to sweat, heat, friction, and occlusion from athletic equipment or clothing. It can be seen in the presence or absence of acne vulgaris. Common sites include the back, shoulders, and chin.

Diagnosis

- The diagnosis of acne is made clinically.
- The types of lesions often help determine the type and grade of acne in an athlete (Table 13-2).

TABLE 13-2 GRADING OF ACNE VULGARIS

Grade	Severity	Description
I	Mild	Open and closed comedones
II	Moderate	Erythematous papules and pustules with or without comedones, often with inflammation
III	Severe	Cystic, often with fluctuant lesions

After Savin R, Donofrio L. Aggressive acne treatment: as simple as one, two, three? Phys Sportsmed 1996;24:41.

- Acne most frequently affects the face, but can also affect the shoulders, back, chest, upper arms, and upper legs.

Treatment

- Treatment of acne involves correcting one or more of the underlying processes that results in acne formation.
- Athletes must be told that there is no quick fix to acne, because it often takes 6 weeks to see the full benefit of each treatment.
- Acne vulgaris responds to several treatments (Table 13-3).
- More recent developments in acne therapy include laser therapy and newer topical retinoids (tazarotene gel).
- Another intervention now being used with good results is photodynamic therapy with aminolevulinic acid.
- Acne mechanica generally responds to the following:
  - Decreasing friction, occlusion, and excessive moisture (cotton under pads, use moisture transfer material).
  - Hygienic practices (immediate postpractice showering and regular washing of undergarments).
  - Topical tretinoin may be considered if acne persists despite nonpharmacologic changes.

Athletic Considerations

- Athletes may present to the office or training room for acne. Advice on predisposing factors and possible treatment is frequently sought.
- Equipment—including chin straps, helmets, sweatbands, and shoulder pads—can serve as a source of friction and occlusion and contribute to acne mechanica.
- Uniforms that do not allow moisture and sweat to evaporate can result in occlusion and increased sweat production.

WARTS

Pathology

Warts are common epithelial tumors that are contagious and are most commonly found on the hands, feet (plantar),

elbows, and knees. Warts are caused by many types of human papilloma viruses. Warts may occur at a single location or at various locations. They can also occur as single or multiple lesion(s). Some of these tumors can become malignant. However, a majority of warts seen among athletes are benign. Transmission is via contact or fomite.

Diagnosis

- Diagnosis is made by history and physical findings.
- The shape and distribution of various warts are characteristic in different subtypes.
- Plantar warts are sharp, well-defined hyperkeratotic lesions (single or in clusters "mosaic warts") with a smooth collar of thickened keratin (Fig. 13-8).
  - Often upon paring or debulking these lesions, pinpoint bleeding may occur.
  - This occurrence helps differentiate plantar warts from calluses or corns.
- Verrucae vulgaris are raised, round, or irregular in shape, and they are sharply demarcated (Fig. 13-9).
  - These lesions usually have a rough surface and are normally from 2 to 10 mm in diameter.
  - This type frequently occurs at sites prone to trauma (e.g., hands, elbows, and knees).
  - It may also occur on the face and scalp.

Treatment

- Verrucae vulgaris respond to numerous modalities:
  - Cryocautery with liquid nitrogen
  - 1% salicylic acid or lactic acid
  - Daily electrodesiccation with curettage
  - Recurrence rates approach 33%
- Verrucae plantaris respond to numerous modalities:
  - 30% to 70% trichloroacetic acid
  - 40% salicylic acid
  - Taping with salicylic tape or duct tape for several days

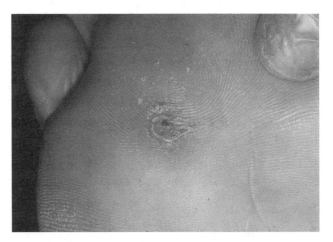

Figure 13-8   Plantar wart (verrucae plantaris). Characteristic punctate bleeding is present after paring. Note the loss of skin markings. (From Goodheart HP. Goodheart's Photoguide of Common Skin Disorders, 2nd ed. Philadelphia: Lippincott Williams & Wilkins, 2003.)

TABLE 13-3 ACNE TREATMENTS

Treatment	Example
Astringents	Benzoyl peroxide
Topical antibiotics	Clindamycin solution
Keratolytics	Salicylic acid, cleansing soaps
Mechanical exfoliates	Loofah sponges
Oral antibiotics	Tetracyclines, macrolides
Retinoic acid[a]	Topical liquid cream or gels, oral preparations
Steroid injections	
Incision and drainage[b]	

[a] Contraindicated during pregnancy.
[b] Potential for scarring exists.

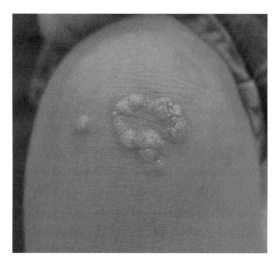

Figure 13-9 Warts (verrucae vulgaris) on the knee. (Image provided by Stedman's Medical Dictionary.)

- Immunologic therapy (candida or measle intralesional injections).

Athletic Considerations

- There are no set rules against participation for athletes with warts.
- Although not necessary for participation, occlusive dressing of the wart if on an exposed area may be considered.

BLISTERS

Pathology

Blisters are intraepidermal skin lesions caused by high moisture (perspiration or water from an outside source) in conjunction with prolonged shearing/frictional forces. Other exacerbating factors are poor shoe fit and/or socks that are not highly absorbent.

Treatment

- Treatment is multifactorial.
- If possible, leave the blister intact.
- If it is too uncomfortable or larger than 5 to 10 mm, then the fluid may be drained using a needle or a scalpel after antiseptic preparation.
- Avoid unroofing the lesion to lower the chances of a secondary infection and decrease the degree of discomfort.

Athletic Considerations

- Although friction blisters are certainly not sport-specific, they occur more frequently and are larger in tennis players than in many other athletes, probably because of the start-and-stop nature of the sport.

- Powder may help, but many athletes use emollient lotion (lubricant).
- Acrylic socks have also been suggested to maintain dryness.

CALLUSES AND CORNS

Pathology

Calluses and corns are the result of hyperkeratosis. They are thickened regions of the skin that are a normal physiologic response to multifactorial stresses. Hyperkeratosis occurs secondary to increased mechanical stresses. Poorly fitting footwear, improper foot mechanics, and high levels of activity are all players in the pathogenesis of these lesions. Corns tend to be more cone-shaped and are usually found on the dorsal and sides of the toes and feet (hard corns; Fig. 13-10). They can also occur between the toes (soft corn). Calluses are usually thicker and larger than corns. They tend not to be as conical and live on the plantar aspect of the foot (Fig. 13-11).

Diagnosis

- This diagnosis tends to be clinical.
- Warts are one of the few other lesions that can mimic calluses and corns.

Treatment

- Decrease friction by avoiding improperly fitted shoes or incremental increases of activity levels.
- After bathing, gently pumice and use lotions with lactic acid or urea to decrease the size and discomfort of calluses.

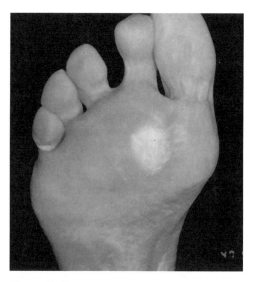

Figure 13-10 Calluses are nonpainful, thickened patches of skin that occur at pressure points. (From Weber J, Kelley J. Health Assessment in Nursing, 2nd ed. Philadelphia: Lippincott Williams & Wilkins, 2003.)

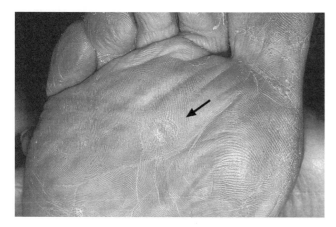

Figure 13-11 Corn (clavus). The circular central translucent core resembles a kernel of corn. (From Goodheart HP. Goodheart's Photoguide of Common Skin Disorders, 2nd ed. Philadelphia: Lippincott Williams & Wilkins, 2003.)

- Symptomatic relief is recommended and can also be accomplished by various methods of padding (i.e., lambs wool, metatarsal pads).
- If conservative therapy fails, there are surgical procedures that can be tried.
- Calluses under the metatarsal heads are best managed conservatively, because metatarsal osteotomies have unpredictable results, and the callous may transfer to an adjacent metatarsal head.

UPPER RESPIRATORY INFECTIONS

STREPTOCOCCAL PHARYNGITIS

Pathology

Sore throat is one of the most common presenting symptoms seen in an outpatient medical practice. Both viral and bacterial agents can lead to acute pharyngitis. It has been estimated that 10% of the cases of sore throat that present to a clinician are related to streptococcal infection.

Streptococcus is a class of bacteria that are characterized as Gram-positive cocci that align in chains. The class of streptococcus is then further subdivided into groups based on surface proteins on the cell wall of the bacterium. Streptococcal pharyngitis is most commonly caused by group A streptococcus but can also be less commonly caused by group C and group G streptococci. The most important task in the evaluation of sore throat is to identify patients infected with group A streptococci so that they may be treated, thereby limiting potential consequences of the infection.

Diagnosis

- Streptococcal pharyngitis occurs most commonly in the winter and spring months.

- It is spread by direct contact with respiratory tract secretions of a person who has the infection.
- There is an incubation period of 2 to 4 days, followed by an abrupt onset of sore throat, fever, malaise, and headache.
- Symptoms of generalized upper respiratory infection—including cough, hoarseness, laryngitis, and runny nose—are usually not present.
- On physical examination, a clinician may find tender anterior cervical lymphadenopathy, tonsillar exudates, or the appearance of pus on the tonsils.
- Because the clinical findings in streptococcal pharyngitis can be nonspecific, laboratory testing is required to definitively make the diagnosis.
- Studies have been done looking at clinical predictors for strep throat to aid clinicians in making the preliminary diagnosis of streptococcal pharyngitis, but the predictive value of these factors is still unreliable.
- The most widely used clinical predictors are looking for tonsillar exudates, tender anterior lymphadenopathy, fever >100°F, and the absence of cough.
  - If three or four of these predictors are present, one can be sure that the throat culture will be positive for streptococcus in 40% to 60% of the cases.
  - If three or four of the predictors are absent, the throat culture will be negative 80% of the time.
- The two main forms of laboratory testing available to make the diagnosis of group A streptococcal pharyngitis are rapid antigen testing (RAT) and the gold standard of throat culture.
  - RAT kits identify streptococcal antigens on pharyngeal swabs and can be used in office settings to obtain an almost immediate result.
  - This form of testing has improved greatly in the last few years but still do not approach the sensitivity and specificity of standard throat cultures.
  - If a RAT kit is used, a positive result can be considered diagnostic and the patient may be treated.
  - If the result is negative, the test must be followed by a standard throat culture to ensure that it was not a false-negative result.

Treatment

- Streptococcal pharyngitis is a self-limited infection that typically resolves on its own within 2 to 5 days after the onset of symptoms.
- There are still a number of reasons to treat the infection, including reduced severity and duration of the illness, reduced risk of complications from the infection, and a reduction in the spread of the illness to others.
  - Complications of group A streptococcal pharyngitis include the development of acute rheumatic fever and poststreptococcal glomerulonephritis.
  - The risk of developing either one of these complications is lowered greatly if the infection is properly treated.
- Cases of group C or group G streptococcal pharyngitis may be treated to decrease the severity of symptoms and to decrease the spread of the illness, but these groups

- are not generally associated with the development of rheumatic fever or glomerulonephritis.
- Group A streptococcus has remained quite sensitive to penicillins.
  - The most cost-effective therapy is Penicillin VK 500 mg by mouth two times a day for 10 days.
  - In cases of penicillin allergic patients, either erythromycin 500 mg four times a day for 10 days, or azithromycin 500 mg by mouth on day 1, with 250 mg by mouth once a day on days 2 to 5 may be used.

Athletic Considerations

- Athletes with streptococcal pharyngitis are allowed to participate in sports, provided that symptoms have resolved to the point that he or she feels physically able to do so.
- Athletes who have fevers, or who are clinically dehydrated by examination, should be disqualified until these symptoms resolve or have been corrected.
- Early detection and treatment can shorten the severity and duration of symptoms, allowing quicker recovery time and return to play.
- In the case of team sports, it is important to stress hand washing and other common infection control measures to help decrease the spread of the infection to teammates.
- The infected athlete should be assigned his or her own water bottle and other personal equipment but need not be quarantined from the team.
- Table 13-4 is a summary of infectious diseases and their treatment.

VIRAL UPPER RESPIRATORY INFECTIONS

Pathology

Upper respiratory tract infections, otherwise known as the "common cold," are caused by a variety of viral agents and are self-limited syndromes. Each of these viral agents cause an indistinguishable clinical syndrome, and the identification of which specific virus is responsible for the patient's symptoms is irrelevant. The most common viral agents involved in causing upper respiratory tract infections are rhinovirus, coronavirus, parainfluenza, respiratory syncytial virus, and adenovirus. Transmission of these agents occurs by aerosolized droplets from the respiratory tract and direct physical contact.

Diagnosis

- The syndrome usually begins with mild malaise, rhinorrhea, nasal congestion, and sore throat.
- Over the next 1 to 2 days, patients may develop laryngitis and cough.
- Fever is unusual and, if present, is of low grade and usually does not exceed 100°F.
- Infectivity is greatest at the time of maximal symptoms.

- Physical examination may reveal boggy nasal mucosa with clear rhinorrhea, serous middle ear effusions without erythema, and an erythematous pharynx without exudate.
- Lung sounds should be clear without any coarseness or focal consolidation.

Treatment

- The mainstay of treatment of viral upper respiratory syndromes is palliative.
  - Acetaminophen or ibuprofen may be used for myalgias and low-grade fever.
  - Nasal congestion may be relieved with oral decongestants such as pseudoephedrine.
- Patients should be sure to maintain adequate hydration and rest.
- In some studies, supplementary vitamin C has been shown to decrease the duration of symptoms related to the common cold and may be a reasonable and safe treatment option.

Athletic Considerations

- Similar to streptococcal pharyngitis, athletes with viral upper respiratory infections may participate if they feel physically able to do so.
- It is important for the participating athlete to ensure good hydration because the illness may lead to dehydration from low-grade fever or poor oral intake.
- Also, it is quite important in team settings that hand washing, reduced finger-to-nose contact, and isolation of water bottles be done to prevent spread of the infection to other teammates.

INFECTIOUS MONONUCLEOSIS

Pathology

Infectious mononucleosis is an illness caused by the Epstein-Barr virus (EBV) and is characterized by the triad of fever, tonsillar pharyngitis, and lymphadenopathy. The infection is most common in those 10 to 19 years of age. There is also a higher incidence of the illness in populations of young adults who are in close contact, such as high school and college students.

EBV is a herpes virus that is primarily spread by saliva and replicates in B lymphocytes. The incubation period of the virus is 4 to 8 weeks, and the virus can persist in the oropharynx of infected individuals for up to 18 months after clinical recovery. Actually, most primary EBV infections are subclinical infections and usually go undetected.

Diagnosis

- The typical presentation of infectious mononucleosis often begins with malaise, headache, and poor appetite.
- It then progresses to the triad of moderate-to-high fever, pharyngitis, and lymphadenopathy.

TABLE 13-4 SUMMARY OF INFECTIOUS DISEASES COMMONLY EXPERIENCED BY ATHLETES

Condition	Symptoms	Exam Findings	Diagnosis	Treatment	Contact Sports Participation
Streptococcal pharyngitis	Sore throat Fever Malaise	Tonsillar exudates Fever >100°F Anterior cervical adenopathy	Rapid antigen testing kits Throat culture	Penicillin VK Erythromycin Azithromycin	Full participation as long as athlete is well hydrated.
Viral upper respiratory infection	Mild malaise Rhinorrhea Cough Laryngitis Sore throat	Boggy nasal mucosa Red pharynx Lungs clear	Clinical based on history and PE	Supportive Tylenol or Motrin Fluids Vitamin C/zinc	Full participation as long as athlete is well hydrated.
Infectious mononucleosis	Severe fatigue Headache Loss of appetite Fever Sore throat	Tonsillar exudates Posterior cervical adenopathy Splenomegaly Clear rhinorrhea	CBC, with atypical lymphocytes + Heterophile antibodies EBV titer	Supportive Tylenol or Motrin Fluids Restriction of activity	No activity for a minimum of 3 weeks from the onset of symptoms, or longer if splenomegaly is present. Then a graded return to activity.
Influenza	Fever Myalgias Cough Malaise Nasal congestion Fatigue Quick onset of symptoms	Fever Rhinorrhea Red pharynx	Clinical *or* Rapid test kits Viral culture/PCR in rare instances	Supportive *or* Amantadine Rimantadine Zanamivir Oseltamivir	May return when symptomatically improved.

CBC, complete blood cell count; EBV, Epstein-Barr virus; PE, physical examination; PCR, polymerase chain reaction.

- Pharyngitis is frequently accompanied by tonsillar exudate and can be confused with the appearance of streptococcal pharyngitis.
- The characteristic lymphadenopathy is symmetric and typically involves the posterior cervical chain, which lies posterior and deep to the sternocleidomastoid muscle.
- Other clinical findings of the syndrome may include severe fatigue, splenomegaly, a generalized maculopapular rash (which is more common with concomitant antibiotic use), hemolytic anemia, and thrombocytopenia.
- Patients with suspected infectious mononucleosis by history and physical examination should have both a complete blood count with differential and heterophile antibody test (monospot) done to confirm the diagnosis.
  - The complete blood count will typically reveal a mildly elevated total white blood cell count composed of 60% to 70% lymphocytes, with greater than 10% being atypical.
    - Atypical lymphocytes are not specific to EBV infections but, when combined with the clinical picture, can be quite suggestive of the diagnosis.
  - Heterophile antibodies are antibodies that react to antigens from unrelated species.
    - In the case of mononucleosis, the test is performed using equine erythrocytes as the substrate.

- The heterophile antibody test is both sensitive and specific for infectious mononucleosis.
- A patient will develop detectable heterophile antibodies within 1 week of the onset of symptoms.
- These antibodies will peak from 2 to 5 weeks and may persist in some patients for up to 1 year.
- A negative heterophile antibody test may occur early in the course of the illness, and if the diagnosis is still in doubt, repeating it later may result in a positive test.
- In a few rare instances, the heterophile antibody test will reveal a false negative.
- In these instances, EBV-specific antibody testing can be obtained, which tests for antibodies directed against antigens on the EBV virus capsid.

Treatment

- Supportive care remains the mainstay in treatment of infectious mononucleosis.
- Acetaminophen or nonsteroidal anti-inflammatory medication can be used for the treatment of fever, myalgias, and throat discomfort related to the infection.
- Adequate rest is also important, but complete bed rest is not necessary.
- Treatment with antiviral agents such as acyclovir has demonstrated suppression of viral shedding from in-

fected individuals but do not affect the clinical course of the illness.

- More recently, attention has been focused on the use of corticosteroids in infectious mononucleosis.
- Study results suggest that prednisone and other corticosteroids may be helpful in decreasing pharyngeal and lymphoid swelling but do not have any significant effect on the course of the infection.

Athletic Considerations

- The two most important factors to consider when deciding an athlete's return to play after infectious mononucleosis are spleen size and the likelihood of a decline from relapse of symptoms.
- Splenic rupture accounts for the greatest risk of both morbidity and mortality in athletes with infectious mononucleosis.
- As the spleen enlarges from the infiltration of lymphocytes, it becomes increasingly fragile and may lead to spontaneous rupture or rupture related to minor abdominal trauma.
- It has been estimated that greater than 50% of patients with primary EBV infection have splenomegaly as part of the illness.
- These changes in the spleen seem to be most prominent from day 4 to day 21 of the illness, with the risk of splenic rupture being highest at this time as well.
- It is recommended that all athletes should have an absolute minimum disqualification of 21 days from the onset of the illness to minimize the possibility of injury to the spleen.
- After day 21 of the illness, a careful physical examination should be performed focusing on assessment of the spleen size.
    - One of the major difficulties in determining spleen status is that the physical examination of the spleen is difficult and, in many cases, the spleen is enlarged even when it is not palpable on physical examination.
    - Abdominal ultrasound is the study of choice to assess spleen size in patients with infectious mononucleosis, but experts differ in opinion on whether an ultrasound is required before allowing an athlete to return to play.
    - If an athlete's spleen status is in question, especially if the athlete participates in a contact sport, the treating physician should not hesitate to obtain an ultrasound to ensure that spleen size is normal.
    - At this time, however, no formal recommendation has been made for the use of abdominal ultrasound in the return-to-play decision for athletes with mononucleosis.
    - If the spleen remains enlarged by either physical examination or ultrasound, an athlete should be held from participation until splenic enlargement resolves.
- Another question to consider when deciding to allow an athlete to return to play is whether the viral syndrome has resolved enough to prevent relapse of the symptoms of the illness.

- The major concern is that too rapid of a return to activity may exacerbate the athlete's symptoms lending to a longer time of recovery.
- In general, all athletes should have a 3-week disqualification period.
- If symptoms of the viral syndrome are resolving, and no further splenic concerns exist, the athlete may begin a graded return to training leading up to full participation.

INFLUENZA

Pathology

Influenza, or the flu, is an acute respiratory disease caused by the influenza virus. The influenza virus is grouped into three types: A, B, and C. Influenza A and influenza B are further divided into various subtypes that cause the typical infection associated with the flu. Influenza causes yearly epidemics from December to March in temperate climates and can cause significant morbidity and mortality. The virus replicates in the epithelial cells of the respiratory tract and is spread via respiratory secretions expelled during coughing, sneezing, or talking. The disease can spread very quickly in close quarters such as schools, nursing home, or locker rooms.

The incubation period for influenza is short, usually 1 to 4 days. Adults are typically infectious 1 day before symptoms appear and, on average, 5 days into the illness. Children may be infectious for slightly longer.

Diagnosis

- The main challenge in diagnosis is differentiating the influenza virus and its symptoms from other common upper respiratory viruses, both of which are very prevalent during the winter months.
- Some of the classic symptoms of influenza are fever (generally 100° to 104°F), myalgias, and cough.
    - These symptoms tend to be more common in influenza than in other viruses that cause colds.
- In addition, a patient may experience congestion, sore throat, anorexia, and malaise similar to symptoms with other common winter viruses.
- Another possible clue to differentiating influenza from other viruses is the acuity of symptoms.
    - The symptoms of influenza tend to occur quickly, whereas other viruses tend to have a more gradual onset with symptoms that occur mildly, and then progress over several days.
    - Flu symptoms also tend to resolve quickly, lasting on average 5 to 7 days; however, malaise can sometimes persist longer.
- Mortalities related to the influenza occur every year typically in individuals over 65 or young children. From 1990 to 1999, there were approximately 36,000 deaths attributed to influenza.
    - The main cause of death is pneumonia, either from the influenza virus or as a result of a coinfection with another virus or bacteria.

- Influenza may also worsen existing cardiac or pulmonary disease, leading to hospitalizations and sometimes death.
- The diagnostic tests available to aid in the diagnosis of influenza include viral culture, serology, polymerase chain reaction, enzyme immunoassay, and direct immunofluorescence.
    - Many of these tests are not practical because the results take too long to return, and some testing methods only occur in specialized laboratories.
    - A viral culture is important epidemiologically, as it can identify the exact subtype of influenza, although it will not aid in treatment decisions because the results usually take 5 to 10 days to return.
    - There are several rapid test kits available that use enzyme immunoassay and immunofluorescence techniques and generally return results anywhere from 10 to 30 minutes. Most of these rapid tests are more than 70% sensitive and more than 90% specific.
- One of the best ways to limit morbidity and mortality related to influenza is widespread vaccination.
    - Each year, the subtypes of influenza thought to be most prevalent in the given year are determined, and vaccines are created against these subtypes.
    - The vaccine is available as inactivated (killed virus), which is available via injection, and live attenuated virus is available via a nasal spray.
    - Typically, those at highest risk for complications—such as infants, the elderly, and individuals with chronic disease, as well as health care workers—are vaccinated as early as the vaccine becomes available.
    - Others can be vaccinated throughout the flu season, depending on the amount of vaccine available in a given year.
    - The main side effect of vaccination is a mild flu-like illness, which can be more pronounced with use of the live attenuated vaccine.

Treatment

- There are medications available that may lessen the time course of influenza symptoms, but these need to be started when the virus is actively replicating usually within the first 48 hours of symptom onset.
- Amantadine and rimantadine have been available the longest; although their mechanism of action is not entirely understood, they are believed to inhibit an ion channel on the influenza A virus.
    - The major drawback is that these medications are effective only against influenza A.
    - They also may cause gastrointestinal or central nervous system side effects that may limit their use.
- In 1999, the U.S. Food and Drug Administration approved the neuraminidase inhibitors zanamivir (Relenza) and oseltamivir (Tamiflu) for the treatment of influenza.
    - Neuraminidase is a viral glycoprotein necessary for the replication of influenza A and B.

- The standard adult dose of oseltamivir is 75 mg twice/day for 5 days.
- Zanamivir is administered by oral inhalation, and so it needs to be used with caution in those with existing asthma or chronic obstructive pulmonary disease, because it may cause bronchospasm.
    - The standard adult dose of zanamivir is 10 mg delivered via an inhalation device twice per day for 5 days.
- The benefit of these medications is that they are effective against both influenza A and B. The main drawback is the cost.
- In addition to their use for treatment of influenza, amantadine, rimantadine, and oseltamivir have been approved for chemoprophylaxis of close contacts of individuals diagnosed with influenza.

Athletic Considerations

- Outbreaks of influenza can spread quickly among teams, so it is important to make the diagnosis early so that the infected individual may be removed from contact with teammates.
- Infected individuals should avoid contact with others for 5 days.
    - However, if treatment is begun within the first 48 hours of symptom onset, the infectious period is likely lessened.
- There are no good data on the duration of the infectious period in a treated individual, but a general rule is 3 days.
- Unvaccinated, close contacts of individuals who are diagnosed with influenza may undergo chemoprophylaxis to prevent infection.
- Infected individuals may return to competition when they are symptomatically improved, which may take 3 to 10 days.
- Again, the malaise from influenza may last longer than 1 week and may be a limiting factor in return to activity.
    - An individual should not be allowed to return if they are still febrile or clinically dehydrated.
- If the supplies of vaccine allow, vaccinating teams who are active in the winter months early in the flu season is the ideal way to prevent team epidemics.

SUGGESTED READING

Aronson, MD. Infectious mononucleosis in adults and adolescents. Up To Date Online. Accessed October 25, 2004.

Bartlett JG. Approach to acute pharyngitis in adults. Up To Date Online. Accessed October 25, 2004.

Bergfeld WF. Dermatologic problems in athletes. Clin Sports Med 1982;1:419–430.

Bisno AL, Peter GS, Kaplan EL. Diagnosis of strep throat in adults: are clinical criteria really good enough? Clin Infect Dis 2002;35:126.

Bisno AL. Acute pharyngitis. N Engl J Med 2001;344:205.

Brandfonbrener A, Epstein A, Wu S, et al. Corticosteroid therapy in Epstein-Barr virus infection. Arch Intern Med 1986;146:337.

Burroughs KE. Athletes resuming activity after infectious mononucleosis. Arch Fam Med 2000;9:1122.

Conklin RJ. Common cutaneous disorders in athletes. Sports Med 1990;9:100–117.

Cooper RJ, Hoffman JR, Bartlett JG, et al. Principles of appropriate antibiotic use for acute pharyngitis in adults: background. Ann Intern Med 2001;134:509.

Dienst WL Jr, Dightman L, Dworkin MS, et al. Pinning down skin infections: diagnosis, treatment, and prevention in wrestlers. Phys Sportsmed 1997;25.

Dommerby H, Stangerup SE, Stangerup M, et al. Hepatosplenomegaly in infectious mononucleosis, assessed by ultrasonic scanning. Laryngol Otol 1986;100:573–579.

Ebell MH. Epstein-Barr virus infectious mononucleosis. Am Fam Phys 2004;70:1279.

Eiland G, Ridley D. Dermatological problems in the athlete. J Orthop Sports Phys Ther 1996;23:388–402.

Fitzpatrick TB, Johnson RA, Wolff K, et al. Color Atlas and Synopsis of Clinical Dermatology. New York: McGraw-Hill, 1997.

Friedman ND, Sexton DJ. The common cold in adults. Up To Date Online. Accessed November 12, 2004.

Habif T. Clinical Dermatology. St. Louis: Mosby, 1996.

Harper SA, Fukuda K, Uyeki TM, et al. Prevention and control of influenza. MMWR 2004;53(RR06):1–40.

Karlowski TR, Chalmers TC, Frenkel LD, et al. Ascorbic acid for the common cold, a prophylactic and therapeutic trial. JAMA 1998; 231:1038.

Kirkpatrick GL. The common cold. Primary Care 1996;23:657.

Landry GL, Chang CJ. Herpes and tinea in wrestling. Phys Sportsmed 2004;32:43–44.

Levy JA. Common bacterial dermatoses. Phys Sportsmed 2004;32: 33–39.

MacKnight JM. Infectious mononucleosis. Phys Sportsmed 2002;30: 27–31.

Montaldo NJ. An office-based approach to influenza: clinical diagnosis and laboratory testing. Am Fam Physician 2003;67:111–118.

Montaldo NJ, Gum KD, Ashley JV. Updated treatment for influenza A and B. Am Fam Physician 2000;62:2467–2476.

Snow V, Mottur-Dilson C, Cooper RJ, et al. Principles of appropriate antibiotic use for acute pharyngitis in adults. Ann Intern Med 2001; 134:506.

Srivastava KP, Quinlan EC, Casey TV. Spontaneous rupture of the spleen secondary to infectious mononucleosis. Intern Surg 1972; 57:171–173.

Tynell E, Aurelius E, Brandell C, et al. Acyclovir and prednisolone treatment of acute infectious mononucleosis: a multicenter, double blind, placebo-controlled study. J Infect Dis 1996;174:324.

York WH. Spontaneous rupture of the spleen: report of a case secondary to infectious mononucleosis. JAMA 1962;179:170–171.

14

ANATOMY AND BIOMECHANICS OF THE SHOULDER

DEREK PLAUSINIS
LAITH M. JAZRAWI
JOSEPH D. ZUCKERMAN
ANDREW S. ROKITO

The shoulder complex consists of four articulations: the glenohumeral joint, the scapulothoracic articulation, the acromioclavicular joint, and the sternoclavicular joint. The coordinated activity of these articulations provides greater motion than any other joint in the body. Bony constraints are limited. To achieve stability during motion, the ligamentous restraints and muscular activity are crucial to shoulder biomechanics.

This chapter discusses the relevant anatomy, kinematics, static stability, and dynamic stability of the four main articulations forming the shoulder complex. Clinical examples of applied biomechanics are provided in each section.

STERNOCLAVICULAR JOINT

Anatomy

The sternoclavicular joint is the synovial joint that is responsible for linking the upper extremity directly to the thorax. The joint consists of the enlarged, saddle-shaped medial end of the clavicle that articulates with the superolateral aspect of the manubrium and a small facet on the first rib. The sternoclavicular joint contains a fibrocartilaginous articular disc, or meniscus, that completely covers the articular surfaces and divides the joint into two compartments. The joint is surrounded by a capsule and the anterior and posterior sternoclavicular ligaments. Joint stability is achieved from the costoclavicular and interclavicular ligaments (Fig. 14-1). The costoclavicular ligaments are lateral to the joint capsule and run between the undersurface of the medial end of the clavicle and the first rib.

The clavicle functions as a bony strut connecting the thorax to the upper extremity and links the sternoclavicular joint to the acromioclavicular joint. The clavicle is an S-shaped bone with the medial two thirds of the body having an anterior convexity and the lateral third having an anterior concavity. These curvatures contribute to the normal appearance and contour of the upper chest. In addition to

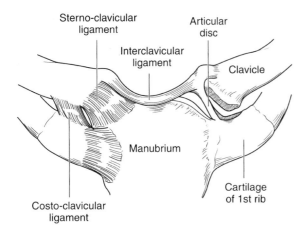

Figure 14-1   Anatomy of the sternoclavicular joint. Note that the articular disc divides the joint into two compartments. (From Squire ME, Esmail AN, Soslowsky LJ. Anatomy and biomechanics of the shoulder. In: McGinty JB, Burkhart SS, Jackson RW et al., eds. Operative Arthroscopy, 3rd ed. Philadelphia: Lippincott Williams & Wilkins, 2003:162.)

Motion

The sternoclavicular joint is capable of protraction-retraction, elevation-depression, and rotation. Elevation and depression result in motion between the clavicle and the disc, and rotary movements in motion between the disc and the sternum. The normal range of motion of the sternoclavicular joint is up to 35 degrees of protraction-retraction (Fig. 14-2A), and 35 degrees of upward elevation (Fig. 14-2B). Rotation along the axis of the clavicle is up to 50 degrees (Fig. 14-2C). In the first 70 degrees of shoulder elevation, motion occurring at the sternoclavicular joint is mostly clavicular elevation with little axial rotation. Beyond approximately 70 degrees of arm elevation, clavicular rotation starts to occur.

Full elevation of the upper extremity requires coordinated motion between the glenohumeral and sternoclavicular joints. For every 10 degrees of arm elevation, there is approximately 4 degrees of clavicular elevation. If the sternoclavicular joint were to be surgically fused, shoulder motion would be significantly impaired with shoulder abduction limited to approximately 90 degrees.

Stability

The sternoclavicular joint itself has little intrinsic bony stability. Stability is provided by the articular disc, in conjunction with the anterior and posterior sternoclavicular ligaments, the costoclavicular ligament, and the interclavicular ligaments (Fig. 14-1). The major constraint to sternoclavicular motion is the costoclavicular ligament,

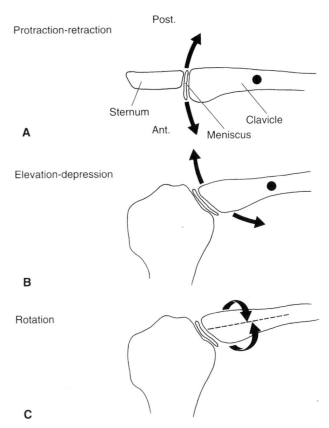

Figure 14-2   Motion at the sternoclavicular joint. A: Axial (transverse) view with clavicular protraction and retraction. B: Coronal view demonstrating elevation and depression. C: Coronal view demonstrating rotation along the longitudinal axis of the clavicle. (From Della Valle CJ, Rokito AS, Gallagher Birdzell M, et al. Biomechanics of the shoulder. In: Nordin M, Frankel VH, eds. Basic Biomechanics of the Musculoskeletal System. Baltimore: Lippincott Williams & Wilkins, 2001:321.)

which resists upward, as well as posterior, displacement of the clavicle. The anterior and posterior sternoclavicular ligaments provide stability to anterior and posterior translations, as well as superior displacement. The interclavicular ligament, connecting the superomedial aspect of the clavicles, becomes taut when the arm is depressed and relaxed when the arm is elevated. The interclavicular ligament assists with restraining the joint superiorly, with the posterior portion also contributing to anterior stability of the sternoclavicular joint. Finally, the articular disc contributes to limiting inferior displacement through articular contact and also prevents medial displacement of the clavicle.

If the costoclavicular ligaments are competent, there is sufficient stability of the proximal clavicle to allow resection of the medial clavicle in cases of arthrosis. However, if the costoclavicular ligaments have been previously injured, as in the case of a sternoclavicular dislocation, then excision of the medial clavicle alone will lead to instability of the proximal clavicle, and consideration must be given to costoclavicular ligament reconstruction.

ACROMIOCLAVICULAR JOINT

Anatomy

The acromioclavicular joint is a synovial joint linking the lateral clavicle to the acromion. The joint lies in an antero-posterior direction and has a variable tilt anywhere from a vertical orientation in the sagittal plane to a 50-degree tilt, with the clavicle overriding the acromion (Fig. 14-3). It is subject to high loads transmitted from the chest muscula-ture and is stabilized by the acromioclavicular joint liga-ments (capsular thickenings) and the coracoclavicular ligaments. The coracoclavicular ligaments consist of the posteromedially directed conoid ligament and the anterolat-erally directed trapezoid ligament. The coracoacromial liga-ment lies anterior and lateral to the acromioclavicular joint and runs from the most lateral aspect of the coracoid to the medial aspect of the acromion.

The acromioclavicular joint has a wedge-shaped articular disc that originates from the superior aspect of the joint and whose function is poorly understood. Unlike the disc of the sternoclavicular joint, the acromioclavicular joint disc usually has a perforation at the center. The joint is com-posed of hyaline cartilage early in life, but transforms to fibrocartilage on the acromial side by age 17 and on the clavicular side by age 23.

Motion

Motion between the clavicle and the scapula is synchron-ous, with little relative motion at the acromioclavicular joint. The majority of scapulothoracic motion occurs with coordinated sternoclavicular joint movement, and thus rigid

fixation or fusion of the acromioclavicular joint produces little loss of overall shoulder function.

Stability

The acromioclavicular joint capsule is the primary restraint to horizontal and rotational stability. Specifically, the supe-rior acromioclavicular ligament is the most important stabi-lizer to anteroposterior translation. With some contribution of the acromioclavicular ligaments, the primary restraint to vertical stability is the coracoclavicular ligaments (conoid and trapezoid), which can be viewed as suspending the sca-pula from the clavicle. The smaller conoid ligament acts to limit superior-inferior displacement of the clavicle. The quadrilaterally shaped trapezoid, lateral to the conoid, is the larger and stronger of the two ligaments and resists axial compression and motion about the horizontal axis. The del-toid and trapezius muscles also help stabilize the acromio-clavicular joint and have fibers that blend with the superior acromioclavicular ligament. The exact contribution of the deltoid and trapezius to stability is not known.

Injury to the acromioclavicular ligaments is a common clinical problem, and an understanding of the anatomy and biomechanics will help guide proper diagnosis and treat-ment. When the acromioclavicular joint ligaments have been disrupted with intact or strained coracoclavicular liga-ments (i.e., a type II injury), physical examination will dem-onstrate horizontal instability but will not demonstrate any vertical stability. When the coracoclavicular ligaments are also injured (i.e., type III to type V injuries), vertical instabil-ity of the acromioclavicular joint will also be clinically evi-dent. Finally, if the deltotrapezial fascia is also injured, lead-ing to complete joint dislocation (type V injury), then—in

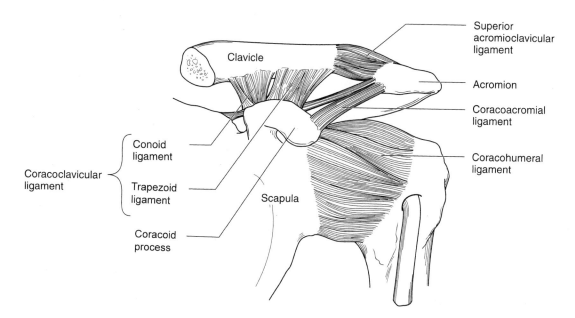

Figure 14-3 Anatomy of the acromioclavicular joint. The coracoclavicular ligaments (conoid and trapezoid) and the primary vertical stabilizer. The superior acromioclavicular ligament is the primary horizontal stabilizer. (From Squire ME, Esmail AN, Soslowsky LJ. Anatomy and biomechanics of the shoulder. In: McGinty JB, Burkhart SS, Jackson RW, et al., eds. Operative Arthroscopy, 3rd ed. Philadelphia: Lippincott Williams & Wilkins, 2003:163.)

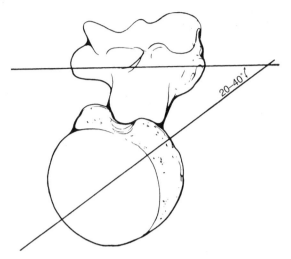

Figure 14-4 Orientation of the humeral head demonstrating retroversion with respect to the transepicondylar axis at the elbow. (From O'Brien SJ, Fealy S, Drakos M, et al. Developmental anatomy of the shoulder and anatomy of the glenohumeral joint. The normal retroversion is usually in the range from 20 degrees to 40 degrees. In: Rockwood CA Jr, Matsen FA III, Wirth MA, et al., eds. The Shoulder, 3rd ed. Philadelphia: Saunders-Elsevier, 2004:13.)

addition to horizontal and vertical instability—the acromion can be passively brought under the distal clavicle with cross-body adduction of the arm.

GLENOHUMERAL AND SCAPULOTHORACIC MOTION

Anatomy

Proximal Humerus

The humeral head is covered with hyaline cartilage and is nearly spherical in shape. The articular surface forms a 120-degree arc and has an upward or medial inclination of 45 degrees. When referenced from the transepicondylar axis of the distal humerus, the humeral head is retroverted, or posteriorly directed, with respect to the intercondylar plane of the distal humerus (Fig. 14-4). There is a wide range of humeral retroversion among individuals, and most surgeons use the range of 20 to 40 degrees of humeral retroversion as a guide during reconstructive procedures.

Rotator Cuff and Glenohumeral Joint Capsule

The rotator cuff tendons are composed of the subscapularis, the supraspinatus, the infraspinatus, and the teres minor (Fig. 14-5). Both the supraspinatus and the infraspinatus

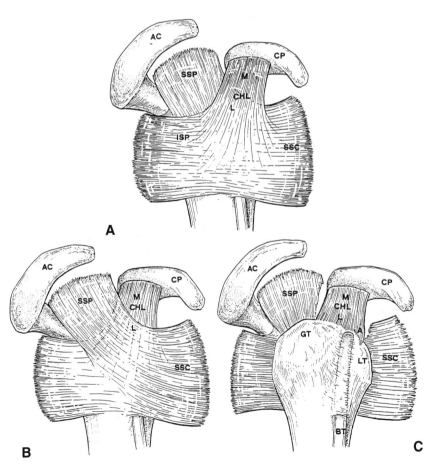

Figure 14-5 Anterolateral view of a right shoulder demonstrating rotator cuff insertions and the rotator interval. **A:** The superficial layer of the rotator interval consists of the superficial fibers of the coracohumeral ligament (*CHL*), which extend to the insertions of the supraspinatus (*SSP*) and subscapularis (*SSC*). **B:** The second layer of the rotator interval showing fibers of SSP and SSC crossing through the interval and uniting with CHL. **C:** The third layer of the rotator interval consists of deep fibers of CHL inserting into the greater tuberosity (*GT*) and lesser tuberosity (*LT*), and forming an anterior covering band (*A*) around the long biceps tendon (*BT*). AC, acromion; CP, coracoid process; ISP, infraspinatus; L, lateral; M, medial. (From Jost B, Koch PP, Gerber C. Anatomy and functional aspects of the rotator interval. J Shoulder Elbow Surg 2000;9:336–341.)

are innervated from the suprascapular nerve, whereas the teres minor is innervated by a branch of the axillary nerve, and the subscapularis is innervated by the upper and lower subscapular nerves. The supraspinatus originates from the supraspinatus fossa of the scapula and inserts on the greater tuberosity on the superior aspect of the proximal humerus. The infraspinatus and teres minor muscles originate from the posterior aspect of the scapula below the scapular spine and insert on the posterior aspect of the greater tuberosity. The subscapularis, which lies on the anterior surface of the scapula, inserts on the lesser tuberosity. The rotator cuff tendons have well-defined, relatively broad insertions on the tuberosities, with the average medial-to-lateral distance across the supraspinatus insertion measuring 12.7 mm.

The glenohumeral joint is surrounded by a capsule with distinct anatomical regions and capsular thickenings (Fig. 14-6). The triangular area bound by the superior edge of the subscapularis, the anterior edge of the supraspinatus,

and the base of the coracoid define the rotator interval. Deep to the capsule of the rotator interval lies the long head of the biceps tendon that exits the glenohumeral joint at the apex of this triangular region.

The rotator interval is made up of the joint capsule, the superior glenohumeral ligament, and the coracohumeral ligament. The middle glenohumeral ligament, which has a great deal of anatomic variability in the anterosuperior quadrant of the joint, may occasionally form part of the rotator interval. Below the rotator interval, the anterior band of the inferior glenohumeral ligament originates from the inferior labrum at the level from midglenoid. Additional detailed anatomy and the specific functions of these ligaments are discussed further under the section on static stability.

The long head of biceps tendon leaves the rotator interval laterally and travels in the bicipital (intertubercular) groove, which is covered by the transverse humeral ligament. The

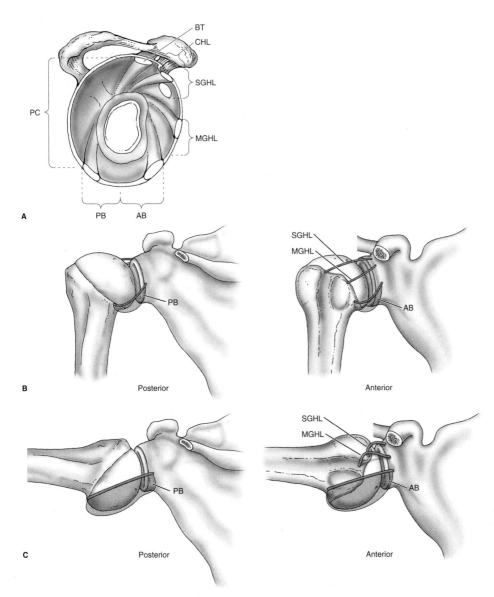

Figure 14-6 **A:** Section through the glenohumeral joint capsule perpendicular to the plane of the scapula. *AB*, anterior band of inferior glenohumeral ligament; *BT*, long head of biceps tendon; *MGHL*, middle glenohumeral ligament; *PB*, posterior band of inferior glenohumeral ligament; *PC*, posterior capsule; *SGHL*, superior glenohumeral ligament. **B:** In adduction and neutral rotation, the SGHL is the primary ligamentous restraint. **C:** In abduction and neutral rotation, the AB and PB tighten to prevent inferior translation. (After Warner JP, Deng XH, Warren RF, et al. Static capsuloligamentous restraints to superior-inferior translation of the glenohumeral joint. Am J Sports Med 1992;20:677, 682–683.)

location of the bicipital groove may be identified by positioning the shoulder with the elbow at the side and the forearm internally rotated approximately 10 degrees. The long head of the biceps should then lie directly anterior and be palpable between the two tuberosities.

Scapula and Glenoid

The scapula is a flat triangular bone supported by ligamentous attachments to the clavicle (see Fig. 14-3) and muscular attachments to the chest wall. It lies on the posterolateral aspect of the thorax between the second and seventh ribs and is angled 30 degrees anterior to the coronal plane of the thorax (Fig. 14-7). In the resting position, the scapula has a slight rotation of the superior border toward the midline of approximately 3 degrees. When referenced to the medial border of the scapula, the glenoid has a slight upward tilt of approximately 5 degrees. The glenoid fossa is retroverted, compared with the scapular plane an average of 7 degrees, although there is sizeable variation among individuals (Fig. 14-8).

The scapula has numerous muscle attachments that include the origin of all the rotator cuff muscles. The serratus anterior, which helps to stabilize the scapula against the chest wall and thus to prevent "scapular winging," attaches to the medial undersurface of the scapula and lies just anterior to the subscapularis. These two muscles glide along one another with scapulothoracic movement. The rhomboids and levator scapulae attach along the medial border of the scapula and assist with elevation. Superiorly, the deltoid and trapezius attach to the scapular spine and acromion process.

Radiographically, the scapular glenoid appears to have a relatively flat surface. However, the articular cartilage is thicker peripherally than it is centrally, which increases the depth of the glenoid. In addition, the glenoid is surrounded

by a fibrocartilaginous rim called the *labrum* (Fig. 14-9). As a result, the humeral head and glenoid are, in fact, quite congruent. The radius of curvature for the glenoid is only slightly larger than that of the humeral head. In 88% of cases, the radius of curvature of the glenoid is no more than 2 mm greater than that of the humeral head, and all cases will have less than a 3-mm mismatch.

Muscles of the Shoulder Girdle

Anatomically, the shoulder musculature can be thought of as an outer layer consisting of the deltoid and pectoralis major muscles, an inner layer consisting of the rotator cuff muscles (subscapularis, supraspinatus, infraspinatus, and teres minor), and the scapular stabilizing muscles (trapezius, levator scapulae, rhomboids, and serratus anterior).

The deltoid gives the shoulder its normal rounded contour and is composed of the anterior, middle, and posterior heads—all of which insert into the deltoid tuberosity on the anterolateral aspect of the humerus. The origin of the deltoid is from the anterior lateral third of the clavicle, the lateral acromion, and the posteromedial scapular spine. The anterior head acts as a strong flexor and internal rotator of the humerus, the middle head as an abductor, and the posterior head as an extensor and external rotator.

The pectoralis major lies over the anterior chest wall and is composed of two heads: the clavicular head originating from the medial two thirds of the clavicle and the sternocostal head originating from the sternum, manubrium, and the upper costal cartilages. The two heads converge at the sternoclavicular joint. The pectoralis major insertion lies just anterior to the long head of the biceps and the intertubercular groove. The prime function of the pectoralis major is to adduct and internally rotate the humerus. The clavicular head also serves as a forward elevator of the humerus, whereas the sternocostal head extends the humerus. Beneath the outer layer of deltoid and pectoralis lies the rotator cuff musculature, which is discussed in the previous section.

The trapezius has a broad origin from the posterior neck and the thoracic vertebra and plays a critical role in scapular motion. The uppermost fibers insert into the lateral third of the clavicle, the middle fibers insert into medial margin of the acromion the spine of the scapula, and the inferior fibers converge near the medial margin of the scapular spine. Deep to the trapezius lies the levator scapulae and the rhomboid major and minor. The levator attaches to the vertebral border of the scapula just above the level of the scapular spine, and the rhomboids attach just below the scapular spine.

The serratus anterior is a sizeable muscle also critical to scapular motion. It originates from digitations of the outer upper eight or nine ribs and runs along the chest wall toward the scapula. The serratus inserts along the full length of the vertebral border of the scapula.

The scapulothoracic articulation is not a synovial joint but rather consists of a series of bursae to permit muscles to glide past one another. The largest and most consistent bursa is the scapulothoracic bursa located between the serratus anterior and the rib cage. Another large bursa, although not always present, is the subscapularis bursa between the subscapularis and the serratus. A consistent, well-defined bursal structure is also present between the

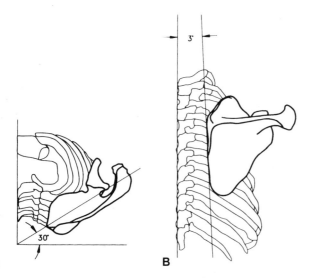

Figure 14-7 Scapular orientation on the chest wall demonstrating the scapular plane angled 30 degrees from the coronal plane **(A)** and with 3 degrees rotation toward the midline **(B)**. (From Itoi E, Morrey BF, An KN. Biomechanics of the shoulder. In: Rockwood CA, Matsen FA, Wirth MA, et al., eds. The Shoulder, 3rd ed. Philadelphia: Saunders-Elsevier, 2004:231.)

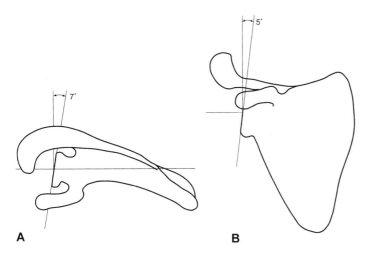

A   **B**

Figure 14-8   **A:** The glenoid fossa is retroverted approximately 7 degrees with respect to the scapular plane. **B:** When referenced to the medial border of the scapula, there is a slight superior tilt to the glenoid of approximately 5 degrees. (From Simon SR, Alaranta H, An KN, et al. Kinesiology. In: Buckwalter JA, Einhorn TA, Simon SR. Orthopaedic Basic Science. Rosemont, IL: American Academy of Orthopaedic Surgeons, 2000:737.)

superomedial angle of the scapula and the undersurface of the trapezius. Finally, a less consistently observed bursa may sometimes be located between the inferior angle of the scapula and the latissimus dorsi.

Motion

Although the glenohumeral joint is the central player in motion of the shoulder complex, coordinated activity of the acromioclavicular, sternoclavicular, and scapulothoracic articulations is vital to the overall function of the shoulder complex. To help understand the function of the shoulder girdle musculature, Jobe and Pink have categorized the shoulder girdle muscles into the glenohumeral protectors, humeral positioners, scapular pivoters, and the propeller

muscles. The rotator cuff muscles are the glenohumeral protectors and primarily function to provide dynamic joint stability. The humeral positioners are composed of the three parts of the deltoid and serve as the prime mover of the glenohumeral joint. The scapular pivoters consist of the serratus anterior, the trapezius, the rhomboids, and the levator scapulae. The pivoter muscles all function to position the glenoid in space for optimal glenohumeral function. Finally, the propellers are made up of the pectoralis major and the latissimus dorsi. The propeller muscles do not attach to the scapula; rather, they run from the torso to the humerus. They assist in transferring energy from the trunk and lower extremities during throwing activities and also serve as powerful interval rotators and adductors.

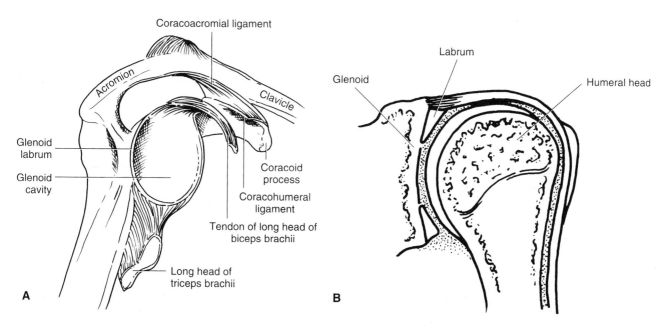

A   **B**

Figure 14-9   **A:** The glenoid labrum attached to the underlying bony glenoid and is continuous with the anchor of the tendon of the long head of the biceps. **B:** In cross section, the labrum has a triangular configuration and helps to deepen the glenoid, thereby, increasing stability of the glenohumeral joint. (From Della Valle CJ, Rokito AS, Gallagher Birdzell M, et al. Biomechanics of the shoulder. In: Nordin M, Frankel VH, eds. Basic Biomechanics of the Musculoskeletal System. Baltimore: Lippincott Williams & Wilkins, 2001:324.)

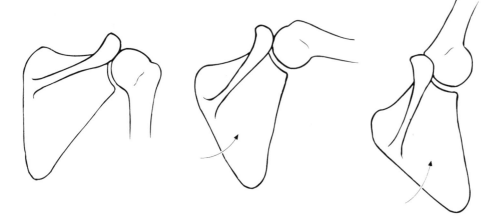

Figure 14-10 With forward elevation or abduction, synchronous rotation of the scapula occurs with an overall 2:1 ratio of glenohumeral to scapulothoracic motion. (From Simon SR, Alaranta H, An KN, et al. Kinesiology. In: Buckwalter JA, Einhorn TA, Simon SR, eds. Orthopaedic Basic Science. Rosemont, IL: American Academy of Orthopaedic Surgeons, 2000:745.)

In the clinical setting, glenohumeral motion can be difficult to assess in isolation since shoulder motion involves contributions from the glenohumeral joint and the scapulothoracic articulation (Fig. 14-10). Glenohumeral and scapulothoracic kinematics are reviewed individually below, followed by a discussion on composite shoulder motion.

Glenohumeral Joint

Within the midrange of motion of the shoulder, the glenohumeral junction functions almost as a ball-and-socket joint. Active motion of the shoulder is also accompanied by obligate humeral head translations that are small and usually in the range of 0 to 2 mm. Pathology of the glenohumeral joint capsule or rotator cuff, however, alters the normal kinematics. With asymmetric capsular contractures, increased translations are observed in the direction opposite to the contracture. For example, when the anterior capsule has been overtightened following an instability procedure, increased posterior translation of the humeral head occurs, and degenerative changes in the joint may follow. In the case of large rotator cuff tears, excessive superior translation may be observed because the rotator cuff can no longer stabilize the humeral head from the upward pull of the deltoid.

When the rotator cuff is not active to stabilize the glenohumeral joint, glenohumeral translations with passive range of motion may be dramatically increased—up to 12 mm in some cases. These higher translations may be observed in the operating room with patients under anesthesia or in the clinical setting, when a patient can relax their shoulder musculature.

Scapulothoracic Articulation

The scapula provides an anatomic link between the trunk and arm. Scapular motion is generated by the scapular pivoters (serratus anterior, upper and lower trapezius, rhomboids, and levator scapulae), with the primary function to position the glenoid in space for optimal glenohumeral function. Appropriate placement of the glenoid in space (a) assists with glenohumeral stability, (b) provides adequate clearance of the rotator cuff tendons under the acromion to prevent impingement, and (c) maintains deltoid tension to allow for optimal power, regardless of arm position. The primary movements of the scapula are elevation, depression, protraction, retraction, and rotation. As previously

noted, scapular motion is almost always coupled with glenohumeral motion.

Scapular stability relies on the activity of force couples: muscle groups acting in opposite directions to provide stability and control movement. In the case of scapular elevation, rotation of the scapula occurs by synergistic contraction of the upper trapezius, the levator scapula, and the upper serratus anterior (Fig. 14-11). To stabilize the scapula, the force of these muscles is balanced by the activity from the scapular depressors, the lower portions of the trapezius, and serratus anterior.

Integrated Motion of the Shoulder Complex

Motion of the shoulder complex involves two integrated components: the glenohumeral joint and the scapulothoracic articulation (see Fig. 14-10). Traditional assessment of motion involved flexion in the sagittal pane, extension and abduction in the coronal plane, and internal/external rotation (axial rotation of the humerus with the arm held in an adducted position) (Fig. 14-12). During most activities, however, the limb is seldom active in these specific planes of motion. For example, abduction in the coronal plane is limited by bony impingement of the greater tuberosity on the acromion. Elevation in the plane of the scapula, therefore, is considered to be a more functional measure; as in this plane, the inferior portion of the capsule is not twisted, and the musculature of the shoulder is optimally aligned for elevation of the arm (Fig. 14-13). For clinical assessment of motion, the American Shoulder and Elbow Surgeons have recommended that four planes of shoulder motion be assessed in the clinical setting: total forward elevation, external rotation with the elbow at the side, external rotation with the arm abducted 90 degrees, and internal rotation behind the back.

Elevation. The average forward elevation is 167 degrees in men and 171 degrees in women. In the first 30 degrees of elevation in the scapular plane, motion occurs mostly at the glenohumeral joint. As the arm is elevated further, scapulothoracic motion plays a larger role, with an equal contribution of glenohumeral and scapulothoracic movement in the last 60 degrees of elevation. Overall, there is a 2:1 ratio of glenohumeral to scapulothoracic motion in elevation. Elevation of the arm also involves a complex rota-

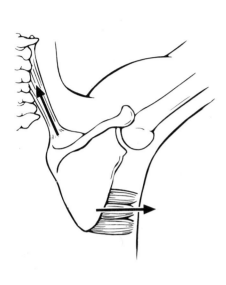
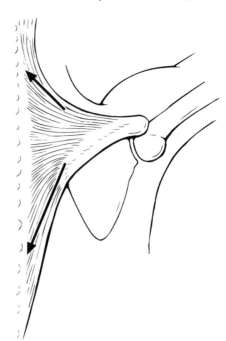

Figure 14-11 Rotation of the scapula is generated by force couples. Synergistic contraction of the levator scapulae and serratus anterior occur, along with synergistic contraction of the upper and lower portions of the trapezius. (From Simon SR, Alaranta H, An KN, et al. Kinesiology. In: Buckwalter JA, Einhorn TA, Simon SR. Orthopaedic Basic Science. Rosemont, IL: American Academy of Orthopaedic Surgeons, 2000:745.)

tory motion of the scapula, with anterior rotation during the first 90 degrees followed by posterior rotation, with a total arc of approximately 15 degrees.

During active shoulder elevation, the deltoid and supraspinatus work synergistically to raise the arm, and electromyographic studies have shown that both muscles are active throughout the range of elevation. With the arm at the side in the resting position, the line of pull of the deltoid is more vertical, whereas the supraspinatus pulls in a more horizontal direction (Fig. 14-14). The supraspinatus, therefore, is thought to play a larger role in initiating abduction. As the arm is progressively elevated from the side, the vertical or shearing component of the deltoid force is lessened, and the direction of pull approximates that of the supraspinatus. The combined function of the supraspinatus and deltoid muscles has been clinically demonstrated with selective anesthetic blocks. With an axillary nerve block and resulting deltoid paralysis, forward elevation is possible, although it is significantly weakened. Similarly, a suprascapular nerve block with resultant supraspinatus paralysis has a similar effect. How-

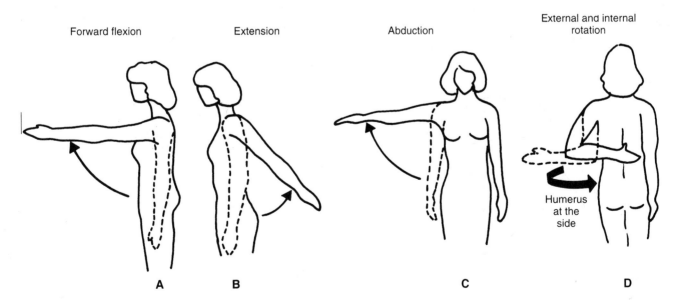

Figure 14-12 Traditional assessment of shoulder motion. Flexion **(A)** and extension **(B)** in the sagittal plane; abduction **(C)** and internal and external rotation **(D)**. (From Della Valle CJ, Rokito AS, Gallagher Birdzell M, et al. Biomechanics of the shoulder. In: Nordin M, Frankel VH, eds. Basic Biomechanics of the Musculoskeletal System. Baltimore: Lippincott Williams & Wilkins, 2001:320.)

Scapular plane elevation

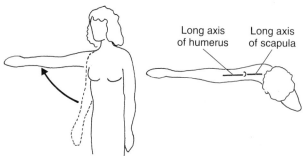

Figure 14-13 Elevation in the scapular plane, usually approximately 30 degrees forward from the coronal plane. (From Della Valle CJ, Rokito AS, Gallagher Birdzell M, et al. Biomechanics of the shoulder. In: Nordin M, Frankel VH, eds. Basic Biomechanics of the Musculoskeletal System. Baltimore: Lippincott Williams & Wilkins, 2001:320.)

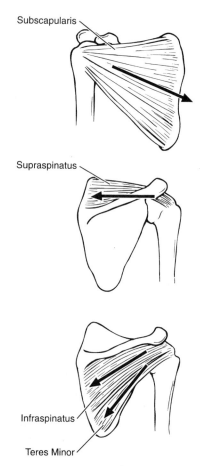

Figure 14-15 The direction of pull of the infraspinatus, teres minor, and subscapularis are in an oblique direction to provide a vertical component of humeral head depression and horizontal compressive force across the joint. The supraspinatus has a more horizontal orientation, therefore, contributing little to humeral head depression. (From Simon SR, Alaranta H, An KN, et al. Kinesiology. In: Buckwalter JA, Einhorn TA, Simon SR. Orthopaedic Basic Science. Rosemont, IL: American Academy of Orthopaedic Surgeons, 2000:744.)

ever, when both the axillary and suprascapular nerves are blocked, there is a substantial loss of arm elevation.

To counteract the tendency for the deltoid to sublux the proximal humerus superiorly under the acromion, the rotator cuff muscles are active to provide a humeral head depressor function. The subscapularis, infraspinatus, and teres minor have an oblique orientation that provides both a compressive force and a downward directed force (Fig. 14-15).

Using electromyography and stereophotogrammetry, the muscles of the shoulder girdle have been grouped according to relative importance with regard to elevation (Box 14-1).

Extension. The average extension (or posterior elevation) of the shoulder is approximately 60 degrees, and the maximum range is limited by capsular tension. The posterior and middle heads of the deltoid are the prime movers for extension of the arm. The supraspinatus and subscapularis are continually active throughout arm extension to stabilize the glenohumeral joint by resisting forces tending to dislo-

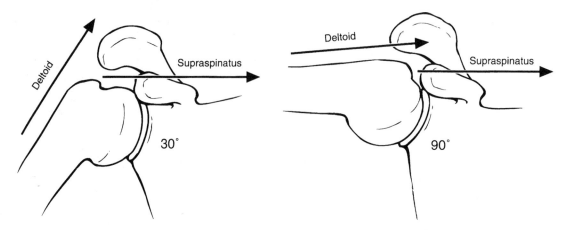

Figure 14-14 In the initial phases of glenohumeral abduction, the deltoid has a more vertically oriented direction of pull, whereas the supraspinatus remains relatively constant throughout motion. (From Simon SR, Alaranta H, An KN, et al. Kinesiology. In: Buckwalter JA, Einhorn TA, Simon SR. Orthopaedic Basic Science. Rosemont, IL: American Academy of Orthopaedic Surgeons, 2000:743.)

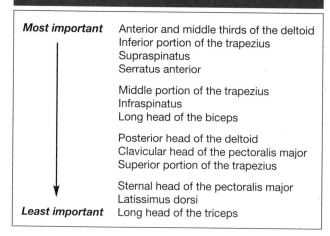

BOX 14-1 MUSCLE ACTIVITY FOR ACTIVE SHOULDER ELEVATION

Most important	Anterior and middle thirds of the deltoid
	Inferior portion of the trapezius
	Supraspinatus
	Serratus anterior
	Middle portion of the trapezius
	Infraspinatus
	Long head of the biceps
	Posterior head of the deltoid
	Clavicular head of the pectoralis major
	Superior portion of the trapezius
	Sternal head of the pectoralis major
	Latissimus dorsi
Least important	Long head of the triceps

cate the humerus anteriorly. The latissimus dorsi and teres major also contribute to extension, and when the elbow is extended, the triceps brachii may also contribute.

External Rotation. The infraspinatus is the primary external rotator of the shoulder with significant contributions made by the posterior deltoid and the teres minor. With progressive shoulder abduction, the posterior deltoid increases in efficiency as an accessory external rotator of the humerus through improvement of its moment arm. The subscapularis is also active but serves an antagonistic role as the main stabilizer, preventing anterior displacement of the humeral head with external rotation.

Internal Rotation. Internal rotation of the shoulder is accomplished by the combined activity of the subscapularis, the sternal head of the pectoralis major, the latissimus dorsi, and the teres major. The subscapularis is active during all phases of internal rotation, with relatively decreased activity toward the limits of abduction. With increasing abduction, the activity of the sternal head of the pectoralis major and the latissimus dorsi also decrease. The posterior and middle heads of the deltoid compensate by increasing eccentric activity in the abducted position.

Adduction. Shoulder adduction is the main function of the pectoralis major, teres major, subscapularis, and latissimus dorsi, with the latissimus dorsi being the most powerful adductor. In the upright position, the weight of the limb also assists with adduction.

Spinal Contribution to Shoulder Motion

Although often overlooked, motion of the thoracic and lumbar spine contributes to the ability to position the upper extremity in space. Movement of the spine in a direction away from an extremity attempting to reach an object enhances the attainable range of motion. In addition, the latissimus dorsi, the pectoralis major, and the periscapular muscles help transmit energy from the lower extremities and trunk to the upper extremity. The spinal contribution enhances the overall motion and function of the shoulder complex, which is of great importance in overhead activities, such as throwing and racquet sports.

GLENOHUMERAL JOINT STABILITY

The glenohumeral joint is the most mobile articulation in the human body and requires contributions from both static structures and musculotendinous activity to maintain stability. Static restraints include the joint capsule and ligaments, the glenoid labrum, the thicker peripheral glenoid cartilage, and a negative intra-articular pressure. In the clinical setting of recurrent instability, the presence of bony glenoid deficiency or humeral head defects (e.g., Hill-Sachs lesions) also become critical factors. Dynamic stability is achieved by the ability of the periscapular muscles to optimally position the glenoid in space, the ability of the rotator cuff muscles to provide stabilizing compressive forces to hold the humeral head in joint (concavity compression), and activity from the long head of the biceps.

Static Stability

Glenoid Fossa

The glenoid is shallow and only able to contain about one third of the diameter of the humeral head. The ability of the glenoid to provide static stability to the glenohumeral joint stems from the relative height of the peripheral glenoid, compared with the central glenoid. Although the bony glenoid appears relatively flat radiographically, the articular cartilage is thicker peripherally than it is centrally to help increase the depth of the glenoid. The glenoid labrum, which is a fibrocartilaginous rim, also serves to augment the height of the peripheral glenoid by providing 50% of the overall depth of the glenohumeral joint (see Fig. 14-9). The labrum is triangular in cross section and has firm attachments inferiorly to the underlying bone. In the anterosuperior portion of the glenoid, the labrum has a more variable and looser attachment. As noted previously, with soft tissues taken into account, the humeral head and glenoid are in fact quite congruent, with less than 3 mm of radius of curvature mismatch.

With recurrent or chronic glenohumeral dislocation, the anteroinferior glenoid bone stock may become deficient. Clinical and laboratory studies have suggested that, when more than 25% of the anteroposterior diameter of the glenoid has been eroded, a soft-tissue reconstruction alone is not sufficient and a structural bone graft is required to achieve stability.

Capsule and Ligaments

The glenohumeral joint capsule has proximal attachments both directly onto the glenoid labrum anteroinferiorly and beyond the glenoid labrum. Laterally, the capsule attaches to the anatomical neck of the humerus. Superiorly, it is attached at the base of the coracoid and envelops the long head of the biceps tendon, making the long head an intra-articular structure. The surface area of the joint capsule is twice that of the humeral head, and the average fluid volume that the capsule can hold is approximately 15 mL in women and 20 mL in men. Thus, there is a significant degree of inherent laxity, and this capsular redundancy allows for a wide range of motion.

Near the terminal range of motion of the glenohumeral joint, portions of the capsule will tighten to limit range of motion and provide stability. With shoulder adduction, the capsule is taut superiorly and lax inferiorly. Conversely, with shoulder abduction, this relationship is reversed and the inferior capsule tightens. With external rotation, the anterior capsule tightens, and in internal rotation, the posterior capsule tightens. As any portion of the shoulder capsule tightens, there is generally a small obligate humeral head translation in a direction opposite the contracture (e.g., at the limit of external rotation, the anterior capsule tightens and a posteriorly directed obligate translation occurs).

The anterior and inferior aspects of the capsule contain three distinct ligamentous extensions critical to shoulder stability and function—the superior, middle, and inferior glenohumeral ligaments (see Fig. 14-4). The superior glenohumeral ligament originates from the anterosuperior labrum, just anterior to the long head of the biceps, and inserts onto the upper part of the lesser tuberosity. It is present in the majority of shoulders but is only well developed in 50%. With the arm positioned at the side in the resting or adducted position, the superior glenohumeral ligament is the primary restraint to external rotation and inferior translation. The inferior glenohumeral ligament also contributes to stability, with abduction up to 50 degrees.

The coracohumeral ligament lies anterior to the superior glenohumeral ligament and originates from the lateral side of the base of the coracoid (see Fig. 14-5). It is composed of two bands that insert above and below the long head of the biceps on the greater and lesser tuberosities. The coracohumeral ligament reinforces the capsule of the rotator interval between the subscapularis and supraspinatus. In terms of static restraint, the coracohumeral ligament has the same function as the superior glenohumeral ligament: stability in adduction and external rotation and resistance to inferior translation.

The middle glenohumeral ligament originates inferior to the superior glenohumeral ligament within the 1 to 3 o'clock position (for a right shoulder) and inserts further inferiorly on the lesser tuberosity. It may also originate from the anterosuperior portion of the labrum, the supraglenoid tubercle, or the scapular neck; several morphologic variants have also been described. Whereas the superior glenohumeral ligament may be difficult to see at arthroscopy, the middle glenohumeral ligament is usually seen to be crossing the subscapularis from superomedial to inferolateral. There is great variability in the anatomy of this structure, and it is absent in as many as 30% of shoulders. It may be present as a cord-like variant (Buford complex) that may be mistaken for a detached anterior labrum or a sheet-like variant blending with the anterior band of the inferior glenohumeral ligament. Although these anatomic variants have been associated with increased glenohumeral internal rotation, the anatomic variants themselves do not appear to predispose to instability. Functionally, the middle glenohumeral ligament is the primary static restraint in external rotation over the range of abduction from 45 to 60 degrees; however, it does demonstrate a contribution to glenohumeral stability throughout the arc of abduction.

The inferior glenohumeral ligament has its greatest clinical and functional significance with regard to anterior shoulder stability. It originates from the inferior labrum and has been shown to have three distinct components inserting on the anatomic neck of the humerus—an anterior band originating from 2 to 4 o'clock (right shoulder), a posterior band originating from 7 to 9 o'clock (right shoulder), and an intervening axillary pouch (see Fig. 14-4). The inferior glenohumeral ligament is the primary anterior stabilizer of the shoulder with the arm in 90 degrees of abduction. As the arm is abducted and externally rotated, the anterior band of the inferior glenohumeral ligament tightens and resists anterior translation. With internal rotation of the abducted arm, the posterior band becomes taut, and posterior translation is resisted. The inferior glenohumeral ligament complex also serves to help resist inferior translation with the arm in the abducted position.

Humeral Head

The integrity of the humeral head articular surface is an important consideration in the clinical setting of instability. In the case of an anterior shoulder dislocation, the posterior aspect of the humeral head may sustain an impaction fracture (Hill-Sachs lesion) as it rests on the anteroinferior glenoid rim after dislocation. Most humeral head lesions are small (less than 20% of the articular surface), and capsulolabral detachments (Bankart lesions) are the most likely causes of recurrent instability in these cases. However, even when the capsulolabral detachments have been repaired, instability may still be problematic with larger humeral head lesions. In these cases, the rotational arc length of the humeral head has now been effectively shortened, with no change to the capsule length. As the shoulder is externally rotated, the posterior humeral head defect may then engage the glenoid rim before the capsule tightens to limit the range of motion, and dislocation follows.

A similar problem with humeral head defects may occur after posterior dislocations. The posterior glenoid rim, in these cases, creates an impaction fracture of the anterior humeral head (reverse Hill-Sachs or McLaughlin lesion). With larger defects (less than 20% of the articular surface), forward flexion and internal rotation may allow the humeral head defect to engage the posterior glenoid rim, leading to recurrent posterior dislocation.

Intra-articular Pressure

In the normal state, the glenohumeral joint contains less than 1 mL of fluid. The synovial fluid adheres to the articular cartilage overlying the glenoid and proximal humerus and lubricates the joint. Cohesive and adhesive forces are present within this lubricating layer, adding some stability to the joint by making it difficult to pull the two articular surfaces apart. The contributions of these cohesive and adhesive forces, however, are relatively small.

Under normal conditions, the pressure in the glenohumeral joint is lower than atmospheric, resulting in the so-called negative intra-articular pressure. This relatively lower joint pressure pulls the overlying capsule and glenohumeral ligaments inward and adds to joint stability. This stabilizing effect will be lost when the intra-articular pressure rises to, or exceeds, the ambient pressure, as occurs with joint effusions or hemarthroses. The intra-articular pressure will also increase if the joint is vented by any capsular injury, leading to increases in glenohumeral translation.

In the laboratory setting, venting the capsule has been shown to have a significant effect on increasing glenohumeral translation. However, the compressive forces generated by active rotator cuff muscles will decrease the allowed glenohumeral translation and are ultimately more important for joint stability.

Dynamic Stability

Rotator Cuff

Although the rotator cuff muscles do directly contribute to shoulder motion, the primary function of the rotator cuff is to stabilize the glenohumeral joint. This stability is achieved through compressive forces generated to hold the humeral head in the glenohumeral joint ("concavity compression") and assists with muscular balance during coordinated shoulder movement.

With shoulder motion occurring in all planes, the rotator cuff muscles are active to stabilize the glenohumeral joint. Because of the inherent lack of bony stability in the glenohumeral joint, the force generated by one muscle requires the activation of an antagonistic muscle, so that a dislocating force does not result. For example, with active internal rotation of the shoulder, forces from the subscapularis and pectoralis will tend to pull the humeral head out anteriorly. The infraspinatus and teres minor are, therefore, also active to help stabilize the glenohumeral joint. The antagonist muscles (the infraspinatus and teres minor in this example) usually provide stability via an eccentric contraction whereby the muscle is lengthened while actively contracting. The antagonist may also act by producing a neutralizing force of equal magnitude, but opposite in direction, as in the case of the periscapular muscles stabilizing the scapula.

The subscapularis, infraspinatus, and teres minor all have functions of providing both shoulder motion and glenohumeral stability. These cuff muscles all have a more oblique orientation compared with the supraspinatus (see Fig. 14-15). The subscapularis and infraspinatus are inferiorly directed approximately 45 degrees and the teres minor approximately 55 degrees. The oblique orientation of the infraspinatus, teres minor, and subscapularis thus provide both compression and a downward directed force (see Fig. 14-15), whereas the horizontally oriented supraspinatus strictly provides a compressive force (see Fig. 14-14). The subscapularis, along with the middle and inferior glenohumeral ligaments, has also been shown to act as an important anterior stabilizer of the glenohumeral joint, particularly with the arm held at 45 degrees of abduction.

The supraspinatus contributes some stability to the glenohumeral joint but has little humeral head depressor function to counteract the tendency for the deltoid to sublux the proximal humerus superiorly under the acromion.

The teres major muscle also originates from the scapula but inserts on the humerus below the surgical neck, posterior to the intertubercular groove, and is not part of the rotator cuff. It functions to assist with arm adduction and internal rotation and does not contribute to glenohumeral stability.

An understanding of the biomechanics of the rotator cuff is a useful tool to assess the clinical presentation of rotator cuff pathology. In cases of massive rotator cuff tears with involvement of the supraspinatus, infraspinatus, and subscapularis, the patient is frequently unable to achieve any functional elevation. As the deltoid activates to elevate the arm, the antagonist action of the infraspinatus and subscap-

ularis are too weak to keep the humeral head centered. As a result, the humeral head migrates superiorly and comes into contact with the acromion.

Long Head of Biceps

The biceps muscle is composed of two heads: a short head, which originates from the tip of the coracoid process, and a long head, which originates from the superior glenoid labrum and supraglenoid tubercle. Although the primary function of the biceps muscle is to supinate the forearm and flex the elbow, the long head plays an additional role in shoulder stability. The clinical importance of the long head of the biceps tendon, however, has been controversial in the nonathlete population.

In cadaveric models, the long head of the biceps has been demonstrated to be an important static restraint to anterior-superior instability. Recently, however, the contribution of the biceps to shoulder function has been questioned. When electromyography has been used to measure biceps activity during active shoulder motion but with the elbow held fixed in a brace, negligible biceps activity was demonstrated. However, almost any purposeful movement of the upper extremity would require both active elbow and shoulder motion, and it is unclear to what extent biceps activity contributes to shoulder stability with combined shoulder and elbow movement.

In the population of throwing athletes, there is little debate as to the importance of the biceps tendon. When the long head of the biceps is loaded in cadaveric models, decreased anterior humeral head translations are observed with the shoulder in a position of 90 degrees of abduction and 60 to 90 degrees of external rotation. The biceps anchor and superior labrum may become detached as a result of trauma or stress, producing an injury to the superior labrum anterior and posterior (SLAP) lesion. In cadaveric models, the creation of a SLAP lesion resulted in an increased strain on the anterosuperior band of the inferior glenohumeral ligament of between 102% and 120%, with the shoulder in abduction and external rotation. When an anterior load is applied to a cadaveric shoulder with an induced SLAP lesion, increases in both the anterior and inferior translations have been observed. This has been described as a "circle concept" in which the increase in humeral head translation, or "pseudolaxity," occurs as a result of injury to the posterosuperior labrum (Fig. 14-16).

Periscapular Muscles

As noted previously in the discussion of scapular motion, the scapula provides a stable socket for the articulation of the humeral head. As the extremity is positioned in space, the periscapular muscles are active to position the glenoid optimally in space. This permits maximizing the rotator cuff compressive forces and glenohumeral joint stability.

GLENOHUMERAL JOINT FORCES

The forces acting on any joint during purposeful activities represent a complex biomechanical problem. Although the descriptive anatomy of a joint may be readily understood, a true understanding of joint forces is a challenging three-

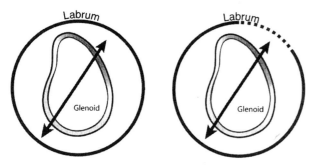

Figure 14-16 "Circle concept of instability," demonstrating how disruption of the labral attachment on one side of the glenoid may create laxity on the opposite side of the ring. (From Burkhart SS, Morgan CD, Kibler WB. The disabled throwing shoulder: spectrum of pathology. Part I: pathoanatomy and biomechanics. Arthroscopy 2003;19:417.)

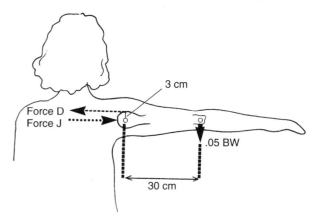

Figure 14-17 Free-body diagram of the static shoulder in 90 degrees of abduction. (From Della Valle CJ, Rokito AS, Gallagher Birdzell M, et al. Biomechanics of the shoulder. In: Nordin M, Frankel VH, eds. Basic Biomechanics of the Musculoskeletal System. Baltimore: Lippincott Williams & Wilkins, 2001:337.)

dimensional spatial problem requiring knowledge of limb position, kinematics, applied loads, and the activity level of each muscle crossing the joint.

The effectiveness of a muscle in moving a joint depends on the force generated by the muscle and the moment arm (or lever arm). The moment arm is defined as a perpendicular line from the center of rotation of the joint to the line of action of a force. The resultant moment is then calculated as the product of the force and the moment arm. Note that in biomechanics, the term *moment* is usually used to characterize bending across a long bone or joint in a direction other than along the axis of a long bone. The term *torque* is used to describe a rotational moment acting along the axis of a bone. In either case, bending moments and torques are equivalent concepts and calculated in the same manner.

A common approach to estimating joint reaction forces is first to consider the joint in a stationary, or static, position, while simplifying the anatomy and geometry. A free-body diagram is then constructed and a force balance carried out. When the limb is not accelerating, the sum of all forces at any point must be equal to zero, and the sum of all moments at any point must also be equal to zero.

For example, consider the case of a shoulder abducted 90 degrees, where we are interested in estimating the force of pull of the deltoid muscle and the glenohumeral joint reaction force. In this example, we will ignore the contribution of the rotator cuff muscles, which would normally be active to help stabilize the humeral head. The analysis begins with a free-body diagram. The extremity is modeled with the glenoid removed from the diagram and replaced by the joint reaction force, J (Fig. 14-17). Similarly, the deltoid is replaced by the force of the deltoid muscle, D, which will be modeled approximately parallel to the arm in the position of 90 degrees of abduction. The perpendicular distance from the force, D, to the center of rotation of the humeral head is taken as 3 cm. We will assume that only the deltoid is active, and no other muscle forces will be considered. The weight of the arm will be estimated to be 0.05 times body weight (BW), and the center of gravity of the limb as 30 cm from the center of rotation of the shoulder. The final free-body diagram is shown in Figure 14-17.

The joint reaction force and deltoid force may now be solved using equilibrium equations. Because the arm is not accelerating, the sum of all forces in any direction must be equal to zero, and the sum of all moments about any point must be equal to zero. We will use the convention that moments acting in a counterclockwise direction are positive, and moments in a clockwise direction are negative. Therefore,

$$\Sigma\,M\,=\,0.$$

Moment generated by deltoid + Moment generated by weight of arm = 0.

$$(D \times 3\ cm) + (-0.05\ BW \times 30\ cm) = 0.$$

$$D = 0.5\ BW.$$

A force balance may now be carried out using the principle that the sum of all forces in any direction must be equal to zero. If the direction to the left is taken as negative, then in the horizontal direction:

$$\Sigma\,F\,=\,0.$$

$$(-D) + J = 0.$$

$$J = D = 0.5\ BW.$$

At 90 degrees of abduction, the joint reaction force and deltoid force are essentially equal and opposite forces. This simple analysis highlights the very high loads transmitted to the relatively small glenoid (J): a force of one half of body weight with the arm simply held out to the side. Loads will increase when a mass is held in the hand a known distance from the shoulder. With an object held in the hand, the analysis can be repeated by including the moment and weight generated by the additional mass.

Note that so far, the analysis has concentrated on predicting the loads that a musculotendinous unit must generate to support a given limb position and applied load. The analysis does not address the physiologic ability of a muscle to produce the required force, nor does it consider the maximum joint forces based on the muscles maximum strength. Knowing the muscle cross-sectional area, an estimate of the maximum muscle forces may be made. Maximal muscle force is dependent on muscle pretension, and estimates from the literature provide a broad range of results that are usually in the range from 4 to 9 kg/cm^2 (57 to 128 lb/in^2).

BIOMECHANICS OF THROWING

Pitching has been divided into six phases: windup, early cocking, late cocking, acceleration, deceleration, and follow-through (Fig. 14-18). During windup, the pitcher places the body in a position to optimize the contribution of all parts of the body toward accelerating the ball. Approximately 50% of the velocity of the overhand throw results from the forward step of the stride leg and the body rotation. The remainder of the ball propulsion is generated from the shoulder, elbow, and wrist. In the windup phase, shoulder muscle activity is low, and few injuries occur during this phase.

In early cocking, the trapezius and serratus anterior muscle show moderate-to-high activity as these muscles protract and upwardly rotate the scapula. The scapular positioning places the glenoid in proper position to avoid the occurrence of impingement and instability. The middle deltoid achieves peak activity during the early cocking phase, and the supraspinatus is active to help stabilize the humeral head. Once the humerus is abducted beyond 90 degrees, humeral head translation is limited by the inferior glenohumeral ligament.

In late cocking, the humerus is externally rotated up to 160 to 185 degrees in professional pitchers. As the anterior capsule tightens in abduction and external rotation, an obligate posterior glenohumeral translation occurs. The scapular protractor (serratus anterior) and the retractors (middle trapezius, rhomboids, and levator scapulae) are all active to support a stable base for rapid humeral external rotation.

The long head of the biceps compresses the humeral head into the glenoid and contributes to anterior stability. The activity of the deltoid diminishes in late cocking, and the rotator cuff muscles become more active. In particular, the teres minor and infraspinatus are primarily responsible for the extreme external rotation. The supraspinatus becomes oriented more posteriorly and becomes less effective in providing a stabilizing superior compressive force. The end of late cocking occurs as the pectoralis major, latissimus dorsi, and serratus anterior muscles show increased activity to generate maximum horizontal adduction.

From the position of maximal external rotation, the shoulder is rapidly internally rotated during the acceleration phase, over a period of 42 to 58 ms in professional players. All scapular muscles remain active to stabilize the scapula during this phase. The latissimus dorsi and the pectoralis major are the primary muscles contributing to the acceleration of the ball, with the latissimus showing the highest activity and oriented anatomically to provide the greatest torque. Energy is also transferred from the lower extremities and the rotation of the trunk. The subscapularis, teres minor, and infraspinatus remain active to stabilize the glenohumeral joint. The acceleration phase is terminated when the ball is released, and the arm then undergoes deceleration and follow-through.

The deceleration phase is responsible for dissipation of the residual kinetic energy in the limb after the ball is released. It has been recognized as the most violent phase of throwing, whereby the shoulder continues its internal rotation while opposing muscles around the shoulder activate simultaneously to control deceleration. The teres minor contracts eccentrically and demonstrates the highest level of activity of all the cuff muscles, whereas the subscapularis also remains active to stabilize the humeral head. The middle and posterior heads of the deltoid are active to dece-

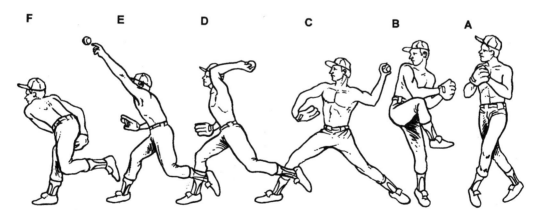

Figure 14-18   The six phases of the pitching motion. **A,B:** Windup begins when the pitcher initiates motion and ends when the ball is removed from the glove. **C:** The stride leg extends toward the batter, and the knee and hip of the pivot leg extend to propel the body forward into the stride. **D:** In late cocking, the trunk rotates forward while the shoulder achieves a position of maximum external rotation. **E:** The shoulder is rapidly internally rotated during the acceleration phase. **F:** After ball release, deceleration forces are applied to the shoulder as it continues to internally rotate. Deceleration is complete when the arm reaches a position of 0 degrees internal rotation. The arm is then adducted across the body in follow-through phase. (From Park SS, Loebenberg ML, Rokito AS, et al. The shoulder in baseball pitching. Biomechanics and related injuries. Bull Hosp Joint Dis 2002–2003;61:81.)

lerate the arm. It was initially proposed that labral injuries occurred most commonly in the deceleration phase; however, recent studies have demonstrated that labral injuries may more commonly occur in the acceleration phase.

In the follow-through phase, the shoulder muscles become less active as the body essentially catches up to the throwing arm. The shoulder adducts and the elbow flexes with all shoulder and upper extremity muscles showing low-to-moderate electromyographic activity.

Throwing activities highlight the complexity and challenges of shoulder anatomy and biomechanics. For optimal shoulder girdle function, coordinated activity of the glenohumeral joint, the scapulothoracic articulation, the acromioclavicular joint, and the sternoclavicular joint is essential. Both static and dynamic stabilizers play critical roles in preventing instability and injury. However, when the shoulder is afflicted by trauma or chronic disease, an understanding of shoulder anatomy and biomechanics enables the physician to prescribe an effective course of treatment and rehabilitation.

SUGGESTED READING

An KN. Muscle force and its role in joint dynamic stability. Clin Orthop Relat Res 2002;403(suppl):S37–S42.

Burkart AC, Debski RE. Anatomy and function of the glenohumeral ligaments in anterior shoulder instability. Clin Orthop Relat Res 2002;400:32–39,

Halder AM, O'Driscoll SW, Heers G, et al. Biomechanical comparison of effects of supraspinatus tendon detachments, tendon defects, and muscle retractions. J Bone Joint Surg Am 2002;84:780–785.

Itoi E, Morrey BF, An KN. Biomechanics of the shoulder. In: Rockwood CA Jr, Matsen FA III, Wirth MA, et al., eds. The Shoulder, 3rd ed. Philadelphia: Saunders-Elsevier, 2004:223–267.

Jobe CM, Coen MJ. Gross anatomy of the shoulder. In: Rockwood CA Jr, Matsen FA III, Wirth MA, et al., eds. The Shoulder, 3rd ed. Philadelphia: Saunders-Elsevier, 2004:33–95.

Jobe FW, Pink M. Classification and treatment of shoulder dysfunction in the overhead athlete. J Orthop Sports Phys Ther 1993;18:427–432.

Kibler WB. The role of the scapula in athletic shoulder function. Am J Sports Med 1998;26:325–337.

Meister K. Injuries to the shoulder in the throwing athlete. Part one: Biomechanics/pathophysiology/classification of injury. Am J Sports Med 2000;28:265–275.

Michener LA, McClure PW, Karduna AR. Anatomical and biomechanical mechanisms of subacromial impingement syndrome. Clin Biomech 2003;18:369–379.

Rao AG, Kim TK, Chronopoulos E, et al. Anatomical variants in the anterosuperior aspect of the glenoid labrum: a statistical analysis of seventy-three cases. J Bone Joint Surg Am 2003;85:653–659.

Renfree KJ, Wright TW. Anatomy and biomechanics of the acromioclavicular and sternoclavicular joints. Clin Sports Med 2003;22:219–237.

Sethi N, Wright R, Yamaguchi K. Disorders of the long head of the biceps tendon. J Shoulder Elbow Surg 1999;8:644–654.

Williams GR Jr, Shakil M, Klimkiewicz J, et al. Anatomy of the scapulothoracic articulation. Clin Orthop Relat Res 1999;359:237–246.

PHYSICAL EXAMINATION TESTS FOR THE SHOULDER AND ELBOW

ROBERT J. NICOLETTA

SHOULDER

The shoulder is a complex structural unit. It is a ball-and-socket joint that links the upper extremity to the axial trunk. Due to its large range of motion, there is an inherent sacrifice in bony stability. The shoulder complex is made up of three bones (the scapula, clavicle, and humerus) with four articulations (the sternoclavicular, acromioclavicular (AC), scapulothoracic, and glenohumeral joints). Major soft-tissue contributors include the muscles of the rotator cuff (supraspinatus, infraspinatus, teres minor, and subscapularis), the glenoid labrum, glenohumeral ligaments, coracoacromial and coracoclavicular (CC) ligaments, long head of the biceps tendon, and scapulothoracic muscles (Figs. 15-1 and 15-2).

The primary function of the rotator cuff is to act as a dynamic stabilizer of the glenohumeral joint and a humeral head depressor. It contributes to the torque that is required in shoulder elevation and internal and external rotation of

the humerus. The supraspinatus, which lies across the top of the glenohumeral joint, provides joint compression by contraction. This counteracts the force generated during shoulder elevation that is provided by the deltoid. The supraspinatus also contributes to shoulder abduction along with the deltoid. The infraspinatus and teres minor muscles both function as external rotators of the arm. The subscapularis function is to provide internal rotation and to act as dynamic barrier to anterior humeral displacement. The long head of the biceps tendon is felt to contribute to dynamic stability of the humeral head in the superior and posterior planes. The supraspinatus arises from the supraspinatus fossa of the scapula, passes beneath the acromion and AC joint, and inserts into the upper portion of the greater tuberosity. It is innervated by the suprascapular nerve. The infraspinatus originates from the infraspinatus fossa of the scapula, inserting into the posterolateral aspect of the greater tuberosity. It is also innervated by the suprascapular nerve. The teres minor, innervated by the axillary nerve, originates from the lateral border of the scapula and inserts on the lower portion of the greater tuberosity. The subscapularis

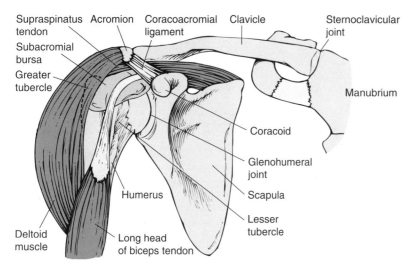

Figure 15-1 Shoulder (right anterior view) joint. (From Weber J, Kelley J. Health Assessment in Nursing, 2nd ed. Philadelphia: Lippincott Williams & Wilkins, 2003.)

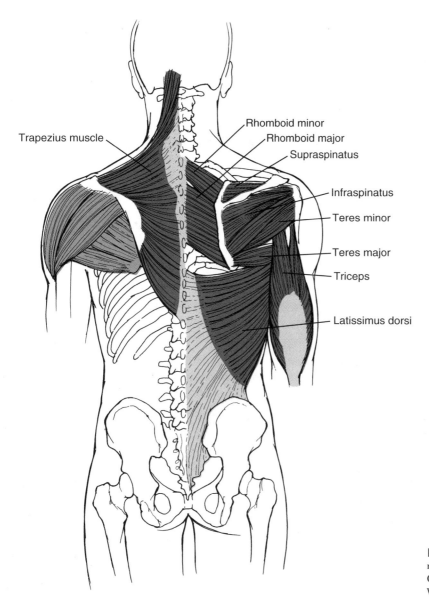

Figure 15-2 Muscles of the posterior shoulder region. (From Hendrickson T. Massage for Orthopedic Conditions. Philadelphia: Lippincott Williams & Wilkins, 2003.)

arises from the anterior surface of the scapula, inserting on the lesser tuberosity. It is innervated by the upper and lower subscapular nerves.

With regard to injuries involving the shoulder, the injury mechanism and arm position are important factors. The patient's age, dominant arm, and chief complaint play a major role in establishing an accurate diagnosis and should not be overlooked. Within the shoulder physical examination, numerous provocative tests have been described. These can be thought of, in a general sense, as belonging to two categories: tests that evaluate the rotator cuff and those that test for shoulder stability. Within these two general categories are numerous specific tests that attempt to isolate specific structures within the glenohumeral joint, subacromial space, AC joint, and surrounding supporting structures.

Physical Examination

- As always, physical examination of the shoulder joint complex should take place only after a detailed and thorough history has been performed.
- The patient should be unclothed and the entire upper extremity—including the front and back of the torso—should be visualized.
- After careful inspection, palpation for areas of bony and soft-tissue tenderness is performed, and documentation of both active and passive shoulder range of motion is noted.
- The following specific provocative physical examination tests can then be used and are utilized to confirm selectively suspicious findings obtained from the history. (If the test is illustrated by a figure, the steps in performing it are in the legend.)

Rotator Cuff

Impingement Tests

In 1972, Neer described three phases of impingement by encroachment on the subacromial space by bursa and spurs leading to rotator cuff irritation (Table 15-1). The following tests are used to evaluate for rotator cuff irritation/injury in the subacromial space.

Jobe's Supraspinatus Test. This test evaluates for subacromial impingement resulting from contact between the rotator cuff and biceps tendon against the coracoacromial

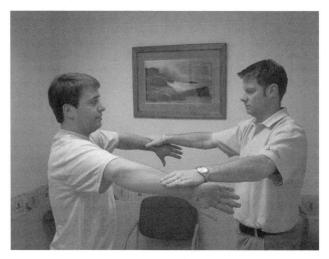

Figure 15-3 Jobe's test is performed with the patient standing with both shoulders abducted to 90 degrees, horizontally adducted approximately 30 degrees, and internally rotated so the patient's thumbs point to the floor. In this position, the examiner resists the patient's attempt to abduct both shoulders.

arch (Fig. 15-3). This contact can cause an inflammatory response, resulting in subacromial bursitis and reducing the space for the rotator cuff tendons to glide underneath the acromion. Also known as the empty can test, the supraspinatus test (or Jobe's test) was first described in 1983. A positive finding produces pain or weakness about the involved shoulder, implicating the supraspinatus muscle or tendon as the site of pathology. Complaints of pain involving the anterior shoulder or anterolateral arm involving the deltoid muscle may also be indicative of tendonitis or impingement of the supraspinatus outlet. Itoi et al. evaluated the empty can test in 143 shoulders of 136 patients with a positive result documented for pain, muscle weakness, or both. Examination results were correlated with follow-up high-resolution magnetic resonance imaging. The empty can test was 70% accurate in predicting a torn supraspinatus tendon when muscle weakness was used as a positive finding. Pain was observed in 71 shoulders (50%).

Neer's Impingement Test. Tests for impingement are intended to either produce pain about the shoulder or reproduce patient-specific symptoms. The Neer test, first described in 1972 and then further in 1983, is another test for subacromial outlet impingement (Fig. 15-4). A positive test will reproduce pain in patients with impingement syndrome and may also be positive in patients with adhesive capsulitis, calcific tendonitis, and AC arthrosis. For those with true impingement pain, the Neer's test can usually be relieved with subacromial local anesthetic injection. The injection is performed under sterile conditions with insert of local anesthetic into the subacromial space. Patient subjective decrease in pain is felt to be indicative of impingement. In an anatomic study evaluating the provocative position of the Neer test, subacromial soft-tissue contact with the medial aspect of the acromion was noted. McDonald et al. demonstrated a 75% sensitivity of this test for subacromial bursitis and 88% for abnormalities of the rotator cuff,

TABLE 15-1 NEER'S THREE PHASES OF IMPINGEMENT OF THE ROTATOR CUFF

Phase	Description
I	Acute inflammation with edema and hemorrhage in the rotator cuff tendon
II	Tendonitis and fibrosis
III	Spur formation and full thickness rotator cuff tear

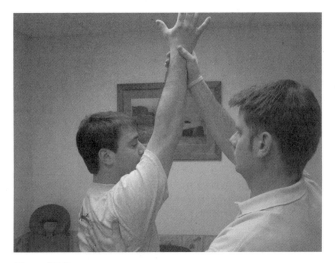

Figure 15-4 Neer's test is performed with the patient seated and the examiner standing. In this position, scapular rotation is prevented by one hand as the other is used to raise the patient's arm in forward flexion causing the greater tuberosity to impinge against the acromion.

with specificities of 48% and 51%. Furthermore, the Neer impingement test was positive in 25% of patients with Bankart lesions and 46% of those with superior labrum anterior and posterior (SLAP) lesions. The test was also positive in 69% of those patients with AC arthritis.

Hawkins' Test. Hawkins and Kennedy described this test in 1980 as an alternative test for supraspinatus outlet impingement (Fig. 15-5). The maneuver brings the greater tuberosity of the humerus farther under the coracoacromial ligament reproducing impingement pain. Shoulder pain and apprehension in this position are felt to be indicative of supraspinatus subacromial impingement. Analysis of this test has demonstrated 88% and 92% sensitivity for rotator cuff abnormalities and subacromial bursitis, respectively, with a specificity of 43% and 44%. Of the patients with AC

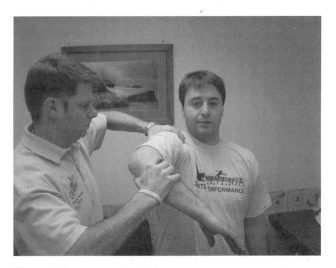

Figure 15-5 For Hawkins' test, the patient is either seated or standing. The examiner forward flexes the patient's humerus to 90 degrees and then internally rotates the shoulder.

joint arthritis, greater than 90% had a positive test result with the Hawkins test.

Yocum's Test. Yocum's test was described in 1983 to selectively test the function of the supraspinatus tendon and appears very similar to the Jobe supraspinatus test. This is another test for supraspinatus outlet impingement. The test is performed with abduction of the patient's arm to 90 degrees, forward flexion to 30 degrees, and maximal internal rotation. In this position, the examiner resists active shoulder abduction, and reproduction of pain and/or weakness in this position implicates the supraspinatus tendon as the site of injury and is felt to be indicative of impingement tendonitis.

Internal Rotation Resistance Stress Test. In 2001, this test was described by Zaslav to differentiate between intra-articular (internal impingement) and classic outlet impingement syndromes (Fig. 15-6). Internal impingement is commonly seen in overhead athletes with subtle glenohumeral instability. These patients have impingement of the posterior rotator cuff along the posterior superior labrum in the late cocking phase of the throwing motion and pain in the region of the infraspinatus insertion with abduction and maximal external rotation on physical examination. If the patient with a positive impingement sign has good strength in external rotation, this test is considered positive and predictive of internal impingement. A negative test (more weakness in external rotation) is suggestive of classic outlet impingement (external impingement). A prospective study of 110 patients yielded a sensitivity of 88% and specificity of 96% in defining these diagnoses. The positive predictive value was 88%, and the negative predictive value was 94%.

Subcoracoid Impingement Test. The subcoracoid impingement test was described to reproduce entrapment of the rotator cuff between the humeral head and the coracoid

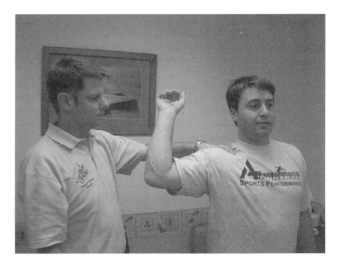

Figure 15-6 The internal rotation resistance stress test is performed with the patient standing and the arm in 90 degrees of abduction in the coronal plane and 80 degrees of external rotation. With the examiner standing behind the patient, a manual isometric muscle test is performed for external rotation and this is compared to one for internal rotation in the same position.

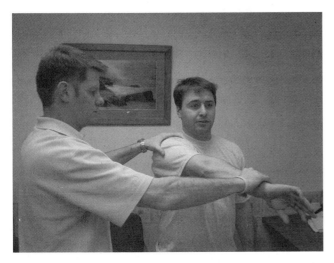

Figure 15-7 The subcoracoid impingement test is performed with the involved arm forward flexed to 120 to 130 degrees and internally rotated, reproducing the patient's symptoms of pain.

identifying those patients with a suspected diagnosis of subcoracoid impingement (Fig. 15-7). Although uncommon, this diagnosis has been described in patients with a long or laterally placed coracoid process and should be considered in patients with negative classic impingement signs that describe anterior/lateral pain with overhead activities and have subjective complaints similar to those with classic outlet impingement. From an anatomic standpoint, these patients have impingement of the coracoid process on the proximal humerus with forward flexion and internal rotation of the arm. Gerber showed that forward flexion to 90 degrees combined with internal rotation was restricted and consistently painful in patients with subcoracoid impingement.

Tests for Rotator Cuff Tears

Numerous tests have been described to evaluate the integrity of the musculotendinous units of the rotator cuff. The following tests attempt to identify weaknesses or deficiencies in rotator cuff strength that signify a tear.

External Rotation Lag Sign. The external rotation lag sign (ERLS) is designed to test the integrity of the supraspinatus and infraspinatus tendons. The test is performed with the patient either seated or standing. The elbow on the side of the involved shoulder is passively flexed to 90 degrees, and the shoulder is held at 20 degrees of elevation (in the scapular plane) and near-maximal external rotation. In this position, the patient is then asked to actively maintain the position of external rotation when the examiner releases the wrist while supporting the limb at the elbow. The sign is considered positive when a lag occurs and the patient is unable to actively maintain the position of external rotation. This should be recorded to the nearest 5 degrees. It is important to take into consideration any loss of passive motion as a result of capsular contracture or subscapularis injury, because this may lead to false-negative or false-positive results. Also, the involved side should be compared with the uninvolved contralateral shoulder. Jobe's test may be more sensitive for posterosuperior rotator cuff tears when compared with the ERLS. Furthermore, the ERLS was more

sensitive than the drop sign (described below). There was found to be no difference in accuracy when comparing the Jobe sign and ERLS, and both were more accurate than the drop sign. Positive predictive value for the Jobe sign was 84%, and the negative predictive value was 58%. The drop sign and ERLS both had 100% positive predictive values, and 56% and 32% negative predictive values, respectively.

Internal Rotation Lag Sign. The internal rotation lag sign (IRLS) is designed to test the integrity of the subscapularis tendon. The test is performed with the patient either standing or seated on the examination table. The involved arm is held at maximal internal rotation by the examiner. The patient's elbow is flexed to 90 degrees, and the shoulder is held at 20 degrees of elevation and 20 degrees of extension. The hand is passively lifted away from the lumbar region until near full internal rotation is accomplished. The patient is then instructed to actively maintain this position as the examiner releases the wrist while maintaining support at the elbow. When a lag occurs and the patient is unable to maintain the arm position, the test is said to be positive for injury to the subscapularis (either partial or full thickness tear) and is recorded to the nearest 5 degrees and compared with the contralateral side. With large tears, an obvious drop of the hand will occur. A slight lag may indicate a partial tear of the superior portion of the subscapularis tendon.

Hertel et al. described the relationship between the lag signs and extent of rotator cuff injury. If the rotator cuff was intact, the IRLS, ELRS, and drop arm tests were negative. In patients with an isolated tear of the supraspinatus tendon, a lag of 5 to 10 degrees was seen in 94% (16 of 17 patients). All patients with combined tears of the infraspinatus and supraspinatus demonstrated a lag of 10 to 15 degrees. Eighty percent (4 of 5 patients) with partial subscapularis tendon tears demonstrated lag signs of 5 degrees. All of those with complete ruptures had lag signs approaching 10 degrees.

Lift-off Test. Described by Gerber and Krushnell in 1991, the lift-off test is used to identify an isolated rupture of the subscapularis tendon (Fig. 15-8). The test is considered positive for a subscapularis tear if the patient is unable to lift the dorsum of his hand off his back.

In 1996, Gerber further described a lift-off test lag sign for subscapularis muscle rupture. The test is performed by bringing the patient's arm passively behind the body into a position of maximal internal rotation. The test is considered normal if the patient is able to maintain maximal internal rotation after the examiner releases the patient's hand. In their series, a normal test was demonstrated in 100 patients who had no shoulder complaints and in 27 patients with a rotator cuff tear that did not involve the subscapularis tendon. Eight of nine patients (88%) tested with full thickness subscapularis tendon tears had positive lift-off test results.

Belly Press Test. Another test that addresses the integrity of and injury to the subscapularis tendon is the belly press test (Fig. 15-9). In this test, the patient is instructed to press his abdomen with the palm of his hand while attempting to keep the arm in maximal internal rotation. If active internal

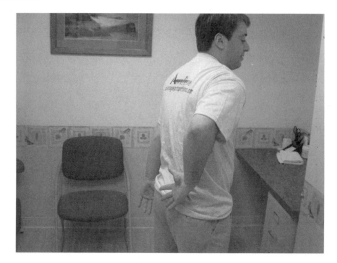

Figure 15-8 The lift-off test is performed with the patient standing and with the involved arm in a position of internal rotation placing the dorsum of the patient's hand against his back. The patient is then asked to actively lift the hand off the back.

rotation is intact, the elbow does not drop backward signifying an intact subscapularis. However, if strength of the subscapularis is impaired, internal rotation cannot be maintained. Thus, the patient notes weakness, and the elbow drops back behind the trunk. This is felt to be an indication of either partial or complete subscapularis tear. In Gerber's series of patients studied in 1996, eight of eight patients had a positive belly press test result with subscapularis tendon tears.

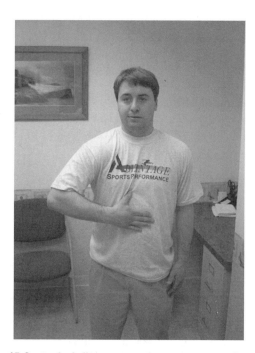

Figure 15-9 In the belly press test, the patient presses the abdomen with the palm of the hand while attempting to keep the arm in maximal internal rotation.

Drop Sign. The drop sign is designed to isolate and test the integrity of the infraspinatus tendon. The test is performed with the patient either standing or seated on the examination table. With the elbow flexed to 90 degrees, the examiner holds the involved arm at 90 degrees of elevation in the scapular plane and near full external rotation. In this position, external rotation is maintained primarily by the infraspinatus. The patient is then instructed to maintain this position as the examiner releases the wrist while supporting the elbow. The sign is considered positive for a tear of the infraspinatus tendon if a lag or drop occurs and is recorded to the nearest 5 degrees and compared with the contralateral side.

Biceps Tendon

The long head of the biceps tendon acts as a humeral head depressor and plays a role in anterior stability of the glenohumeral joint by increasing the resistance of the shoulder to torsional forces in the positions of abduction and external rotation. In the presence of a rotator cuff tear, the biceps may also be torn or become enlarged by increased functional requirements if the tear involves the anterior superior rotator cuff or subscapularis. The following tests attempt to identify injury to the long head of the biceps tendon.

Speed's Test

Described in 1966 by Crenshaw and Kilgore, this test attempts to isolate the long head of the biceps tendon as the source of shoulder pain (Fig. 15-10). The test is positive if the maneuver produces tenderness or pain localized to the bicipital groove and may represent such pathologic findings as biceps tendonitis or SLAP lesions.

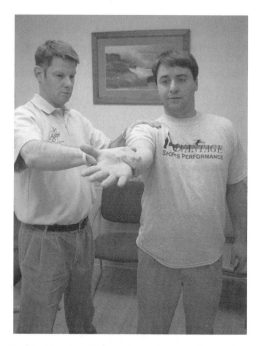

Figure 15-10 For Speed's test, the patient is either in the sitting or standing position. The involved shoulder is flexed to 90 degrees with the elbow fully extended and the forearm supinated. The examiner then places one hand along the volar aspect of the patient's forearm and resists the patient's attempt to actively forward flex the shoulder.

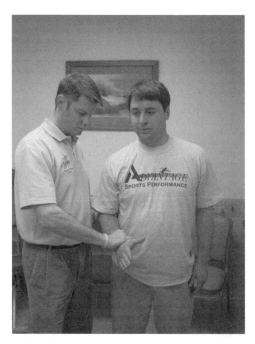

Figure 15-11 Yergason's test is performed with the patient either sitting or standing and the elbow flexed to 90 degrees while stabilized against the side of the body. The forearm begins in a pronated position. The examiner then holds the patient's wrist to resist active supination, then instructs the patient to attempt to actively supinate the forearm/wrist.

Yergason's Test

Yergason's test was originally described in 1931 as the "supination sign" (Fig. 15-11). The test is considered positive if the maneuver reproduces pain in the region of the proximal bicipital groove and may indicate proximal bicipital tendonitis.

Acromioclavicular Joint

The AC joint is a diarthrodial joint between the concave surface of the anteromedial aspect of the acromion and the convex surface of the distal clavicle. A fibrocartilaginous disc exists within the AC joint. The main function of the joint is to serve as a connection between the scapula and clavicle supporting the shoulder on the chest wall. The AC joint is exposed to mainly compressive forces. The stability of the AC joint is provided by two sets of ligaments: the CC ligaments (conoid and trapezoid) and AC capsuloligamentous complex. The superior and inferior AC ligaments act as the primary restraints to posterior clavicular displacement. The CC ligament provides restraint to anterior and superior displacement of the clavicle.

Crossover Impingement Test

The crossover impingement test attempts to evaluate the AC joint as the source of anterior/superior shoulder pain and is positive in patients with AC arthritis or those with recent diagnosis of AC separation (Fig. 15-12). When the maneuver is performed, superior shoulder pain (specifically pain localized at the AC joint) is indicative of AC joint pa-

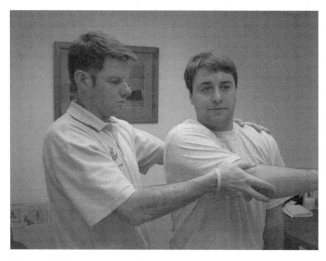

Figure 15-12 For the crossover impingement test, the patient is in the sitting position with the examiner standing with one hand on the posterior aspect of the patient's shoulder to stabilize the trunk and the other hand holding the patient's elbow on the involved side. The examiner then maximally adducts the involved shoulder across the patient's body.

thology. Pain not felt specifically at the AC joint and more involving the anterior shoulder may indicate supraspinatus, long head of the biceps, or subscapularis pathology. Complaints of posterior shoulder pain with this maneuver may relate to posterior capsule or posterior rotator cuff pathology. One study demonstrated a 77% sensitivity using this test to evaluate AC joint pathology.

Acromioclavicular Joint Distraction Test

The AC joint distraction test is used to diagnose AC and or CC ligament sprain (Fig. 15-13). A positive finding is

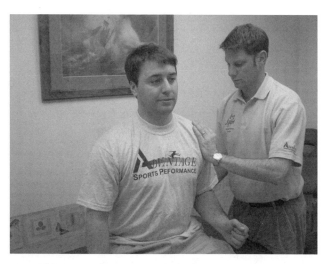

Figure 15-13 For the AC joint distraction test, the patient sits with the involved arm at the side and the elbow flexed to 90 degrees. The examiner stands on the patient's involved side, and with one hand holds the patient's arm just above the elbow, while the examiner's other hand is placed over the involved AC joint. In this position, the examiner applies gentle downward pressure on the arm and notes any movement at the AC joint.

described as pain and/or movement of the scapula inferior to the clavicle indicating injury to the AC and or CC ligament.

Acromioclavicular Joint Compression Test

The AC joint compression test is performed with the patient in the sitting position and arm relaxed at the side. The examiner stands on the involved side and places one hand on the patient's clavicle and the other on the spine of the scapula. In this position, the examiner gently squeezes the hands together, noting any movement at the AC joint. Pain or movement of the clavicle is felt to represent a positive finding in AC or CC ligament injuries.

Piano Key Sign

The piano key sign further evaluates potential injury involving the AC joint. The test is used in patients suspected of sustaining AC sprain or separation with injury to the AC joint and/or CC ligaments. The patient sits with the involved limb relaxed at the side. In this position, the examiner applies direct downward pressure to the patient's distal clavicle to depress it into its normal resting position in a patient with AC ligament and CC ligament disruption. This should be compared with the involved contralateral side.

Shoulder Instability

Just as there are the aforementioned numerous tests to evaluate the rotator cuff, biceps tendon, AC, and sternoclavicular joints, there are special focused tests used to evaluate for shoulder instability, laxity, and labral tears, including SLAP tears.

Apprehension Test

The apprehension test is used to evaluate for glenohumeral anterior laxity/instability (Fig. 15-14). A positive finding is

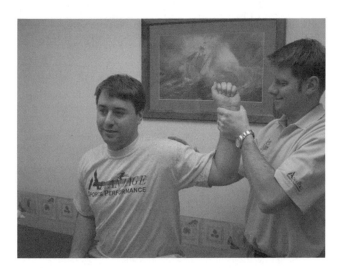

Figure 15-14 The apprehension test for glenohumeral anterior laxity/instability is performed with the patient sitting on the examination table. The involved shoulder is placed in 90 degrees of abduction with the elbow in 90 degrees of flexion. The examiner then slowly passively externally rotates the shoulder.

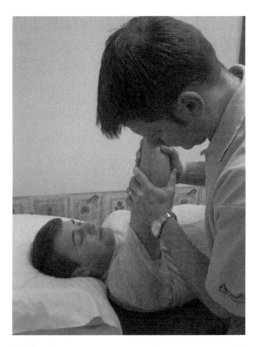

Figure 15-15 The apprehension test for posterior instability is performed with the patient lying supine on the examining table. The examiner places the patient's involved shoulder in 90 degrees of forward flexion and internal rotation while applying a posterior force through the long axis of the humerus.

described as one in which the patient looks or feels apprehensive or expresses feelings of pain or apprehension if the shoulder were to be externally rotated further.

The apprehension test can also be performed to evaluate for posterior instability (Fig. 15-15). A positive finding is felt to be present if the patient expresses apprehension toward further movement in the posterior direction.

Jobe's Apprehension-relocation Test

This test is used in conjunction with the preceding apprehension test. It is performed with the patient supine and the arm in 90 degrees of abduction and external rotation. During the apprehension portion of the test, the examiner pushes anteriorly on the posterior aspect of the humeral head. This maneuver may produce a sense of apprehension and at times also associated with pain in patients with recurrent instability/dislocation. Patients with anterior subluxation are felt to experience pain but not apprehension with this test, and patients with a normal shoulder will be asymptomatic with the maneuver. The relocation test is then performed (Fig. 15-16). Patients with instability or subluxation and secondary outlet impingement will have pain relief and can tolerate maximal external rotation with the posteriorly directed force applied to the proximal humerus. Patients with primary impingement alone will have no change in their pain. Sensitivity for this test has been described at 68%; specificity, 100%; positive predictive value, 100%; negative predictive value, 78%; and accuracy, 85% when apprehension was the determinant of a positive test result.

Sulcus Sign

Testing for the sulcus sign attempts to produce inferior subluxation of the humerus on the glenoid (Fig. 15-17). If a depression is observed with this maneuver between the lateral edge of the acromion and the humeral head, the sulcus sign is said to be positive, indicating injury to the rotator interval and contributing to inferior glenohumeral instability. This should be compared with the uninvolved contralateral side. The amount of depression should be lessened with the same downward traction applied with the arm in external rotation. The sulcus sign is graded 1+ when a gap is less than 1 cm, 2+ when the gap is between 1 and 2 cm, and 3+ when the gap is more than 2 cm. In 1997, Henry et al. found the sulcus sign to have a sensitivity of 97% and specificity of 99% in evaluation of inferior glenohumeral laxity.

Anterior Drawer Test

The anterior drawer test assesses for anterior glenohumeral laxity/instability (Fig. 15-18). The relative movement of the humerus relative to the scapula can then be graded and compared with the contralateral side. Grading reflects the degree of humeral head translation anterior to the glenoid rim. A grade of 1+ is given for translation of the humeral head to the edge of the glenoid; 2+ if the humeral head can be subluxated over the glenoid rim but reduces spontaneously; and 3+ if a frank dislocation of the humeral head over the glenoid rim does not reduce spontaneously.

Posterior Drawer Test

The posterior drawer test assesses posterior glenohumeral laxity/instability (Fig. 15-19). During the test, the examiner

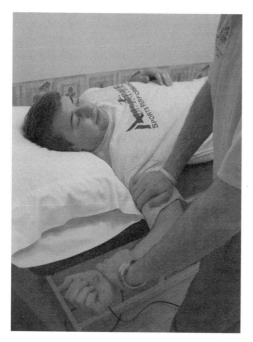

Figure 15-16   The relocation test is used in conjunction with the apprehension test for posterior instability. It is performed by administering a posteriorly directed force on the humeral head with the arm in the abducted, externally rotated position.

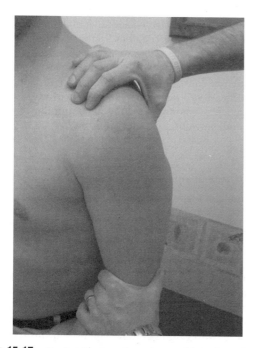

Figure 15-17   Testing for the sulcus sign can be performed with the patient sitting or lying supine. The examiner applies downward traction on the involved arm with the scapula stabilized.

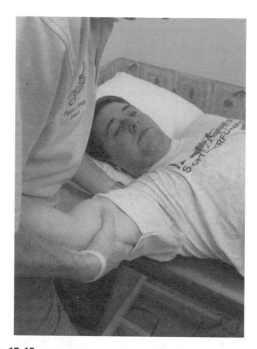

Figure 15-18   For the anterior drawer test, the examiner faces the involved shoulder with the glenohumeral joint positioned at the edge of the examining table. The involved shoulder is held in 80 to 120 degrees of abduction, 0 to 20 degrees of forward flexion, and 0 to 30 degrees of lateral rotation. The examiner holds the patient's scapula with one hand, pressing the scapular spine forward with the index and middle fingers, the thumb exerting counter pressure on the coracoid process. With the other hand, the examiner grasps the patient's upper arm and attempts to draw it anteriorly.

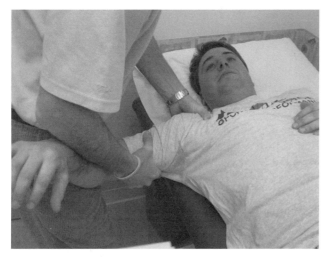

Figure 15-19 For the posterior drawer test, the patient is supine, and the examiner stands next to the involved side, positioning the shoulder in 80 to 120 degrees of abduction and 20 to 30 degrees of forward flexion. The patient's elbow is flexed in a relaxed position. The examiner then stabilizes the scapula by placing the other hand posterior to the shoulder joint capsule with the thumb over the coracoid process. In this position, while stabilizing the scapula, the examiner internally rotates the humerus, applying downward pressure and pushing the humeral head posteriorly.

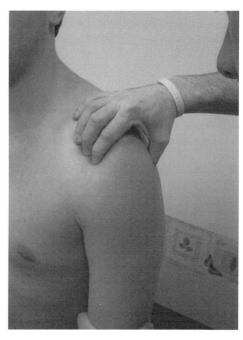

Figure 15-20 The load and shift test is performed with the patient in the sitting position and the examiner behind him or her on the involved side. The examiner stabilizes the clavicle and scapula with one hand and with the other hand grasps the humeral head. The examiner then places an axial load along the shaft of the humerus in an attempt to compress the humeral head into the glenoid fossa.

notes the extent of posterior movement of the humeral head and compares this to the uninvolved contralateral side. This may also be graded, as is done with the anterior drawer test.

Load and Shift Test

In the load and shift test, both anterior and posterior stresses are applied, and the amount of translation of the humerus on the glenoid is noted (Fig. 15-20). An anterior or posterior translation of the humeral head greater than 25% of the diameter of the humeral head when a load is applied is considered a positive test. This test should always be repeated bilaterally with comparison to the contralateral shoulder. Translation between 25% and 50% has been described as being a grade I positive test. Greater than 50% translation with subsequent reduction is considered grade II. The same amount of translation without reduction is described as grade III. Tzannes et al. have described a 100% specificity for both the anterior and posterior load shift tests in diagnosing anterior/posterior instability. However, the sensitivity has been described as 50% and 14% for the anterior and posterior tests respectively.

Glenoid Labrum

The glenoid labrum is a fibrous ring that is attached to the glenoid articular surface through a fibrocartilaginous transition zone. It is an anchor point for capsuloligamentous structures, thereby deepening the glenoid concavity and reducing excessive glenohumeral translation. The labrum functions to increase the depth and surface area of the glenoid. It has been noted that labrum excision decreases the depth of the glenohumeral socket by 50%, reducing resistance to instability by 20%.

The following special tests attempt to isolate tears of the glenoid labrum.

Grind Test

In association with instability, the grind test may help detect a glenoid labral tear. The test is performed with the patient lying supine and the affected shoulder abducted 90 degrees with the elbow flexed 90 degrees. In this position, the examiner grasps the patient's elbow with one hand and the proximal humerus with the other hand and applies compression to the glenoid labrum while attempting to circumduct the humeral head 360 degrees around the surface of the glenoid. A positive finding of a clunking or grinding sensation may be indicative of a glenoid labrum tear.

Clunk Test

Another way to evaluate for labral tears is the clunk test. With the patient supine, the examiner places one hand on the posterior aspect of the patient's humeral head and the other hand proximal to the patient's elbow joint. In this position, the examiner passively abducts and externally rotates the patient's arm overhead applying an anterior force to the humerus. The arm may also be brought into internal rotation. The examiner then circumducts the humeral head around the glenoid labrum. A positive finding of a clunking or grinding sensation is felt to be indicative of a glenoid labral tear. In a study by Stetson evaluating the test in 65 patients with shoulder pain comparing physical examination results with findings from diagnostic arthroscopy, the crank test was 56% specific, 46% sensitive, and had a positive predictive value of 41% and a negative predictive value of 61%.

SLAP Tests

SLAP lesions were first described by Snyder in 1990. Since then, there have been a number of tests developed to detect this lesion by physical examination. The following tests attempt to isolate the superior labrum biceps anchor complex and identify injury to this area.

Biceps Tension Test.   Snyder's biceps tension test is performed with resisted shoulder flexion with the elbow extended and forearm supinated. A positive test result (felt to be indicative of a SLAP lesion) was defined as deep anterior shoulder pain reproduced with this maneuver. In 1993, Field and Savoie observed the biceps tension test to be positive in 20 consecutive patients with a diagnosis of SLAP lesion.

Compression-rotation Test.   Snyder also described the compression-rotation test performed with the patient supine, shoulder abducted 90 degrees, and the elbow flexed 90 degrees. In this position, a compression force is applied to the humerus, which is then rotated in an attempt to trap the suspected torn labrum. A positive test will demonstrate a catch or snap of the torn superior labrum.

O'Brien Active Compression Test.   The O'Brien active compression test was described to distinguish between SLAP lesions and AC joint pathology (Fig. 15-21). The test is considered positive for a SLAP lesion if deep shoulder pain is present in the internally rotated position and reduced in the second position (forearm supinated). Pain localized to the AC joint or on top of the shoulder was considered to be diagnostic of AC joint abnormalities. In a series of more than 300 patients, this test demonstrated a sensitivity of 100%, a specificity of 99%, a positive predictive value of 95%, and a negative predictive value of 100% for labral abnormalities.

Biceps Load Test.   The biceps load test was described for the evaluation of SLAP lesions in patients with and without recurrent anterior instability. This test is performed with the patient in the supine position and the examiner on the side of the affected shoulder. The involved shoulder is then abducted 120 degrees and maximally externally rotated with elbow in 90 degrees of flexion and the forearm supinated. The patient is then instructed to flex the elbow while this is restricted by the examiner. The test is considered positive if the patient complains of pain during the resisted elbow flexion. In 1999, Kim assessed this test in 75 patients, with a reported specificity of 97%, a sensitivity of 91%, a positive predictive value of 83%, and a negative predictive value of 98%.

Other Tests Involving the Shoulder

Other important tests in the category of shoulder examination, but not isolated to the shoulder, include tests for thoracic outlet syndrome and the brachial plexus.

Brachial Plexus Stretch Test.   The brachial plexus stretch test is performed with the patient sitting. The examiner stands behind the patient and places one hand on the side of the patient's head and the other hand on the shoulder on the same side. In this position, the examiner laterally flexes the patient's head while applying gentle downward pressure on the shoulder. Pain that radiates in the patient's arm opposite to the laterally flexed neck is described as a positive finding. If pain is in the neck on the side toward lateral flexion, this may represent cervical spine facet joint impingement.

Adson's Maneuver.   Adson's maneuver attempts to evaluate for thoracic outlet syndrome (Fig. 15-22). An absent or diminished radial pulse is felt to be indicative of thoracic outlet syndrome secondary to subclavian artery compression by the scalene muscles.

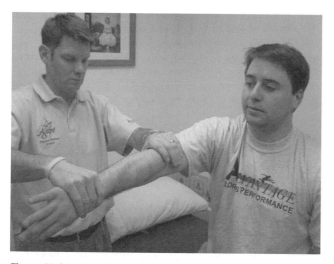

Figure 15-21   The O'Brien active compression test is performed with the patient either sitting or standing. The involved shoulder is placed in 90 degrees of forward flexion, and 30 to 45 degrees of horizontal adduction and maximal internal rotation. The examiner then applies a downward force to the arm against the patient's manual resistance. With the arm in the same position, the palm is then fully supinated and the maneuver repeated.

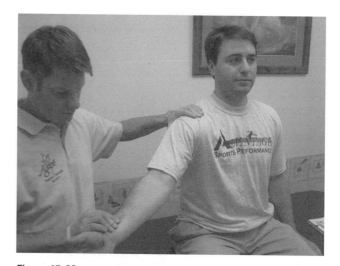

Figure 15-22   In Adson's maneuver, the patient is either standing or sitting, and the examiner places his fingers over the radial artery at the wrist. The examiner then externally rotates and extends the patient's involved arm while palpating the radial pulse. The patient then extends and rotates the neck toward the involved arm and inhales.

ELBOW

The elbow complex is made up of three separate articulations: the ulnohumeral joint, humeroradial (radiocapitellar) joint, and the radioulnar joint. The medial epicondyle of the distal humerus serves as the attachment site of the ulnar collateral ligament (UCL) and the flexor-pronator muscles of the forearm (flexor carpi radialis, flexor carpi ulnaris, flexor digitorum superficialis, pronator teres, and palmaris longus) (Fig. 15-23). The lateral epicondyle of the distal humerus provides attachment for the lateral UCL along with the extensor muscles of the forearm (extensor carpi radialis longus and extensor carpi radialis brevis, extensor carpi ulnaris, extensor digiti minimi, anconeus, and supinator) (Fig. 15-24). The bony stability of the joint is provided by the capsule, the UCL, the radial collateral ligament, and the annular ligament. The elbow allows flexion and extension along with supination and pronation. This enables the hand to be placed in a variety of positions in space.

History and Physical Examination

- Although elbow injuries are not as common as those involving the shoulder, they may be difficult to diagnose.
- A complete and thorough history and a full and systematic physical examination are required for correct diagnosis.
- Along with this, knowledge of elbow anatomy and the abnormal conditions that may affect the joint are crucial.
- A history should include a description of the patient's onset of symptoms (acute or chronic), location of pain, duration of symptoms, dominant arm, and associated activities.
    - Information gained will help to focus the physical examination.
- Examination of the elbow joint should begin with inspection.

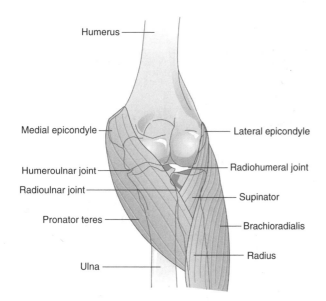

Figure 15-23   Anterior view of the left elbow joint. (From Bickley LS, Szilagyi P. Bates' Guide to Physical Examination and History Taking, 8th ed. Philadelphia: Lippincott Williams & Wilkins, 2003.)

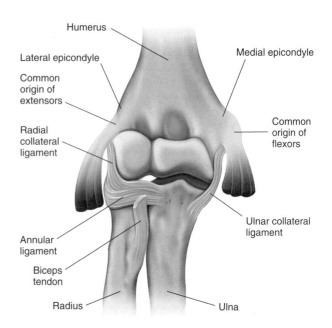

Figure 15-24   Anterior view of the right elbow joint, radius, and ulna, showing the ligaments. (From Premkumar K. The Massage Connection Anatomy and Physiology. Baltimore: Lippincott Williams & Wilkins, 2004.)

- As with the shoulder, the patient should be unclothed to the waist for the examination.
- The elbow is a superficial joint, and many of its disorders can be detected by simple inspection.
- Inspection should involve the entire upper extremity along with comparison with the uninvolved contralateral extremity.
- After inspection, the examination should proceed with palpation of bony landmarks, including the medial and lateral epicondyles, radiocapitellar joint, medial joint line, medial and lateral collateral ligaments, distal biceps, and triceps tendons.
- Range of motion in the flexion/extension and pronation/supination planes should be measured and recorded and compared to the contralateral side.
- Information obtained from the history and initial physical examination will provide clues toward the diagnosis and direct the examiner to proceed further with necessary provocative tests.

Lateral Epicondylitis

One of the most common diagnoses involving the elbow is lateral epicondylitis or tennis elbow. There have been numerous tests described to evaluate this entity, which involves angiofibroblastic tendinosis of the extensor carpi radialis brevis origin at the lateral humeral epicondyle. The following special tests are used to aid in this diagnosis.

Cozen's Test

Cozen's test is also known as the resistive tennis elbow test (Fig. 15-25). A report of pain along the lateral epicondyle

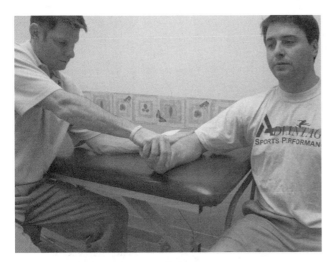

Figure 15-25   Cozen's test is performed with the patient sitting. The examiner stabilizes the involved elbow with one hand and places the palm of the other hand on the dorsal aspect of the subject's hand just distal to the proximal interphalangeal joint of the patient's long finger. The patient is then instructed to extend the long finger against the examiner's resistance.

or radiation along the extensor-supinator muscle compartment is considered a positive finding for lateral epicondylitis. This test can also be performed with resisted wrist extension when the elbow is fully extended. Pain with this maneuver along the lateral epicondyle is considered a positive finding.

Passive Tennis Elbow Test

In the passive tennis elbow test (Fig. 15-26), a report of pain along the lateral epicondyle may be indicative of lateral epicondylitis.

Golfer's Elbow Test

In evaluating medial epicondylitis or golfer's elbow, the golfer's elbow test has been described (Fig. 15-27). The test is

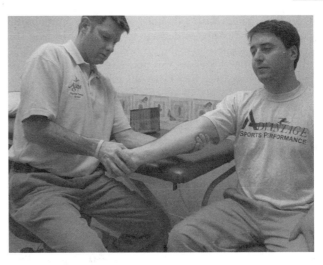

Figure 15-27   The golfer's elbow test is performed with the patient either sitting or standing. The examiner faces the subject and palpates along the humeral medial epicondyle. While the patient makes a fist on the involved side, the examiner passively supinates the forearm and extends the elbow and wrist.

considered positive if pain or complaints of discomfort are elicited along the medial aspect of the elbow (especially pain at the medial epicondyle).

Instability

Valgus Stress Test

Pain along the medial epicondyle region may also be caused by injury to the ulnar nerve or structural damage to the UCL. As such, it is important to assess these structures individually. The valgus stress test has been described to evaluate injury to the UCL (Fig. 15-28). Medial or increased

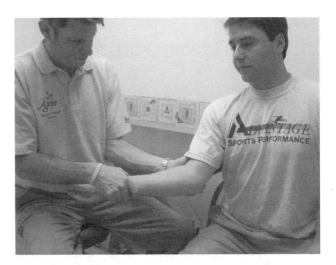

Figure 15-28   Valgus stress test. The test is performed with the patient sitting and the involved elbow flexed to 20 to 30 degrees. The examiner stands with the distal hand around the subject's wrist (medially) and the proximal hand over the patient's elbow joint (laterally). In this position, with the patient's wrist stabilized, the examiner applies a valgus stress to the elbow with the proximal hand.

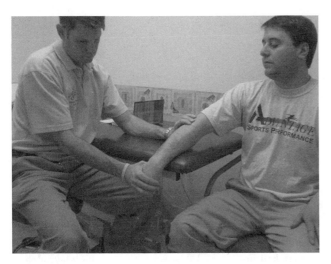

Figure 15-26   The passive tennis elbow test is performed with the patient sitting and the involved elbow in full extension. In this position, the examiner passively pronates the patient's forearm and flexes the patient's wrist.

valgus movement with a diminished or absent end point is considered indicative of damage to the UCL. During this test, it is imperative that the humerus not be internally or externally rotated because this may give a false-positive result. A recent study by O'Driscoll et al. demonstrated a 100% sensitivity and 75% specificity utilizing a valgus stress test for the diagnosis of UCL injury in the elbow.

Milking Test

The milking test is another provocative maneuver for evaluating UCL injury and subtle valgus instability (Fig. 15-29). A positive test reproduces the patient's symptoms of medial elbow pain and may indicate UCL injury.

Varus Stress Test

Injury to the radial (lateral) collateral ligament may be evaluated with the varus stress test (Fig. 15-30). Lateral elbow pain or increased varus movement with an absent or diminished end point is felt to be indicative of injury to the radial (lateral) collateral ligament.

Lateral Pivot Shift Test

The posterolateral rotatory-instability test, or lateral pivot shift test, assesses laxity of the ulnar portion of the lateral collateral ligament (Fig. 15-31). Apprehension in the awake patient indicates a positive test—injury to the ulnar portion of the lateral collateral ligament. However, displacement of the ulna from the trochlea usually can only be performed with the patient under general anesthesia.

Nerve Compression or Entrapment

Elbow Flexion Test

The elbow flexion test is performed with the patient either sitting or standing. The patient is instructed to maximally flex the elbow and hold this position for 3 to 5 minutes. Radiating pain in the median nerve distribution in the pa-

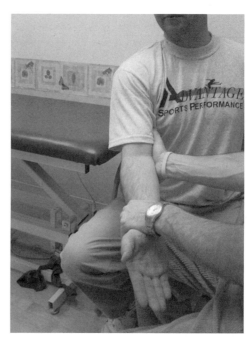

Figure 15-30 In the varus stress test, the patient is sitting and the involved elbow is flexed to 20 to 30 degrees. The examiner sits facing the patient with the distal hand around the patient's wrist (laterally) and the proximal hand around the patient's elbow (medially). In this position with the patient's wrist stabilized, the examiner applies a varus stress to the elbow.

tient's arm or hand (lateral forearm or tip of thumb, index and middle finger, ulnar half of ring finger) is considered a positive finding indicative of cubital fossa syndrome. This test may also be indicative of ulnar nerve compression in the ulnar groove if radiating pain extends in an ulnar nerve distribution (the small finger and radial half of the ring fin-

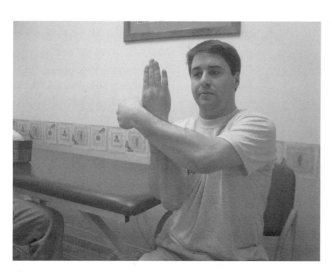

Figure 15-29 In the milking test, the patient is seated. With the patient's forearm fully supinated, the thumb is grasped and a valgus stress is applied to the elbow as the joint is passively flexed greater than 90 degrees.

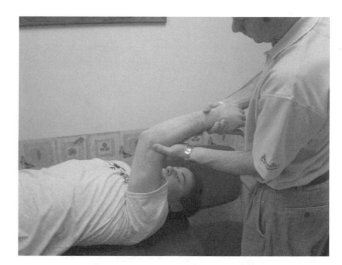

Figure 15-31 In the lateral pivot shift test, the patient is supine. The involved arm is extended back over the patient's head and the shoulder externally rotated. The examiner stands at the head of the table and supinates the patient's forearm while simultaneously applying a valgus stress and axial compression and flexion of the elbow.

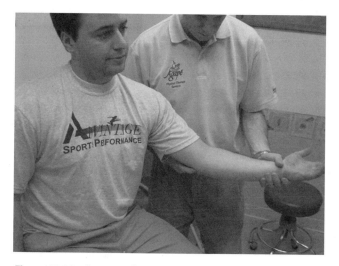

Figure 15-32 In testing for Tinel's sign, the patient is seated with the elbow in slight flexion. The examiner grasps and stabilizes the patient's wrist with one hand and taps the ulnar nerve between the medial epicondyle and olecranon with the other hand.

digitorum profundus). It may be performed with the patient sitting or standing. The patient is instructed to pinch the tips of the thumb and index finger together. The inability to touch them together is described as a positive finding, indicating potential pathology of the anterior interosseous nerve between the two heads of the pronator muscle.

ger). In 1998, Rosati et al. evaluated the validity of this test for diagnosing ulnar nerve compression at the cubital tunnel. The percentage of positive tests was only 3.6% at 1 minute and increased to 16.2% at 3 minutes.

Tinel's Sign

Tinel's sign is used to evaluate for ulnar nerve compromise about the elbow (Fig. 15-32). A positive finding is described as subjective tingling along the ulnar nerve distribution of the forearm, hand, and fingers. This test should be repeated on the contralateral side for comparison. In 1994, a study by Novak examined 44 extremities with cubital tunnel syndrome. Of those, 31 had Tinel's sign and sensitivity of 70%.

Pinch Grip Test

The pinch grip test has been described to evaluate the anterior interosseus nerve (a branch of the median nerve that innervates the pronator quadratus, flexor pollicis longus, and the first and second components of the flexor

SUGGESTED READING

Bennett WF. Specificity of the Speed's test: arthroscopic technique for evaluating the biceps tendon at the level of the bicipital groove. Arthroscopy 1998;14:789–796.

Bigliani LU, Morrison DS, April EW. The morphology of the acromion and its relationship to rotator cuff tears. Orthop Trans 1986;10:228.

Ellenbacker TS, Boeckmann RR. Interrater reliability of manual valgus stress testing of the elbow joint and its relation to an objective stress: radiography technique in professional baseball pitchers. J Orthop Sports Phys Ther 1998;27:95.

Field LD, Savoie FH III. Arthroscopic suture repair of superior labral detachment lesions of the shoulder. Am J Sports Med 1993;21:783–790.

Gerber C, Hersche O, Farron A. Isolated rupture of the subscapularis tendon. J Bone Joint Surg 1996;78A:1015–1023.

Hawkins RJ, Kennedy JC. Impingement syndrome in athletes. Am J Sports Med 1980;8:151–158.

Neer CS II. Anterior acromioplasty for the chronic impingement syndrome in the shoulder: a preliminary report. J Bone Joint Surg 1972;54A:41–50.

Neer CS II. Impingement lesions. Clin Orthop 1983;173:70–77.

O'Brien SJ, Pagnani MJ, Fealy S, et al. The active compression test: a new and effective test for diagnosing labral tears and acromioclavicular joint abnormality. Am J Sports Med 1998;26:610–613.

O'Driscoll, SW, Lawton, RL, Smith A. The "moving valgus stress test" for medial collateral ligament tears of the elbow. Am J Sports Med 2005;33(2):231–239.

Silliman JF, Hawkins RJ. Classification and physical diagnosis of instability of the shoulder. Clin Orthop 1993;291:7–19.

Snyder SJ, Karzel RP, Del Pizzo W, et al. SLAP lesions of the shoulder. Arthroscopy 1990;6:274–279.

Tennent DT, Beach WR, Meyers JF. A review of the special tests associated with shoulder examination. Part I: The rotator cuff tests. Am J Sports Med 2003;31:154–160.

Tennent DT, Beach WR, Meyers JF. A review of the special tests associated with shoulder examination. Part II: laxity, instability and superior labral anterior and posterior (SLAP) lesions. Am J Sports Med 2003;31:301–307.

Yergason RM. Supination sign. J Bone Joint Surg 1931;13:160.

16

SHOULDER INJURIES IN THROWING ATHLETES

ANDREAS H. GOMOLL
GEORGE F. HATCH
PETER J. MILLETT

Shoulder injuries, both traumatic and chronic, are a relatively common occurrence in overhead athletes. Shoulder injuries can be career-changing, or even career-ending events, especially for overhead athletes such as baseball pitchers, football quarterbacks, tennis players, and swimmers. Efficient throwing requires a coordinated effort that progresses from the toes to the fingertips, and this has been described by Kibler as the kinetic chain concept. The sequence of body segment motions begins with the lower body and moves to the upper body and arm. Energy is generated in the legs and trunk and is then transferred through the shoulder to the arm, which delivers the force to the ball. Any condition that affects a component of the chain, especially those located more proximally in the kinetic chain, may produce changes in later segments, possibly resulting in the development of pathology.

Due to ongoing controversy regarding the exact causes of injury in the thrower's shoulder, the authors will not attempt to provide a single unifying theory. Instead, we will provide an overview clarifying the terminology and describing common pathologic findings, and presenting the various theories on injury in the throwing shoulder. The purpose of this chapter is to discuss the biomechanics, presentation, diagnosis, and treatment of common shoulder injuries in overhead athletes.

SHOULDER BIOMECHANICS AND KINEMATICS

Overhead athletes perform a majority of their upper extremity activity in the inherently unstable position of maximal abduction and external rotation. A thorough understanding of the biomechanics and joint kinematics of the shoulder is a necessary prerequisite to diagnose and treat shoulder injuries successfully in these athletes. Due to the frequency of shoulder injuries in baseball pitchers, we will review the mechanics of throwing.

During a baseball pitch, ball velocities frequently exceed 90 miles per hour, and the shoulder of a professional player will rotate at speeds of up to 7,000 degrees per second, with distractive forces equal to body weight. These are among the fastest angular velocities created in all of sport. Throwing has been divided into six phases (Table 16-1 and Fig. 15-18 in Chapter 15), and the entire throw usually takes

TABLE 16-1 THE SIX PHASES OF THE BASEBALL PITCH

PHASE	ACTION	DESCRIPTION
1	Wind-up	Readying phase
2	Early cocking	Concluding with the shoulder positioned in 90 degrees of abduction, with the elbow positioned slightly behind the plane of the body
3	Late cocking	Arm reaches maximum external rotation
4	Acceleration	Internal rotation of the arm with highest angular velocity
5	Deceleration	Eccentric contraction of all muscle groups to slow the arm results in greatest loads across the joint
6	Follow-through	Rebalancing phase

less than 2 seconds. The first three phases occupy 1.5 seconds, acceleration occupies only 0.05 seconds, and the last two occupy approximately 0.35 seconds. Also see Chapter 15 for further details on the kinematics of throwing.

A model of the throwing shoulder during the baseball pitch has been created through a combination of in vitro biomechanical studies, electromyographic analysis, and clinical observation. Although football throwing follows the same basic phases, there are slight differences, imparted by the greater weight of the football, and mainly resulting in lower angular velocities of approximately 5,000 degrees per second.

ADAPTATION

Generally, most upper extremity throwing sports require repetitive motion of the shoulder under high loads at the extremes of motion. Because of these loads, adaptive changes occur in the dominant extremity of overhead athletes. These changes affect passive stabilizing structures such as the capsule, ligaments, and bone, as well as dynamic stabilizers such as the rotator cuff, shoulder girdle, and chest wall musculature. It is widely believed that repetitive subfailure loads can lead to acquired laxity of the shoulder, and this has been demonstrated in cadaveric models.

In throwing athletes, the ability to rotate the humerus externally to generate high ball velocities is paramount. Studies have shown a direct correlation between the amount of external rotation of the abducted arm and the subsequent speed of the pitched ball. With repetitive throwing in a developing skeleton, adaptation of the osseous and ligamentous anatomy occurs, which results in increased humeral retroversion and acquired ligamentous laxity, allowing increased external rotation in the throwing arm.

Examination of the dominant arm of asymptomatic high-level overhead athletes (baseball pitchers and tennis play-

ers) has shown increased external rotation and decreased internal rotation in the abducted shoulder. It is commonly accepted that the majority of these changes result from laxity in the anterior inferior glenohumeral ligament and contracture of the posterior capsule. In the throwing position, the anterior inferior glenohumeral ligament is the primary restraint to external rotation. Therefore, it appears likely that this ligament would be repetitively stressed and could develop laxity, allowing for increased external rotation. Interestingly, baseball pitchers commonly have an increased sulcus sign on physical exam, which may be related to laxity of the coracohumeral ligament, another restraint to external rotation in both the abducted and adducted arm.

Another factor contributing to increased external rotation in the throwing arm is acquired retroversion of the humeral head. Multiple studies have associated this with throwing. This osseous adaptation has been described in professional handball and baseball players, especially when intense training was started before skeletal maturity. An average increase in humeral retroversion of 10 to 20 degrees was observed compared with the nondominant arm.

As a result of the adaptive changes—both ligamentous and osseous—range of motion (ROM) is altered. Some authors suggest that increased humeral retroversion is the predominate cause of this altered ROM. Others believe that laxity of the anterior inferior glenohumeral ligament is the main factor and recommend capsular plication as part of the surgical treatment. Still, other studies suggest that the posterior capsular contracture is the initiating and primary cause of pathology and recommend release of the posterior capsule as part of surgical treatment. Clearly, this area remains in need of additional study.

In addition to bony and ligamentous adaptation, throwing athletes typically demonstrate muscular asymmetry between the dominant and nondominant arm as a result of muscle adaptation. It is not uncommon for athletes to develop hypertrophy of the shoulder girdle musculature, humeral head, cortex, and arm musculature of the throwing arm. In chronic shoulder conditions such as suprascapular nerve dysfunction or rotator cuff pathology, however, subtle atrophy can sometimes be found, especially in the infraspinatus and supraspinatus fossa. Overhead athletes, particularly volleyball players, can demonstrate significant atrophy of the infraspinatus with weakness in external rotation as a result of suprascapular neuropathy. This neuropathy is thought to represent a repetitive traction injury, with constriction occurring at the spinoglenoid notch (often associated with labral cysts) or more proximally at the scapular notch.

Several investigators have examined muscle strength in the overhead throwing athlete with varying results and conclusions. External rotation strength as a function of the infraspinatus and teres minor muscles in the dominant shoulder of professional baseball pitchers has been found to be significantly weaker than the nonthrowing shoulder. The shoulder abductors, the deltoid, and supraspinatus muscles usually do not demonstrate marked hypertrophy in throwers, and some studies have even demonstrated significantly weaker supraspinatus strength in the throwing arm of pitchers compared with the nondominant arm.

Conversely, testing of internal rotation in the dominant shoulders of pitchers has demonstrated significantly increased strength of the internal rotators and adductor muscles. The subscapularis, latissimus dorsi, pectoralis major, teres major, coracobrachialis, and the long head of the triceps act in concert to internally rotate and adduct the arm during the acceleration phase of throwing.

EVALUATION

History

■ A detailed history is the basis for a successful diagnosis and treatment.
■ Duration, location, and timing of symptoms, as well as associated symptoms, provide essential clues to the diagnosis.
■ Patient age and history of other injuries are also important in creating a differential diagnosis.
  ■ Patient age is relevant in that certain diagnoses are more common in particular age groups.
  ■ For example, shoulder pain in young athletes should raise concerns for physeal injury.
  ■ Younger athletes are also more likely to have problems with laxity.
  ■ Older players, especially pitchers, are more likely to suffer from rotator cuff pathology.
  ■ Pitchers in the middle of their careers may experience both laxity and rotator cuff pathology.
■ Timing of symptoms during the throwing cycle is important in formulating a differential diagnosis (Table 16-2).
  ■ Pain during cocking can suggest labral pathology, internal impingement, laxity, and/or instability.
  ■ Pain during late cocking or the early acceleration phase is seen with anterior instability.
  ■ Pain after ball release or during deceleration is frequently associated with rotator cuff pathology.
  ■ Posterior instability typically presents with pain during follow-through.
■ Timing of symptoms during a game is also important.
  ■ Symptoms occurring late in the game or after repeated pitching starts suggest fatigue, typically of the rotator cuff. These symptoms may respond well to rest and rehabilitation.
■ History of associated symptoms and/or other nonshoulder injuries should also be obtained.

TABLE 16-2 RELATIONSHIP OF PHASE OF THROW WITH DIFFERENTIAL DIAGNOSIS

Phase in Throwing Cycle	Possible Differential Diagnosis
Wind-up	
Early cocking	
Late cocking	Labral pathology
Acceleration	Internal impingement
	Anterior instability
Deceleration	Rotator cuff pathology
Follow-through	Posterior instability

■ It is important to consider the kinetic chain concept, as injuries to the lower extremities, spine, and other areas may alter throwing mechanics and in turn cause shoulder pain.
■ A history of numbness, tingling, or discoloration in the fingers should raise concern for a neurologic or vascular problem.
■ Distal paresthesias or "dead arm" may also be associated with shoulder instability.

Physical Examination

Observation

■ The majority of injuries seen in the throwing athlete will present with an insidious onset; therefore, the examiner must be attuned to the presence of vague complaints and subtle findings on physical exam, as opposed to gross deformity and overt distress.
■ Inspection of both symptomatic and asymptomatic throwing athletes at rest will typically reveal some asymmetry—frequently, hypertrophy of the dominant shoulder and arm.
■ Chronic shoulder conditions can present with very subtle atrophy that can be detected with careful inspection of the supraspinatus and infraspinatus fossa, in addition to the scapular stabilizers bilaterally.
■ Atrophy within the infraspinatus fossa can signal the presence of suprascapular neuropathy, which occurs in overhead and throwing athletes presumably from traction.
■ General posture and alignment of the shoulder girdle should also be noted.

Palpation

■ Many throwing athletes with shoulder pathology will hold the scapula in a depressed and protracted position.
■ Palpation can be helpful in distinguishing between disorders of the subacromial space or supraspinatus, the long head of the biceps, and the teres major tendons.
■ All bony prominences around the shoulder should be palpated, especially the acromioclavicular (AC) joint, where tenderness and swelling can indicate degeneration.
■ Acute AC joint disruptions are uncommon unless there has been a history of trauma.
■ Attention should also be directed to the bicipital groove and coracoid process.
■ Tenderness of the bicipital groove is typical for biceps tendonitis, whereas pain with deep palpation of the coracoid can indicate an impingement process.
■ The exam should always include palpation of the posterior joint line, where pain from both rotator cuff and labral pathology can sometimes be elicited.
■ Additionally, pain from the presence of posterior glenoid osteophytes (e.g., Bennett's lesions) can be appreciated with deep palpation of the posteroinferior glenohumeral joint.

Range of Motion

■ ROM, both glenohumeral and scapulothoracic, must be evaluated.
■ Scapulothoracic motion should be smooth and symmetrical.

- Asymmetry or winging of the scapula should alert the examiner to the presence of periscapular muscle weakness and overuse or, less commonly, nerve injury or tightness of the pectoralis minor muscle.
- Painful crepitus with scapulothoracic motion may suggest inflammation of the scapulothoracic bursa.
- Rotation of the abducted arm in overhead athletes typically shows loss of internal rotation and increased external rotation due to posterior capsular tightness and stretching of the anterior structures.
- Posterior capsular tightness is best assessed in the prone position, where maximum internal rotation of the shoulder can result in inferior scapular winging.
- Frequently, there is a net loss in ROM due to a comparatively larger loss of internal rotation than gain of external rotation.
- Limitations in internal rotation beyond the normal-but-shifted range may place the athlete at risk for the development of shoulder problems, which will be discussed in more detail later in the chapter.

- Any discrepancy between active and passive ROM may be a sign of muscle dysfunction or inhibition by pain.

Strength Testing

- Strength testing of the rotator cuff, deltoid, and periscapular muscles should always be performed.
- Internal (subscapularis and pectoralis major muscles) and external rotation (infraspinatus and teres minor muscles) should be evaluated with the arm at the side and in 90 degrees of abduction.
- The supraspinatus may be evaluated with resisted abduction with the 90 degrees in the plane of the scapula and the thumbs pointing to the ground.
- The subscapularis is evaluated with the lift-off test and the belly press test.
- Any pain elicited during testing will help identify the source of the patient's symptoms.
- More subtle muscular dysfunction can frequently be detected by using specific tests (Table 16-3).

TABLE 16-3 SUMMARY OF FUNCTIONAL TESTS

Muscle and Test	Description
Supraspinatus	
Jobe	Patient asked to bring arm to 90 degrees of flexion and full pronation with thumbs pointing to floor, and examiner compares resistive strength to downward directed force; pain and/or weakness indicates supraspinatus dysfunction (see Fig. 14-3 in Chapter 14). Sensitivities range from 0.8 to 0.9; specificities from 0.5 to 0.6[a].
Drop arm sign	Patient asked to bring arm to 90 degrees of flexion and full pronation with thumbs pointing to floor; examiner lifts arm and lets drop; unable to maintain position in supraspinatus dysfunction. Sensitivity of 0.2; specificity of 1.0[a].
Infraspinatus and teres minor	
Gross strength	Resisted external rotation with arm by the side and at 90 degrees of abduction.
Hornblower's sign	Patient asked to externally rotate arm from a position of 90 degrees of abduction; unable to maintain position in infraspinatus dysfunction.
External rotation lag sign	Patient asked to maintain position of maximum passive external rotation; unable to maintain position in infraspinatus dysfunction. Sensitivity quoted as 0.7; specificity as 1.0[a].
Biceps	
Speed's test	Patient asked to forward elevation from 90 degrees of forward flexion; pain indicates bicep tendonitis (see Fig. 14-10 in Chapter 14).
Subscapularis	
Gross strength	Resisted internal rotation with arm by the side.
External rotation	Increased passive external rotation, compared with contralateral side—suspicious for subscapularis rupture.
Lift-off test	Patient places back of hand on buttock; unable to lift hand off in subscapularis dysfunction (see Fig. 14-8 in Chapter 14).
Lift-off lag test	Patient places back of hand on buttock. Examiner lifts hand maximally away from buttock; unable to maintain position in subscapularis dysfunction.
Belly press	Useful in patients with limited internal rotation. Patient firmly pushes hand into lower abdomen with elbow held forward of body; while maintaining forward position of elbow in subscapularis dysfunction (see Fig. 14-9 in Chapter 14).

[a] Sensitivity and specificity provided were available from Dinnes (2003); these figures are sometimes based on a single study and may not be completely accurate.

Stability

- Glenohumeral joint translation should be evaluated in all directions (anterior, posterior, and inferior).
- This should be done in multiple positions with the athlete standing, sitting, and lying supine.
- Although increased laxity in the dominant arm may not necessarily be the source of pathology, reproduction of pain with any of these maneuvers is helpful in identifying the presence and direction of glenohumeral instability.

Provocative Tests

- Provocative tests are a very important tool when trying to determine the source of a patient's shoulder pain.
- The Neer and Hawkins' impingement tests are routinely used to evaluate the subacromial space and supraspinatus muscle (Table 16-4).
- The apprehension and relocation tests are sensitive tools in diagnosing classic anterior instability if true apprehension is elicited.
  - They are less specific when only pain is produced.
- Placing the arm in abduction and external rotation reproduces the symptoms of pain in many throwing athletes.
- A positive relocation test—in which posterior shoulder pain is diminished when a posteriorly directed force is applied to the maximally abducted and externally rotated arm—may be a sensitive means of diagnosing occult anterior instability and internal impingement, which can contribute to rotator cuff disease and posterior-superior labral pathology.
  - Some have speculated that, rather than testing true instability, the anterior-posterior force used in the relocation test may represent an "unlocking" of internally impinged tissues.
- A variety of provocative tests for the superior labral pathology have been described (Table 16-5).
  - Although these tests may be sensitive for detecting labral tears, none have shown great specificity, and therefore may also be positive in other pathology.
- We prefer the active compression test.

TABLE 16-4 COMMONLY USED TESTS FOR IMPINGEMENT

Test	Description
Neer's impingement sign	Pain with forced forward elevation (see Fig.14-4 in Chapter 14).
Hawkins impingement sign	Pain with internal rotation from a position of 90 degrees of forward elevation and 90 degrees of elbow flexion (see Fig. 14-5 in Chapter 14). Sensitivities range from 0.8 to 0.9; specificities from 0.2 to 0.6[a].
Neer's impingement test	Repeated Neer's sign after subacromial injection—increases specificity of impingement diagnosis. Sensitivities range from 0.7 to 0.9; specificities from 0.23 to 0.60[a].

[a] Sensitivity and specificity provided were available from Dinnes (2003); these figures are sometimes based on a single study and may not be completely accurate.

TABLE 16-5 COMMONLY USED TESTS FOR SUPERIOR LABRAL LESIONS

Test	Description
Clunk test	With the shoulder in maximum elevation, circumduct the humeral head. A clunk that recreates the symptoms is a positive test.
Anterior slide test	The patient places hand on hip. The examiner places one hand on top of the acromion, the other behind the elbow to create a superior force, which the patient resists. Pain in the anterior shoulder constitutes a positive test.
O'Brien's test (active compression test)	Arm is forward flexed to 90 degrees and adducted 10 degrees (see Fig.14-10 in Chapter 14). A positive test demonstrates pain with resisted downward pressure on the internally rotated arm, whereas external rotation alleviates the pain.

Other Tests

- Examination of the cervical spine is a necessary part of any shoulder exam due to the high frequency of referred pain from this location.
- Furthermore, the lower extremities and trunk should also be carefully examined.

Imaging Studies

- Imaging should start with plain radiographs, adding cross-sectional studies such as computed tomography (CT) or magnetic resonance imaging (MRI) as needed to obtain additional information about the bony anatomy and condition of soft tissues.

Radiography

- Basic radiographs should include a true anteroposterior, axillary, and outlet views of the shoulder, with specialized radiographs for the detection of specific lesions added as needed.
- The Stryker notch view is useful in the evaluation of posterior humeral lesions and in the diagnosis of a Bennett's lesion (exostosis of the posterior glenoid).

- A West Point view can be used to identify bony Bankart lesions, whereas specialized views are available to evaluate the AC joint for arthritic or traumatic changes.

Computed Tomography
- CT scans have specific but limited applications in the evaluation of the thrower's shoulder.
- It is the study of choice for the evaluation of glenoid abnormalities, such as bony Bankart lesions and, in conjunction with a contrast arthrogram, it allows for the evaluation of labral tears.

Magnetic Resonance Imaging
- In addition to plain radiographs, MRI is the imaging modality of choice for most conditions of the thrower's shoulder.
- Ideally suited for soft-tissue imaging, MRI is particularly useful in evaluating rotator cuff pathology and injury to the glenoid labrum.
- MRI, when used in conjunction with gadolinium arthrography, has reached a sensitivity of 90%, even for the evaluation of partial thickness rotator cuff tears.
- It also allows for the assessment of muscle degeneration, an important consideration before surgical treatment of chronically retracted rotator cuff tears, and the evaluation of labral cysts.
- To detect intra-articular pathology such as labral tears, the sensitivity of MRI can be augmented by the intra-articular injection of gadolinium. It is important to note that even MRI scans of asymptomatic throwing athletes commonly show pathologic changes; therefore, the MRI findings should be used primarily to support a diagnosis suggested by the history and physical exam findings, rather than as a screening tool.

Diagnostic Arthroscopy
- Diagnostic arthroscopy remains the gold standard for the diagnosis of pathology in the thrower's shoulder.
- Intra-articular pathology can be clearly defined, and the integrity of the rotator cuff and biceps–labral anchor complex can be directly tested.
- By using what some have termed "dynamic-assessment arthroscopy," the diagnosis of internal impingement can be made.
- Viewed from the posterior portal with the shoulder in the ABER (abduction-external rotation) position combined with extension, contact between the undersurface of the rotator cuff and the posterior-superior labrum is easily identified, along with any associated lesions of these and other surrounding structures.
- Diagnostic arthroscopy should be reserved, however, for the throwing athlete who has failed conservative management for 3 to 6 months and still continues to have an unclear diagnosis.

CONDITIONING, TRAINING, AND NONOPERATIVE TREATMENT

- With very few exceptions, the treatment of shoulder injuries, especially in professional athletes, should start with a conservative program.

- Conservative management is divided into four phases: rest, stretching, strengthening, and a throwing program.
  - The first phase consists of activity restriction or modification, nonsteroidal anti-inflammatory drugs, ice, massage, and gentle passive ROM exercises.
  - Once the acute pain has diminished, the program should aim to increase motion with the goal of full motion before advancing to the next phase.
    - Focus is typically on contracted structures, such as the posterior capsule and pectoralis minor muscle in throwers.
  - Only after full motion has been restored, the athlete should begin strengthening, with an emphasis on dynamic stabilizers at first but also including trunk and lower extremity musculature in the program.
- The goal is to return to full throwing velocity over the course of 3 months.
- Lack of significant improvement after 3 months, or the inability to return to competitive play within 6 months, constitutes failure of conservative management, and should prompt additional diagnostic tests and consideration of surgical intervention.
- Certain diagnoses such as acute rotator cuff tears or dislocations may warrant earlier and more aggressive surgical intervention on a case by case basis.

SHOULDER CONDITIONS AND SURGICAL CONSIDERATIONS

Laxity and Instability

The development of laxity in the athlete was first described by Neer (1990), was thought to be "acquired," and as such, thought to be a distinct entity separate from traumatic and atraumatic instability. Neer theorized that this acquired laxity resulted from repetitive injury and microtrauma. This concept of acquired laxity gained widespread acceptance. However, there was no solid evidence to demonstrate whether laxity represented a failed repair mechanism or a remodeling response.

Glenohumeral instability and associated internal impingement are probably the most studied but least understood components of pathology in the thrower's shoulder. The definitions of laxity and instability are often blurred in the literature leading to much confusion. Although the terms are related, they are distinct entities. Laxity does not equal instability. Laxity is excessive motion for a particular direction or rotation for a particular joint. It may represent a normal inherent property of the soft tissues or it may be an adaptation for a given sport. For many authors, the term "instability" is generally reserved for the sensation of humeral head translation in the glenoid, associated with pain and discomfort. Taking this into account, the nomenclature of "subtle instability" may have led to some confusion. Others have called this microinstability. Kuhn (2002) recommended that a better description might have been "pathologic laxity."

Although it is obvious that some laxity is essential to compete in high-level overhead sports, excessive laxity may be responsible for the development of shoulder pathology.

For example, excessive laxity of the glenohumeral ligaments could predispose the athlete to injury to the labrum and/or rotator cuff. However, this athlete may not have a sensation of instability. This pathologic laxity is the "subtle instability" described by Jobe et al. (1983). It presents as pain with certain motions, but does not result in true apprehension or a feeling of impending dislocation.

Instability presents either as primary, posttraumatic, or microinstability. Primary instability is the result of generalized ligamentous laxity, whereas posttraumatic instability is caused by a distinct traumatic event. Microinstability is the result of repetitive stresses, especially in shear, during the cocking and acceleration phases. Initially, the stretching of anterior structures permits athletes to attain higher degrees of external rotation, thus allowing them to perform at a higher level. Over time, increasing loads lead to further stretching and failure of the anterior capsule. Microinstability develops with increased anteroposterior translation of the humeral head that can lead to labral fraying, subacromial impingement, and rotator cuff tears.

Superior Labrum Anterior-posterior Lesions

The labrum is a fibrocartilaginous lip surrounding and deepening the glenoid. It also serves as the attachment site for the long head of the biceps and the superior and middle glenohumeral ligaments. Labral tears are common in athletes and can be quite debilitating, especially tears of the superior labrum affecting the biceps anchor. Superior labral tears have received increased attention and have been termed *superior labrum, anterior–posterior*, or SLAP lesions. The original reference describes four types of SLAP lesions (Figs. 16-1 through 16-3; Table 16-6).

Type I SLAP lesions of the superolabral complex are common in throwers, whereas true avulsions of the biceps anchor (type II SLAP lesions) are less frequent. Several theories exist regarding their etiology. Classically, SLAP lesions were thought to be the result of traction or compressive mechanisms, such as sudden pulling on the arm or falls on the outstretched arm. It was thought that traction on the biceps was likely responsible for the development of these lesions during the deceleration phase of throwing, but recent biomechanical studies and arthroscopic observations have suggested the extreme external rotation seen in the thrower's shoulder as the causative factor. Increased strain at the biceps anchor during the late cocking phase with the arm in maximum external rotation results in a "peel-back" effect, which has been suggested as the mechanism behind

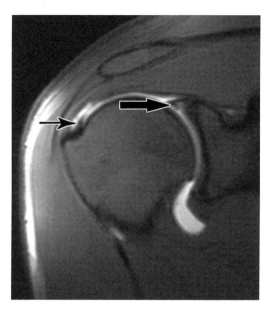

Figure 16-2   Shoulder MRI demonstrating partial thickness rotator cuff tear (*small arrow*) and SLAP tear (*large arrow*). (From Magee T, Williams D, Mani N. Shoulder MR arthrography: which patient group benefits most? Am J Roentgenol 2004;183:969–974.)

the development of SLAP lesions in throwers (see Fig. 16-5). This is supported by laboratory studies that have shown the long head of the biceps to be an important dynamic restraint to external rotation of the abducted arm. As part of the "peel-back" theory, the authors have noted an increased incidence of SLAP lesions in patients with decreased total arc of motion, such as seen in baseball pitchers who often have internal rotation deficits greater than the concomitant gain in external rotation (Fig. 16-4). Burkhart and Morgan (1998) have developed a theory regarding the association between decreased glenohumeral internal rotation and the development of pathology in the shoulder. This model is known as glenohumeral internal rotation deficit (GIRD) and will be discussed in more detail later in the chapter.

Diagnosis

- SLAP lesions present with vague pain, which sometimes localizes to the posterosuperior joint line and can be exacerbated with overhead activities.
- They can produce symptoms of locking or snapping and, depending on tear size, instability.

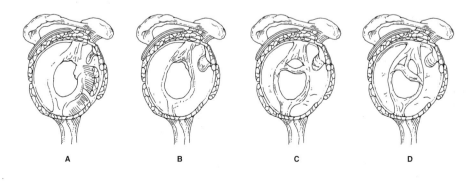

A   B   C   D

Figure 16-1   SLAP types. **A:** Type 1. **B:** Type 2. **C:** Type 3. **D:** Type 4.

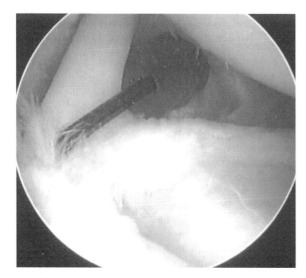

Figure 16-3 Shoulder arthroscopy, view from posterior portal, demonstrating the biceps anchor with a SLAP tear.

- Throwers frequently report pain in the late cocking phase and loss of velocity.
- Posterior tightness and positive provocative tests are common physical findings.
- Radiographic workup should include conventional radiographs and MRI arthrogram to delineate the lesion further.

Treatment

- Treatment of SLAP lesions is typically conservative at first, with many players responding to rest and rehabilitation in the acute period.
- If the acute inflammation in the shoulder has subsided, and the player has completed a course of rehabilitation

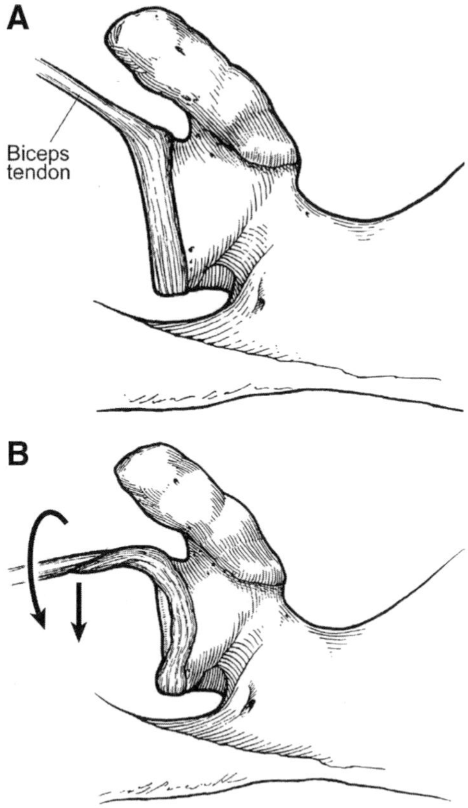

Figure 16-4 Peel-back effect. **A:** Superior view of the biceps and labral complex of a left shoulder in a resting position. **B:** Superior view of the biceps and labral complex of a left shoulder in the abducted, externally rotated position, showing peel-back mechanism as the biceps vector shifts posteriorly. (From Burkhart SS, Morgan CD, Kibler WB. The disabled throwing shoulder: spectrum of pathology. Part I: pathoanatomy and biomechanics. Arthroscopy 2003;19:404–420; with permission from the Arthroscopy Association of North America.)

but is still unable to resume throwing, serious consideration should be given to surgical intervention.

- Surgical treatment of symptomatic SLAP lesions consists of shoulder arthroscopy, which frequently demonstrates a positive "drive-through" sign, a displaceable biceps vertex and, in up to 60% of cases, associated rotator cuff pathology, mostly partial-thickness undersurface tears.
- If the biceps-labral anchor is avulsed, it is partially debrided and secured back to the glenoid with suture anchors, followed by a postoperative rehabilitation program for posterior capsular stretching.
- If minor tearing and fraying are present, but no true avulsion of the biceps anchor, a simple labral debridement can be performed.
- Although thermal capsulorrhaphy has fallen into disfavor in most cases, there have been some favorable results in the throwing athletes with superior labral tears.
  - When thermal capsulorrhaphy was combined with labral repair, better results were seen than with labral repair alone, and 87% of overhead athletes were able to return to play.

TABLE 16-6 SLAP LESIONS

Type	Description
I	Fraying of the labrum with a stable biceps anchor
II	Detachment of the biceps anchor from the superior glenoid in addition to the fraying observed in type I lesions
A	Anterior
B	Posterior
C	Combined
III	Bucket-handle tear of the superior labrum with a preserved biceps anchor
IV	Extension of the bucket-handle tear into the biceps tendon but no instability of the anchor itself

- After formal repair of the biceps–labral complex, throwers undergo a brief period of immobilization, followed by a rehabilitation program that focuses on throwing mechanics.
- Return to play is typically 4 to 6 months postoperatively, although return to elite throwing may take closer to 1 year.
- Patients with a stable biceps anchor at the time of surgery who have undergone only limited labral debridement are not immobilized after surgery and can typically resume play after 4 to 6 weeks of rehabilitation.
  - Authors have reported on the outcome of this type of program, with return to preinjury performance levels in more than 80% of pitchers.

Rotator Cuff Disorders and Impingement

- Most rotator cuff tears in this population are partial-thickness, articular-sided tears.
- Some result from acute tensile overload but more commonly the cause is repetitive microtrauma and eccentric failure of the fibers.
- Whereas cuff tears may occur in the setting of impingement, in this population they are more commonly the result of subtle instability.
- Subacromial decompression alone has not been effective in the athletic population, with return to previous activity levels in only half the patients.
- Similarly, simple debridement of partial tears, a largely effective procedure in lower-demand patients, produces less consistent results especially in the overhead athlete.
- Full-thickness rotator cuff tears are a rare event in the overhead athlete but have a very poor prognosis even when repaired, with only half of all players able to return to play.
- Several types of impingement have been described in the literature:
  - "Classic" subacromial or outlet impingement
  - "Secondary" or nonoutlet impingement
  - Subcoracoid impingement
  - Internal impingement

Classic Subacromial Impingement or External Impingement

- The "classic" form of impingement as described by Neer (1983) is the result of compression of the rotator cuff between the coracoacromial arch and the humeral head.
- Anatomical variants such as a hooked acromion, acromioclavicular joint arthritis with osteophyte formation, and a laterally sloping acromion have been proposed as predisposing factors.
- Subacromial impingement is typically diagnosed in the older throwing athlete who has a stable shoulder.
- These overhand athletes will often have loss of internal rotation without concomitant increase in external rotation as seen in many younger throwers.
- Adaptive bony changes may also play a role in this loss of internal rotation.
- Subacromial impingement can be further exacerbated by weakness of the rotator cuff from fatigue or improper technique, leading to superior migration of the humeral head.

- These patients have a painful arc, positive impingement maneuvers, and will typically respond well to subacromial injections.
- Radiographs in older throwers usually show varying degrees of an acquired, or congenitally prominent anterior acromion that predisposes to outlet stenosis.
- Many patients improve with anti-inflammatory medications combined with a well-supervised physical therapy program focusing on rotator cuff rehabilitation and scapular dynamics.
- Arthroscopy with subacromial decompression is reserved for those who fail conservative management.
- Unlike the subacromial space of a younger thrower, which is typically smooth and white in appearance, the older thrower can demonstrate an irritated and thickened bursa with fraying, matched excoriation and hypertrophy of the coracoacromial ligament.
- If a significant bursal-sided partial or full-thickness rotator cuff tear is present, consideration for repair is recommended, either through a "mini-open" or arthroscopic approach.
- It is imperative to inform patients before surgery, however, that a return to the same premorbid level of competition is unlikely.
- External impingement as the sole source of pain appears to be relatively uncommon in throwing athletes, with the exception of the older thrower.
  - This may help explain why a high failure rate of almost 80% was seen in early reports for throwing athletes being treated with subacromial decompression for apparent impingement.

Secondary Impingement

- Secondary, or nonoutlet, impingement is a dynamic process in which a normal subacromial arch is present but there is abnormal proximity between the arch and the underlying rotator cuff.
- There is a strong association between scapulothoracic dyskinesia and impingement symptoms.
  - Weakness in the scapular stabilizers leads to lack of proper rotation of the scapula during humeral elevation.
  - As a result, the space available for the rotator cuff is acutely narrowed and thus causes impingement symptoms.
- Posterior capsular tightness can also create a vector imbalance resulting in posterior-superior migration of the humeral head with secondary rotator cuff symptoms.
- Malunion from displaced fractures of the greater humeral tuberosity, and massive rotator cuff tears with loss of the humeral head depressors, can also result in secondary impingement.
- Treatment recommendations are based on the primary pathology.
  - If the secondary impingement is associated with a partial-thickness rotator cuff tear affecting more than half the cuff thickness, the recommended treatment includes a formal open, mini-open, or arthroscopic cuff repair.
  - When scapular dyskinesia is the cause of secondary impingement, rehabilitation of the periscapular musculature is typically successful.

- When impingement is caused by tightness involving the capsule, as in adhesive capsulitis, or by adhesions in the subacromial space, as seen in trauma or postsurgical cases, surgical correction with lysis of adhesions is recommended.

Coracoid Impingement

- Coracoid impingement occurs when the subscapularis tendon is compressed between the lesser tuberosity and the coracoid tip.
- Possible causes include postoperative changes (e.g., Bristow procedure), previous trauma, anterior instability, and idiopathic impingement.
- Coracoid impingement is typically a diagnosis of exclusion.
    - Patients present with localized anterior shoulder pain, which can mimic or occur in combination with subacromial impingement.
    - The test most often cited in the literature is pain localized to the coracoid when the shoulder is passively forward flexed, adducted, and internally rotated.
        - This test differs from O'Brien's test, because the latter requires active resistance in this position.
- Injections in the subcoracoid space have been recommended to aid in the diagnosis and treatment of the condition.
- A shortened coracohumeral distance, the distance between the coracoid and the lesser tuberosity with the arm in maximum internal rotation (average 11 mm in normal vs. 5.5 mm in symptomatic shoulders) has been described in association with subcoracoid impingement. This, however, is not specific to this problem.
- If conservative measures fail, a coracoidplasty is the next appropriate step in treatment.
    - This has been described both open and arthroscopically, with the goal being to debride the tip of the prominent coracoid to increase the space between the coracoid and the lesser tuberosity.

Internal Impingement

Walch et al. (1992) first described internal impingement as a physiologic phenomenon in which the undersurface of the rotator cuff contacts the posterior-superior labrum when the arm is placed in maximum external rotation and abduction (Fig. 16-5). Halbrecht et al. (1999) demonstrated this phenomenon in college baseball players and showed that internal impingement can occur even in the absence of symptoms. This is thought to result from recurrent microtrauma, which can ultimately lead to rotator cuff tearing and destabilization of the biceps–labral complex. Internal impingement presents as a spectrum of pathologies with significant overlap that typically involves SLAP lesions, partial thickness rotator cuff tears, hyperlaxity of the anterior glenohumeral ligaments, and posterior capsular contractures.

Several authors have postulated that internal impingement is most likely caused by shoulder girdle muscle fatigue resulting from a lack of conditioning or overthrowing and/or anterior capsular stretch resulting in anterior capsular insufficiency. The authors believe that, during the acceleration phase of throwing, the humerus should be aligned in the plane of the scapula and that with fatigue of the shoulder girdle muscles the humerus drifts out of the scapular plane. This has been termed "hyperangulation" and is called "opening up" by many pitching coaches. This hyperangulation of the humerus in turn stresses the anterior capsule (Fig. 16-6). Loss of anterior capsular integrity compromises the normal posterior rollback of the humeral head, leading to anterior translation, therefore causing the undersurface of the rotator cuff to abut against the margin of the glenoid and labrum. Reducing the laxity in the anterior inferior glenohumeral ligament seems to improve outcome significantly in the throwers with internal impingement.

Glenohumeral Internal Rotation Deficit

Burkhart et al. (2003) have recently questioned whether or not internal impingement actually occurs. They described their own model (GIRD) as the primary cause behind the pathologic changes seen in the "internal impingement" patient. The Morgan-Burkhart model is based on the frequency of posterior capsular contractures in throwers. Combined with the possibility of acquired humeral retroversion, the tight posterior capsule shifts the center of rotation of the humerus in the posterior-superior direction. This permits greater clearance of the greater tuberosity. Because of

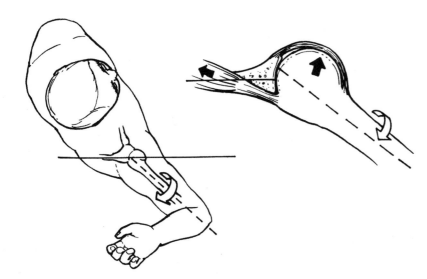

Figure 16-5 Internal impingement of the undersurface of the rotator cuff against the posterior labrum in maximum external rotation/abduction. (From Meister K. Injuries to the shoulder in the throwing athlete. Part I: biomechanics/pathophysiology/classification of injury. Am J Sports Med 2000;28:265–275.)

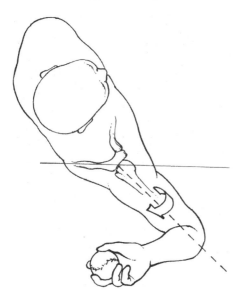

Figure 16-6 Hyperangulation of the humerus.

the diminished "cam" effect, the anterior capsule becomes functionally lengthened (Fig. 16-7). With a functionally lengthened anterior capsule allowing clearance of the greater tuberosity, excessive external rotation is achieved. As a result, the biceps anchor is "peeled back" under tension, causing injury to the posterior-superior structures, most notably to the posterosuperior labrum. The progres-

sion of the "peel-back" mechanism allows further "pseudo-laxity" of the anterior capsule to occur. The pathologic cycle culminates in torsional failure of the rotator cuff, not compressional failure as in the internal impingement model. The end results are articular-sided partial rotator cuff tears and SLAP lesions typically seen in the throwing shoulder.

The GIRD model attempts to quantify the internal rotation deficit to identify those players at risk for pathology. Defined as a greater than 25-degree loss of internal rotation of the dominant shoulder, compared with the contralateral side, GIRD is a common phenomenon in throwing athletes. Some studies have found average deficits of up to 50 degrees when compared with the contralateral side, with concomitant increases in external rotation on the order of 30 degrees. Shoulders with a total arc of motion less than 180 degrees and an internal rotation deficit of greater than 25 degrees seem to be at risk for developing SLAP lesions as a result of increased posterosuperior "peel-back" forces.

Verna (1991) is credited with first recognizing the relationship of GIRD with the development of shoulder dysfunction. By following 39 professional pitchers over a single season, he demonstrated that the development of shoulder problems occurred in more than half of the players with GIRD greater than 35 degrees.

In a similar study by Kibler (1998), high-level tennis players were divided in two groups and prospectively followed for 2 years. One group performed daily posteroinferior capsular stretching to minimize GIRD, whereas the control group continued their routine exercise program. Over the course of the study period, those in the stretching group

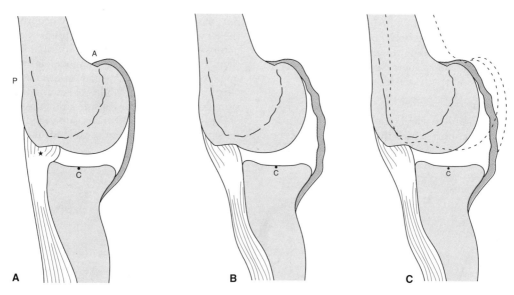

Figure 16-7 Cam effect. **A:** With the arm in a position of abduction and external rotation, the humeral head and the proximal humeral calcar produce a significant cam effect of the anteroinferior capsule, tensioning the capsule by virtue of the space-occupying effect. **B:** With a posterosuperior shift of the glenohumeral contact point, the space-occupying effect of the proximal humerus on the anteroinferior capsule is reduced (reduction of cam effect). This creates a relative redundancy in the anteroinferior capsule that has probably been misinterpreted in the past as microinstability. **C:** Superimposed neutral position (*dotted line*) shows the magnitude of the capsular redundancy that occurs as a result of the shift in the glenohumeral contact point. (After Burkhart SS, Morgan CD, Kibler WB. The disabled throwing shoulder: spectrum of pathology. Part I: pathoanatomy and biomechanics. Arthroscopy 2003;19:404–420.)

had a 38% decrease in the incidence of shoulder problems compared with controls.

Approximately 90% of throwers with GIRD respond to a physical therapy program focused on stretching of the tight posterior capsule, with a concomitant decrease in shoulder-related problems. The remaining 10%, frequently older elite players, who are unresponsive to conservative treatment can be treated by selective arthroscopic postero-inferior capsulotomy in the zone of the posterior band of the inferior glenohumeral ligament.

Increased Humeral Retroversion

Recent studies have investigated the issue of acquired humeral retroversion, its contribution to throwing, and its relevance to internal impingement. Increased humeral retroversion allows for increased external rotation with an obligate loss of internal rotation. Interestingly, Riand et al. (1998) reported that a loss of normal humeral retroversion (normally 25 to 35 degrees) to less than 10 degrees total humeral retroversion will increase the risk of contact between the greater tuberosity and the posterior-superior glenoid labrum (e.g., internal impingement). In patients with a loss of humeral retroversion (as opposed to throwing athletes who typically have increased retroversion), the subsequent internal impingement was corrected with humeral osteotomy.

Scapular Dyskinesia

The work of Kibler (1998) has added greatly to our understanding of scapular dynamics and its role in preventing injuries in the throwing athletes. The scapula functions to provide a stable platform for the humeral head during rotation and elevation, while transferring kinetic energy from the legs and trunk to the upper extremity. It has been estimated that only half of the kinetic energy imparted to the ball results from arm and shoulder action. The remaining half is generated by leg and trunk rotation, and is transferred to the upper limb through the scapulothoracic joint, making it an important, but frequently overlooked part of the kinetic chain.

Scapular dyskinesia results from imbalances of the periscapular musculature secondary to fatigue, direct trauma, or nerve injury (e.g., the long thoracic nerve). It can negatively impact shoulder function in several ways. To reach the extremes of motion needed in overhead athletics, elevation of the acromion is required or else impingement results. Normal function of the serratus anterior, trapezius, and rhomboid muscles is required to achieve the necessary scapular positioning. Loss of function from nerve injury, weakness, and/or fatigue leads to scapular hyperangulation and a relative increase in glenoid anteversion, placing the anterior capsular structures at risk. Associations between scapular dyskinesia and anterior instability and impingement have been documented by several authors.

Because the scapula transfers energy derived from trunk rotation to the pitching arm, destabilization of the scapula results in energy losses that decrease velocity. In an attempt to compensate for the loss of power, the pitcher tries to regain velocity by increasing the effort of the shoulder muscles, which results in increased strain on the shoulder. For these reasons, rehabilitation of the throwing athlete must

have a strong emphasis on strengthening and conditioning the scapular stabilizers.

- The vast majority of scapula-related issues can be resolved by a physical therapy program directed at the scapular stabilizers.
- Sometimes, however, surgical intervention can be required for entities such as scapular bursitis or a snapping scapula, which can be treated by excision of the offending tissues at the inferior and/or superior margin of the scapula.

Bennett Lesion

- The Bennett lesion is a mineralization at the posteroinferior glenoid present in approximately 20% of major league pitchers, best seen on the Stryker-Notch view.
- The lesion is thought to be the result of enthesopathic changes of the posterior capsule and inferior glenohumeral ligament.
- It is an infrequent cause of pain in the overhead athlete and can be associated with tears of the posterior labrum and rotator cuff.
- The diagnosis of a symptomatic Bennett lesion is difficult but frequently presents with posterior shoulder pain during throwing, especially in the follow-through phase.
- Tenderness to palpation of the posteroinferior glenohumeral joint is common, whereas resolution of pain with local injection can be both diagnostic and therapeutic.
- Symptomatic Bennett lesions can be treated by arthroscopic debridement.

Chondral Injuries

- True osteochondritis dissecans of the shoulder is a very rare occurrence, with less than 20 cases described in the literature.
- Traumatic osteochondral defects are seen more frequently as impression fractures of the humeral head (Hill-Sachs lesion), and fractures involving the glenoid rim (Bankart lesion) after anterior glenohumeral dislocation.
- Both can be the cause of recurrent dislocations, in which case they should be corrected by grafting of the Hill-Sachs lesion and fixation of the glenoid fracture.

Neurovascular Conditions

Vascular Injuries
- Vascular compromise after shoulder injury is rarely seen outside major trauma such as scapulothoracic dissociation injuries.
- Presenting predominantly as arterial thrombosis rather than transection, these injuries occur in less than 1% of shoulder dislocations and proximal humerus fractures.

Effort Thrombosis
- Effort thrombosis is a rare entity presenting with symptoms of tiredness, heaviness, and gradual development of swelling over the course of a few days.
- It has been described in a wide range of activities, including baseball, softball, hockey, swimming, wrestling, and backpacking.

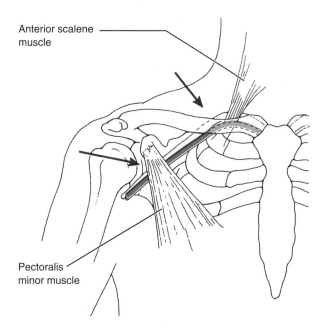

Anterior scalene
muscle

Pectoralis
minor muscle

Figure 16-8 Common compression sites in thoracic outlet
syndrome. (After Meister K. Injuries to the shoulder in the throwing
athlete. Part 2: evaluation/treatment. Am J Sports Med 2000;28:
587–601.)

■ Exam findings include slight discoloration, venous en-
gorgement, and size difference, compared with the contralateral extremity.

■ Venography or more modern CT or MRI-based imaging
typically demonstrate thrombosis of the subclavian vein
at the level of the first rib.

■ The cause, although still not conclusively proven, is
likely compression of the vascular structures between
the first rib and the clavicle, especially with the arm in
maximum abduction.

■ Treatment options include catheter-directed thrombolysis, balloon venoplasty, and staged resection of the first
rib with good results and return to preinjury level of play
within 6 to 36 months.

Thoracic Outlet Syndrome (TOS)

■ This term describes the compression of neurovascular
structures that traverse the thoracic outlet, which is
formed by the clavicle, first rib, and the anterior scalene
muscle (Fig. 16-8).

■ A subset of patients has an identifiable cause for the
compression such as cervical ribs, exostosis of the first
rib, or malunions of the first rib or clavicle.

   ■ In most cases, however, no such abnormality can be
   identified.

■ Presenting complaints are neurological in greater than
90% of patients, and include pain, paresthesias, and
weakness—especially in a lower plexus distribution.

■ Vascular symptoms occur rarely and commonly present
as activity-related claudication, pulse, or blood-pressure
deficits.

■ The workup is complicated by the lack of any specific
diagnostic tests.

■ Several provocative tests have been described, such as
placing the affected extremity in maximum abduction
and external rotation, which leads to recreation of symptoms in more than 80% of patients.

■ Management should be conservative initially, with activity modification, nonsteroidal anti-inflammatory drugs,
strengthening of the shoulder girdle, and scapular stabilizers. This is successful in more than 70% of patients.

■ Surgical treatment is reserved for those severely affected
or for those with refractory pain after conservative management.

■ Studies have demonstrated a greater than 90% success
rate with surgical decompression, frequently by resection of the first rib through a transaxillary approach.

Quadrilateral Space Syndrome

■ Quadrilateral space syndrome is defined as compression
of the axillary nerve and posterior humeral circumflex
artery as they traverse the quadrilateral space.

   ■ This space is defined by the humerus laterally, the
   long head of the triceps medially, and the teres
   minor and major muscles superiorly and inferiorly,
   respectively.

■ This rare condition presents in overhead athletes with
nonspecific symptoms such as dull, aching, or burning
pain in the posterolateral aspect of the shoulder, exacerbated by activity, especially with repetitive exercise with
the arm abducted and externally rotated.

■ Physical findings include deltoid weakness and wasting,
pain to palpation over the quadrilateral space, and reproduction of symptoms with the arm in the flexion-
abduction-external rotation (FABER) position.

■ Angiography frequently demonstrates occlusion of the
posterior humeral circumflex artery when the arm is
placed in the FABER position, whereas electromyographic studies can demonstrate denervation in the deltoid and teres minor muscles.

■ Due to the rarity of the syndrome, no definite treatment
guidelines have been established, but current recommendations include conservative treatment initially,
with surgical exploration and release of the neurovascular structures reserved for refractory cases.

SUMMARY

The etiology of injuries seen in the thrower's shoulder is
multifactorial. Overlapping signs and symptoms exist, as
well as numerous causes of disability. The problems appear
to be a combination of abnormal mechanics, muscle fatigue
and imbalance, scapular dyskinesia, increased humeral retroversion, posterior capsular contractures, anterior capsular laxity, and repetitive microtrauma. As a result, throwers
commonly develop multiple areas of pathology involving the
posterior superior labrum, the articular surface of the rotator cuff, cartilage lesions and bony exostoses of the posterior
glenoid, cystic changes at the insertion of the rotator cuff,
thickening of the posterior capsule, and redundancy of the
anterior capsule.

The etiology and exact pathomechanics of throwing remain controversial and are complicated by the difficulty of recreating an accurate in vitro model of the complex kinetic chain. Different schools of thought exist regarding the initiating event for many of the problems seen in the thrower's shoulder—whether it is anterior capsular laxity or posterior capsular tightness. Fortunately, for the practitioner, regardless of the conflicting theories regarding the pathomechanics at work in the throwing shoulder, the evaluation and treatment algorithms of the injured athlete are, with few exceptions, very similar.

Regardless of the specific cause, the repetitive stresses experienced typically during the late cocking and early acceleration phase result in damage to the posterior glenoid, the biceps-labral complex, and the articular surface of the rotator cuff. The forces acting on these posterior structures are a combination of compressive, tensile, and torsional forces, which culminate in actual fiber failure of both the biceps–labral complex and the rotator cuff. Conditioning of the entire kinetic chain, and respecting adequate recovery periods between games, is imperative, and it is the responsibility of the coaches, trainers, and physicians to educate the players.

SUGGESTED READING

Bigliani LU, Codd TP, Connor PM, et al. Shoulder motion and laxity in the professional baseball player. Am J Sports Med 1997;25:609–613.

Burkhart SS, Morgan CD. The peel-back mechanism: its role in producing and extending type II SLAP lesions and its effect on SLAP repair and rehabilitation. Arthroscopy 1998;14:637–640.

Burkhart SS, Morgan CD, Kibler WB. Current concepts: the disabled shoulder: spectrum of pathology. Part I: pathoanatomy and biomechanics. Arthroscopy 2003;19:404–420.

Burkhart SS, Morgan CD, Kibler WB. Current concepts: the disabled shoulder: spectrum of pathology. Part II: evaluation and treatment of SLAP lesions in throwers. Arthroscopy 2003;19:531–546.

Fleisig GS, Andrews JR, Dillman CD, et al. Kinetics of baseball pitching with implications about injury mechanisms. Am J Sports Med 1995;23:233–239.

Halbrecht JL, Tirman P, Atkin D. Internal impingement of the shoulder: comparison of findings between throwing and non-throwing shoulders in college baseball players. Arthroscopy 1999;15:253–258.

Jobe FW, Jobe CM. Painful athletic injuries of the shoulder. Clin Orthop Relat Res 1983;173:117–124.

Jobe FW, Kvitne RS. Shoulder pain in the overhand or throwing athlete. Orthop Rev 1989;18:963–975.

Jobe FW, Tibone JE, Perry J, et al. An EMG analysis of the shoulder in pitching and throwing. Am J Sports Med 1983;11:3–5.

Kibler WB. The relationship of glenohumeral rotation deficit to shoulder and elbow injuries in tennis players: a prospective evaluation of posterior capsular stretching. In: Annual Closed Meeting of the American Shoulder and Elbow Surgeons. New York: ASES, 1998.

Kibler WB. The role of the scapula in athletic shoulder function. Am J Sports Med 1998;26:325–337.

Kuhn JE. Comprehensive evaluation and treatment of the shoulder in the throwing athlete: biomechanics, pathomechanics, clinical evaluation, and diagnostic testing. Arthroscopy 2002;18:74–81.

Neer CSI. Impingement lesions. Clin Orthop Relat Res 1983;173:70–77.

Neer CSI. Shoulder Reconstruction. Philadelphia: WB Saunders, 1990.

Snyder SJ, Karzel RP, Del Pizzo W, et al. SLAP lesions of the shoulder. Arthroscopy 1990;6:274–279.

Verna C. Shoulder flexibility to reduce impingement. In: 3rd Annual Professional Baseball Athletic Trainers Society. Mesa, AZ: PBATS, 1991.

Walch G, Boileau P, Noel E, et al. Impingement of the deep surface of the supraspinatus tendon on the posterosuperior glenoid rim: an arthroscopic study. J Shoulder Elbow Surg 1992;1:238–245.

Warner JJP, Micheli LJ, Arslanian LE, et al. Scapulothoracic motion in normal shoulders and shoulders with glenohumeral instability and impingement syndrome. Clin Orthop Relat Res 1992;285:191–199.

ANTERIOR INSTABILITY OF THE SHOULDER

JAMES BICOS
AUGUSTUS D. MAZZOCCA
ROBERT A. ARCIERO

The shoulder is one of the most unconstrained joints in the human body. With 6 degrees of freedom, the shoulder has the unique ability of positioning the hand in space and gives us the mobility of performing many tasks, from activities of daily living to high-end sports activities. The shoulder needs normal "laxity" to function. Laxity refers to the translation of the humerus within the glenoid fossa. Many individuals are extremely lax on physical examination but are asymptomatic in terms of shoulder complaints. It is when this laxity causes abnormal shoulder function that we refer to instability of the shoulder. Therefore, laxity does not equate to instability, and instability refers to the *symptomatic* complaint of instability and dysfunction.

PATHOGENESIS

Classification

Instability of the shoulder is a common problem. The reported incidence is difficult to estimate because of the large range in variability of presentation. Instability should be viewed as a spectrum of pathology from unidirectional traumatic instability on one end of the spectrum to atraumatic multidirectional instability at the other end. The three basic categories of instability are traumatic, acquired, and atraumatic.

Traumatic

Traumatic instability is further subcategorized into anterior and posterior instability.

- *Anterior instability* usually results from a fall with the arm in an abducted and externally rotated position or an anterior force with the arm in abduction and external rotation (i.e., arm tackling in football, falling while skiing).
- *Posterior instability* results from a posteriorly directed force with the arm forward elevated and adducted (motor vehicle accident or pass blocking in football). A grand mal seizure or electrical shock can also produce a traumatic posterior dislocation.

Acquired

This type of instability, usually microinstability, is subtle and is associated with pain in a throwing athlete or associated with rotator cuff tendinosis/dysfunction. The instability can occur from repetitive stretching of the shoulder ligaments from activity or sports requirements.

214

Atraumatic

Atraumatic instability is multidirectional, and these patients have symptomatic glenohumeral subluxation or dislocations in more than one direction. Many patients will present with severe pain as an initial complaint and not overt instability. For treatment purposes, it is important to differentiate atraumatic multidirectional instability by the *primary* direction of instability.

- Primary anterior: pain associated with the arm in an abducted, externally rotated position.
- Primary posterior: pain when pushing open a heavy door.
- Primary inferior: pain associated with carrying heavy objects at the side.

Other Factors

Shoulder instability can be further classified by the degree, chronology, and/or direction of the instability.

- *Degree of instability*—Patients can complain of the feeling of apprehension about the shoulder, subluxation episodes, or full dislocation of the shoulder.
- *Chronology of instability*—It is important to elucidate in the medical history of the patient complaining of shoulder instability whether the instability is congenital, acute (usually less than 3 weeks from injury), chronic (usually more than 3 weeks from injury), recurrent, or some combination. The importance of this classification system relates to the treatment options available to the patient.
- *Direction of instability*—anterior, posterior, inferior, and superior.

Pathophysiology

Understanding the anatomy and biomechanics of the lesions that are observed in patients with traumatic anterior instability will facilitate repair of these lesions, which is essential for a successful clinical outcome.

The overall stability of the glenohumeral joint involves passive and active mechanisms. Passive or static factors include joint conformity, adhesion/cohesion, finite joint volume, and ligamentous restraints, including the labrum. The ligaments and capsule are aided by receptors that provide proprioceptive feedback. When capsuloligamentous structures are damaged, alterations in proprioception occur that are partially restored with operative repair. Static stabilizers are also affected by congenital factors that include glenoid hypoplasia and disorders of collagen structure that result in excessive joint laxity. The active mechanisms involved with glenohumeral stability are primarily provided by the rotator cuff muscles. The severity of the instability pattern may be influenced by patient age, seizure disorder, and psychological or secondary gain factors.

The Bankart Lesion

The inferior glenohumeral ligament (IGHL) complex is the primary ligamentous restraint to anterior glenohumeral translation, specifically with the arm in an abducted and

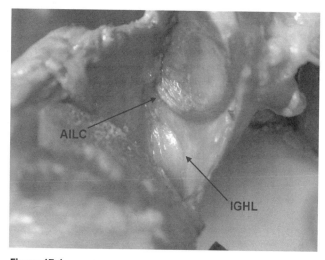

Figure 17-1   Cadaveric image of the inferior glenoid humeral ligament *(IGHL)* and anterior-inferior labral complex *(AILC)*.

externally rotated position (Fig. 17-1). The specific anatomy of the IGHL has been described as having anterior and posterior bands with an intervening axillary pouch. Detachment of the anterior-inferior labrum and capsule (comprising the anterior band of the IGHL as a capsulolabral complex) is considered one of the major pathoanatomical features of traumatic anterior shoulder instability. In fact, up to 85% of traumatic anterior shoulder dislocations can be associated with detachment of the anterior-inferior labrum and capsule. Broca and Hartman first described the lesion in 1890, followed by Perthes in 1906, and Bankart in 1923. This lesion has subsequently been named the Perthes-Bankart lesion (Fig. 17-2).

The mechanism of how the Bankart lesion leads to instability has been studied extensively. The detachment of the labrum from the anterior-inferior glenoid is the essential lesion leading to anterior instability. By displacing the anterior labrum, glenoid depth is decreased by up to 50% and

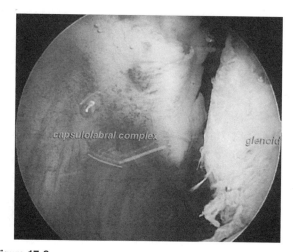

Figure 17-2   Arthroscopic view of a Bankart lesion, left shoulder, sitting position viewed from posteriorly.

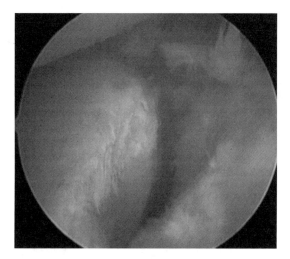

Figure 17-3 Arthroscopic view of an anterior labrum periosteal sleeve avulsion lesion. Anterior view of the left shoulder with the lesion being mobilized.

passive restraints, such as the concavity-compression mechanism discussed earlier, are also lost.

Detachment of the anterior-inferior labrum and capsule from the glenoid has been shown to nearly double anterior translation. Performance of Bankart repair, repairing the anterior IGHL and labrum back to the glenoid, restores glenohumeral stability. Plastic deformation of the capsule is a fundamental component of anterior instability. This is an important concept in treatment of anterior instability, because in addition to repair of the glenoid labrum, a capsular plication must be performed.

There is evidence to suggest age plays a role in the type of pathology seen with anterior dislocations. IGHL detachment tends to occur in young shoulders, and the capsular ligaments tend to tear in the older ones. Avulsion of the anterior glenoid labrum has been found in 100% of young patients and 75% of those older than 50. Associated fractures, tears of the rotator cuff, and capsular injuries are more common in those patients more than 50 years of age. Literature states a 30% incidence of rotator cuff tears in patients greater than 40 years old, increasing to 80% in patients greater than 60 years old with associated anterior dislocation.

A differentiation has been made between the Bankart lesion and an anterior labral ligamentous periosteal sleeve avulsion lesion (ALPSA) (Fig. 17-3). In both acute and chronic anterior dislocations, the anterior scapular periosteum does not rupture as in a Bankart lesion, but the anterior IGHL, labrum, and the anterior scapular periosteum are stripped and displaced in a sleeve-type fashion medially on the glenoid neck. This is an important diagnostic variant to recognize because in a chronic situation, a cursory inspection of the anterior-inferior quadrant of the glenoid may not reveal evidence of trauma. However, closer inspection more medially will show a large, medially displaced scarred labrum on the anterior portion of the glenoid neck.

Superior Labrum Extension

An arthroscopic shoulder examination frequently leads to observations of additional lesions associated with anterior instability. Occasionally, the injury may extend inferiorly into the capsule or the axillary pouch (Fig. 17-4A). Injuries may also extend superiorly into the attachment of the biceps tendon, producing a concomitant superior labrum anterior-posterior (SLAP) lesion (Fig. 17-4B). This lesion is generally observed when the dislocation involves an extreme type of trauma.

In a variation of the anterior-superior labrum lesion, the anterior supraspinatus can have partial or complete tears resulting in various amounts of instability. This has been called the superior labrum, anterior cuff (SLAC) lesion. This can be caused by both acute and chronic trauma.

Humeral Avulsion of Glenohumeral Ligament Lesions

A third type of lesion that can be observed is a lateral detachment of the IGHL from the humeral neck. This was subsequently described as a humeral avulsion of glenohumeral ligament (HAGL) lesion (Fig. 17-5). Continued forced ab-

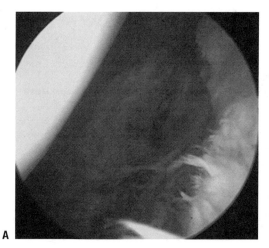
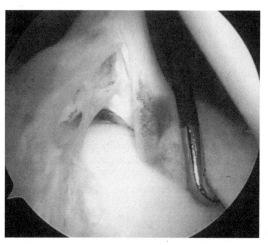

A   B

Figure 17-4 **A:** Arthroscopic capsular repair. **B:** Sitting position, left shoulder, viewed from posterior. Arthroscopic SLAP lesion, type IV.

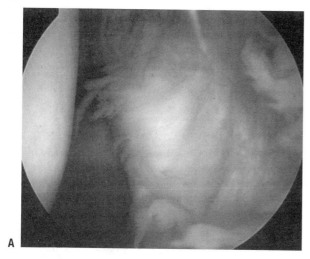
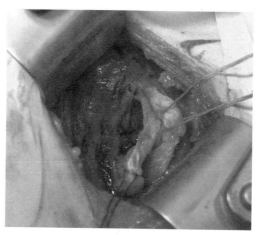

Figure 17-5 **A:** Arthroscopic view of a humeral avulsion glenohumeral ligament lesion (HAGL), sitting position, posterior left shoulder. The subscapularis muscle is seen as a shadowed area in the background. **B:** Open example of HAGL lesion, right shoulder. The subscapularis is tagged with a suture to the right. The HAGL lesion is tagged with sutures inferiorly.

duction (i.e., a force started in abduction of 90 to 105 degrees) supplemented by impaction tears the capsule from the neck of the humerus. Both open and arthroscopic repair techniques have been described. In arthroscopic repair, a standard anterior-inferior portal is made, and the bone at the anterior-inferior aspect of the humeral neck is burred through this portal. An anterior-lateral portal is created 2 cm lateral and 2 cm inferior to the coracoid process. A suture hook is used to place monofilament absorbable suture through the capsule, and these are tied through the anterior-lateral portal over the subscapularis tendon. Although relatively rare, this lesion must be sought on any anterior instability arthroscopic examination. HAGL lesions have also been seen after acute anterior dislocations.

Traumatic Bone Deficiency

Fractures or various bony deficiencies can exist that involve both the glenoid and humeral surfaces (Fig. 17-6). The

anatomy of the glenoid and proximal humerus is consistent. The articular surface of the proximal humerus is similar to that of a sphere. It is composed of cartilage and subchondral and trabecular bone that is relatively soft, even in young athletes. The glenoid has a consistent morphology as well. It is pear-shaped with the inferior portion approximating that of a true circle. The average superior/inferior glenoid diameter range is 30.4 to 42.6 mm in males and 29.4 to 37.0 mm in females. Bony lesions of the glenoid or humeral head place greater demand on the integrity of soft-tissue repairs and have been shown to cause recurrent anterior instability of the shoulder.

Humeral Bone Deficiencies. The Hill-Sachs lesion is found on the humerus and is an impression fracture caused by the humeral head being dislocated anteriorly and impacting on the anterior glenoid. This is generally located at the posterior-superior portion of the humeral head. An "engaging" Hill-Sachs lesion, which catches and locks the humeral head in a functional position of abduction and external rotation, has also been reported. The long axis of the Hill-Sachs lesion is parallel to the glenoid and engages its anterior corner. A nonengaging Hill-Sachs lesion is when the impression fracture from the anterior dislocation catches and locks the humeral head with the arm in a nonfunctional position (i.e., shoulder abduction of less than 70 degrees). The nonengaging Hill-Sachs lesion passes diagonally across the anterior glenoid with external rotation so there is continual contact between the articular surfaces. These shoulders are reasonable candidates for arthroscopic Bankart repair. It is important to realize, however, that the Hill-Sachs lesion is created by the position of the arm when the dislocation occurs. A Hill-Sachs lesion that develops with the arm at the side with some extension of the shoulder will be located more vertically and superiorly than the lesion that occurs with the shoulder abducted and externally rotated. The Hill-Sachs lesion that develops with the arm at the side is generally a nonengaging lesion.

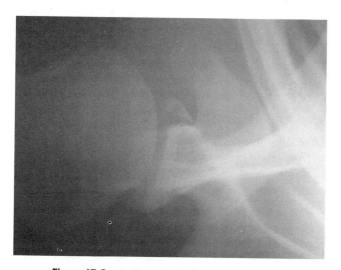

Figure 17-6 Radiograph of a bony Bankart lesion.

There are three ways of addressing the engaging Hill-Sachs lesion. The first is an open capsular shift procedure that restricts external rotation, thus not allowing the lesion to engage. The second approach, which is reserved for large defects of the humeral head, is filling the impression fracture with a size-matched humeral osteoarticular allograft. The third is a proximal rotational humeral osteotomy that internally rotates the articular surface of the humerus and effectively prevents the impression fracture from engaging the glenoid rim.

Glenoid Bone Deficiencies. Two types of fractures occur involving the anterior-inferior glenoid: the impression fracture or the avulsion fracture. The compression Bankart lesion is secondary to compression of the anterior-inferior bony articulation of the glenoid by the humeral head. Repeated episodes of instability create the "inverted pear" lesion, as well as a typical bony Bankart. Investigators in the past have recommended a coracoid transfer if the glenoid rim fracture comprised 25% of the anterior-posterior diameter of the glenoid. Burkhart et al. (2002) described the containment of the humeral head by the glenoid as a result of two geometric variables: (a) the deepening effect of a wire glenoid due to the longer arc of its concave surface and (b) the arc length of the glenoid itself. They caution that if the bony fragment is excised or if there is an inverted pear-shaped glenoid, arthroscopic techniques without a bone augmentation procedure may be predisposed to failure (Fig. 17-7).

Evidence of a bony glenoid lesion can be seen by placing the arthroscope in the anterior-superior portal, looking inferiorly at the glenoid. The bare spot of the glenoid is roughly in the center of the glenoid and with a calibrated probe, the distance from the anterior rim of the glenoid to the bare spot is measured, as well as the distance from the bare spot to the posterior glenoid rim. A bone augmentation procedure is indicated when there is a 25% reduction in the length from the anterior glenoid to the bare spot compared with the posterior glenoid to the bare spot.

Glenoid Retroversion and Hypoplasia. Increased glenoid retroversion and glenoid hypoplasia have been implicated in posterior or multidirectional instability.

Etiology and Epidemiology

Studies have shown the overall incidence of traumatic shoulder instability in the general population to be approximately 1.7%. After an anterior shoulder dislocation, the risk of recurrent shoulder instability has been related to the following factors:

- *Age at primary dislocation*—There is a significantly higher rate of recurrent anterior shoulder instability in younger patients with acute traumatic anterior shoulder dislocations. The majority of the recurrent instability episodes occur in the first 2 years after the primary incident.
- *Number of anterior shoulder instability recurrences*, with a positive correlation between a higher number of recurrences and an increased risk of instability.
- *Future athletic participation*—For first-time contact sport athletes, an 80% recurrence rate was seen with conservative treatment and return to contact sport. On the other hand, there was a 16% recurrence rate with arthroscopic treatment of the Bankart lesion and return to contact sport.
- *Bone loss* (glenoid or Hill-Sachs lesion).

The risk of recurrent anterior shoulder dislocation has not been found to be related to the type and duration of immobilization. One long-term (10-year follow-up) study on immobilization outcomes after anterior shoulder dislocations found no effect on recurrence rates related to the length of immobilization. Of the primary anterior shoulder dislocators, 50% had a recurrent dislocation at 10 years out. Of the recurrent dislocators, 50% had surgery, and of those with surgery, 50% were stable at 10-year follow-up. Interestingly, degenerative joint disease was found in both surgical and nonsurgical candidates, with 11% of the patients who underwent surgery having mild secondary degenerative joint disease at the 10-year follow-up.

DIAGNOSIS

Physical Examination and History

Clinical Features
- A comprehensive evaluation of anterior shoulder instability should start with a focused but detailed history of the instability episode.
- The onset, circumstances, direction of dislocation, frequency of dislocations/subluxations, and magnitude of the instability episodes should be delineated.
- The age of the patient is important. As a general guideline, patients less than 35 years old with shoulder pain often have an instability diagnosis, whereas patients

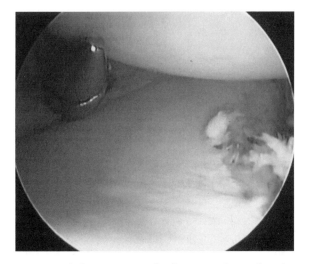

Figure 17-7 Arthroscopic example of an inverted pear-shaped glenoid. Left shoulder, anterior-superior viewing portal, lateral posterior. Note the bony deficiencies of the anterior-inferior glenoid to the right.

older than 35 years usually suffer from some type of impingement diagnosis.

- The patient should be asked about the location of the shoulder pain because this will give clues with regard to the type of pathology present.
  - Pain at the anterior-lateral deltoid may represent supraspinatus tendon injury.
  - Pain at the posterior joint line may represent injury to the posterior labrum or infraspinatus pathology.
  - Anterior joint line pain or pain over the coracoid points to a subscapularis tendon injury, a biceps tendon injury, or a capsulolabral tear.
  - Pain can also be referred from other sites in the body and be perceived as shoulder pain. Referred areas of pain to the shoulder that should be remembered include cervical radiculopathy, cardiac ischemia or pericarditis, thoracic outlet syndrome, and bone or soft-tissue tumors.
- A thorough review of symptoms may reveal other medical conditions that manifest as shoulder pathology.
  - Patients with diabetes mellitus have an increased risk of frozen shoulder and infection.
  - Renal failure predisposes to avascular necrosis.
  - A significant alcohol or seizure history may point to a posterior shoulder dislocation.
- Before physical examination, a differential diagnosis of shoulder pathology should be formulated. The differential diagnosis of traumatic injury to the shoulder can be divided into three categories:
  - Osseous lesions include clavicle fractures, proximal humerus fractures, fracture dislocations of the greater tuberosity, and scapular fractures (glenoid, coracoid, and acromial).
  - Soft-tissue lesions include contusions of the deltoid or trapezius muscles (i.e., myositis ossificans), acromioclavicular joint sprain, glenohumeral dislocations, and traumatic rotator cuff tears (rare in athletes <35 years old).
  - Nerve lesions include injury to the axillary nerve, suprascapular nerve traction injury, and long thoracic nerve injury. The axillary nerve has been found to be injured in approximately 9% to 18% of anterior shoulder dislocations. The sensation is usually preserved, and motor weakness must be sought for the diagnosis. Injury to the long thoracic nerve causes scapular winging from the weakened serratus anterior muscle.
- The physical examination of the shoulder should follow a systematic approach to avoid missing concurrent pathology.
- The shoulder should be inspected for muscular atrophy or asymmetry from a posterior viewpoint. For example, atrophy of the infraspinatus fossa may be secondary to disuse or suprascapular neuropathy.
- The cervical spine should be palpated posteriorly for bony tenderness along the spinous processes.
  - Cervical range of motion should be noted, and a neurovascular examination of the upper extremities should be performed. Reflexes and long-tract signs should be evaluated when necessary.
  - Spurling's test should be checked to rule out referred shoulder pain from cervical spinal nerve impingement.
- All bony prominences about the shoulder should be palpated.
  - Coracoid or acromioclavicular joint tenderness should be noted in the initial physical examination.
  - The soft tissues about the shoulder should be palpated for tenderness.
  - Specific locations of pathology include pain over the bicipital groove anteriorly (i.e., biceps tendon pathology) and pain at the greater tuberosity area.
- Overall ligamentous laxity should be sought in patients with shoulder instability complaints.
  - Thumb or finger hyperextension can be tested, and a sulcus sign might be seen.
  - Patients with ligamentous laxity have an increased risk of multidirectional instability.
- Active and passive range of motion in all scapular planes (forward flexion, extension, abduction, external rotation with the arm at the side and in 90 degrees of abduction, and internal rotation up the back and with the arm in 90 degrees of abduction) should be recorded.
  - Increased external rotation in the dominant shoulder may be a normal finding.
  - Loss of internal rotation may be secondary to a contracture of the posterior capsule/cuff.
- Strength testing should include the supraspinatus (empty beer can sign), infraspinatus (resisted external rotation with the arm at the side), subscapularis (lift-off test), trapezius/rhomboids (shoulder shrug), deltoid (resisted abduction with arm at the side), and the serratus anterior (check for scapular winging).
- One of the most important tests for documentation of anterior shoulder instability is the apprehension and relocation test (see Fig. 15-15 in Chapter 15).
  - The patient is told to lie supine with the affected arm and shoulder hanging off the edge of the examining table. The arm is brought into 90 degrees of abduction and slowly externally rotated.
    - With a positive test, the patient will experience pain or the feeling that the shoulder is about to dislocate.
  - In the second part of the examination, the relocation test (see Fig. 15-16 in Chapter 15), the examiner applies an anterior force to the proximal humerus (i.e., in an attempt to center the humeral head).
    - With a positive relocation test, the patient either has a decrease in the anterior shoulder pain or a decrease in the sense that the arm is about to dislocate.
- Anterior to posterior translation of the humerus should also be documented using the load and shift test (see Fig. 15-20 in Chapter 15).
  - In the same position as the apprehension test (supine with affected shoulder hanging off the side of the exam table), the shoulder is abducted to 70 degrees, forward flexed to 45 to 50 degrees, and axially loaded so that a compressive force is applied across the glenohumeral joint. The humeral head is then

TABLE 17-1 GRADING SYSTEM FOR SHOULDER TRANSLATION

Grade	Description
1+	Increased translation compared with the contralateral shoulder but no subluxation over the labrum is felt
2+	Humeral head subluxes over the glenoid rim but spontaneously returns to the reduced position
3+	Humeral head locks over the glenoid rim

(Adapted from Altchek DW, Warren RF, Wickiewicz TL, et al. Arthroscopic labral debridement: a three-year follow-up study. Am J Sports Med 1992;20:702–706.)

grasped anteriorly and posteriorly by the examiner between the index and thumb, and the humeral head is translated anteriorly and posteriorly. The amount of translation is recorded and a grade assigned (Table 17-1).

- Patients with a grade 2+ or 3+ anterior translation, compared with the contralateral normal extremity, are good candidates for arthroscopic stabilization.

Posterior instability of the shoulder should be examined by forward flexing the arm to 90 degrees, with approximately 20 to 30 degrees of adduction. By applying a posteriorly directed force to the arm, the posterior labrum and capsule are stressed.

- Any pain with this maneuver alerts the surgeon to posterior capsular pathology.

With any examination for instability, rotator interval lesions must be sought. The sulcus sign tests for rotator interval pathology (see Fig. 15-17 in Chapter 17).

- With the patient in the seated or standing position and the arm hanging at the side, a downward force is applied to the arm. The amount of inferior translation that occurs is documented in comparison with the contralateral extremity. The grading system is given in Table 17-2.
  - The sulcus sign should decrease with external rotation of the arm.
  - If there is a sulcus sign at neutral rotation that persists in external rotation or if there is a >2+ sulcus with 2+ to 3+ anterior shoulder transla-

TABLE 17-2 GRADING OF THE SULCUS SIGN

Grade	Inferior Translation (cm)
1+	≤1
2+	1–2
3+	>2

(Adapted from Neer CS, Foster CR. Inferior capsular shift for involuntary and multidirectional instability of the shoulder. J Bone Joint Surg Am 1980;62:897–908.)

tion on the load and shift test, there is an increased risk of a large rotator interval lesion.

- The biceps anchor should also be examined for a SLAP tear. This can be evaluated with O'Brien's test (see Fig. 15-21 in Chapter 15).
  - A positive test reproduces the shoulder pain with resistance of a downward force when the arm is forward flexed to 90 degrees, adducted, and internally rotated. The pain is reduced with resistance to a downward force with the arm forward flexed to 90 degrees, adducted, and externally rotated.
  - A false-positive test may occur, however, with acromioclavicular joint pathology because of the amount of adduction that the arm is placed into for the test.

Radiologic Examination

Radiographs

- Radiographic evaluation is required in the assessment of shoulder instability. Shoulder anatomy, as well as any fractures associated with the dislocations, is critical to document before treatment and may significantly change the overall treatment plan.
- A standard anterior-posterior view of the arm in slight internal rotation is used to identify a fracture of the greater tuberosity.
- A true scapular anterior-posterior radiograph permits evaluation of a glenoid fossa fracture, if present.
- The West Point axillary view is used to assess bony avulsions of the attachment of the IGHL, bony Bankart lesions, or anterior-inferior glenoid deficiency.
- The Hill-Sachs lesion can be quantified and evaluated by examining the Stryker notch view.

Computed Tomography Scan

- A computed tomography (CT) scan can be an accurate means of determining glenoid version and overall glenoid morphology. It has the ability to reconstruct the anatomy of the glenoid in three dimensions and it can also isolate the glenoid for viewing by subtracting the humerus from the image.
- The shape of the articular surface can aid the surgeon in preoperative planning.
- Substantial bone loss may be a contraindication to arthroscopic stabilization.

Magnetic Resonance Imaging.

- Magnetic resonance imaging (MRI) is used for assessment of associated pathology.
- Contrast enhancement improves the diagnostic ability to detect labral tears (both superior and anterior-inferior), rotator cuff tears (both partial and full thickness), and articular cartilage lesions.
- In identification of HAGL lesions, MRI in the midsagittal coronal oblique plane shows the detachment of the inferior glenoid labrum (IGL) and that the axillary pouch is converted from a full distended U-shaped structure to a J-shaped structure, as the IGL drops inferiorly (Fig. 17-8).

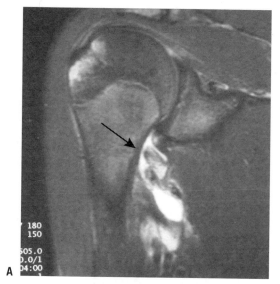
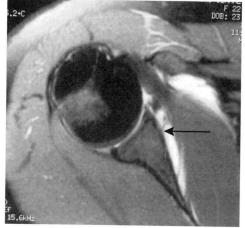

Figure 17-8   A: MRI example of the HAGL lesion. B: MRI example of a Bankart lesion.

- The appearance of a HAGL lesion with MRI has been described as an avulsion fracture from the neocortex in the humeral neck. A thin radiolucency is observed inferior to the anatomic neck of the humerus, and once again the fluid-filled distended U-shaped axillary pouch is converted into a J-shaped structure by the extravasation of contrast material. The presence of this lesion may also be a relative contraindication to an arthroscopic shoulder stabilization procedure.
- Algorithm 17-1 summarizes the diagnostic workup of shoulder instability.

TREATMENT

Surgical Treatment

Decision Making

The controversy surrounding open versus arthroscopic techniques for anterior labral stabilization is almost 20 years old. Both open and arthroscopic procedures have involved the use of bone tunnels, staples, transglenoid sutures, rivets, bioabsorbable tacks, and suture anchors. Initial studies reported recurrence rates of arthroscopic techniques from 0% to 44%. Earlier arthroscopic techniques with higher failure rates were attempted on many types of instability patterns and used techniques that did not follow the principals of established open methods.

The major advantage of arthroscopic repair for anterior shoulder instability is the ability to accurately identify and treat the specific pathoanatomy found in the glenohumeral joint. Other advantages of arthroscopic repair include less iatrogenic damage to normal tissues (subscapularis), reduced postoperative pain, and improved cosmesis. Easier functional recovery and improved range of motion than with the open repair method have also been reported. Decision making for arthroscopic versus open techniques can be variable, depending on the surgeon's experience. Ideal indications for arthroscopic stabilization include a traumatic uni-

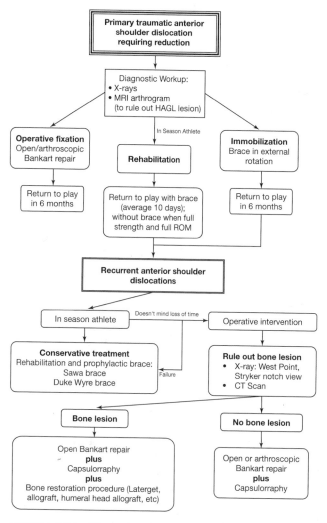

Algorithm 17-1   Diagnosis and management of anterior instability of the shoulder.

directional anterior shoulder dislocation with a Bankart lesion, a first-time dislocator, minimal sulcus sign, no generalized laxity, thick robust ligaments, minimal plastic capsular deformation, and an exam under anesthesia revealing a grade 2+ to 3+ pure anterior translation deformity.

Contraindications to arthroscopic repair include a Hill-Sachs lesion involving greater than 20% to 30% of the articular surface that engages the glenoid rim with the arm in a position of abduction and external rotation, a bony abnormality such as an "inverted pair" glenoid, or a glenoid rim defect >25% of the articular surface. A multiple dislocator (i.e., greater than 5 dislocations or subluxations) is a relative contraindication to arthroscopic repair. Some surgeons still advocate an open procedure in high-demand athletes. An argument can be made that as arthroscopic techniques continue to improve and closely mimic what is done in open procedures, arthroscopic recurrence rates will equal or surpass those of open procedures.

Surgical Technique

A surgical technique is described that is based on the idea of a 180-degree repair (Fig. 17-9). This involves an inferior capsular plication, an anterior shift, a Bankart lesion repair with suture anchors, and a rotator interval closure. In operative treatment of an acute anterior dislocation within 3 weeks, only the Bankart lesion or the anterior-inferior glenoid labrum tear is repaired with suture anchors. The inferior capsular plication and rotator interval closure are reserved for the late repair of a recurrent dislocator.

In the late repair (greater than 3 weeks after the acute dislocation), capsular imbrication and rotator interval closure will be required, because it is thought that there is capsular plastic deformation associated with the repetitive microtrauma of subluxation. With any type of capsular failure, there is a significant amount of elongation, suggesting that plastic deformation of the capsule has occurred. Therefore, some type of capsular shortening is required to return the capsule to its anatomic configuration.

Patient Position and Portal Placement

- The beach chair or lateral decubitus position can be used for instability surgery.
  - The beach chair position offers the advantage of being able to convert to an open procedure easily. When the beach chair position is used, a sterile arm holder is helpful for both holding a desired arm position and for applying a distraction force to the arm.
  - For the lateral decubitus position, a three-point distraction device is used that allows both longitudinal and vertical traction and enables the humeral head to be lifted reproducibly from the glenoid (Fig. 17-10). A beanbag is used to stabilize the patient, with a hip-holder also used just below the scapula posteriorly to stabilize the beanbag, in case air is accidentally liberated. The patient is positioned in a 30-degree backward tilt, which places the glenoid in a parallel orientation to the floor.
- In most cases, general endotracheal intubation is used for anesthesia with an interscalene block for pain control.
  - The beach chair position is amenable only to an interscalene block for the procedure and, as a result of the uncomfortable nature of the lateral position,

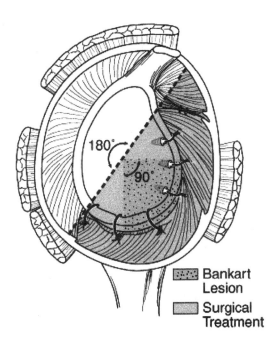

Figure 17-9   Illustration of a surgical reconstruction with an 180-degree arthroscopic repair with three inferior plication sutures, three anchors repairing the labrum, and a rotator interval closure.

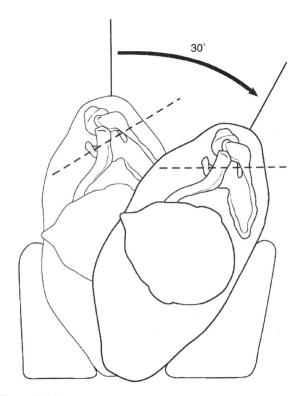

Figure 17-10   Positioning of the patient with the lateral traction device and a 30-degree posterior tilt.

we advocate general anesthesia with or without the regional block.

- Preoperative antibiotics are administered intravenously before skin incision.

- An examination under anesthesia of both shoulders in the supine position is performed documenting forward elevation, external and internal rotation with the arm at the side, as well as external and internal rotation with the arm abducted to 90 degrees.
    - The examination under anesthesia is used to confirm and add further information and/or other pathology that may be present, *not* to make the diagnosis.
    - An anterior load and shift, a posterior "jerk" test, and a sulcus test are performed to assess instability. When performing the load and shift test, care should be taken to compare both shoulders for the amount of humeral head translation.
    - The amount of translation should be noted for each arm position with respect to the degree of humeral rotation and the position of the arm in relation to the plane of the scapula. Arm rotation and position will influence the degree of translation because of the changes that they have on ligament length.

- A standard posterior portal should be placed slightly more laterally than the joint line. If the portal is placed medial to the joint line, this will require the surgeon to lever the arthroscope against the glenoid, making the stabilization procedure quite difficult.
    - An 8- to 10-mm incision is made, and the blunt arthroscope sheath and trocar are inserted atraumatically into the space between the glenoid rim and humeral head.

- The anterior series of portals are then made using spinal needles for localization.
    - The first anterior portal made is superior and lateral in the rotator interval, as high in the anterior-superior quadrant of the shoulder as possible, while still allowing the cannula to be placed anterior to the biceps tendon. Medial placement of the cannula will compromise access to the glenoid. Care should be taken to prevent placement of the cannula posterior to the biceps tendon to avoid entrapment of the tendon with sutures. In general, a 7 mm × 7 cm cannula, smooth or ridged, is placed for suture shuttling.
    - The second portal is the anterior-inferior portal; because of the instruments used through this portal, it is usually an 8.25 mm × 7 cm cannula. Two different portal types can be made.
        - The first type is a transsubscapular portal at the 5 o'clock position. Although this allows accurate and easy anterior-inferior anchor placement, it can be difficult to place because it is going through subscapularis tendon. In this case, to accomplish this as atraumatically as possible, a pointed switching stick is used to pierce the subscapularis tendon first, followed by a dilator system.
        - The second type of anterior-inferior portal is made at the superior rolled edge of the subscapularis and angled inferiorly. Once again, this is also made with spinal needle localization but avoids the trauma of going through the subscapularis tendon. Potential difficulties with this portal placement involve inferior anchor placement because the angle for placing the anchor is more oblique. To overcome this, a stab incision can be made at the 5 o'clock position and the anchor placed through the subscapularis tendon without a cannula. The sutures from the anchor are then shuttled through the anterior-inferior cannula located above the rolled edge of the subscapularis.

    - The final portal that is made is the 7 o'clock portal. This is a posterior-inferior portal, allowing inferior capsular plication. This portal is made roughly 2 cm lateral and 1 cm inferior to the standard posterior portal. An 18-gauge spinal needle is used under direct visualization to assess the position, and an 8.25 mm × 9 cm cannula is then placed. This portal allows a very accurate inferior capsular plication under direct visualization, because the arthroscope is kept in the posterior portal, and suture shuttling devices are used and placed through the large 7 o'clock cannula (Fig. 17-11).

- Care should be exercised in creating portals and in evaluating pump pressure.
    - Shoulder overdistention is compounded by improper portal development and a lengthy procedure.
    - It is important always to establish accurate and small portals, to use cannulas at all times to create a seal in the glenohumeral joint, and to monitor the amount of fluid pressure to decrease the amount of fluid extravasation. An ideal pressure to perform arthroscopic stabilization has not been reported. However, analysis and evaluation of pressure and

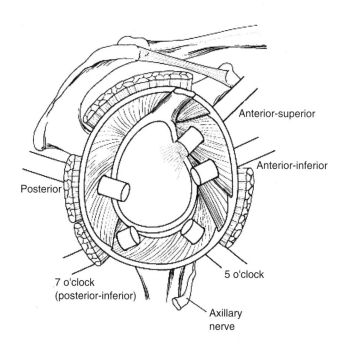

Figure 17-11 Portals that can be used for the "180-degree" repair technique.

shoulder distension as the procedure progresses are critical.

Preparation

- Preparation of the capsule before plication has been advocated to "excite the synoviocytes." This has not been scientifically proven but makes logical sense and can be accomplished with either a shaver or a hand-held burr from the anterior or poster inferior (7 o'clock position) portals.
- Preparation of the glenoid bed for the labrum is also critical. A sharp elevator combined with an arthroscopic shaver or tissue ablation device is used to dissect and liberate the entire labrum, IGHL, and periosteum of the glenoid neck off until the subscapularis muscle is seen through this interval.
- The anterior-inferior labrum should be released so that it "floats" to the glenoid rim.
- With the arthroscope in the posterior portal, the soft tissue and cortical surface of the anterior glenoid rim can be removed using a small burr to create a bleeding surface on the anterior glenoid neck.
- To evaluate this preparation of the glenoid bed, the arthroscope is placed in the anterior-superior or anterior-inferior portal, allowing excellent visualization of the labral complex and bone preparation (Fig. 17-12).

Inferior Plication

- Inferior plication is accomplished by imbricating the axillary pouch. As previously stated, capsular plication (capsulorraphy) is necessary due to the irreversible plastic deformation of the capsule that occurs during an anterior dislocation.
- Arthroscopically, the capsulorraphy can be completed with suture, suture anchors, or thermal energy.
- There are multiple methods for capsulorraphy. The pinch-tuck method involves a suture-passing device in a

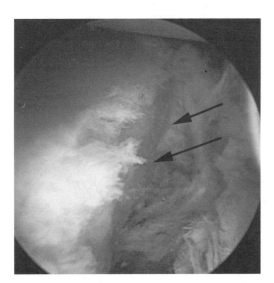

Figure 17-12 Arthroscopic example of anterior glenoid preparation, left shoulder, lateral position, viewed from the anterior-superior portal.

"corkscrew configuration" that can penetrate the tissue approximately 1 cm away from the labrum and then penetrate the labrum itself (Fig. 17-13). When this knot is tied, it creates a blind pouch that scars in. If the labrum is friable or an adequate bite cannot be secured, a suture anchor can be placed into the labrum. The suture can then be shuttled through the inferior capsule and tied. Two to three of these inferior capsular plication sutures are then placed from the posterior-inferior to the anterior-inferior position (positions 8, 7, and 6 o'clock, respectively, on a right shoulder). An accessory posterior portal can be used (7 o'clock portal) or the camera can be changed to the anterior-superior portal and a cannula placed in the posterior portal.

- Suture management at this stage is important.
  - The surgeon can tie each individual suture sequentially after being placed, which makes suture management more straightforward, but this can run the risk of "closing yourself out."
  - The second method for suture management involves shuttling the suture out the anterior cannula, removing the cannula, and replacing it, thus removing the suture pair from within and placing the suture pair on the outside of the cannula. All pairs can then be shuttled back into the joint at the end of throwing all of the plication stitches for tying.
- Once two or three inferior capsular plication sutures are made, attention is turned to the anterior-inferior Bankart lesion.

Bankart Repair with Suture Anchors

- Repair of the Bankart lesion is the critical step in this procedure.
- The suture anchor repair is similar to the open repair technique and is extremely versatile and reproducible.
- There are three variations of this technique: the suture-first method, the anchor-first method, and the Knotless Suture Anchor (Mitek, Inc., Norwood, MA) method. Clinically, there have been no reported differences between any of these techniques in the literature, and their use is based on surgeon preference.
- The anchors themselves can be either metal or bioabsorbable. There are no differences reported clinically on the basis of the material of the anchor.
  - We recommend bioabsorbable anchors because most instability patients are young, and we attempt to avoid the theoretical possibility of migration.
- Proper anchor placement is the most critical step, and no material can help an improperly placed anchor.

Anchor-first Technique

- The anchor-first technique involves placing an anchor through the anterior-inferior cannula first and then shuttling the suture limb second (Fig. 17-14). It is important to note at this time the position of the anterior-inferior cannula and the position in which the anchor should be placed into the glenoid. There are times when the position of the cannula is appropriate for suture shuttling but not for placement of the anchor. In this case, a percutaneous approach can be used to insert an anchor into the glenoid at the 5:30 position.

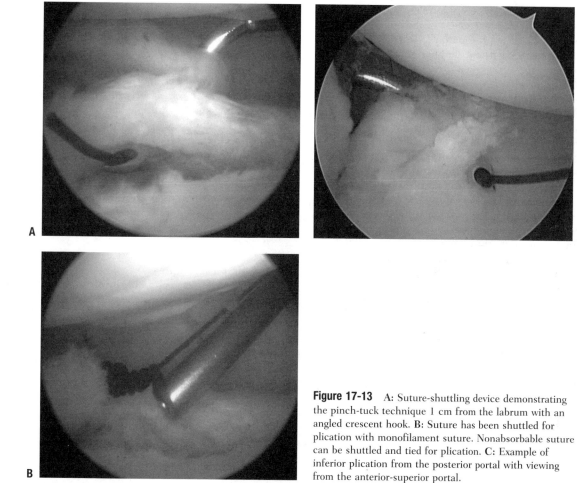

Figure 17-13 **A:** Suture-shuttling device demonstrating the pinch-tuck technique 1 cm from the labrum with an angled crescent hook. **B:** Suture has been shuttled for plication with monofilament suture. Nonabsorbable suture can be shuttled and tied for plication. **C:** Example of inferior plication from the posterior portal with viewing from the anterior-superior portal.

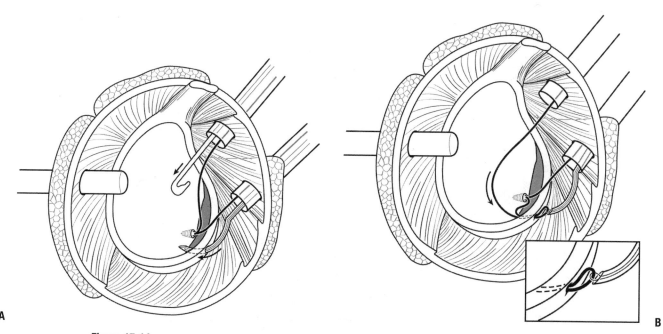

Figure 17-14 **A:** Example of an anchor first shuttling technique with a tissue penetrator inferior to the anchor. **B:** Nonabsorbable suture shuttled through the inferior labrum and inferior glenohumeral ligament complex.

■ The advantage of this technique is a more appropriate perpendicular placement of the anchor into the glenoid face at approximately 2 to 3 mm over the articular service without "bubbling" or causing articular damage.

■ After the anchor has been successfully inserted, one of the suture limbs is passed out of the anterior-superior cannula. This limb, if using a metal anchor or an anchor with a fixed eyelet, is the limb on the tissue side of the suture. The eyelet should be perpendicular to the labrum. A tissue penetrator or suture shuttling device is used to place a passing suture into the tissue inferior to the anchor. The end of the suture is then grasped and pulled out the anterior-superior cannula. A small square knot is tied in the passing suture, serving as a dilating knot. This is followed by tying the nonabsorbable braided suture to the monofilament suture line further distal and pulling the passing stitch through the anterior-inferior cannula, hence shuttling the suture through labrum, inferior-glenoid ligament, and scapular–periosteal complex.

■ On tightening this suture with proper arthroscopic knot-tying techniques, a shift of tissue from inferior to superior should be observed. If the tissue bite was not placed inferior enough to the anchor, then this step should be repeated before continuing the operation. To tie the knot, the knot pusher is placed on the suture limb that is on the tissue side. This will be the post. A sliding or nonsliding (multiple half hitches) knot can be tied at this time. It has been determined that after placement of a sliding knot or multiple half hitches that three alternating half hitches, while switching the post, are the most secure final fixation. The knot should end up on the tissue side so that the labrum can create a bumper effect. The next two or three anchors are then placed approximately 5 to 7 mm apart from each other in the same the fashion as previously described. On completion of the procedure, a "bumper" should be observed at the anterior-inferior glenoid between the 3 and 6 o'clock positions.

Suture-first Technique

■ The suture-first technique involves placing a passing suture initially to ensure adequate soft tissue shift, followed by placement of the anchor (Fig. 17-15). A suture-passing device is placed through the anterior-

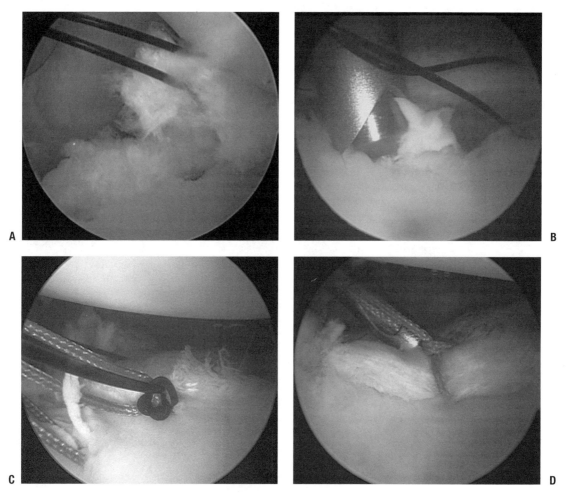

Figure 17-15   A: Arthroscopic view of suture-first technique. Zero PDS placed inferiorly and traction applied. B: Anchor placement more cephalic to suture, so that with eventual knot tying, the labrum and capsule are shifted superiorly. C: Nonabsorbable suture being shuttled with zero PDS. D: Knot-tying.

inferior cannula. The capsular tissue is imbricated inferior to what would be the 5 o'clock anchor position, thus enabling the tissue from anterior-inferior glenohumeral ligament to be shifted superiorly. The passing suture is passed through the tissue and shuttled through the anterior-superior portal. The suture-passing device is removed, and the suture limb that is in the anterior-inferior portal is switched to the anterior-superior portal. Tension is placed on this suture to observe the amount of shift that can be accomplished by placement of the anchor at the appropriate position.

■ If it is determined that this suture is not inferior enough, a second suture can be placed.

■ When an appropriate amount of tissue tension is established, the anchor is placed through the anterior-inferior portal and onto the glenoid rim. As was described previously, once the anchor is placed, the two limbs of the suture are separated—one through the anterior-superior cannula and the other limb is shuttled through the tissue.

■ The same steps are repeated two or three times, depending on the repair quality and amount of injury (Fig. 17-16).

Extension of the Anterior-inferior Labrum Tear into the Superior Labrum

■ If the labral tear extends from the anterior-inferior glenoid up into the superior labrum, the same anterior cannula can be used to continue placing suture anchors.

■ We recommend two or three suture anchors for superior labrum tears, with one placed in front of the biceps tendon anchor and one or two suture anchors placed behind the biceps tendon anchor, depending on the amount of biceps instability.

■ The anchor placed in front of the biceps tendon anchor is guided through the anterior-superior cannula. The one or two anchors placed posterior to the biceps anchor can be placed percutaneously via the "Port of Wilming-

ton." This portal is 1 cm lateral and 1 cm anterior to the posterior-lateral corner of the acromion, through the musculotendinous junction of the rotator cuff.

The Rotator Interval

■ The rotator interval is an important anatomic region with respect to anterior shoulder stability. This anatomic region is defined as the articular capsule bounded superiorly by the anterior portion of the supraspinatus tendon, inferiorly by the superior portion of the subscapularis tendon, medially by the base of the coracoid process, and laterally by the long head of the biceps tendon. The capsular tissue is reinforced by the coracohumeral ligament (CHL) and the superior glenohumeral ligament (SGHL).

■ The rotator interval is of variable size and is present in the fetus and in the adult. Sectioning the rotator interval in cadaveric specimens has resulted in increased glenohumeral translation in all planes tested. Imbrication of rotator interval lesions results in decreased posterior and inferior glenohumeral translation when compared with the intact state. Repair of the rotator interval is a critical factor in shoulders treated arthroscopically for anterior-inferior glenohumeral instability and may contribute to improved clinical outcomes

■ Many authors have reported techniques on closing the rotator interval, but there is no literature comparing what type of suture material will ensure success. One technique for rotator interval closure involves removing the anterior-inferior cannula and placing all instrumentation through the anterior-superior cannula. The medial glenohumeral ligament and/or a small portion of the subscapularis tendon is pierced with either a spinal needle or suture shuttling device, and a monofilament suture is deployed (Fig. 17-17A). The SGHL/CHL complex is pierced with a penetrator and grasps the monofilament suture (Fig. 17-17B). This tissue then can be tied through a cannula internally or externally and cut with a guillotine knot cutter (Fig. 17-17C).

■ The final repair for anterior traumatic shoulder instability with a Bankart lesion involves capsular plication, anterior-inferior labral repair, and rotator interval closure (see Fig. 17-9).

Postoperative Management

■ The first goal to postoperative success is maintenance of anterior-inferior stability.

■ The second goal is the restoration of adequate motion, specifically external rotation.

■ The third goal is a successful return to sports or physical activities of daily living in a reasonable amount of time.

■ The biological healing response of the repaired and imbricated tissue must be respected. One observation that may have led to some of the earlier arthroscopic failures for anterior instability is that because of the significant reduction in postoperative pain, these patients want to move their shoulders earlier, imparting more stress to the repair site. This early cyclic stress and motion eventually fatigues the plication stitches and causes a failure of the repair.

■ The University of Connecticut postoperative protocol

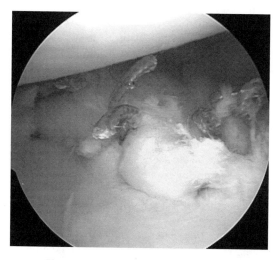

Figure 17-16   Complete Bankart repair.

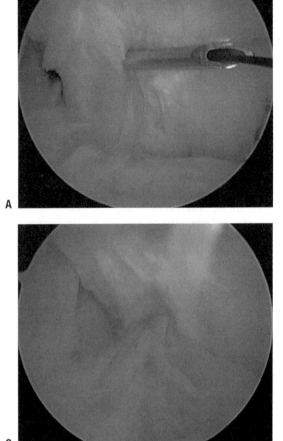

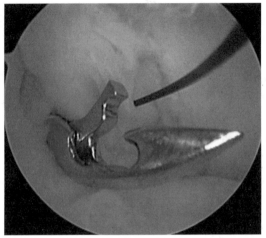

Figure 17-17   **A:** Suture shuttling device through the middle glenohumeral placing a monofilament suture into joint. **B:** Tissue penetrator through superior glenohumeral ligament and coracohumeral ligament retrieving monofilament suture. **C:** The rotator interval is closed extra-articularly.

for anterior-inferior shoulder instability treated by ar-throscopic means involves immobilization immediately postoperatively in an abduction arthrosis.

- This allows the arm to be fixed in a slight amount of external rotation. Codman exercises, combined with pendulum exercises, are started immediately. Active assisted range-of-motion exercises, external rotation (0 to 30 degrees), and forward elevation (0 to 90 degrees) are also started at this time. This regimen is maintained for the first 6 weeks.
- The use of cold therapy devices has been successful in reducing postoperative pain.
- From weeks 6 to 12, active assisted as well as active range-of-motion exercises are started with the goal of establishing full range of motion.
- No strengthening exercises or any type of repetitive exercises are started until after full range of motion has been established.
- Early resistance exercises with aggressive early post-operative rehabilitation do not appear to offer sub-stantial advantages and could compromise the re-pair.
- Strengthening is begun once there is full, painless, active range of motion. Strengthening is begun at 12 weeks, with sports-specific exercises started at 16 to 20 weeks.

- Final contact athletic training is started between 20 and 24 weeks postoperatively.
- Pagnani and Dome (2002) reported on open stabiliza-tion in American football players. Their postoperative program was quite similar to that previously described.
  - At 0 to 4 weeks, the arm is immobilized with a sling and internal rotation; double range-of-motion and pendulum exercises are begun.
  - From 4 to 8 weeks, passive and active assisted shoul-der range of motion with external rotation limited to 45 degrees is done.
  - Rotator cuff strengthening and internal and external rotation strengthening with the arm at low abduc-tion angles are begun when 140 degrees of active forward elevation is obtained.
  - From 8 to 12 weeks, deltoid isometric exercises are started with the arm in low abduction angles, as well as body blade exercises. Abduction is slowly in-creased during rotator cuff and deltoid strengthen-ing exercises. In addition, scapular stabilizer strengthening and horizontal abduction exercises are also begun.
  - From 12 to 18 weeks, restoration of terminal exter-nal rotation is achieved. Proprioceptive neuromus-cular feedback patterns are used, and plyometric ex-

ercises—as well as sports-specific motion using pulley, wand, or manual resistance—are begun.

- After 18 weeks, conventional weight training is begun, and rehabilitation is orientated toward return to sports, progressing from field drills to contact drills. An abduction harness can be used for selected football positions (linemen).
- Full-contact sports are instituted when abduction and external rotation strength are symmetrical on manual muscle testing.

Complications

- Postoperative glenohumeral noise is an inconsistent physical examination finding that occasionally plagues the postoperative course. It is caused by a knot that rubs against the humerus and glenoid with motion.
  - Normally, there is synovialization of the sutures (Fig. 17-18).

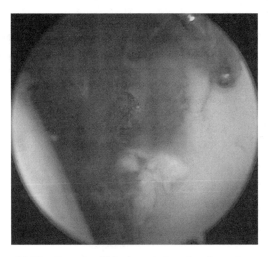

Figure 17-18　Example of labral repair 3 weeks after arthroscopic repair.

TABLE 17-3 RESULTS OF ARTHROSCOPIC BANKART REPAIR

Author	No. of Patients	Mean Follow-up (mo)	Recurrence Rate (%)	Comments
Arciero et al. (1995)	19	19	0	Repair within 10 days; Suretac device
Speer et al. (1996)	52	42	21	Seven atraumatic and two traumatic failures; Suretac device
Laurencin et al. (1996)	19	24	10	Suretac device
Segmuller et al. (1997)	31	12	3.2	Noted that recurrence rate only for pure anterior-inferior dislocation; Suretac device
Resch et al. (1997)	98	35	9	Suretac device
Karlsson et al. (1998)	82	27	10	Suretac device
Jorgensen et al. (1999)	21	36	10	No difference in Rowe or constant score between open or arthroscopic; suture anchor technique
Cole et al. (2000)	37	54	16	Recurrence secondary to contact sports or traumatic fall; Suretac device
Karlsson et al. (2001)	66	28	15	Compared open versus arthroscopic repair; Suretac device
Thal (2001)	27	29	0	No episodes of subluxation or dislocation; 74% regained full range of motion; knotless anchor fixation device
DeBerardino et al. (2001)	52	38	14	Average Rowe score 90; 5-degree loss of external rotation; Suretac device
Kim et al. (2003)	167	44	4	Average Rowe score 96%; suture anchor technique
Fabbriciani et al. (2004)	30 (in arthroscopic group)	≥24	0	No difference in Rowe scores between open and arthroscopic techniques; suture anchor technique

TABLE 17-4 RESULTS OF OPEN BANKART REPAIR

Author	No. of Patients	Mean Follow-up (mo)	Recurrence Rate (%)	Comments
Thomas et al. (1989)	37	66	3	97% good or excellent results (Rowe); open modified Bankart repair
Gill et al. (1997)	56	144	5	93% good or excellent results; average loss of external rotation was 12 degrees
Jorgensen et al. (1999)	20	36	10	See Table 17-3
Fabbriciani et al. (2004)	30 (in open group)	≥24	0	See Table 17-3

- If this does not happen, a squeak can be detected that may necessitate the removal of the knot after healing has been established.

Results

- Arthroscopic stabilization for anterior-inferior instability has evolved over the past 25 years. It is difficult to compare redislocation rates and subluxation rates with techniques used in the past. This discussion will attempt to focus on techniques that are similar to what have been described previously.
- It is important to note when evaluating the literature whether recurrences are classified as subluxations that prevent the athletes from returning to their sport versus redislocations. Our definition of recurrence is any subluxation event that causes the athlete to lose a day of practice. It is then noted if the athlete required further stabilization or if they returned to play unencumbered.
- Traumatic anterior instability treated by suture anchor reconstruction has been associated with a stabilization rate of 95% for 2 years.
- The recurrence rate after arthroscopic repair is about 15%.
- Current arthroscopic stabilization techniques use suture anchors, permanent suture, and address capsular redundancy with plication techniques. The arthroscopic technique now more closely mirrors the open method, and more recent reports demonstrate results that are comparable with the open techniques.

- The rates of recurrence (dislocation and subluxation) in at-risk collision athletes are similar with both methods. Tables 17-3 and 17-4 are compilations of studies addressing the open versus arthroscopic issues.

SUGGESTED READING

Arciero RA, Wheeler JH, Ryan JB, et al. Arthroscopic Bankart repair versus nonoperative treatment for acute, initial anterior shoulder dislocations. Am J Sports Med 1994;22:589–594.

Bach BR Jr, Warren RF, Fronek J. Disruption of the lateral capsule of the shoulder: a cause of recurrent dislocation. J Bone Joint Surg Br 1988;702:274–276.

Bankart ASB. The pathology and treatment of recurrent dislocation of the shoulder joint. Br J Surg 1938;26:23–29.

Burkhart SS, DeBeer JF, Tehrany AM, et al. Quantifying glenoid bone loss arthroscopically in shoulder instability. Arthroscopy 2002;18:488–491.

Buss DD, Lynch GP, Meyer CP, et al. Nonoperative management for in-season athletes with anterior shoulder instability. Am J Sports Med 2004;32:1430–1433.

Harryman DT, Ballmer FP, Harris SL, et al. Arthroscopic labrum repair to the glenoid rim. Arthroscopy 1994;10:20–30.

Itoi E, Hatakeyama Y, Kido T, et al. A new method of immobilization after traumatic anterior dislocation of the shoulder: a preliminary study. J Shoulder Elbow Surg 2003;12:413–415.

Matson FA, Thomas SC, Rockwood CA, et al. Glenohumeral instability. In: Rockwood CA, Matson FA, eds. The Shoulder, Vol. 2, 2nd ed. Philadelphia: WB Saunders, 1990:633–639.

Pagnani MJ, Dome DC. Surgical treatment of traumatic anterior shoulder instability in American football players. J Bone Joint Surg Am 2002;84:711–715.

Perthes G. Über operationen bei: habitueller schulterlusation. Dtsch Ztschr Chir 1906;85:199–227.

POSTERIOR AND MULTIDIRECTIONAL INSTABILITY OF THE SHOULDER

CARLOS A. GUANCHE

Evaluation of shoulder instability can be fraught with difficulties in making the appropriate diagnosis. Anterior instability due to a macrotraumatic event is simple to diagnose and treat. With more subtle events, in which the direction of instability is not readily obvious, treatment is significantly more complex. The problem is usually created by the existence of multidirectional instability (MDI) in an individual. The balance of stability versus mobility in the glenohumeral joint is what allows a wide range of motion and performance of overhead activities. Finding this balance, however, is especially difficult in cases of posterior and MDI. The axiom of exhausting conservative management is critically important in this population, especially as it applies to those whose instability is proportional to their leisure activity level. The disability associated with posterior subluxation is variable. Typically, activities of daily living and work functions are not limited by recurrent posterior subluxation. Participation in sports is generally more troublesome, often requiring modification or complete elimination of the activity. Even though it is not appropriate to terminate someone's hobbies as they affect instability, it certainly should be taken into consideration in situations where there is a significant vulnerability to further injury.

Adherence to the principles of rehabilitation and surgery, as well as genetics, should be practiced in these cases. Problems with posterior and MDI may be attributable not only to activity level but also to inherited anatomy and laxity. In Neer and Foster's original 1980 study describing the capsular shift procedure, all 40 shoulders had inferior instability, with generalized ligamentous laxity noted in 17 patients.

There are many cases of posterior instability that are straightforward and easily solved by addressing the posterior structures only. This chapter will discuss MDI as a separate entity in most sections.

PATHOGENESIS

Epidemiology

The incidence of posterior instability has been underestimated historically, likely because of difficulties in diagnosis. The incidence of posterior instability has been estimated at 5% of all instability, with the majority being anterior. Recently, with increasing use of shoulder arthroscopy, the incidence has risen. The understanding of the condition has also increased significantly.

Likewise, MDI was previously thought to occur on an infrequent basis. This form of instability results from some combination of excessive tissue compliance, muscular dyscoordination, and occasionally inadequacy of the glenoid concavity. With increasing understanding of the pathophysiology of instability—and especially understanding problems about the rotator interval—the incidence has increased in proportion to other instabilities, with many surgical failures being attributed to a lack of recognition of an additional direction of instability.

Pathophysiology

Selective Ligament-cutting Studies

The influence of any one variable leading to shoulder instability is difficult to ascertain. Several studies are available that summarize the impact of selective cutting of various sections of the glenohumeral joint capsule and its intrinsic ligaments. The influence of passive and active stabilizers of the shoulder in the most clinically relevant position of 90 degrees of forward flexion and varying degrees of rotation has been studied. Of the muscles tested, the subscapularis contributed the most to resisting a subluxation force. The coracohumeral ligament was an effective contributor in neutral humeral rotation, and the posterior-inferior glenohumeral ligament was an effective contributor in internal humeral rotation. The long head of the biceps was found to reduce the subluxation force in neutral rotation and internal rotation but became less important with external rotation.

With respect to inferior translation, in the neutrally rotated and adducted shoulder, the superior glenohumeral ligament (SGHL) is the most important stabilizer. At 45-degree abduction, the anterior band of the inferior glenohumeral ligament is the primary restraint to inferior translation in neutral or internal rotation, whereas the posterior band of the inferior glenohumeral ligament is the primary restraint in external rotation.

In another study, a constant internal rotation torque of 1.5 Nm was applied while selective sectioning was performed. With regard to the posterior structures, the infraspinatus and teres minor were the primary stabilizers to internal rotation for the first 45 degrees of abduction, with the lower half of the posterior capsule active from 45 to 90 degrees. In addition, no cases of posterior subluxation occurred with intact anterior structures, thus giving credence to the circle concept of instability.

Other Factors

In some situations, bony deficiency of the glenoid can be a contributory factor in the etiology of the instability pattern. In addition, the concept of static posterior subluxation with the possible contribution to later degenerative arthritis has also been espoused. Patients with this diagnosis who have been followed for the longest period of time appear to progress from subluxation to degenerative joint disease at a relatively young age (Fig. 18-1).

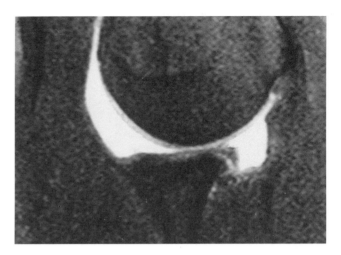

Figure 18-1   MRI with gadolinium arthrogram depicting static posterior subluxation in a 30-year-old patient.

Muscle inhibition or weakness is common in glenohumeral abnormalities, whether from instability, labral lesions, or arthrosis. The musculature most susceptible to this includes the serratus anterior and trapezius. Scapular instability has been found in as many as 100% of instability problems. The abnormalities in muscle function are thought to occur as a result of a decreased ability of the musculature to exert torque and stabilize the scapula, as well as a disorganization of the normal muscle firing patterns.

Rotator Interval

One of the most important developments in the understanding of shoulder instability, especially MDI, has been the delineation of the pathophysiology associated with lesions of the rotator interval. This area is a triangular space, with its apex centered at the transverse humeral ligament over the biceps sulcus, having its greatest dimension at the base of the coracoid process. The interval is a section of the glenohumeral joint capsule that is bordered superiorly by the anterior margin of the supraspinatus tendon and inferiorly by the superior border of the subscapularis tendon. The coracohumeral ligament (CHL) strengthens the interval, as does the SGHL, which courses from the anterosuperior labrum deep to the substance of the rotator interval capsule and the CHL to insert near the lesser tuberosity (Fig. 18-2).

The presence of an enlarged interval has been shown to contribute to humeral head translations, as well as play a significant role in posterior stability of the joint. In one cadaveric study, a radio frequency probe was used to perform a thermal capsuloplasty of the rotator interval. An electromagnetic tracking device was used to measure anterior and posterior glenohumeral translations. Anterior translation was decreased by 31.5%, whereas posterior translation was decreased by 43.1% while applying a 10 N load. Clinical studies have also documented the beneficial effect of rotator interval closure in supplementing open stabilizations, as well as in selected cases of MDI.

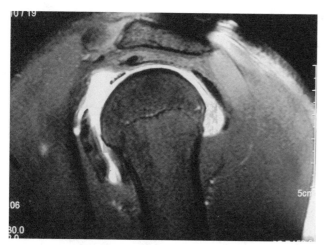

Figure 18-2 Wide rotator interval in an active overhead athlete with signs of MDI.

Mechanism of Injury

Posterior Instability

Historically, posterior instability was thought to be associated with electrical shocks and seizure disorders. The effect of an excessive electrical charge and a tonic seizure is to predominantly activate the posterior rotator cuff musculature. This can cause a posterior dislocation, which is missed by physicians and other health care providers upon first presentation in up to 50% of cases.

More recently, the scope of the problem has been expanded to include other mechanisms. A common mode involves a posterior force applied to the arm while it is in a forward flexed, adducted, and internally rotated position. Most commonly, this problem is noted in football players who block with their arms in such a position. For that reason, offensive linemen appear to have the largest incidence of this problem relative to other positions.

Multidirectional Instability

The development of symptomatic MDI appears to be a gradual phenomenon that is a spectrum of pathologies. Most commonly, patients have evidence of subtle laxity in both shoulders. This subtle congenital laxity, superimposed on the performance of repetitive overhead activities, leads to a gradual stretching of the restraining structures and symptomatic instability. A critical distinction is the separation of laxity from instability. In many situations, the contralateral, asymptomatic shoulder exhibits significant laxity but not symptomatic instability. This needs to be carefully considered in the treatment.

Congenital factors also play a role in many shoulder instability patterns; however, in MDI patients, this preexisting laxity may be more significant. Samples of shoulder capsule and skin from 25 patients with anterior instability, MDI, failed MDI surgery, as well as patients with no history of instability were analyzed for collagen characteristics and elastin density. Patients in the anterior instability and MDI groups were not statistically different; however, patients who failed MDI surgery had smaller fibrils and decreased density of collagen, as well as an increase in elastin density.

This lends credence to a genetic predisposition to shoulder laxity in this subgroup.

In addition to the variability in the collagenous makeup of the patients, there are variations in the anatomic findings that may impact the degree and type of instability. In a study of 10 adult glenohumeral cadaveric joints sectioned in the abducted, externally rotated position, 80% had a capsular origin from the labrum, whereas in 20% it originated solely from the glenoid neck. This correlated closely to an embryological study in which 77% of the glenohumeral ligaments originated from the labrum and 23% from the glenoid neck. These variables are important to note because they may impact not only laxity and/or instability but also surgical repair. Repair of a normal anatomic variant would regrettably result in an equivocal surgical outcome.

DIAGNOSIS

History

- A thorough history and physical examination are imperative in patients with recurrent instability.
- The report of the initial episode of instability is key to determining the direction(s) of pathology.
- Factors that determine the direction and type of instability are: the position of the arm when symptoms occur, the intensity of the force leading to the episode, and the number and types of recurrences.
- In addition, radiographs from any of the earlier events are helpful to confirm the direction of instability.

Posterior Instability

- The type and mechanism of the inciting event in the patient's instability are critical to the diagnosis.
- The less traumatic the episode, the more likely there is generalized ligamentous laxity and perhaps bony glenoid deficiency or malposition.
- In many cases, the initial trauma associated with posterior instability occurs with the arm held in forward flexion, adduction, and internal rotation.
- In most studies, evaluating the presentation of posterior instability pain appears to be a prominent factor.
- Although the pathologic cause of subluxation can be capsular laxity and/or a labral tear, the majority of patients present with either posterior or diffuse pain in their shoulder.
- Commonly, the athletes suffering from this problem are weight lifters, throwers, racquet sport athletes, swimmers, and football players.
  - Football players deserve special attention because their specific position appears to play an important role in the diagnosis. Most commonly, offensive lineman are affected.
  - With the current blocking techniques allowing for the players to "punch out" with their arms in a forward flexed position, the capsule sustains intense posterior stress.
- The additional cumulative trauma associated with weight lifting may contribute to the problem.

Multidirectional Instability

- The usual presentation of MDI is that of vague shoulder pain, often global in nature, and occasionally severe and debilitating.
  - This is in contradistinction to most cases of anterior instability, in which the instability itself is typically the reason for the patient's initial office visit.
- In patients with MDI, the most obvious diagnosis is often scapular dyskinesia.
- Patients with atraumatic instability may have a family history of similar findings and a history of other joint problems, most notably recurrent patellofemoral instability.

Physical Examination

- Both shoulders are carefully examined so that the symptomatic and asymptomatic sides can be compared.
- It is helpful to begin on the normal side to assess for general laxity and strength and to gain the patient's confidence.
- Regardless of the type of instability, a thorough evaluation includes assessment of motion, laxity, and stability.
- Often, the presenting complaint from patients with either symptom complex is scapular winging.
  - Scapular dyskinesis or loss of control of scapular motion during arm elevation is seen by observing the patient from behind and by asking him or her to slowly elevate and lower the arms.
  - The motion of the scapulae on the chest wall is then observed for asymmetry.
  - Several repetitions may be necessary before this is observed.
  - Winging can also be better demonstrated by asking the patient to push against a wall to accentuate the problem.
- In most cases of dyskinesia associated with posterior or MDI, the static observation of the scapulothoracic joint is normal, whereas the active evaluation reveals marked scapulothoracic motion asymmetry (Fig. 18-3).

Posterior Instability

- Posterior instability is best evaluated with the jerk test, which involves placing the patient's arm in 90 degrees of elevation and 90 degrees of internal rotation.
- The maneuver can be performed with the patient in the seated or supine position.
  - The supine position is simpler and preferred because it puts the patient at ease and gives the examiner some mechanical advantage.
- In either position, the arm is then moved from the coronal to the sagittal plane and back, whereas an axial load is applied to the humerus.
- If posterior instability is present, the humeral head subluxes over the glenoid rim and reproduces the patient's symptoms.
- Reduction of the humeral head when the arm returns to the coronal plane is often accompanied by a palpable and audible clunk.

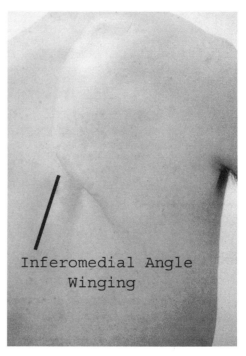

Figure 18-3 Scapulothoracic dyskinesia with winging in an active thrower with MDI.

- The competence of the glenoid concavity and the integrity of the soft-tissue structures about the shoulder should also be assessed with the load and shift test.
- The supine patient's arm is positioned in 20 degrees of abduction and 20 degrees of forward flexion with neutral rotation.
- The humeral head is loaded axially into the glenoid fossa and translated both posteriorly and anteriorly.
- An assessment with respect to the degree of translation is made.
- The extent of translation is described relative to the ability to translate the humeral head out of the glenoid fossa (Table 18-1).
- In addition to the aforementioned signs of excessive translation, using signs of labral pathology (such as the crank, O'Brien's, and Kibler maneuvers) can help assess the integrity of the labral structures.
- These tests are delineated in other sections of this chapter, or in review articles on the topic.

Multidirectional Instability

- The assessment of MDI includes the examination maneuvers described earlier, as well as all of the maneuvers that apply to anterior instability. These are described in greater detail in other parts of this textbook.
- Specific maneuvers that delineate MDI further include the assessment of a sulcus sign, an indicator of inferior shoulder translation, as well as determination of generalized signs of ligamentous laxity—including elbow and knee hyperextension, the ability to place the thumb to the forearm, and metacarpophalangeal joint hyperextension.

TABLE 18-1 GRADING OF TRANSLATION OF THE HUMERAL HEAD OUT OF THE GLENOID FOSSA IN POSTERIOR INSTABILITY

Grade	Description
0	No translation from the center of the glenoid
I	<50% of the humeral head across the glenoid fossa (normal)
II	Translation of the humeral head onto the glenolabral rim
III	Translation over the glenolabral rim
IV	Translation with complete dislocation requiring manual reduction

(Adapted from Antoniou J, Harryman DT II. Posterior instability. Op Tech Sports Med 2000;8:225–233.)

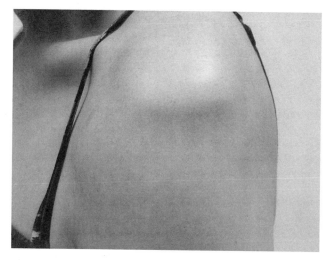

Figure 18-4 Sulcus sign in a patient with failed anterior instability repair.

- The sulcus test is performed with the patient in the seated position.
  - A distraction force is applied to the arm at the side of the body with the shoulder in neutral rotation. The degree of separation between the acromion and humeral head is then determined.
  - Grading is shown in Table 18-2 and Figure 18-4.
- Inferior laxity should always be assessed in both shoulders because a large number of asymptomatic shoulders will have a positive sulcus sign.
- Additionally, the degree of inferior instability should be assessed with the arm in an externally rotated position while maintaining neutral abduction.
- An obliteration of the sulcus sign in this position indicates competence of the rotator interval or the SGHL complex.
  - The importance of this factor cannot be underestimated because simple rotator interval closure is often enough to stabilize a shoulder with MDI.

Radiologic Examination

- Although the diagnosis of instability can be made without any further imaging studies, a number of imaging modalities may be helpful in delineating the anatomical factors involved, as well as associated pathological entities, especially in older individuals whose incidence of rotator cuff pathology is increased with instability.

TABLE 18-2 GRADING OF THE SULCUS SIGN IN MULTIDIRECTIONAL INSTABILITY

Grade	Description
I	Translation of <1 cm
III	Translation of 1–2 cm
III	Translation of >2 cm

- The use of routine radiographic imaging, especially in patients who will require surgical intervention, should be used.
- In some cases, simple soft-tissue reconstructions may not suffice to stabilize a joint.
  - Surgical discussion with the patient should include the possibility of bony reconstruction, as described later in this chapter and in other areas of this text.
- The standard radiographs that should be obtained include an anteroposterior view (made perpendicular to the scapular plane), an axillary view, and a lateral or Y view.
- It is important to detect lesions such as glenoid deficiencies, glenoid retroversion, erosion of the posterior glenoid, and extra-articular ossifications of the posterior glenoid margin (Bennet lesions).
- In cases in which a significant bony deficit is either seen or suspected, more specialized views can be obtained, such as the Stryker notch view or the Bernageau view.
- In continued questions of bony deficiency, the use of computed tomography scanning is certainly useful and indicated.
- The use of routine magnetic resonance imaging (MRI) studies is not advocated in most situations.
- The clinical indications for MRI include suspected rotator cuff pathology.
- In cases of MDI, the arthrogram portion of an MRI may shed light on the capsular volume.
- The posterior-inferior glenoid labrum is difficult to visualize in many MRI studies and as such is not useful in determining the treatment algorithm in many cases.
- In repetitive overhead athletes, an MRI study with gadolinium enhancement should be considered because superior labrum anterior-posterior (SLAP) lesions frequently occur and may impact the surgical approach.
- In addition, the evaluation of capsular volume and labral injury is made more definitive with the use of MRI (Fig. 18-5).

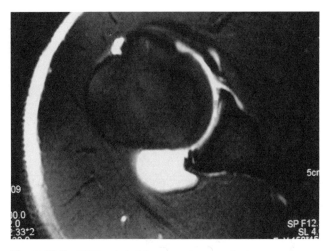

Figure 18-5 MRI with gadolinium arthrogram depicting a posterior labral tear in a patient with significant posterior capsular redundancy.

TREATMENT

Surgical Indications and Contraindications

Posterior Instability

- The initial treatment of any instability remains nonsurgical, with the emphasis on supervised strengthening of the rotator cuff muscles and special attention to the infraspinatus and teres minor, deltoid strengthening, and scapulothoracic stabilization in posterior instability.
- This treatment regimen has proven particularly successful in atraumatic instability and has allowed 80% of patients to function effectively as opposed to 16% of those with the traumatic variants of instability.
- It is paramount to separate those patients with voluntary instability from this group of patients.
- It is important to differentiate between patients who are able to sublux their shoulders by positioning and muscular activation and those who do so for secondary gain.
  - Patients who actively attempt to either sublux or dislocate their shoulders, most commonly in a posterior direction, are clearly poor candidates for surgical reconstruction of any kind.
  - One way to separate these individuals is to assess their instability (or its reproducibility by the patient) with the arm both at the side and at 90 degrees of flexion.
  - In those whose humeral head subluxes posteriorly with flexion and cross body adduction, a better response is seen with surgical intervention.
  - With that said, there is substantial evidence to support surgical intervention in patients who can voluntarily sublux their shoulders, fail conservative management, and cannot participate in activities at their desired level.
- In summary, patients who have posterior instability of the shoulder should not be condemned to nonoperative management solely because they are able to subluxate the shoulder voluntarily.

- The judicious use of psychiatric evaluations for determination of confounding variables is suggested.

Multidirectional Instability

- This is probably the most complex patient population seen in instability problems.
- The basic idea is to maintain mobility while limiting excessive translation.
- Surgical stabilization is considered for recurrent posterior traumatic instability and for persistent atraumatic posterior instability.
- The indications for stabilization of a shoulder with MDI are continuing instability that persists despite concerted rehabilitation and activity modification.
  - The caveat here is that this is feasible for the patient.
- The determination of which surgical procedure to opt for can be a challenge.
  - A particular technique is chosen on the basis of the quality of the soft tissues and the bony anatomy and, most importantly, by the experience of the surgeon.
  - Unfortunately, these procedures are performed on an infrequent basis by most surgeons.
  - This can lead to insecurity by the surgeon, and occasionally to poor decision making as a result of inexperience with the nuances of posterior and MDI.

Examination under Anesthesia

- The most important decision regarding the surgical intervention of a shoulder with any form of instability is the examination of the shoulder under anesthesia. The importance of this single maneuver cannot be overstated.
- The final decision with respect to the order of repair, the direction of repair, and the type of repair should be predicated on simple anatomical principles.
- Translation under anesthesia can be significantly different than that while the patient is conscious.
  - In a study of 50 patients, using the load and shift test before and after the induction of anesthesia, 92% were found to have anterior translation at least one grade higher during anesthesia than while awake.
- The typical findings associated with a specific injury to any given anatomical structure within the shoulder are well defined.
- A simple and thorough examination covering all of the known stabilizing elements should delineate the consequent steps to be taken in a surgical procedure.
- Table 18-3 demonstrates the common areas involved in instability and the subsequent findings noted on physical examination.
  - This table can be used to determine the necessity of repair of each specific anatomical structure at the time of surgical intervention.
- Finally, the contralateral shoulder should also be examined to assess for signs of generalized laxity.

Surgical Treatment

Posterior Instability (Table 18-4)

- There is no consensus with regard to the procedure of choice for the patient with posterior instability who fails a conservative course of treatment.

TABLE 18-3 ANATOMICAL STRUCTURES RESPONSIBLE FOR SPECIFIC AREAS OF STABILITY

Structure	Responsible Translation
Rotator interval	Inferior subluxation[a]
Middle glenohumeral ligament	Translation at 45 degrees
Anterior, inferior glenohumeral ligament	Translation at 90 degrees
Axillary recess	Inferior (abduction)
Posterior, inferior glenohumeral ligament	Posterior translation at 90 degrees
Midposterior capsule	Posterior translation at 45 degrees

[a] Done with the arm at the side in neutral and external rotations. Inferior translation normally significantly decreases with external rotation. Failure to change inferior translation indicates incompetent interval.

- Open surgical stabilization techniques for the treatment of recurrent posterior instability include soft-tissue and bony procedures.
- A variety of arthroscopic techniques have also been described.
- The bony procedures include posterior bone block, posterior glenoid osteotomy, and humeral rotational osteotomy; bony pathology, however, is rare.
  - In most situations, the use of soft-tissue procedures is sufficient.
  - The indications for posterior bone block procedures are reserved for those situations in which a soft-tissue procedure has failed.

- In the case of glenoid osteotomy, the indications for the procedure are excessive posterior glenoid version greater than 10 degrees.
  - In one study, the average glenoid version angle was altered from 9.35 to 4.62 degrees. However, 25% of the patients showed postoperative degenerative changes in the glenohumeral joint at 5 years.
- The use of humeral osteotomy for the treatment of recurrent instability does not have strong support in the literature.
- In general, the outcome of bony procedures has been inconsistent and difficult to justify in shoulders without definite bony deformity.
- Soft-tissue procedures that have been well described include those that address the capsule either from a posterior approach or from an anterior approach.
  - Labral pathology is also addressed, if present.
  - The success rates for these repairs have been as high as 96% in primary repairs.
  - The amount of pathologic laxity present in any given patient has been difficult to quantify. In most studies, however, the posterior inferior margin of the capsule appears to be the critical area that needs to be addressed with the repair.
- The CHL and SGHL complexes play a significant role in posterior instability.
  - Several authors have adopted an anterior surgical approach to correct posterior instability. Nobuhara and Ikeda (1987) reported 96% good and excellent results with rotator interval reconstructions in 78 patients with posteroinferior instability. Recurrent instability occurred in only 4%.
- Other soft-tissue procedures seek to excessively tighten internal rotation by buttressing the capsular imbrication with muscle tissue.

TABLE 18-4 SUGGESTED TREATMENT FOR POSTERIOR INSTABILITY

Problem	Management
Normal radiographs (axillary view)	
Posterior translation in 45 degrees abduction only	Posterior (midcapsular) imbrication
Posterior translation in 90 degrees abduction only	Posterior inferior imbrication
Posterior translation in both positions	Pancapsular plication + assessment as below for rotator interval closure
Posterior translation in 0 degrees abduction only	Rotator interval closure
Abnormal radiographs (axillary view)	
Abnormal axillary view with >10 degrees retroversion	CT scan
Normal CT (within 5 degrees side-to-side difference)	As for normal radiographs
CT scan with >10 degrees difference side to side	Glenoid osteotomy (posterior intracapsular approach)

CT, computed tomography.
Evaluate for superior labrum anterior-posterior (SLAP) lesion either arthroscopically or with gadolinium-enhanced MRI.

- A posterior capsular plication and overlapping of the infraspinatus tendon (reverse Putti-Platt repair) has been reported but has shown a large percentage of unsatisfactory results.
- Arthroscopic techniques for the treatment of posterior instability are well described in the literature (Fig. 18-6).
  - Many studies, however, are limited in usefulness as a result of the limited sample sizes.
  - In one study, the capsule was prepared by gentle abrasion of the synovial surface of the posterior capsule then advanced by about 1 cm to the posterior glenoid labrum and sutured in place using three to eight nonabsorbable sutures (Fig. 18-5). At a minimum 2-year follow-up, 12 of 14 patients treated with arthroscopic posterior capsular plication had 12 excellent results, and 2 had fair results.
  - Another study delineated the pathologic findings in 41 patients with posterior instability and noted that there were four types of labral lesions: a labral split or flap tear (32%), synovial and capsular stripping (22%), chondral or labral erosion (17%), and Bankart-type detachment (12%).

- A study assessing the outcomes of traumatic posterior instability shed light on the fact that posterior disruptions occur more frequently than previously thought and can be managed arthroscopically in a straightforward fashion.
  - It was concluded that arthroscopic repair of the posterior capsulolabral complex was an effective means of management.
- In a study that used a variety of techniques designed to address the multiple factors responsible for instability, it was shown that a 90% success rate with 1- to 7-year follow-up in the maintenance of stability can be achieved.
  - Sixty-one patients were treated with six failures, two of which responded to rehabilitation and did not require further surgery.
  - The treatment algorithm included the use of absorbable tacks for posterior labral repairs in conjunction with arthroscopic rotator interval plication. In cases with more extensive capsular laxity, a suture punch capsulorrhaphy with an extensive vertical shift was also used. A mini-open capsulorrhaphy was used in

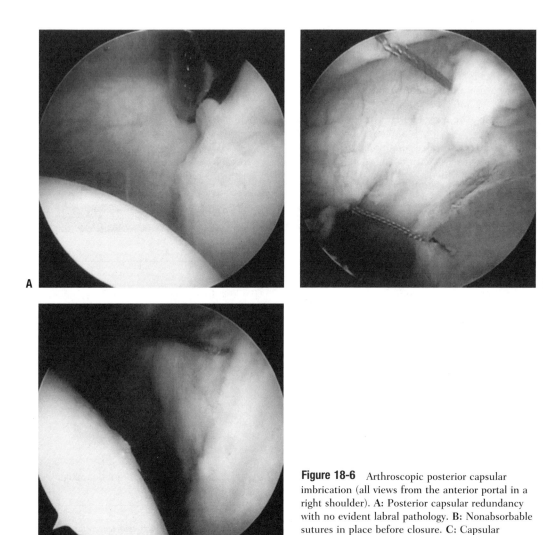

Figure 18-6 Arthroscopic posterior capsular imbrication (all views from the anterior portal in a right shoulder). **A:** Posterior capsular redundancy with no evident labral pathology. **B:** Nonabsorbable sutures in place before closure. **C:** Capsular volume reduced after suture tying.

cases of diffuse posterior capsular damage, whereas thermal capsulorrhaphy was used in simple diffuse stretching of the entire capsular complex.

■ Laser and radio frequency–induced capsular shrinkage (thermal capsulorrhaphy) has also been used in an attempt to imbricate the capsule.

▫ The lack of basic science to validate the use of these devices, along with the lack of long-term clinical outcomes, makes it difficult to recommend these treatment modalities.

▫ The basic science studies available indicate that with the use of an yttrium-aluminum-garnet laser the amount of glenohumeral joint translation may be decreased. A decrease in posterior translation from 7.2 to 4.4 mm was noted with a 15-N load, whereas a 20-N load allowed translation of 10.4 mm before and 6.5 mm after ablation. In addition, the response to heat-induced shrinkage is proportional to the collagen density of the area.

▫ Areas with high collagen density, such as the middle and inferior glenohumeral ligaments, will respond more dramatically than the posterior capsule and rotator interval.

▫ There is a paucity of peer-reviewed literature to justify the use of heat capsulorraphy. A limited number of non-peer-reviewed articles show promising results thus far, but none deal exclusively with posterior instability.

Multidirectional Instability (Table 18-5)

■ The basic principle of MDI surgery is to reduce the volume of the capsule and therefore provide some restraint to the humeral head, reducing the load on the shoulder musculature.

■ This can be accomplished with a variety of procedures, including the traditional open inferior capsular shift through arthroscopic means or by thermal shrinkage.

■ Neer and Foster introduced the concept of MDI and its treatment in 1980.

TABLE 18-5 SUGGESTED TREATMENT FOR MULTIDIRECTIONAL INSTABILITY[a]

Problem	Management
Excessive anterior translation, coupled with a positive sulcus	Anterior capsulorrhaphy with rotator interval closure
Excessive posterior translation, coupled with a positive sulcus	Posterior capsulorrhaphy with rotator interval closure
Excessive translation in the anterior, posterior, and inferior directions	Pancapsular plication and rotator interval closure (anterior if done open)

[a] Predicated on proficiency with arthroscopic surgical techniques. Otherwise, surgical intervention in open fashion is well founded in the literature.

▫ The inferior capsular shift was described as a procedure for the symptomatic patient who had been unresponsive to nonoperative therapy.

▫ In their study, 36 patients (40 shoulders) with involuntary inferior and multidirectional subluxation and dislocation and who had failed standard operations underwent an open inferior capsular shift, in which a flap of the capsule was shifted to reduce capsular and ligamentous redundancy on all three sides.

▫ Their results revealed that one shoulder began subluxing again within 7 months after operation, but no other unsatisfactory results were noted for at least 2 years.

■ A subsequent study by Cooper and Brems (1992) using the identical surgical procedure corroborated Neer and Foster's findings.

▫ The postoperative range of motion in this population was well maintained with a mean forward elevation of 172 degrees; external rotation was 77 degrees, and internal rotation was to the level of the eighth thoracic vertebra. Ninety-one percent of the patients continued to function well without evidence of recurrence, whereas four had disabling, recurrent instability.

▫ In a study analyzing the results in a contact athlete population after surgical intervention, the overall recurrence rate for a traditional open inferior capsular shift was 8%, with successful return to sports occurring in 82% of the patients.

■ In addition to the traditional shift procedure, further refinements in the technique have been made as a result of increasing understanding of the rotator interval capsule (Fig. 18-7).

▫ A study of 10 shoulders using closure of the interval—as well as imbrication of the anterior, inferior, and posteroinferior aspects of the capsule through an anterior approach—produced good or excellent results in 90% of patients.

■ In the more recent literature, arthroscopic-only techniques have attempted to imbricate the capsule in a variety of ways.

▫ In a study by Treacy et al. (1999), 25 patients were treated with an arthroscopic transglenoid capsular shift. At an average 5-year follow-up, 88% had satisfactory results, with no patient experiencing loss of external rotation and 7 of 11 returning to sports at their preinjury level.

▫ In the 2001 prospective study by Gartsman et al., of 47 patients, 94% rated their results as good to excellent according to the Rowe scale at 35-month average follow-up. One patient was considered a failure of the index operation as a result of persistent instability and underwent a second operative procedure, whereas two others had persistent pain. In essence, 44 of 47 patients were treated successfully.

■ In addition to the previously described techniques, attempts to treat this problem with heat capsulorrhaphy have been made, but heat therapies have thus far shown poor results, compared not only with traditional open methods but also with the newer arthroscopic procedures.

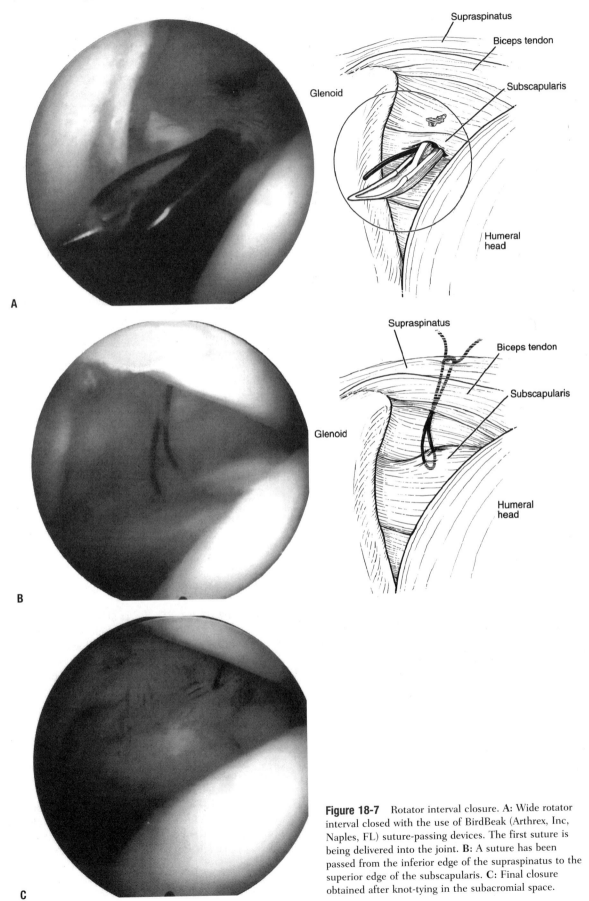

A

B

C

Figure 18-7   Rotator interval closure. **A:** Wide rotator interval closed with the use of BirdBeak (Arthrex, Inc, Naples, FL) suture-passing devices. The first suture is being delivered into the joint. **B:** A suture has been passed from the inferior edge of the supraspinatus to the superior edge of the subscapularis. **C:** Final closure obtained after knot-tying in the subacromial space.

Postoperative Management

- The most critical aspect of surgical treatment for posterior and MDI appears to be the rehabilitation.
- These patients often have long-standing instability that has not been addressed with adequate rehabilitation.
- The scapulothoracic articulation is frequently dysfunctional and needs to be addressed.
- It is important to develop a stable platform for the shoulder positioners (rotator cuff) to be effective.

Posterior Instability

- Although the specific rehabilitation program varies on the basis of the procedure performed, some general recommendations can be made.
- Any surgery for posterior instability seeks to reduce excessive laxity in the posterior capsule.
- These patients should avoid stress to this area in the early phases of recovery.
- As with any other surgical procedure, early passive range of motion is highly beneficial to enhance circulation within the joint to promote healing.
- The overall goals of the surgical procedure and rehabilitation are to control pain and inflammation and to regain normal upper extremity strength, endurance, and normal motion while maintaining the desired level of function.
- In most cases, the patient should be placed in a splint/sling that protects the individual from excessive internal rotation.
    - Many apply an abduction splint, but other devices that allow 15 to 30 degrees of abduction and neutral internal rotation are adequate in most situations. The UltraSling (DJ Ortho, Vista, CA) device is one such apparatus.
- Physical therapy should be initiated within the first week after surgery.
- Supervised rehabilitation is to be supplemented by a home fitness program in which the patient performs the given exercises at home or at a gym facility.
- The first 1 to 3 weeks involve the gradual return of motion, especially external rotation, which in many cases is not addressed with a posterior reconstruction.
    - Passive motion is instituted, with active-assisted motion in the scapular plane.
    - Motion should be limited in internal rotation to a maximum of 30 degrees, with external rotation on an as-tolerated basis.
    - Pendulum exercises are instituted.
    - Submaximal and pain-free isometrics in all planes can also be instituted.
- Beginning at 3 weeks postoperatively, the patient is advanced to unlimited internal rotation, while avoiding the extremes of motion.
- Strengthening is instituted with neutral tubing and prone horizontal adduction exercises with a limit of 45 degrees.
- Scapular stabilization is begun at this time, as well as rhythmic stabilization in proprioceptive neuromuscular facilitatory patterns.
- Immobilization is discontinued between 4 and 6 weeks, depending on the degree of capsular laxity and the extent of the surgical procedure.

- At 6 weeks, posterior capsular stretching is instituted and titrated, depending on the degree of original laxity and the existing internal rotation contracture.
- Strengthening is increased with the use of an upper extremity ergometer.
- Dynamic stabilization exercises are also advanced such that, at the end of 12 weeks, the patient should have a full, painless range of motion with normal arthrokinematics.
- Between 12 and 24 weeks, a light plyometric program is begun with a gradual return to sport-specific and functional drills.
    - An interval throwing program can also be instituted.
- Return to activity requires both time and clinical evaluation.
- To most safely and efficiently return to normal or high-level functional activity, the patient requires adequate strength, flexibility, and endurance.
- Functional evaluation, including strength and range-of-motion testing, is one method of evaluating a patient's readiness to return to activity.
- Symptoms such as pain, swelling, or instability should be closely monitored both by the patient and physician.
- In general, a return to contact sports is allowed at about 4 months and full unrestricted throwing at 6 months.

Multidirectional Instability

- Historically, after surgery for MDI, 6 weeks of postoperative immobilization was recommended, followed by heat and gentle assisted exercises.
    - The goal was for range of motion to be 20 degrees less than the opposite shoulder.
    - Isometrics was advocated at 8 weeks and progressive resistive exercises beginning at 12 weeks.
    - Sports and lifting more than 20 lb were restricted for 9 months, and certain swimming strokes (back and butterfly), heavy overhead use of the arm, and contact sports were advised against for 12 months after surgery.
    - This protocol has fallen out of favor as a result of the excessive tightness and severe muscle weakness that followed the regime.
- The current postoperative stabilization protocol for MDI involves about 6 weeks of immobilization.
- The patient is able to perform elbow and hand range of motion only for at least 3 weeks and sometimes for the first 6 weeks.
- After the initial immobilization, the patient begins supine stretching exercises, followed by wand exercises as tolerated. Flexion and internal rotation are increased beginning on postoperative week 2. External rotation is mobilized to neutral, then increased 10 degrees per week; abduction is allowed to 45 degrees, then increased 10 degrees per week after 6 weeks.
- Isometrics are instituted as soon as possible to limit muscle atrophy.
- Beginning at 6 weeks, strengthening is initiated, including the rotator cuff and scapulothoracic musculature.
- Range of motion is returned to within normal limits with stretching and joint mobilization programs.

■ Eccentric exercise programs and proprioceptive neuromuscular facilitation techniques are started at 12 weeks postoperatively. In addition, sports such as swimming can now be resumed. An interval throwing program may also begin at this time, with a gradual return to unrestricted activities at 4 to 6 months.

■ The one muscle that deserves particular attention with respect to open procedures is the subscapularis.

  ■ In open surgery, that is typically the only muscle detached and subsequently repaired.

  ■ It is paramount to obtain a solid repair of that tendon.

  ■ Also important is the protection of that muscle in the physical therapy that follows.

■ To protect the repair, internal rotation strengthening should not be instituted until 6 weeks postoperatively.

RESULTS

■ The many reasons for failure in the rehabilitation and reconstruction of patients with posterior or MDI can be divided into incorrect diagnosis (direction), surgical error, and rehabilitation error.

■ The episode leading to recurrence is likely to offer some idea as to the etiology.

  ■ An atraumatic event leading to recurrence in a patient may indicate failure to address some component of the instability, whereas a more significant trauma may indicate simple recurrence from a macrotraumatic event.

■ The patient should be questioned with regard to their postoperative satisfaction with the procedure.

  ■ If the patient indicates that functional return had not occurred before a subluxation event, then he/she is likely to have undergone inadequate rehabilitation or in more extreme cases experienced a surgical failure.

Diagnostic Failure

■ The most common errors are incorrect diagnosis and failure to address the primary (and often, secondary) component of instability in cases of MDI.

  ■ A reason for this is the vagueness of symptoms in most patients.

  ■ Commonly, the patient presents with only vague pain and inability to perform activities.

  ■ The variety of positions that cause the instability vary from adduction to internal rotation and possibly extension, further adding to the confusion.

■ The all-important examination under anesthesia may have been neglected or not performed at all.

  ■ This step should be the final determining factor with respect to the surgical intervention undertaken, as previously stated.

■ The patients themselves often dictate the appropriate course of action.

  ■ Frequently, in many cases of simple posterior or MDI, the best course of action is nonoperative.

■ The concept of "conservative" therapy is easy to misuse.

■ In cases in which patients either can modify their activities to reduce their instability or present with congenital soft-tissue laxity, no surgery is the best therapy.

■ Failure of repair in these patients can lead to a cascade of events culminating in multiple failed procedures, with a nonfunctional extremity and no obvious good salvage option.

Surgical Failure

■ Beyond misdiagnosis of the type of instability, failures are attributable to a lack of understanding of surgical principles.

■ In some situations, a labral detachment is properly addressed, but the remaining capsular redundancy is not.

■ In most cases, surgeons are more comfortable with anterior approaches to the shoulder. Although in many cases traditional open procedures work well, they are clearly inadequate in others.

■ Judicious use of the arthroscope and a thorough examination under anesthesia go a long way toward preventing those unfortunate decisions.

■ In cases in which bony procedures are performed, the likelihood of complications increases.

■ Procedures redirecting the glenoid are fraught with technical difficulty and carry with them the complications of poor position of the osteotomy; nonunion, avascular necrosis; and prominent hardware.

■ All of these are devastating complications that may lead to salvage operations, including glenohumeral arthrodesis.

■ Overtightening of the joint and consequent degenerative changes are also fairly common problems.

Rehabilitation Failure

■ The typical patient will spend 2 hours in the operating room but many days in the therapist's office.

■ This fact is simply forgotten by many, not the least of which is the surgeon.

■ To that end, the most common rehabilitation error is that of failure to complete the process (and in some cases, not to institute it at all).

■ A thorough rehabilitation focus, beginning with scapulothoracic stabilization and strengthening with a progression to proprioceptive neuromuscular facilitation, is integral to returning patients to their preoperative activity level.

SUMMARY

The treatment of posterior and MDI continues to be a challenging clinical problem with more questions than answers. Nonoperative treatment with concerted physical therapy remains the cornerstone of treatment in most patients, with excellent results obtained in most patients in the available literature.

Some, however, will fail nonoperative measures. The important principles to apply with respect to operative intervention are to adequately assess the patient for all possible directions of instability and then to address these areas during the procedure. The use of arthroscopy in these situations allows for a thorough diagnosis and should be used in most cases.

The surgical approach undertaken obviously varies from case to case. Either traditional open means or newer arthroscopic techniques appear to produce good to excellent results in the majority of patients, when done properly.

Appropriate return to activities is guided by the surgical approach. In nearly all cases, the most important aspect is the postoperative rehabilitation that takes into account not only the glenohumeral joint but also the periscapular area.

SUGGESTED READING

Antoniou J, Harryman DT II. Posterior instability. Op Tech Sports Med 2000;8:225–233.

Blasier RN, Soslowsky LJ, Malicky DM, et al. Posterior glenohumeral subluxation: active and passive stabilization in a biomechanical model. J Bone Joint Surg Am 1997;79:433–440.

Burkhart SS, De Beer JF. Traumatic glenohumeral bone defects and their relationship to failure of arthroscopic Bankart repairs: significance of the inverted-pear glenoid and the humeral engaging Hill-Sachs lesion. Arthroscopy 2000;16:677–694.

Burkhead WZJ, Rockwood CAJ. Treatment of instability of the shoulder with an exercise program. J Bone Joint Surg Am 1992;74:890–896.

Choi CH, Ogilvie-Harris DJ. Inferior capsular shift operation for multidirectional instability of the shoulder in players of contact sports. Br J Sports Med 2002;36:290–294.

Cooper RA, Brems JJ. The inferior capsular shift procedure for multidirectional instability of the shoulder. J Bone Joint Surg Am 1992;74:1516–1522.

Curl LA, Warren RF. Glenohumeral joint stability: selective cutting studies on the static capsular restraints. Clin Orthop 1996;330:54–65.

Eberly VC, McMahon PJ, Lee TQ. Variation in the glenoid origin of the anteroinferior glenohumeral capsulolabrum. Clin Orthop 2002;400:26–31.

Gartsman GM, Roddey TS, Hammerman SM. Arthroscopic treatment of multidirectional glenohumeral instability: 2- to 5-year follow-up. Arthroscopy 2001;17:236–243.

Harryman DT, Sidles JA, Harris SL, et al. The role of the rotator interval capsule in passive motion and stability of the shoulder. J Bone Joint Surg Am 1992;74:53–66.

Kibler WB. The role of the scapula in athletic shoulder function. Am J Sports Med 1998;26:325–337.

Mair SD, Zarzour RH, Speer KP. Posterior labral injury in contact athletes. Am J Sports Med 1998;26:753–758.

Miniaci A, McBirnie J. Thermal capsular shrinkage for treatment of multidirectional instability of the shoulder. J Bone Joint Surg Am 2003;85:2283–2287.

Neer CS II, Foster CR. Inferior capsular shift for involuntary inferior and multidirectional instability of the shoulder: a preliminary report. J Bone Joint Surg Am 1980;62:897–908.

Nobuhara K, Ikeda H. Rotator interval lesion. Clin Orthop Relat Res 1987;223:44–50.

Rodosky MW, Harner CJ, Fu FH. The role of the long head of the biceps muscle and superior glenoid labrum in anterior instability of the shoulder. Am J Sports Med 1994;22:121–126.

Rowe CR, Pierce DS, Clark JG. Voluntary dislocation of the shoulder: a preliminary report on a clinical, electromyographic and psychiatric study of twenty-six patients. J Bone Joint Surg Am 1973;55:445–460.

Rowe CR, Zarins B. Recurrent transient subluxation of the shoulder. J Bone Joint Surg Am 1981;63:863–872.

Savoie FH, Field LD. Arthroscopic management of posterior shoulder instability. Oper Tech Sports Med 1997;5:226–232.

Treacy SH, Savoie FH III, Field LD. Arthroscopic treatment of multidirectional instability. J Shoulder Elbow Surg 1999;8:345–350.

Uhthoff HK, Piscopo M. Anterior capsular redundancy of the shoulder: congenital or traumatic? An embryological study. J Bone Joint Surg Am 1985;67:363–366.

Warner JJP, Micheli LJ, Arslenian LE, et al. Scapulothoracic motion in normal shoulders and shoulders with glenohumeral instability and impingement syndrome. A study using Moire topographic analysis. Clin Orthop 1992;285:191–199.

Wirth MA, Groh GI, Rockwood CA. Capsulorrhaphy through an anterior approach for the treatment of atraumatic posterior glenohumeral instability with multidirectional laxity of the shoulder. J Bone Joint Surg Am 1998;80:1570–1578.

Zabinsky SJ, Callaway GH, Cohen S, et al. Revision shoulder stabilization: 2- to 10-year results. J Shoulder Elbow Surg 1999;8:58–65.

DISORDERS OF THE ROTATOR CUFF

ALAN S. CURTIS
ABRAHAM T. SHURLAND

The treatment of rotator cuff disorders is currently an area of intensive research with advances continually being made. Our understanding of the causes of rotator cuff disease in the athlete has grown enormously, as have surgical techniques. This chapter is intended to provide an introduction to rotator cuff disorders. A general overview of the anatomy and biomechanics of the rotator cuff will be presented, followed by an overview of some of the major disorders of the rotator cuff, including impingement, rotator cuff tears, and calcific tendinopathy.

ANATOMY

Although the basic structure of the rotator cuff has long been known, advancements are still being made to our knowledge of the details of its structure. Most recently, the size and shape of the insertions of the rotator cuff into the humeral head have been described, which has implications for the treatment of rotator cuff repairs.

The rotator cuff is a blending of the tendinous insertions of four muscles: the supraspinatus, infraspinatus, subscapularis, and teres minor. These muscles originate on the scapula and insert into the tuberosities of the humeral head. The supraspinatus originates on the supraspinatus fossa and passes under the acromial arch to insert on the superior aspect of the greater tuberosity. It is innervated by the su-

prascapular nerve, which courses under the transverse scapular ligament in the suprascapular notch. The supraspinatus allows abduction of the humerus. The infraspinatus originates on the infraspinatus fossa and inserts on the posterior aspect of the greater tuberosity. It is innervated by the continuation of the suprascapular nerve after the nerve courses around the spinoglenoid notch. The teres minor runs just inferior to the infraspinatus, inserts on the posterior inferior aspect of the tuberosity, and is innervated by the axillary nerve. Both the infraspinatus and the teres minor are external rotators of the shoulder. Finally, the subscapularis originates on the anterior surface of the scapula and inserts on the lesser tuberosity. It is the most powerful of the rotator cuff muscles, and it allows internal rotation. The subscapularis is composed of two parts: (a) the upper portion, which is multipennate and the greater force generator; and (b) the lower portion, which has a parallel arrangement of fibers. The upper portion of the muscle is innervated by the upper subscapular nerve, and the lower portion of the muscle is innervated by the lower subscapular nerve. The tendons of these four muscles all blend with each other and with the underlying capsule before inserting into the humerus.

The microscopic anatomy of the supraspinatus and infraspinatus tendons has been studied and broken into five layers (Table 19-1 and Fig. 19-1). The space between the su-

TABLE 19-1 LAYERS OF THE SUPRASPINATUS AND INFRASPINATUS TENDONS

Layer	Description
1	On the cephalad surface or bursal surface; composed of fibers of the coracohumeral ligament
2	Primary load-bearing layer. Consists of a parallel arrangement of collagen fibers
3	Collagen fibers smaller and more randomly oriented than layer 2
4	Deep extension of the coracohumeral ligament. Fibers in this layer run transverse to the direction of the fibers in layer 2. Thought to tie the other layers together and distribute forces from one part of the cuff to the other. The major component of layer 4 can be seen arthroscopically from the undersurface of the cuff as a crescent-shaped thickening known as the "rotator cuff cable."
5	Capsular layer

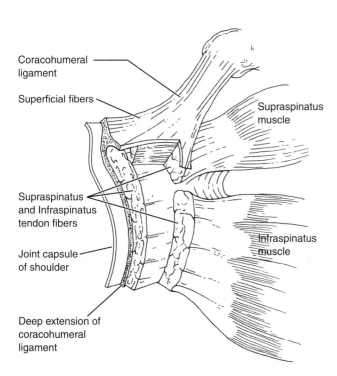

Figure 19-1   Schematic diagram of a transverse section through the supraspinatus and infraspinatus tendons and capsule of the shoulder. (After Clark JM, Harryman DT II. Tendons, ligaments, and capsule of the rotator cuff: gross and microscopic anatomy. J Bone Joint Surg Am 1992;74:713–725. © 1992 The Journal of Bone and Joint Surgery.)

praspinatus and the subscapularis is known as the rotator interval. This interval is pierced by the tendon of the long head of the biceps. The rotator interval is composed of a complex interweaving of fibers of the leading edge of the supraspinatus, the superior edge of the subscapularis, and the coracohumeral and superior glenohumeral ligaments. The coracohumeral ligament forms layer 1 of the supraspinatus tendon as shown in Figure 19-1. This layer continues anteriorly to form the roof of the interval and the superior aspect of the biceps tendon sheath. The floor of the sheath is composed of fibers of the superior glenohumeral ligament and subscapularis tendon.

The muscle bellies of the rotator cuff muscles transition into the tendinous cuff, and this inserts into the bone of the humeral head. The humeral head is made up of the articular surface, the greater and lesser tuberosities, and the bicipital groove that separates the tuberosities. The shape and size of the footprint of insertion of the rotator cuff tendons have received interest recently because arthroscopic techniques have allowed the diagnosis and treatment of partial undersurface cuff tears. Knowledge of the insertional footprint allows the surgeon to estimate the size of a partial tear.

- The subscapularis has the largest of the footprints. It is, on average, comma-shaped, 40 mm long, and 19 mm wide. The insertion initially blends with the capsule then tapers to a well-defined tendon that is discrete from the capsule as it crosses the joint and becomes the subscapularis muscle.
- The supraspinatus footprint is rectangular, 23 mm long, and 16 mm wide.
- The infraspinatus has the second largest footprint. It wraps and interdigitates with supraspinatus superiorly and is 28 mm long and 18 mm wide.
- The teres minor has the smallest insertion. The footprint measures 28 mm × 10 mm.
- If the right proximal humerus is viewed from the perspective of the glenoid, the subscapularis extends from 7 to 11 o'clock. The supraspinatus goes from 11:30 to 1 o'clock. The infraspinatus then continues from 12:30 to 3 o'clock and is followed by the teres minor, which goes from 3 o'clock to 5 o'clock.

The acromial arch is composed of the acromial process, which is a continuation of the spine of the scapula. The arch is completed by the coracoacromial ligament, which extends from the coracoid to the anterior inferior edge of the acromion. The supraspinatus tendon passes under the acromial arch on its way to its insertion on the greater tuberosity. The acromial arch and the humeral head can be thought of as forming a container. The contents of the container are the supraspinatus tendon, the biceps tendon, and the subacromial bursa. Reduction in the size of the container or increases in the volume of its contents can result in there being insufficient space for the supraspinatus tendon—a condition called "impingement."

BIOMECHANICS

The rotator cuff has two main functions: to provide stability to the glenohumeral joint and to allow shoulder motion.

Absence of a fully functioning subscapularis has been shown to result in increasing internal rotation weakness as the limit of motion is approached. The subscapularis also acts as a restraint to anterior subluxation of the humerus and a restraint to passive external rotation. The infraspinatus and teres minor have been shown to provide 80% of external rotation force, and the supraspinatus provides 50% of abduction torque output for shoulder elevation.

The main function of the rotator cuff has traditionally been thought to produce motion of the glenohumeral joint. However, recent biomechanical studies have thrown light on the stabilizing function of the rotator cuff, and many now believe that this may be its primary role. The bony architecture of the shoulder provides little stability to the glenohumeral joint. Most of its stability is provided by the soft tissues that surround it, including the capsuloligamentous structures. The rotator cuff provides dynamic stability to counteract the potentially destabilizing effect of the other muscles of the shoulder girdle, such as the effect of the deltoid muscle in abduction of the shoulder. In the absence of the stabilizing effect of the cuff, the deltoid will cause the humerus to migrate proximally. This destroys the fulcrum of glenohumeral rotation, making abduction more difficult. The rotator cuff muscles are located close to the joint. This is ideal for performing their stabilizing function. The infraspinatus and subscapularis co-contract to provide compression across the glenohumeral joint. The supraspinatus works as a humeral head depressor. Contraction of this muscle changes the resultant vector across the joint to a more inferiorly directed force and thus counteracts the force of the deltoid, which is directed superiorly.

TENDON DEGENERATION

There are two major theories for the development of rotator cuff disease, the intrinsic and extrinsic theories. The intrinsic theory holds that tendon degeneration is the result of changes in the mechanical properties of the tendons. This may be because of several factors, including aging and poor vascularity. The abnormal cuff is no longer able to perform its function to stabilize the glenohumeral joint, which can result in a high-riding humeral head and subacromial impingement. This then adds further trauma to the tendons and leads to further degeneration.

The extrinsic theory suggests that factors external to the tendons are the primary cause of the disorder. Factors such as repetitive overuse, tensile overload, and impingement begin the process of tendon degeneration, which results in destabilization of the joint and then further impingement. Today, we understand tendon degeneration to be multifactorial and dependent on both intrinsic and extrinsic causes.

SPECIFIC DISORDERS

Impingement

In the past decade, the concept of impingement has grown from the classic subacromial process to a broad category of extrinsic sources of injury to the rotator cuff. Impingement can now be broken down into two main categories, external and internal.

- *External impingement* refers to pathologic contact between the rotator cuff and structures outside the shoulder joint.
  - Subacromial impingement is the most common form of external impingement. In this disorder, the undersurface of the acromion and structures in the subacromial space are the offending agents.
  - Anterior impingement is another form of external impingement. It occurs when the coracoid process comes into contact with the subscapularis with internal rotation maneuvers.
- *Internal impingement* involves abnormal contact between the rotator cuff and structures within the shoulder joint itself.
  - Posterior impingement is a form of this and is primarily a disorder of overhead athletes. In these individuals, abnormal contact is made between the posterior supraspinatus and infraspinatus and the posterior superior glenoid when the arm is in the fully cocked position.

Subacromial Impingement

Epidemiology and Pathophysiology. Subacromial impingement is by far the most common form of impingement. As the supraspinatus tendon travels from the supraspinous fossa to the greater tuberosity of the humerus, it travels under the acromial arch. This arch limits the upward excursion of the tendon. Under normal circumstances, the humeral head remains located on the glenoid, and there is sufficient room for the tendon to travel without impingement. In pathologic states, however, the size of the "container"—and thus the space for the tendon—is diminished (Fig. 19-2).

Neer coined the term "impingement syndrome" in 1972. In his classic article, he implicated the anterior acromion, the coracoacromial ligament, and the acromioclavicular joint. He classified impingement into three stages: tendon inflammation, fibrosis, and cuff tear. Bigliani showed in cadaveric studies that there is a relationship between the morphology of the acromion and the presence of cuff tears. He defined three acromial shapes: type 1 (flat), type 2 (curved), and type 3 (with an anterior hook; Fig. 19-3), which occurred in 17%, 43%, and 40% of the specimens, respectively. Of the specimens with rotator cuff tears, 75% of these had type 3 acromial morphology.

In older patients, primary factors such as acromial shape and coracoacromial ligament hypertrophy lead to impingement. In the younger athletic population, secondary impingement as a result of instability is much more common. Subtle glenohumeral laxity can allow superior migration of the humeral head with overhead activities. Another factor that should not be overlooked in the young patient presenting with impingement is the possibility of an os acromiale. The acromion is formed by the union of three ossification centers that are usually fused by age 22—the preacromion, the mesacromion, and the metacromion (Fig. 19-4). Persistent nonunion of these centers of ossification is called an "os acromiale." The incidence of os acromiale in the general

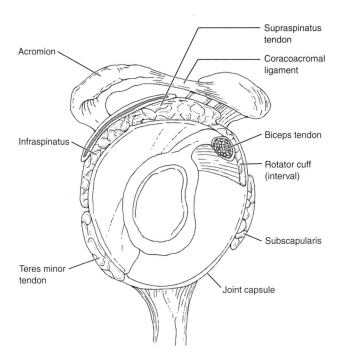

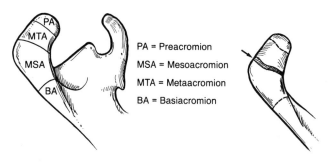

Figure 19-4 Ossification centers of the acromion. The most common site of failure of ossification is between the mesoacromion and the meta-acromion. (From Butters KP. Fractures of the scapula. In: Bucholz RW, Heckman JD. Rockwood and Green's Fractures in Adults, 5th ed. Baltimore: Lippincott Williams & Wilkins, 2001:1079–2263.)

Figure 19-2 Bigliani classification of acromion shape as determined on the outlet view. (After Curtis AS, Wilson P. Shoulder pain in the workplace. Orthop Clin North Am 1996;27:763–781.)

population is estimated to be between 2.7% and 6%. As many as 60% of these cases are bilateral. Norris and Bigliani (1993) noted an association between persistent os acromiale and impingement. The most common site of persistent nonunion is the growth plate between the mesacromion and the metacromion.

Injury to the rotator cuff or its innervation can result in an inability of the cuff to generate the normal compressive forces across the glenohumeral joint. This causes an imbalance to occur between the stabilizing forces of the rotator cuff and the destabilizing forces of the powerful deltoid muscle, which can result in subacromial impingement with elevation of the arm. The loss of the scapular stabilizing

muscles, as is seen with winging of the scapula, can cause the normal scapular rotation to be lost. The scapula will then fail to rotate out of the way, when the arm is brought overhead, which may also result in impingement.

Diagnosis

History and Physical Examination

- Patients with subacromial impingement will complain of shoulder pain, usually over the anterior-lateral deltoid and exacerbated by overhead activity.
- The pain can radiate down the arm but usually not below the elbow.
- Night pain is an almost constant feature of subacromial impingement, and patients will avoid sleeping on the affected shoulder.
- The Neer impingement sign and the Hawkins test are both provocative tests intended to reproduce the patient's impingement by reducing the subacromial space.
  - With a positive Neer impingement sign, the patient's pain is elicited by forced abduction of the humerus while stabilizing the scapula (see Fig. 15-4 in Chapter 15).

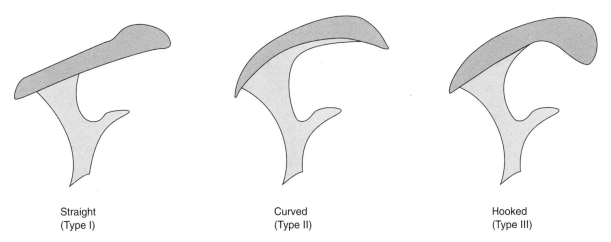

Straight (Type I)   Curved (Type II)   Hooked (Type III)

Figure 19-3 Anatomy of impingement. (After Curtis AS, Wilson P. Shoulder pain in the workplace. Orthop Clin North Am 1996;27:763–781.)

■ In the Hawkins test, the patient is made to grasp the contralateral shoulder and the arm is abducted by elevating the elbow (see Fig. 15-5 in Chapter 15). This forces the greater tuberosity into the acromion, causing pain.
■ In the Neer impingement test, the patient's shoulder pain goes away with a subacromial injection of lidocaine.
  ■ A recent study has shown the value of this test. Results of subacromial decompression in patients with a positive impingement test were compared with those that were negative. Patents with a positive impingement test were 28% more likely to be improved by subacromial decompression 12 months after surgery than those with a negative result.

Radiologic Examination
■ Radiographs are all that is required for evaluation of subacromial impingement.
■ Standard anteroposterior x-ray is useful for assessing the bony architecture of the glenohumeral joint.
■ Calcific tendonitis can be seen in this view as can arthritis of the acromioclavicular joint.
■ A lateral downslope in the acromion can also be seen in this view.
■ The supraspinatus outlet view is taken with the x-ray beam directed 10 degrees caudally. This shows the acromial morphology best.
■ Magnetic resonance imaging (MRI) can be performed when a rotator cuff tear is suspected but is usually unnecessary for isolated impingement. MRI allows an enlarged coracoacromial ligament to be evaluated. Rotator cuff tears and tendonitis can also be seen.

Treatment
Nonsurgical Treatment
■ Treatment of impingement begins with therapy, rest, ice, and nonsteroidal anti-inflammatory drugs.
■ Therapy consists mainly of rotator cuff strengthening exercises to better enable the rotator cuff to counteract the proximally directed force of the deltoid and depress the humeral head.
■ Steroid injections into the subacromial space can also be used.

Surgical Treatment. Should nonoperative management fail, operative treatment with subacromial decompression is indicated. Radical acromionectomy was performed early in the treatment of impingement. This often resulted in disability for the patient because the deltoid was rendered incompetent by the procedure.

Neer believed that the architecture of the acromion should be preserved. He proposed anterior acromioplasty, which requires the removal of a wedge of bone from the acromion, with most of the resected bone coming from the undersurface of the acromion. A high degree of success was reported with this procedure in older patients with percentage success in the 1980s and 1990s. In younger pitchers, one study showed that a good functional result was achieved in only 22% of patients, likely pointing to the different etiology of impingement in this subset of patients.

■ Arthroscopic acromioplasty was first described by Ellman (1987). The arthroscopic approach provides many advantages.
  ■ The deltoid attachment is not disturbed, so the patient can undergo more aggressive rehabilitation early on.
  ■ The acromioclavicular (AC) joint can be inspected and co-planed if needed.
  ■ At the same time, the glenohumeral joint can be inspected and any other pathology can be treated if warranted.
  ■ Rotator cuff tears, biceps tendon pathology, and glenohumeral arthritis can all be diagnosed.
  ■ Results of arthroscopic decompressions are equivalent to the open procedures with few complications.
■ Our preferred method of acromioplasty is based on the technique described by Snyder.
  ■ The supraspinatus outlet view is used to plan the procedure.
  ■ The thickness and shape of the acromion are determined.
  ■ The arthroscope is introduced through a standard posterior portal.
  ■ The glenohumeral joint is arthroscoped first and any intra-articular pathology treated.
  ■ The undersurface of the rotator cuff is inspected.
  ■ The arthroscope is then introduced into the subacromial space.
  ■ A lateral portal is established in line with the posterior edge of the clavicle.
  ■ A shaver and arthroscopic Bovie are used to remove bursal tissue.
  ■ The undersurface of the acromion is then cleared of soft tissue, and the coracoacromial ligament is peeled off of the anterior inferior edge of the acromion but not completely detached.
  ■ A 4.0-mm arthroscopic burr is introduced through a lateral portal, and a line is made in the undersurface of the acromion just behind the acromioclavicular joint, running from medial to lateral.
  ■ This line marks the posterior edge of the resection and acts as a guide to further work.
  ■ Removal of bone begins laterally and progresses medially with the 30-degree arthroscope oriented toward the undersurface of the acromion.
  ■ A flat surface is created, starting at the guide line and working forward (Fig. 19-5).
  ■ Care is taken not to detach the deltoid fascia.
  ■ The scope is then switched to the lateral portal, and the burr is brought in posteriorly.
  ■ Using the posterior acromion as a template, the transition zone between the posterior acromion and the anterior is smoothed.
  ■ Care is taken to remove the acromial facet all the way to the AC joint.
  ■ If the AC joint is hypertrophic, the undersurface of the clavicle can be co-planed to prevent impingement at this location.

Internal Impingement

Epidemiology and Pathophysiology. Internal impingement is a disorder primarily of overhead athletes such as

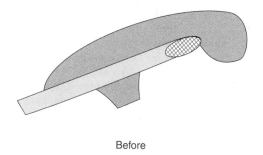 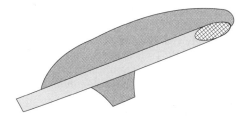

Before   After

Figure 19-5   Converting a type 3 to a type 1 (flat) acromion. (After Curtis AS, Wilson P. Shoulder pain in the workplace. Orthop Clin North Am 1996;27:763–781.)

pitchers. It involves the coming into contact of the undersurface of the posterior supraspinatus and infraspinatus with the posterior superior glenoid labrum when the arm is in the fully cocked throwing position. The cause of this disorder is a source of controversy with two competing theories currently under investigation.

One theory is that the anterior capsule becomes stretched out with overuse, allowing the impingement to occur with the arm fully externally rotated and abducted to 90 degrees.

The other theory suggests that the primary lesion is the posterior capsule that becomes tight through scar tissue formation as a result of the eccentric overload of the posterior cuff as it decelerates during follow-through. This tightness forces the humeral head to rise up when the athlete assumes the cocked throwing position.

Diagnosis
- Patients complain of pain, usually in the posterior shoulder. There is a loss of internal rotation and excessive external rotation.
- A careful physical examination is important to document the patient's arc of motion.
  - The examination is performed with the patient supine on the examining table and both arms abducted to 90 degrees.
  - The elbows are bent to 90 degrees, and the examiner rotates the humerus of each arm to the position of maximal internal and external rotations and compares the motion of the two arms.
  - Normally, the patient will be able to touch his hand to the table in both internal and external rotations.
  - Inability to reach the table in internal rotation and excessive external rotation are the hallmarks of a positive physical examination.

Treatment
- The first line of treatment for internal impingement is physical therapy.
  - The athlete must work aggressively to regain the lost internal rotation.
  - This should be done under the supervision of a therapist experienced in the problems of overhead athletes.
- For the few athletes who fail conservative treatment, arthroscopy is necessary.

- Examination of the undersurface of the rotator cuff may exhibit wear and tear from continued contact with the labrum and the superior labrum may be frayed or detached.
- Repairs of the cuff and any superior labrum anterior-posterior (SLAP) lesions should be performed as indicated.
- The glenohumeral motion problems can be addressed with posterior capsule releases and anterior capsulorraphy as needed to balance the shoulder.

Partial-thickness Rotator Cuff Tears

Classification
Partial-thickness rotator cuff tears (PTRCTs) are a well-defined clinical entity. Our understanding of these tears is quite recent and owes much to the development of arthroscopic surgical techniques. Ellman classified these tears using Neer's classification of rotator cuff disease as a starting point. Neer stage III rotator cuff disease represents the torn rotator cuff, so all partial rotator cuff tears are classified as stage III. Ellman further describes the partial-thickness tear by location: type A is an articular surface tear, type B is a bursal surface tear, and type C is an interstitial tear. The tears are also classified by grade, with grade 1 including tears less than 3 mm deep, grade 2 including tears between 3 and 6 mm deep, and grade 3 including tears deeper than 6 mm.

Pathophysiology
Rotator cuff tears most often begin on the articular side of the cuff. This is believed to be due to the relative hypovascularity of the cuff on the articular side. Histologic studies have shown that the collagen structure on the articular surface of the tendon is less organized and the bundles are smaller, thus resulting in lower mechanical strength. PTRCTs can result from severe cuff tendinosis in which the cuff degenerates over time and then tears when subjected to biomechanical forces. Articular surface tears in overhead athletes can be due to internal impingement. Bursal surface tears are often related to direct attrition of the cuff by subacromial impingement.

Diagnosis
- Clinical findings with PTRCTs cover a spectrum from the findings of simple impingement to those associated with significant rotator cuff tears.

- In overhead athletes, subtle anterior instability of the shoulder may exist.
- MRI is the preferred imaging modality but it has been unreliable for PTRCTs because it can be difficult to differentiate subtle tearing and tendinosis.
- The addition of intra-articular gadolinium can improve the results of MRI significantly.

Treatment

- Surgical options should be entertained when nonsurgical management has failed. Surgical approaches include debridement of the frayed cuff or completion of the tear and repair of the cuff through either arthroscopic or open methods.
- Tendon that is partially torn on the articular surface can be repaired though an arthroscopic transtendonous approach. These tears are known as partial articular supraspinatus tendon avulsion (PASTA) lesions. There are a few generally agreed-on principles to guide the surgeon:
- Bursal surface tears should be treated with subacromial decompression, whereas articular surface tears may be treated with decompression if the clinical situation warrants it.
  - Tears that are more than 50% of the thickness of the tendon should be repaired.
  - If the tendon is torn more than 75%, the tear should be completed and repaired.
- Arthroscopic techniques have a distinct advantage in the treatment of these lesions in that a much better evaluation of articular surface tears can be accomplished by direct visualization of the rotator cuff from under the surface.
  - The extent of the rotator cuff tearing can be estimated on the basis of knowledge of the footprint of insertion of the rotator cuff.
  - When the cuff is viewed arthroscopically, the normal edge of insertion of the cuff (just off the articular surface) can be clearly seen.
  - Knowing that the supraspinatus insertion is 12 to 16 mm wide, the width of the exposed footprint can be measured using a probe, and an estimate of the percentage of the cuff involved can be made.
- Our approach to partial thickness rotator cuff tears is to evaluate the patients under anesthesia for stability. The glenohumeral joint is arthroscoped and the following performed:
  - Frayed cuff is debrided back to healthy tissue.
  - The tear can then be graded for size.
  - In grade 1 and 2 tears, the shoulder is examined for associated pathologies, especially in overhead athletes.
- Grade 3A tears are treated with a PASTA repair.
  - A marking suture is placed through the lesion in articular-sided tears so the other side of the rotator cuff can be examined. This is done by locating the lesion with a spinal needle from the lateral acromion.
  - A portal is then made, and an anchor is placed right through the lesion into the footprint.

- Sutures are then passed retrograde through the cuff 1 cm anterior and posterior to the midline and slightly medially.
- The sutures are tied from the bursal side of the cuff.
- Tears more than 75% of the tendon or with depths of 9 to 12 mm are completed into a V-shaped tear and repaired from the bursal side using arthroscopic techniques.

Results

Results of debridement and decompression of grade 1 and 2 tears have been good.

- Cordasco et al. compared 105 patients at a mean of 4.5 years after surgery. Patients had either no tear or grade 1 and 2 tears. They found patients with and without tears did equally well, with the exception of grade 2B tears, which had a failure rate of 38%. They suggested that grade 2B tears might be better served by primary repair.
- Weber reported on 65 patients with grade 3 tears. Thirty-three tears were repaired by a miniopen approach, and 32 tears were repaired by debridement and decompression. The University of California–Los Angeles shoulder score was 32 for the repaired cuffs and 25 for the decompressed cuffs, with 6 failures. This study supported the concept of repairing cuff tears greater than 50% of the tendon.

Full-thickness Rotator Cuff Tears

Classification

Rotator cuff tears can be classified in many ways. They can be classified by the age of the tear as acute or chronic. They may be classified as partial or full thickness. When a rotator cuff tear becomes full thickness, it often assumes a recognizable pattern that is determined by the amount of detachment of the tendon and propagation along the adjacent intervals. In many cases, the apex of the tear does not represent the actual point of maximal retraction but instead represents the point of maximal interval propagation. The most common patterns are as follows:

- The crescent-shaped tear is pure detachment of the tendons of the supraspinatus and infraspinatus without interval propagation.
- The L-shaped tear is lateral detachment of the supraspinatus—and sometimes the infraspinatus as well—with propagation along the biceps interval so that the apex of the tear points at the base of the biceps (Fig. 19-6).
- The reverse L-shaped tear is detachment of the tendon laterally but this time with propagation posteriorly, between either the supraspinatus and infraspinatus or infraspinatus and teres minor. The apex of this tear points to the base of the scapula spine.
- With chronicity, many of these large tears, or L-shaped tears, assume a V-shaped pattern, making recognition of the original tear pattern difficult.

Diagnosis

History and Physical Examination

- Rotator cuff tears can occur in healthy tissue as the result of a traumatic event or as the end point in a process of tendon degeneration.

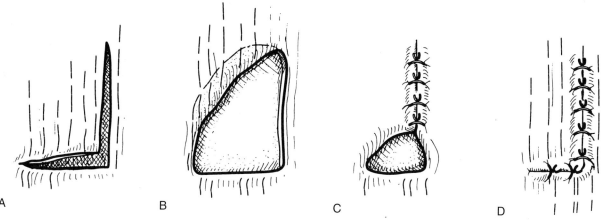

Figure 19-6 **A:** L-shaped rotator cuff tear. **B:** Elasticity of the tendon causes deformation of the L-shaped tear into a U-shaped tear. **C:** Closure of the vertical limb of the tear by side-to-side sutures. **D:** Closure of the horizontal limb of the tear by tendon to bone sutures. (From Burkhart S. Arthroscopic management of rotator cuff tears. In McGinty J, ed. Operative Arthroscopy, 3rd ed. Philadelphia: Lippincott Williams & Wilkins, 2003:512.)

- The diagnosis is usually made clinically and then supported by diagnostic studies.
- Factors such as the age of the tear can complicate the diagnosis.
- A tear that has slowly progressed in size over a period of years may not present with the disabling weakness that an acute tear of the same size would show.
- Patients with small supraspinatus tendon tears will present with complaints similar to those of subacromial impingement, but as the size of the rotator cuff tear increases, weakness usually becomes more profound.
- Strength of the supraspinatus is tested with the arm in 90 degrees of abduction. The patient is asked to resist a downward force by the examiner.
- External rotation strength may be affected in larger tears if the infraspinatus and teres minor are involved. Strength is tested by having the patient hold his or her arms at the side with the elbows bent to 90 degrees and the hands straight out in front. The patient is then asked to rotate externally against the resistance of the examiner.
- Subscapularis testing is done with the liftoff test, in which the patient is asked to place his or her hand behind the back and then lift it off of the back.
- This can be difficult for many patients, even without a subscapularis tear. A simpler test called the belly press test has become more popular and has been shown to isolate the subscapularis equally well. The patient is asked to press his or her hand against the abdomen with the wrist locked in 0 degrees of flexion. Patients with a weak subscapularis will cheat and flex the wrist, allowing the elbow to drop to the side. This allows the patient to recruit accessory muscles to the task.
- Occasionally, patients will present with pain and stiffness, as well as weakness. These patients may have developed a frozen shoulder after an acute rotator cuff tear. This should be carefully noted because the arthrofibrosis should be addressed before any surgical treatment of the rotator cuff can be successful.

Radiologic Examination
- MRI has become the standard imaging modality for the diagnosis of rotator cuff tears.
  - The sensitivity and specificity of the test are reported to be above 90%.
  - MRI allows the surgeon to estimate the shape and size of the tear.
  - The entire shoulder can be evaluated, including the AC joint and the biceps tendon, which are commonly sources of pain.
- Occasionally, patients cannot undergo MRI testing because of metallic implants that could be dislodged by the magnetic field or due to claustrophobia. Ultrasound has been shown to be an excellent alternative to MRI for the diagnosis of rotator cuff tears, although it is somewhat operator-dependent.

Treatment

Indications. The decision to select operative versus nonoperative management of rotator cuff tears involves several factors: the age and health of the patient, the size and acuteness of the tear, and the extent of pain and disability. The clinician must attempt to estimate the risk of progression of the tear and what the effect of progression will be.

- Young and active patients with any size tear are candidates for operative management.
- Any patient with an acute tear should be considered for surgical repair.
- Older patients and patients with chronic massive tears may benefit from a course of nonoperative treatment and have less to lose by delaying surgical intervention.

Surgical Treatment. When operative management is indicated, three options are available to the surgeon: the open approach, the miniopen approach, and the arthroscopic approach.

- The open approach is the traditional method for repairing rotator cuffs, with an excellent track record.
  - It allows good visualization of the rotator cuff and mechanically strong fixation of the tendon to bone through bone tunnels.
  - The main drawbacks of open surgery are the detachment of the deltoid and post operative pain. Partial detachment of the deltoid is inherent to open rotator cuff surgery. Failure of the deltoid repair to heal is a serious complication that can result in disability for the patient.
- The miniopen technique uses arthroscopy to evaluate the rotator cuff tear and perform the acromioplasty if indicated.
  - Once this is completed, the repair is performed through a deltoid-splitting approach that usually involves a simple extension of the lateral portal.
  - This method provides good visualization and spares the deltoid.
  - The surgeon has the option to use bone tunnels, anchors, or a combination of both for fixation.
- The arthroscopic technique has the lowest postoperative pain and preserves the deltoid.
  - It is not faster than the other methods and has a long learning curve associated with it.
  - It relies on anchors for fixation.
  - The technique is relatively new and still evolving. It is gaining increased acceptance in the orthopaedic community.

Our technique of rotator cuff repair is the arthroscopic one. We begin by creating a posterior portal and by introducing the arthroscope into the glenohumeral joint. An anterior portal is established to allow probing of structures and debridement if necessary. The undersurface of the rotator cuff is examined for tears, and some debridement of tears can be performed from within the shoulder joint. The tear is characterized from the undersurface as to its size and if it is partial or full thickness. The scope is than taken into the subacromial space and a lateral portal is established. A subacromial decompression is performed if warranted and an extensive bursectomy to expose the bursal rotator cuff surface. The rotator cuff tear is then classified by tear propagation pattern. This enables the surgeon to develop a strategy for rotator cuff repair. The goal is a tension-free repair. If there is a tear propagation interval as exists in L- and reverse L-shaped tears, the interval can be closed with side-to-side sutures. If this is done correctly, the tear will be reduced back to the footprint of insertion on the tuberosity or close to this. The final steps of the repair involve the use of anchors to repair the torn lateral edge of the cuff back to bone (Fig. 19-6C,D).

Rotator Cuff Tear Arthropathy

Pathophysiology
When rotator cuff disease goes unchecked and massive tears develop, the ability of the rotator cuff to stabilize the glenohumeral joint is lost. Over time, the humeral head, under the force of the deltoid muscle, may begin to migrate proximally until it comes to rest on the under surface of the coracoacromial arch. Degenerative arthritis develops in the shoulder as abnormal pressures are exerted on the cartilage by the incongruent joint. This is a painful, disabling condition.

Treatment
- No treatment of shoulder arthropathy is ideal.
- Relief of pain is the primary goal.
- Debridement of the remaining cuff tissue can provide temporary relief.
- Care must be taken not to take down the coracoacromial ligament because this may be all that is supporting the humeral head as it migrates into the acromion.
- Arthroplasty has been used to treat this condition but without the stabilizing effect of the rotator cuff the glenoid component tends to wear out quickly and so total shoulder arthroplasty has been discouraged in the past. New total shoulder replacement options now exist that show some promise in treating this disorder.

Calcific Tendonitis

Classification and Pathophysiology
Calcific tendonitis of the shoulder is an acute or chronically painful condition that is caused by inflammation around calcium deposits located in the rotator cuff tendons.

The cause of the calcific deposits is unknown but, it is believed to be a cell-mediated process. Sarkar and Uthoff described the natural history as being composed of three stages (Table 19-2 and Fig. 19-7).

TABLE 19-2 NATURAL HISTORY OF CALCIFIC TENDONITIS

Stage	Name	Description
1	Precalcific	Fibrocartilaginous metaplasia of cuff tissue occurs, usually near the undersurface. Patients are asymptomatic at this stage.
2	Calcific	Calcium deposits are laid down and resorbed. The resorptive portion of the calcific stage is marked by the ingrowth of vascular channels and the phagocytosis of the calcium deposits by macrophages. Early in the calcific phase, the deposits are chalky in consistency but as resorption begins to occur, they become toothpastelike and can be under pressure. This tends to be the most painful time in the disease process.
3	Postcalcific	Tendon healing occurs.

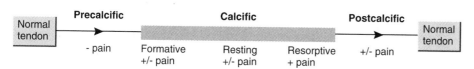

Figure 19-7 Progressive stages of calcific tendonitis. (After Uhthoff HK, Loch JW. Calcific tendinopathy of the rotator cuff: pathogenesis, diagnosis and management. J Am Acad Orthop Surg 1997;5:183–191. ©1997 American Academy of Orthopaedic Surgeons.)

Treatment

- Treatment is nonoperative in the majority of cases.
- Nonsteroidal anti-inflammatory medications, subacromial injections, therapy, and ultrasound have a role in the reduction of symptoms.
- Extracorporeal shock-wave therapy has demonstrated a 70% success rate.
  - Most of the operative treatment of calcific tendonitis is done by arthroscopy.
  - The articular surface of the cuff is examined first.
  - A strawberry-colored lesion often indicates the location of the deposit.
  - The lesion can be tagged with a suture so that it can be accessed from the bursal surface of the rotator cuff.
  - The arthroscope is then introduced into the subacromial space in which a bursectomy is performed.
  - Needling of the deposit with an 18-gauge spinal needle decompresses the lesion.

SUGGESTED READING

Altcheck DW, Dines DM. Shoulder injuries in the throwing athlete. J Am Acad Orthop Surg 1995;3:159–165.

Bigliani L, Norris TR, Fischer J, et al. The relationship between the unfused acromial epiphysis and subacromial impingement lesions. Orthop Trans 1983;7:138.

Bigliani LU, Morrison DS, April EW. The morphology of the acromion and its relationship to rotator cuff tears. Orthop Trans 1986;10:228.

Burkhart SS, Morgan CD, Kibler WB. Shoulder injuries in overhead athletes: the "dead arm" revisited. Clin Sports Med 2000;19:125–158.

Clark JM, Harryman DT II. Tendons, ligaments and capsule of the rotator cuff: gross and microscopic anatomy, J Bone Joint Surg Am 1992;74:713-725.

Cordasco FA, Backer M, Craig EV, et al. The partial-thickness rotator cuff tear: is acromioplasty without repair sufficient? Am J Sports Med 2002;30:257–260.

Ellman H. Arthroscopic subacromial decompression: analysis of one to three year results. Arthroscopy 1987;3:173–181.

Ellman H. Diagnosis and treatment of incomplete rotator cuff tears. Clin Orthop 1990;254:64–74.

Hurt G, Baker CL. Calcific tendonitis of the shoulder. Orthop Clin North Am 2003;34:567–575.

Izquierdo R, Stanwood WG, Bigliani LU. Arthroscopic acromioplasty: history rationale and technique. Instr Course Lect 2004;54:13–20.

MacDonald PB, Clark P, Sutherland K. An analysis of the diagnostic accuracy of the Hawkins and Neer subacromial impingement signs. J Shoulder Elbow Surg 2000;9:299–301.

Neer CS II. Anterior acromioplasty for the chronic impingement syndrome in the shoulder: a preliminary report. J Bone Joint Surg Am 1972;54:41–50.

Snyder SJ. Subacromial Decompression. Shoulder Arthroscopy. New York: McGraw-Hill, 1994:153–155.

Tibone JE, Jobe FW, Kerlan RK, et al. Shoulder impingement syndrome in patients treated by anterior acromioplasty. Clin Orthop 1985;198:134–140.

Weber SC. Arthroscopic debridement and acromioplasty versus mini-open repair in the treatment of significant partial thickness rotator cuff tears. Arthroscopy 1999;15:126–131.

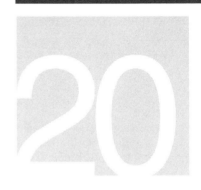

DISORDERS OF THE ACROMIOCLAVICULAR AND STERNOCLAVICULAR JOINTS

MARK J. LEMOS
KELTON BURBANK
JENNIFER TANIGUCHI

ACROMIOCLAVICULAR JOINT

The acromioclavicular (AC) and sternoclavicular (SC) joints serve as the primary links in the suspension of the upper extremity from the axial skeleton. Despite its requisite strength, the AC joint is one of the most commonly injured structures in the athletic population, particularly in young males involved in collision sports. It is also susceptible to overuse injury in the overhead athlete. More than 60 different procedures have been described to treat these injuries, indicative of the lack of consensus historically. More recently, however, the treatment of AC joint pathology has evolved dramatically, especially with the introduction of arthroscopic techniques. This chapter will first describe the anatomy and biomechanics of the AC joint to clarify the complex pathophysiology of injuries to this area. This will facilitate an understanding of the diagnosis and treatment options, which are then reviewed.

Anatomy and Biomechanics

The AC joint is a diarthrodial joint formed by the distal clavicle and the medial facet of the acromion with an ex-

tremely variable orientation. A fibrocartilaginous disk of variable size, shape, and composition resides within the joint. A complete disk is seen in less than 10% of the general population. The frequency with which it is found decreases dramatically with age; nevertheless, it becomes nonfunctional in most individuals after about age 40.

The AC joint first appears at 3 to 5 years of life. The clavicle, which is one of the first bones to ossify, appears first at intrauterine week 5. It increases in diameter via intramembranous ossification. Two epiphyses, one on the medial end and one on the lateral end, contribute to the longitudinal growth via enchondral activity. The medial epiphysis is responsible for the majority of this growth, appearing at about age 18 and fusing between ages 22 and 25. The lateral epiphysis is less consistent and is often mistaken for a fracture in young adults. The acromion has between 2 and 5 ossification centers that appear at puberty. They fuse by age 25. Failure of any of these apophyses to fuse is known as an "os acromiale," which can also be mistaken for a fracture.

The AC joint has a relatively thin capsule, which is supported by the strong AC ligaments, as well as the fascia from the deltoid and the trapezius muscles. The superior,

BOX 20-1 PRIMARY LIGAMENT RESTRAINTS OF THE AC JOINT

Conoid
- Anterior
- Superior

Trapezoid
- Compression

Acromioclavicular ligaments
- Posterior
- Distraction

inferior, anterior, and posterior AC ligaments provide resistance to horizontal translation (Box 20-1). Of these, the superior ligament is the strongest, providing 56% of the resistance to horizontal translation of the clavicle in serial sectioning studies, followed by the posterior ligament, which provided 25%. The insertion of these ligaments on the clavicle averaged about 1.5 cm from the AC joint. This is important when considering distal clavicle resection for AC joint arthrosis (Fig. 20-1).

The coracoclavicular (CC) ligaments—the conoid and the trapezoid—which provide resistance to vertical displacements, further stabilize the AC joint. The more lateral trapezoid is a broad ligament that runs obliquely from the superior surface of the coracoid process to the inferior aspect of the clavicle about 1 cm medial to the AC joint. The more medial conoid ligament is conical in shape and arises along the posteromedial side of the coracoid process. It inserts posteriorly along the undersurface of the clavicle at the junction of the lateral and middle thirds. Both are posterior to the insertion of the pectoralis minor on the coracoid. There is often a bursa separating these two limbs of the CC ligament. The average distance between the coracoid and the clavicle is 1.1 to 1.3 cm, which is important in the diagnosis of complete disruptions of the joint. Sectioning studies have shown the importance of these ligaments is a function of both the direction and the magnitude of the deforming force.

The coracoacromial (CA) ligament runs from the lateral aspect of the coracoid to the undersurface of the acromion. Its function in the stability of the AC joint was originally thought to be important; however, more recent studies imply that it does not have a significant role with forces at or equal to 70 N. It is an important secondary glenohumeral stabilizer, particularly in the presence of a complete rotator cuff tear.

The AC joint has 6 degrees of freedom in allowing motion in the anterior/posterior and superior/inferior planes. Originally, studies by Inman (1944) hypothesized 20 degrees of motion at the AC joint, with forward elevation and abduction of the arm and 40 degrees of clavicular rotation in total. This led many to the conclusion that arthrodesis of the AC joint would limit motion of the shoulder. Subsequent work by Rockwood and Kennedy and Cameron (1954) demonstrated "synchronous scapuloclavicular rotation." Thus, as the clavicle rotates upward, the scapula rotates simultaneously downward. There is 40 to 50 degrees of clavicular rotation but only 5 to 8 degrees at the AC joint. The majority of the rotation occurs at the SC joint.

Epidemiology

Injuries to the AC joint are very common in the athletic population. In an early study, Thorndike and Quigley (1942) noted AC joint injuries in 223 of 578 (39%) athletes with shoulder injuries. Since then, AC joint injuries have been reported to be one of the most common traumatic injuries in rugby, football, ice hockey, skiing, cycling, and snowmobiling. Overuse injuries of the AC joint are also commonly seen in players of golf, baseball, and tennis. AC injuries are much more common in males than females (5 to 10:1) and in young adults. In a review of dislocations of the shoulder complex, dislocations of the glenohumeral joint occurred in 85%, the AC joint in 12%, and the SC joint in 3% (Cave, 1958). However, incomplete injuries are twice as common as complete injuries. As the population ages (and more specifically the athletic population), there will likely be an increase in acute injuries to the AC joint in older individuals as well as an increase in AC joint arthrosis, which has been correlated with previous traumatic injury.

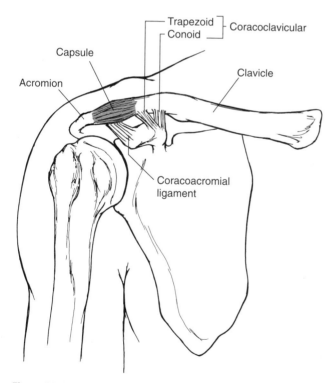

Figure 20-1 The AC joint is supported by the capsule, AC ligaments, and the CC ligament. (From Oatis CA. Kinesiology: The Mechanics and Pathomechanics of Human Movement. Baltimore: Lippincott Williams & Wilkins, 2004.)

Etiology

Either direct or indirect forces can injure the AC joint. The most common etiology is a fall onto the anterior, superior edge of the acromion ("point of the shoulder") with the arm in an adducted position. This drives the acromion downward, away from the fixed clavicle. The resulting appearance of the shoulder is secondary to this movement, not an upward displacement of the clavicle, despite its prominence. Injury can also occur indirectly, via a fall onto an adducted, outstretched arm or elbow, which can cause the humerus to translocate superiorly, forcing the humeral head up and into the acromion. Another indirect mechanism that has been described is a sudden downward force on the upper extremity, such as a change in the position of a heavy load, which pulls the scapula downward. Both of these indirect mechanisms are rare, compared with direct trauma from a fall onto the acromion.

Pathophysiology and Classification

Tossy (1963) and Allman (1967) originally classified AC joint injuries into types I, II, and III on the basis of x-rays and clinical examination. This was later revised by Rockwood (1989) to account for differences he saw within "type III" injuries. He added types IV, V, and VI to account for these differences (Fig. 20-2 and Table 20-1).

Trauma to the AC joint initially injures the AC ligaments (type I). When the force continues, further energy is absorbed by the CC ligaments (type II) and may result in even greater displacement of the joint as these ligaments rupture

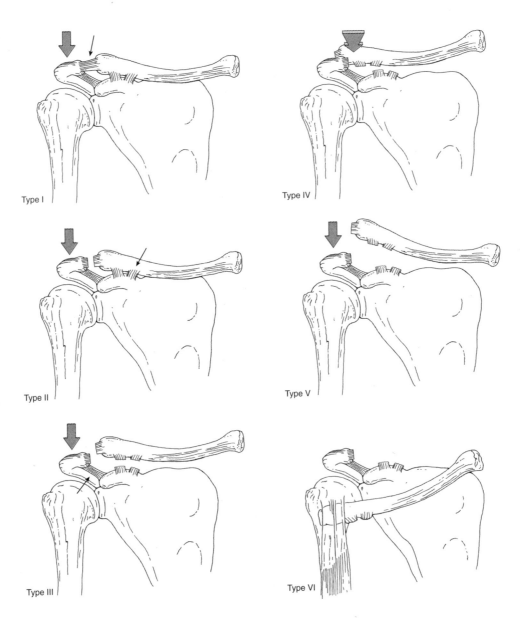

Type I

Type II

Type III

Type IV

Type V

Type VI

Figure 20-2 Classification of AC joint instability.

TABLE 20-1 CLASSIFICATION OF AND CLINICAL FINDINGS FOR AC JOINT INJURIES

Type	Description	Classification
I	The AC ligaments are sprained, but intact. The CC ligaments and the deltotrapezial fascia are uninjured. The AC joint is intact.	No obvious deformity of the shoulder girdle; pain at the AC joint with palpation and some mild swelling. ROM of the shoulder is comfortable and full, except cross-shoulder adduction.
II	The AC ligaments are torn. The CC ligaments are sprained, but intact. The deltotrapezial fascia is typically uninjured. The AC joint is subluxed, unstable in the horizontal plane.	Slight prominence of the clavicle; swelling at the AC joint; pain to palpation over the AC joint and in the costoclavicular interspace. ROM is painful. There is some horizontal instability to the clavicle noted with testing.
III	The AC ligaments are torn. The CC ligaments are torn. The deltotrapezial fascia is sprained. The AC joint is subluxed (<100%), and unstable in the horizontal and vertical planes.	The clavicle is again prominent with marked swelling. There is significant pain at rest and with palpation, ROM testing, which usually cannot be tolerated. The clavicle feels unstable in both the horizontal and vertical planes.
IV	Same as type III, except the clavicle is 100% displaced posteriorly into or through the trapezius muscle.	Typically, the patient has more pain than in type III. The displacement of the joint may not be as apparent as in type III because it is posterior, nor does the clavicle feel "free floating." ROM is not tolerated well.
V	Same as type III, but with >100% displacement of joint in the vertical plane. The deltotrapezial fascia is torn.	Very similar to type III in presentation, except level of pain is greater and the clavicle seems to be more prominent (Fig. 20-3). Skin is likely tented.
VI	Same as type III, but the clavicle is displaced inferior to the coracoid process and posterior to the conjoined tendon. This is very rare and usually the result of severe trauma.	Shoulder appears to be flatter as the clavicle is displaced downward. The acromion is more prominent. There may be an associated neurological injury. Careful assessment for other injuries (rib fracture, pneumothorax, SC joint dislocation) is critical.
VII	Complete dislocation of the AC and SC joints. It is a severe form of a type IV, with a posterior clavicle dislocation.	

AC, acromioclavicular; CC, coracoclavicular; ROM, range of motion; SC, sternoclavicular.

(type III). An even more severe injury may occur with larger forces that result in the disruption of the deltotrapezial fascia, as well as the ligaments (type V). If the deforming force is directed posteriorly and is of sufficient magnitude, the clavicle can be displaced into or through the trapezius muscle (type IV). Type VI is a subcoracoid dislocation of the clavicle. It is associated with extreme trauma and is rare. A type VII, which is complete dislocation of the AC and SC joints, has been described but is extremely rare.

Diagnosis

History and Physical Examination

- The diagnosis of an AC joint disruption is usually made by history and confirmed by physical examination and x-ray.
- With acute traumatic injuries, the diagnosis can be obvious.
- Classification of injury (e.g., Rockwood type II vs. III) and assessing for other concomitant injuries can be more difficult (see Table 20-1).

- In general, palpation of the area and assessment of joint stability are important.
- X-ray analysis is also important (see below).
- In patients without a history of acute trauma, localization of the pathology to the AC joint can be more involved.
- The innervation of the AC joint is provided by the lateral pectoral nerve anteriorly and the suprascapular nerve posteriorly.
- Gerber (1998) evaluated patterns of pain for both AC joint and subacromial pathologies. Irritation of the AC joint produced pain directly over the joint, in the anterolateral neck, and over the anterolateral deltoid—areas that were subtly distinct from the subacromial irritation.
- The cross-shoulder adduction test, performed with the arm elevated to 90 degrees and the elbow bent 90 degrees, can be helpful if it produces pain localized to the AC joint because the arm is adducted across the chest, thereby compressing the joint.
- O'Brien's test can also be helpful in differentiating AC joint pathology from soft-tissue lesions within the gleno-

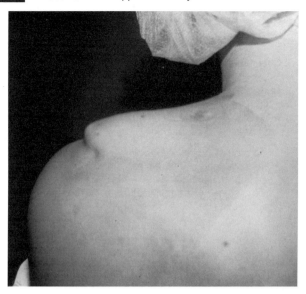

Figure 20-3 Physical examination findings in acute injury: type V.

humeral joint, especially the superior glenoid labrum or proximal biceps attachment.
- In general, a triad of point tenderness—positive cross-shoulder adduction test and relief of symptoms with an injection of a local anesthetic into the AC joint—is indicative of AC joint pathology.
- Clinical features for each type are summarized in Table 20-1. See also Figure 20-3.

Radiologic Examination
- The assessment of the AC joint can be done well with only plain films, but special views and technique are required.
- Because of its relatively superficial location, less penetration strength of the beam (approximately 50%) is needed compared with standard views.
- A Zanca anteroposterior (AP) view, which tilts the beam 15 degrees cephalad, can visualize the AC joint better than a standard AP view by preventing the scapular spine from being superimposed on the AC joint and should be routinely performed.
  - Normal x-ray findings on a Zanca AP view and an axillary lateral include a joint space of 1 to 3 mm, which diminishes significantly with age to about 0.5 mm by age 60.
  - A space of greater than 7 mm in males and 6 mm in females is abnormal.
  - A CC distance of 1.1 to 1.3 cm is normal.
  - Although an incongruent AC joint can be seen in as many as 30% of controls, an increase of 25% to 50% in the CC distance, compared with the unaffected side, can signify complete AC joint dislocation.
- An axillary lateral is critical to assess horizontal displacements, especially in a type IV injury, and should also be done routinely.

- To assess for a coracoid fracture, the Stryker notch view is helpful if indicated.
- Previously, stress views were recommended to differentiate type II, type III, and type V injuries.
  - These were typically done in the AP plane with a 5-lb weight attached to each arm.
  - However, several studies have questioned the efficacy of the routine use of these x-rays.
- Of historical interest, Alexander (1949), described the lateral stress view or "shoulder-forward" view.
  - It is taken from both the uninjured and injured sides as a scapular Y view, with the patient thrusting his or her shoulders forward.
  - On the injured side, the displacement of the acromion anteriorly and inferiorly can be seen.
- Computed tomography (CT) and magnetic resonance imaging are not used routinely, although each may be utilized as an adjuvant in more complicated situations.

Treatment
- The goals of both nonoperative and operative management of AC injuries are full pain-free strength and motion and restoration of normal anatomy and appearance.

Nonsurgical Treatment
- Type I and II injuries are treated nonoperatively, with a sling for up to 2 to 3 weeks, ice, and nonsteroidal medications.
  - The sling is used only as needed for comfort, with gradual return to regular daily activities.
  - A type I injury is treated purely symptomatically, and the patient is usually back to unrestricted activities within 2 weeks.
  - With a type II injury, the patient is not allowed to do any heavy lifting, pushing, pulling, or contact sports for up to 8 to 12 weeks to allow the ligaments to heal.
  - Continued, unrelieved pain can be treated with an injection of steroid into the AC joint.
- The management of type III injuries is controversial; however, there has been no shown benefit of surgery and should be treated in the same way as a type II injury with a sling use of up to 4 weeks for comfort.
  - When in doubt, opt for nonoperative management and treat on the basis of symptoms.
  - Many devices have been described to try to reduce the AC joint with pressure, such as braces, straps, harnesses, and casts.
  - The problems with these devices include skin breakdown from continuous pressure, discomfort, inconvenience, noncompliance, and joint stiffness.
  - Many authors use a sling for simplicity and comfort, and accept the minimal deformity of the injury.
- In type VII injuries, the SC dislocation is treated nonoperatively with good results, and treatment of the AC joint is controversial.
- Physeal injuries and pseudodislocation through an intact periosteal sleeve, as well as base of the coracoid

process fractures associated with AC joint separation, can be treated nonoperatively with good results.

Results and Complications

- On radiographs, there is calcification of ligaments post-injury in 40% of patients but it does not correlate with function.
  - This occurs whether or not the patient has an operation.
  - It can be an isolated bone structure or bridge between the coracoid and clavicle.
- The prognosis for patients with type I and II injuries is good, but they may be more prone to degenerative disease and osteolysis.
- X-ray changes seen in the distal clavicle may include osteoporosis, osteolysis, tapering, or osteophytes.
- Dull aches usually resolve within a year on their own.
- If the joint is still painful, then excision of the distal clavicle can be performed.
- Nonunion of a coracoid base fracture can be very painful.
  - This should be treated with bone graft and stabilization.
- Neurologic injuries may occur early or late, such as brachial plexopathy.
- Fractures of the clavicle, acromion, or coracoid can occur with the initial injury.

Surgical Treatment

- Persistent pain in the AC joint after a stable type I or II injury may be due to osteolysis of the distal clavicle or interposed tissue, such as torn ligaments, loose cartilage, or meniscus.
  - This should be treated with distal clavicle excision and joint debridement.
- With stable type I and II injuries, the CC ligament is intact and thus the AC joint is stable.
- There is some discussion about "unstable" type II injuries.
  - These may be under diagnosed type III injuries.
- There is also a group of patients who have increased AP instability without superior migration.
  - These do not respond well to a distal clavicle resection.
- Operative management of acute (<6 weeks) type III injuries is often reserved for open injuries, brachial plexopathy, severe type III dislocations, and rarely high-level overhead athletes.
- Operative management of chronic (>6 weeks) type III injuries is indicated for failure of nonoperative treatment with continued AC joint pain and instability.
- Type IV, V, and VI injuries require early operative reconstruction because of the severe displacement of the joint, pain, and deformity.

Procedures

- Many surgical procedures have been described for the management of AC separations. There is controversy over the proper surgical technique, and no treatment has emerged as ideal.
  - These procedures can be broken down into five groups: excision of the distal clavicle, dynamic muscle transfer, reconstruction of the CC ligaments, fixation between the clavicle and coracoid, and fixation across the AC joint.
  - With most operative techniques, authors recommend debridement of the AC joint and repair of the deltotrapezial fascia.

Excision of the Distal Clavicle

- This is used mainly for degenerative but stable AC joints that have failed nonoperative management.
- The procedure can be done open (Mumford) or arthroscopically (Flatow).
  - Follow-up studies on open and arthroscopic distal clavicle excisions yield similar results, with 80% to 90% success rates.
  - Surgeons who are comfortable with arthroscopic techniques have the opportunity to also visualize the glenohumeral joint and look for undiagnosed superior labral anterior–posterior (SLAP) tears.
    - Berg and Ciullo noted that, of 20 patients who had a failed distal clavicle excision with presumed osteoarthritis of the AC joint, 15 of these patients had superior labral tears on arthroscopic evaluation at repeat procedure, and 9 of the 15 patients improved after definitive management of this problem.
- The patients who undergo distal clavicle excision should be warned about weakness of the bench press motion but no other significant long-term disability.
- The amount to resect is controversial, with some authors recommending 5 to 7 mm and some 20 to 25 mm.
- The resection should be even and the superior capsule and ligament, as well as the CC ligament should be protected.
- Inferior osteophytes on the distal clavicle should be excised.
- Patients with unstable AC joints and distal clavicle fractures are not good candidates for excision.
- Using distal clavicle excision alone fails to address instability if it exists.
- Postoperatively, the patients are placed in a sling and allowed to do active and passive range of motion.
- They are encouraged to use the arm for everyday activities but to refrain from overhead activities until the pain has subsided.
- At 1 week postoperatively, strengthening exercises are begun and patients are allowed to return to all activities as tolerated.

Dynamic Muscle Transfer

- This procedure involves transferring the tip of the coracoid process and the attached coracobrachialis and short head of the biceps to the undersurface of the clavicle, fixing in place with a screw.
- The muscles then act as an active depressor of the clavicle.
- There is a risk of injury to the musculocutaneous nerve.

- Another problem with this technique is that it reconstructs a static restraint with dynamic tissue, allowing motion and leading to continued pain.

Reconstruction of the Coracoclavicular Ligaments
- In the Weaver-Dunn technique (Fig. 20-4), the distal clavicle is excised, and the acromial end of the CA ligament is transferred to the remaining distal clavicle as a reconstruction for the CC ligaments.
    - A problem with this technique is weak initial fixation to the clavicle, which is via sutures.
    - Another issue is that the AC joint is not anatomically reduced in this procedure.
- These problems have been addressed by Morrison and Lemos via a Modified Weaver-Dunn technique, which consists of passing an augmentation device through the clavicle and through or around the coracoid, anatomically reducing the clavicle and stabilizing the reconstruction while the CA ligament transfer matures.
    - The augmentation device can wear through the bone, amputating the clavicle or coracoid, and may produce a foreign body response in the local tissue, leading to a hypertrophic scar and osteolysis.
- The CA ligament has an important role in shoulder stability, preventing superior migration of the humeral head.
    - Lee et al. showed that the CA ligament also restrains anterior and inferior translations of the humeral head through an interaction with the coracohumeral ligament.
- Jones and Lemos have described reconstructing the CC ligaments by passing a semitendinosus tendon autograft or tibialis anterior tendon allograft around the base of the coracoid and through a 6-mm drill hole in the anterior third of the clavicle.
    - This has been done both in revision and primary procedures.
    - This reconstruction is augmented by suture fixation between the coracoid and clavicle to prevent early failure of the graft while it is healing.

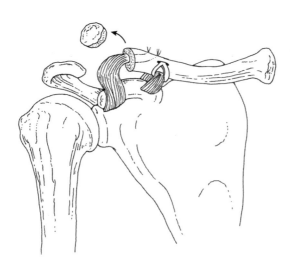

Figure 20-4 Modified Weaver-Dunn technique for reconstruction of the CC ligaments.

- Revascularization of the graft, as with anterior cruciate ligament reconstructions, is assumed and the graft may stretch out over time.
- Lee et al. performed a biomechanical study on cadaveric shoulders, comparing the strength of the native CC ligaments with reconstructions using CA ligament transfer, suture repair, tape repair, and tendon grafts.
    - They found that tendon grafts had the same peak load as the native ligaments, were stronger than the CA ligament transfers and suture repairs, and were stiffer than CA ligament transfers.

Fixation between the Clavicle and Coracoid
- The goal of this technique is to keep the clavicle and coracoid in a reduced position long enough to allow primary healing of the CC ligaments, assuming that the ligaments will heal at the preinjury length and strength.
- Bosworth described placing a screw through the clavicle into the base of the coracoid process, which requires later surgical removal.
    - A stab wound is made 4 cm medial to the distal end of the clavicle.
    - A drill hole is made in the clavicle.
    - The clavicle is depressed and reduced to the coracoid, an awl is used to make a hole in the superior aspect of the base of the coracoid, and a screw is inserted.
- Others have placed cerclage material around the clavicle and coracoid, such as wire or Dacron tape, which can lead to similar problems with the augmentation device used in the modified Weaver-Dunn, such as coracoid or clavicle amputation, scar, and osteolysis.

Fixation across the Acromioclavicular Joint
- Fixation has been described using pins, suture, suture wires, and hook plates.
- Any hardware, like CC screws, requires later removal at 6 to 8 weeks.
- Usually, reconstruction of the AC or CC ligaments is also done.
- The pin is inserted laterally to the AC joint, across the joint, and into the clavicle.
    - Alternatively, the pin can be drilled retrograde from the joint through the acromion, then drilled antegrade across the joint into the clavicle.
- With pin fixation, there is a risk of breakage and migration of the pins into the lung, heart, great vessels, spinal cord, mediastinum, and many other vital structures, which leads to serious consequences, including death.
    - There is also a reported increased risk of AC arthritis.
- Hook plates violate the joint, requires later surgical removal, have a risk of infection, and may bend or dislocate.
    - This fixation is rarely used now a result of the complications; however, there have been recent reports of bioabsorbable devices not requiring later removal.
- More recently, several authors have discussed arthroscopic reconstruction of the AC joint.

Authors' Operative Technique

- We prefer a combination of an autograft CA ligament transfer or a tibialis anterior tendon allograft around the coracoid and through the clavicle with a synthetic augmentation between the clavicle and the coracoid.

Incision and Exposure

- The patient is placed in the modified beach chair position.
- A large radiograph cassette is placed under the patient's AC joint.
- Routine prepping and draping of the extremity are carried out.
- A horizontal skin incision is made, 5 cm long, beginning 1 cm lateral to the AC joint and taken medially along the anterior edge of the clavicle.
- Similarly, a vertical skin incision just lateral to the coracoid may be used.
- Subcutaneous flaps are developed superior and inferior to the AC joint to allow adequate exposure of the deltotrapezial fascia and distal 6 cm of clavicle.
- The deltotrapezial fascia is incised, exposing the lateral clavicle and AC joint.
- Next, the clavicular periosteum is incised along the anterior edge, and subperiosteal dissection is done, exposing the distal 3 cm of clavicle.

Distal Clavicle Excision

- In cases in which the articular surfaces of the clavicle and acromion are normal, distal clavicle excision need not be performed. This is rare in our experience.
- In most cases in which there is damage to the articular cartilage (or in revision cases), 5 to 8 mm of the lateral clavicle is resected with a sagittal bone saw.
- This is done in line with the AC joint, slightly obliquely, from superior lateral to posterior medial.

Coracoid Preparation

- The coracoid is identified.
- The deltoid is split along the line of the fibers using electrocautery.
- The CA ligament is identified and kept intact.
- Using electrocautery, a subperiosteal incision is made on the superior aspect of the coracoid base, and the coracoid is exposed medially and laterally.
- A looped suture passer is passed around the base.
- An augmentation device is passed through or around the coracoid and tagged for later use.

Clavicle and Graft Preparation

- The clavicle is identified.
- Any sharp edges are beveled.
- A 2 × 6 mm burr hole is placed in the clavicle at the junction of its anterior and middle third, 3 cm medial to the AC joint, and directly above the base of the coracoid.
- Medial placement of this drill hole allows the graft to provide tension along the same vector as the normal CC ligaments, and an anatomic reduction of the clavicle can be obtained.

- Two smaller drill holes are placed medial and lateral to the burr hole for later passing of the augmentation sutures.
- If a CA ligament transfer is performed, the acromial insertion of the ligament is identified and harvested with a small 3 to 5 mm wafer of acromion.
- The coracoid attachment is left intact.
- The acromial side is sutured with a no. 2 nonabsorbable braided material.
- This construct is then passed through the end of the clavicle.
- The ends of the tibialis anterior allograft are secured with a no. 2 suture using a tendon suture technique.
- Many different synthetic augmentations have been used.
- The graft and augmentation sutures are placed into the previously placed suture loops around the coracoid base and then passed around the base of the coracoid.
- The augmentation suture is passed through the two smaller drill holes in the clavicle.
- The clavicle is overreduced by 5 mm to the acromion.
- A knot is tied under tension inferior to the clavicle to prevent knot prominence.
- The augmentation suture will provide provisional fixation while the graft reconstruction reorganizes.
- The graft is passed through the inferior aspect of the burr hole in the clavicle and reapproximated.
- The sutures are tied together, then supplemented with additional no. 2 sutures.
- Residual graft tissue is excised.

Closure

- Copious irrigation is performed.
- The deltotrapezial fascia is carefully reapproximated with a no. 2 suture using a mattress suture technique.
- Routine closure of the subcutaneous tissue and skin then follows.
- A compressive dressing, sling, and swathe are applied.

Postoperative Treatment

- The patient is placed in a sling and swathe postoperatively.
- For activity, the patient starts gentle, active-assisted range of motion on postoperative day 1.
- The swathe can be removed in a few days, and the sling is used for 6 weeks.
- At 6 weeks, the patient may progress to active range of motion and strengthening.
- No heavy lifting or pushing is allowed for 6 months.
- Any hardware should be removed at 6 to 8 weeks.

Results

- Morrison and Lemos looked at 14 patients with minimum 2-year follow-up, with a 34 of 36 University of California–Los Angeles (UCLA) score.
  - Similarly good to excellent results can be obtained using allograft reconstruction.
- Harris et al. did a cadaver study comparing various methods of reconstruction.

■ They found that CC slings and suture anchors provided good strength but with greater deformations.

■ Screw fixation provided good stiffness and strength but only if bicortical purchase was obtained.

■ CA transfers were the weakest, the least stiff, and required augmentation.

Complications

■ There are many complications related to operative treatment, including wound and bone infection, hardware migration or failure, erosion or fracture due to augmentation devices, arthritis, and recurrent pain and deformity.

■ Death from migrating pins from the AC joint to the lungs, chest, heart, and mediastinum has been described.

Other Entities

Physeal Injuries

■ Physeal injuries and pseudodislocation through an intact periosteal sleeve occur in children and adolescents.

■ Radiographs show a large increase in the CC interspace.

■ This can be a Salter Harris I or II injury, in which the epiphysis remains congruous with the acromion while the distal clavicle metaphysis is displaced.

■ The CC ligament is intact and attached to the periosteal sleeve.

■ This is treated nonoperatively with good results.

Coracoid Process Fractures

■ Coracoid process fractures, usually of the base, can occur with AC joint dislocation but are an uncommon injury.

■ Usually, the CC ligaments remain attached to the coracoid process fragment.

■ The fracture through the coracoid base allows the clavicle to become high-riding, compared with the acromion.

■ Axillary and Stryker notch views can be helpful with showing this fracture, or a CT scan can be done.

■ Both operative and nonoperative treatments have been described, with similar results.

Acromioclavicular Joint Osteoarthritis

■ Any AC joint injury can lead to posttraumatic osteoarthritis of the AC joint.

■ Osteoarthritis can also occur in conjunction with rotator cuff tears and glenohumeral osteoarthritis.

■ The patient will present with shoulder pain.

■ On physical examination, the patient will have tenderness to palpation over the AC joint and have pain with crossed-body adduction.

■ Radiographs will reveal narrowing of the AC joint, cystic changes, and osteophytes.

■ Conservative therapy is the first line of treatment and consists of nonsteroidal anti-inflammatory medications, activity modification, passive range of motion, strengthening exercises, iontophoresis, and ice.

■ An intra-articular steroid injection can also be done as both a diagnostic and therapeutic test, taking care not to inject the subacromial space.

■ If symptoms persist after 12 months of conservative treatment, then excision of the distal clavicle can be performed either openly or arthroscopically.

STERNOCLAVICULAR JOINT

Traumatic injuries to the SC joint are rare and usually associated with significant trauma. The spectrum of injury includes SC subluxation and dislocation, injuries to the medial clavicular physis, and degenerative joint arthritis. These injuries carry potential risks due to the proximity of the great vessels and mediastinal structures (such as the trachea and esophagus) that lie directly beneath the SC joint.

Anatomy and Biomechanics

Clavicle

The clavicle forms via intramembranous ossification at intrauterine week 5 and is the first long bone to ossify. However, the medial clavicular physis is the last to appear, the last to ossify at age 18 to 20 years old, and fuses with the shaft of the clavicle at age 23 to 25 years old. A complete union may not even be present until age 31. This is important to remember because an SC joint dislocation in a young patient may actually represent a fracture through the medial clavicle physis.

Sternoclavicular Joint

The SC joint is a diarthrodial joint. It is the only articulation between the upper extremity and axial skeleton and, as a result of this, almost any motion of the upper extremity is transferred to the SC joint. The articular surfaces are covered with fibrocartilage. The medial end of the clavicle is large, bulbous, concave front to back, and convex vertically. It articulates with the clavicular notch of the sternum to form a saddle-shaped joint. Less than 50% of the clavicle articulates with the sternum, and the joint surfaces are not congruent, leading to the least amount of osseous stability of any joint in the body. In 2.5% of patients, the medial clavicle has an inferior facet that articulates with the first rib. The SC joint has motion in all planes (Fig. 20-5).

Although the SC joint is small, incongruous, and subject forces with all movements of the upper extremity, it is rarely dislocated because of the stout ligaments supporting it. The SC ligaments are important in preventing downward displacement of the distal clavicle. This includes the intra-articular disc ligament, the costoclavicular ligament, the interclavicular ligament, and the capsular ligament.

Intra-articular Disc Ligament

The intraarticular disc ligament originates from the synchrondral junction of the first rib and sternum, passes through the SC joint dividing it into two spaces, and attaches to the superior and posterior aspects of the medial clavicle. The disc then blends in with the capsular ligament. It is a dense fibrous structure that rarely has a perforation

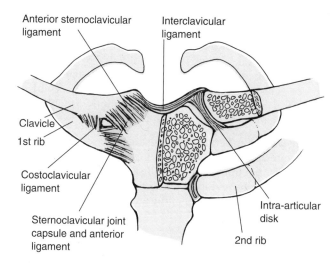

Figure 20-5 SC joint. (From Oatis CA. Kinesiology: The Mechanics and Pathomechanics of Human Movement. Baltimore: Lippincott Williams & Wilkins, 2004.)

connecting the two spaces. It acts to prevent medial displacement of the inner clavicle.

Costoclavicular Ligament

The costoclavicular ligament, also known as the rhomboid ligament, has a twisted appearance and anterior and posterior fasciculi with a bursa between the two. The anterior fasciculus originates from the anteromedial aspect of the first rib and passes upward and laterally to attach to the clavicle. The anterior fibers act as a checkrein against upward rotation and lateral displacement of the clavicle. The posterior fasciculus fibers are shorter, arise laterally to the anterior fasciculus fibers on the first rib, and pass upward and medially. The posterior fibers resist downward rotation and medial displacement of the clavicle. The costoclavicular ligament is short and strong, and the crossing of the fasciculi provides stability to the joint, similar to the CC ligament.

Interclavicular Ligament

The interclavicular ligament connects the superomedial aspect of the clavicle with the capsular ligaments and the upper sternum and also helps to hold up the shoulder.

Capsular Ligament

The capsular ligament consists of thickenings of the capsule anteriorly and posteriorly, and the clavicular attachment is mainly onto the epiphysis. The capsular ligament has been shown to be the most important ligament in preventing anterior, posterior, and upward displacement of the medial clavicle, as well as downward displacement of the distal clavicle.

Surrounding Anatomy

Before operating on the SC joint, it is important to know that anatomy well because there are vital structures in this area. Posterior to the SC joint and medial clavicle is a curtain of muscles—the sternohyoid, sternothyroid, and scale-

nes—which covers the vital structures. The vital structures include the brachiocephalic artery, brachiocephalic vein, vagus nerve, phrenic nerve, internal jugular vein, trachea, and esophagus. The arch of the aorta, superior vena cava, and right pulmonary artery are also very close to the SC joint. The anterior jugular vein also runs between the curtain of muscles and the clavicle, and can vary in size up to 1.5 cm.

Epidemiology, Mechanism, and History

SC injuries are rare and said to account for 3% of all shoulder injuries. Bilateral dislocations are reported infrequently. A significant amount of force is needed to produce a traumatic dislocation of the SC joint. This can be direct or indirect. With a direct force to the anteromedial clavicle, the clavicle is displaced posteriorly into the mediastinum. An indirect force to the anterolateral or posterolateral aspect of the shoulder can lead to a posterior or anterior dislocation of the SC joint, respectively. An indirect mechanism is more common than direct.

Motor vehicle accidents account for 40% of SC injuries, and sports account for 21%. The dislocation usually occurs anteriorly because the posterior capsular ligaments are stronger than the anterior. Atraumatic subluxation of the SC joint has been described in individuals with generalized ligamentous laxity and in a patient with pseudarthrosis of the first and second ribs.

Diagnosis

History and Physical Examination

- A patient with an SC joint injury will complain of severe pain with any movement of the arm.
- The head may be tilted toward the injured side.
- The injured arm will be held across the trunk and supported by the uninjured arm.
- With a dislocation, the affected shoulder is shortened and thrust forward.
  - The pain is worse when supine.
  - With an anterior SC joint dislocation, the medial end of the clavicle is prominent and palpable anterior to the sternum.
  - With a posterior dislocation, the medial clavicle is posterior to the sternum, not palpable, and less prominent, whereas the sternum is more easily palpable.
  - With a posterior dislocation, the subclavian and mediastinal structures may be compressed, leading to venous congestion in the neck or upper extremity, breathing difficulties, choking sensation, decreased blood flow to the arm, and even hypotension and shock.
- Clinically, it can be difficult to tell the difference between an anterior and posterior dislocation.

Radiologic Examination

- An SC dislocation can sometimes be picked up on a routine chest x-ray.
- Rockwood described the serendipity view, which is a 40-degree cephalic tilt view of both SC joints.

- With an anterior dislocation, the clavicle will appear to be superiorly displaced compared with the uninjured side.
- With a posterior dislocation, the clavicle will lie inferiorly.
- CT is the best radiographic study for evaluating SC joint injuries (Fig. 20-6).
  - It can show fractures of the medial clavicle, physeal injuries, and subtle subluxations.
  - It is important to compare the uninjured side with the injured side.
- With chronic posterior SC dislocations, other imaging modalities have been described.
  - Dynamic ultrasound of the subclavian artery has been used to show compression of the artery during elevation of the arm.
- Nerve conduction studies can also confirm a suspected brachial plexus neuropathy.

Classification and Treatment

Physeal Injuries

- Because the medial clavicular physis is the last to ossify at age 18 to 20 years of age and fuses with the shaft of the clavicle at age 23 to 25 years old, an SC joint dislocation in a young 20-year-old may actually be a physeal injury to the medial clavicle.
- Closed reduction of posterior physeal injuries should be performed if they are less than 10 days from the injury.
- After 10 days, if there are no signs of mediastinal compromise, the injury should be treated symptomatically, because the majority of physeal injuries will heal with time without surgery and remodeling will eliminate any deformity.
- If there are symptoms from pressure on the subclavian vessels and mediastinum—such as difficulty breathing, difficulty swallowing, arm swelling, or poor circulation—a closed reduction should be attempted, no matter how far out from the injury and an open reduction is indicated if there is failure of closed reduction.
- At the time of surgery, the intra-articular disk and the more lateral epiphysis have been found to stay with the sternum and be held in place by the capsular ligament.
  - This is important to note because the epiphysis should not be excised with the intra-articular disk ligament.

Sternoclavicular Sprain or Subluxation

- Acute sprains of the SC joint can be mild or moderate.
  - With a mild sprain, the ligaments are all intact and the joint is stable.
    - This can be painful and is treated with ice, a sling for 3 or 4 days, and then gradual use of the arm as tolerated.
  - With a moderate sprain, the joint is subluxated anteriorly or posteriorly and the ligaments may be partially disrupted.
    - This should be treated by holding the shoulders back with a clavicle strap to keep the joint reduced and a sling and swathe to prevent arm motion for 4 to 6 weeks.
- Atraumatic subluxation of the medial clavicle usually occurs in adolescents and young adults.
  - It can be due to generalized ligamentous laxity or a pseudarthrosis between the first and second ribs.
  - This is treated nonoperatively.
  - If the patient continues to be symptomatic, a CT scan should be performed to look for any bony anomalies.
  - Surgery should be reserved for patients with persistent pain, instability, or limitation in activities of daily living.

Anterior Sternoclavicular Joint Dislocation

- It can be difficult to differentiate between an anterior and posterior dislocation of the SC joint on physical examination only.

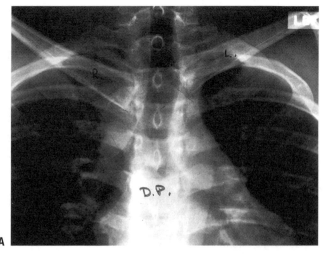
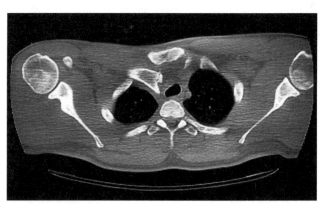

A

B

Figure 20-6 **A:** Routine AP x-ray of posteriorly dislocated right SC joint. **B:** The AP view is suggestive of a posterior dislocation. However, the CT scan clearly demonstrates the posteriorly displaced right medial clavicle. Note the displacement of the trachea. (From Bucholz RW, Heckman JD. Rockwood and Green's Fractures in Adults, 5th ed. Lippincott Williams & Wilkins, 2001.)

- A CT scan is recommended to further evaluate SC joint injuries.
- There is controversy over the treatment of anterior dislocations.
- Although most acute anterior dislocations are unstable after reduction, it is nonetheless recommended that closed reduction be attempted if the patient presents less than 10 days from the injury (Fig. 20-7).
  - This can be done under local or general anesthesia.
  - The patient is placed supine with a 3- to 4-inch roll between the scapulae.
  - Gentle pressure over the anteriorly displaced medial clavicle may reduce the dislocation; however, when the pressure is released, the joint usually redislocates.
- If the patient already has fusion between the medial clavicle physis and the clavicular shaft, then the anterior clavicle would be expected to have an anterior prominence of the medial clavicle.
  - This does not seem to cause problems, even with heavy manual labor.

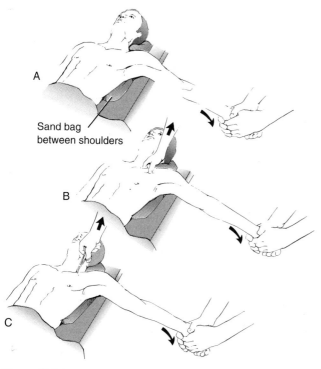

Sand bag between shoulders

Figure 20-7   Technique for closed reduction of the SC joint. **A:** The patient is positioned supine with a sandbag placed between the two shoulders. Traction is then applied to the arm against countertraction in an abducted and slightly extended position. In anterior dislocations, direct pressure over the medial end of the clavicle may reduce the joint. **B:** In posterior dislocations, in addition to the traction, it may be necessary to manipulate the medial end of the clavicle with the fingers to dislodge the clavicle from behind the manubrium. **C:** In stubborn posterior dislocations, it may be necessary to prepare (sterilely) the medial end of the clavicle and use a towel clip to grasp around the medial clavicle to lift it back into position. (From Bucholz RW, Heckman JD. Rockwood and Green's Fractures in Adults, 5th ed. Lippincott Williams & Wilkins, 2001.)

- If the SC joint remains reduced with the shoulders held back, a figure-eight strap can be used.
  - Some authors have recommended a bulky pad over the anteromedial clavicle to hold it reduced.
  - The shoulder should be immobilized for 6 weeks, and strenuous activities should not be done until 8 weeks.
- If the SC joint redislocates after the immobilization is discontinued, a figure-eight strap or sling can be used until the patient is comfortable.
- Open operative procedures should not be done for an anterior SC joint dislocation because the complications are too great, end results are unsatisfactory, and the patient usually does fine with residual prominence.

Posterior Sternoclavicular Joint Dislocation

- A posterior dislocation of the SC joint requires prompt examination and reduction, either closed or open.
- Because of pressure on the hilar structures, it has been associated with respiratory distress, venous congestion, arterial insufficiency, brachial plexus compression, and myocardial conduction abnormalities.
- Damage to the pulmonary and vascular systems needs to be ruled out.
  - When indicated, aortography, pulmonary consult, and vascular consult should be obtained before reduction.
- If the patient presents within 10 days of the injury, closed reduction should be attempted.
  - The reduction should be done as early as possible because there have been reports of greater difficulty reducing dislocations more than 48 hours from the injury.
  - Once the joint is reduced, it is almost always stable.
  - General anesthesia is usually needed because of pain and spasm.
- There are two techniques used for closed reduction: abduction traction and adduction traction.
  - With the abduction-traction technique, the patient is placed supine with the injured shoulder near the edge of the table.
    - A 3- to 4-inch roll is placed between the scapulae.
    - The arm is abducted and lateral traction is applied.
    - The arm is then brought into extension, the clavicle reduces with an audible pop, and it is almost always stable.
    - It may be necessary to grasp the medial clavicle with one's fingers to dislodge it from behind the sternum.
    - If this fails, then the skin is prepped and a sterile towel clamp or reduction tenaculum is used to grasp the medial clavicle and apply anterior traction, whereas lateral traction is applied to the arm.
- With the adduction-traction technique, the patient is also placed supine with a 3- to 4-inch roll between the scapulae.

- The arm is held adducted, whereas downward pressure is exerted on the shoulders, and the medial clavicle is levered over the first rib back into place.
- After closed reduction, the patient should be placed into a figure-eight strap for 4 to 6 weeks.
- If closed reduction fails, open reduction should be done for a posterior SC joint dislocation.
  - Most patients cannot tolerate the symptoms associated with pressure on the mediastinal structures, and even patients who are initially asymptomatic develop symptoms later on.
  - It is important to be totally familiar with the anatomy all around the SC joint. It is also recommended that a thoracic surgeon be available in the case of rupture of a major vessel.
- Wirth and Rockwood recommend resection of the medial clavicle with maintenance, repair, or reconstruction of the costoclavicular ligaments to stabilize the joint. This can be done using suture, internal fixation across the joint, fascia lata, or subclavius tendon.
  - First, the medial clavicle is resected.
  - Next, two or three nonabsorbable sutures are placed around the remaining medial end of the clavicle and through the stump or scar of the costoclavicular ligaments, taking care not to tighten the medial clavicle down to the first rib too much.
  - If present, the capsular and intraarticular disk ligaments can also be sutured to the medial clavicle for stabilization.
  - Last, the periosteal sleeve is closed, which will stabilize the medial clavicle.
  - Metallic pin fixation should be avoided because these have been reported to migrate and cause serious complications, including death.
- For a chronic posterior SC dislocation with an associated thoracic outlet syndrome, resection of the first rib has been performed with good success.
  - This approach avoids iatrogenic damage to the mediastinal structures and instability of the medial clavicle after resection, and leads to a cosmetic scar in the axillomammary skin crease.

Intra-articular Disk Ligament Injury

- This is an uncommon injury but can be quite disabling, and it should be considered in any patient with an acute or chronic injury of the SC joint.
- A patient with an intra-articular disk injury will present with complaints of clicking, grating, and popping in the SC joint similar to a knee meniscal tear but have a stable joint.
- CT scan and arthrography have been used in diagnosis.
- Keep in mind that 6% of intra-articular disks are incomplete and may be read as a tear.
  - These injuries are treated conservatively with ice and rest.
- If symptoms persist, a local injection can be done as both a therapeutic and diagnostic test.
- If the injection relieves the symptoms, then the patient may benefit from an operation with an arthrotomy to remove the disk and resect the medial clavicle if it is degenerative, because this can also be a source of pain.

Degenerative Arthritis of the Sternoclavicular Joint

- Degenerative arthritis of the SC joint results from a traumatic injury.
- Conservative treatment with heat, anti-inflammatory medications, and rest is usually successful.
- If the patient has persistent pain after 6 to 12 months of conservative treatment, a local injection can be done as both a therapeutic and diagnostic test.
  - If the pain is relieved temporarily, then resection of the SC joint is indicated.
- The medial clavicle is resected, being careful to leave the costoclavicular ligament intact.
- The residual stability of the distal clavicle should be constantly checked.
- If too much of the medial clavicle is resected, the patient will have recurrence of pain due to loss of stability of the clavicle.
- This can lead to limited shoulder mobility, neurologic symptoms, thoracic outlet syndrome, and fatigue.

Dislocations of Both Ends of the Clavicle

- This problem presents as an anterior dislocation of the SC joint and a posterior dislocation of the AC joint.
- Wirth et al. reviewed 22 cases of dislocations of both ends of the clavicle.
  - Most patients with this problem have been treated conservatively with satisfactory results.
  - One patient developed a brachial plexus neuropathy treated with excision of part of the clavicle.
  - Four patients had persistent pain localized to the AC joint and were treated with AC joint reconstruction.

Complications

Nonsurgical Treatment

- Complications related to pressure on hilar structures are mainly seen with posterior SC joint dislocations; however, there is some concern for these problems late with posterior physeal injuries.
- The only complications occurring after an anterior dislocation are cosmetic deformity and late degenerative changes.
- The incidence of complications has been reported at 25%; however, only two deaths have been reported as a result of this injury.
- Early complications after a posterior dislocation can affect the trachea, esophagus, or great vessels.
  - These can be very serious and include pneumothorax, laceration of the superior vena cava, respiratory distress, neck venous congestion, rupture of the esophagus with abscess and osteomyelitis of the clavicle, fatal tracheoesophageal fistula, pressure on the subclavian artery, occlusion of the subclavian artery, heart conduction abnormalities, compression of the right common carotid artery, brachial plexus compression, and voice changes.
- Late complications after nonreduced retrosternal injuries can occur in patients who were initially asymptomatic.
  - These include thoracic outlet syndrome, brachial plexopathy, subclavian artery compression, exer-

tional dyspnea, and even fatal sepsis after development of a tracheoesophageal fistula.

Surgical Treatment

- Metallic pin fixation across the SC joint should be avoided because these have been reported to migrate and cause serious complications, including death.
- Smooth pins, threaded Kirschner pins, pins with bent ends, and Hagie pins have all been reported to migrate either intact or broken into the heart, pulmonary artery, innominate artery, aorta, spinal cord, breast, subclavian artery, and base of the neck.

SUGGESTED READING

Allman FL Jr. Fractures and ligamentous injuries of the clavicle and its articulation. J Bone Joint Surg Am 1967;49;774–784.

Bowen MK, Nuber GW. Acromioclavicular and sternoclavicular injuries. Clin Sports Med 2003:22:301–317.

Lee SJ, Nicholas SJ, Akizuki KH, et al. Reconstruction of the coracoclavicular ligaments with tendon grafts. Am J Sports Med 2003;31: 648–659.

Lemos MJ. The evaluation and treatment of the acromioclavicular joint in athletes. Am J Sports Med 1998;26:137–144.

Wirth MA, Rockwood CA Jr. Acute and chronic traumatic injuries of the sternoclavicular joint. J Am Acad Orthop Surg 1996;4: 268–278.

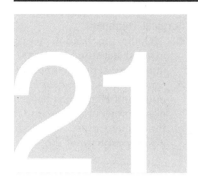

UPPER EXTREMITY NERVE INJURIES

RICHARD M. WILK

There are a variety of injuries to the upper extremity that can occur during participation in sports activities. The most common injuries experienced by athletes include contusions, sprains, fractures, and dislocations. Less frequently, an athlete may suffer from neurologic problems of the upper extremity, either in association with the more common injuries noted previously, or as an isolated entity. This chapter will discuss the various neurologic injuries that may be encountered when providing care for an injured athlete.

ANATOMY

The peripheral nervous system is composed of a highly organized array of structures that function to transmit electrical impulses to and from the central nervous system as the body performs its everyday activities. Sensory and motor nerves facilitate the transmission of impulses in response to visual, auditory, and physiologic stimuli from the environment. The components of the peripheral nerves include the *axon*, as the main conduit to and from the spinal cord, and the *Schwann cell*, which surrounds the axon as it courses throughout the body. Each Schwann cell is composed of myelin and is surrounded by *endoneurium*, with multiple axons forming a *fascicle*. Each fascicle is surrounded by

perineurium, with multiple fascicles being surrounded by *inner epineurium*, and the entire nerve trunk is surrounded by the *outer epineurium* (Fig. 21-1). The significance of this organizational structure will become more relevant as we discuss the nature of nerve injuries.

A brief review of the neurologic anatomy of the upper extremity is helpful in understanding the patterns of injury that can occur during sports participation. The *brachial plexus* is the foundation for any discussion of the neurologic anatomy of the upper extremity. The brachial plexus is formed by the cervical nerve roots (from C5 to T1) as they exit the spinal cord in the cervical spine. The roots combine to form trunks, then divisions, cords, and finally the terminal branches (Fig. 21-2). The terminology is based on the anatomical relationships to the vascular anatomy of the shoulder and the clavicle as the nerves course distally in the upper extremity. The manifestation of a nerve injury is determined by the nature and location of the insult.

PATHOGENESIS

Etiology

Neurologic injuries can result from several different causes. During sports activities, athletes are subjected to numerous

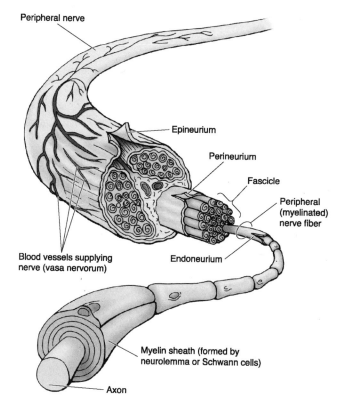

Figure 21-1   Nerve anatomy of axon, Schwann cell, epineurium, endoneurium, and perineurium. (From Moore KL, Dalley AF II. Clinical Oriented Anatomy, 4th ed. Baltimore: Lippincott Williams & Wilkins, 1999.)

stresses that can result in traumatic injuries to the upper extremity, including contusions, fractures, and dislocations. As the popularity of "extreme" sports increases, physicians may see a rise in the number of traumatic injuries, including those involving the peripheral nervous system. Depending on the forces involved, nerves can be damaged by blunt or penetrating trauma, traction from dislocations, or laceration from fracture fragments. Peripheral nerves depend on their surrounding microcirculation for normal function. Neurologic dysfunction in the upper extremity can result from compression of a nerve by cysts, ganglions, or entrapment from other soft-tissue or bony structures. The local compression of a nerve can disrupt the normal microcirculation, leading to ischemia and altered nerve conduction. Athletes who participate in repetitive activities of the upper extremity can experience nerve problems as an overuse injury. In that setting, the recurrent stresses of a particular sport such as tennis or baseball can cause damage to a nerve through traction on the nerve during the motions of the activity. Several investigators have demonstrated conduction abnormalities in rabbit tibial nerves that are stretched 6% of their length, and that the intraneural vascular supply is occluded at 15% lengthening. Finally, there is always the potential for iatrogenic injury to the peripheral nerves that can occur during surgical treatment of orthopaedic disorders of the upper extremity.

Epidemiology

There is limited information in the literature regarding the epidemiology of nerve injuries in sports. In a retrospective review of 346 athletes involved in 27 different sports who were referred for evaluation of neurologic problems, 86% of the injuries involved the upper extremity. Most injuries occurred playing football, with "burners" being the most common diagnosis. In a 5-year study of sports injuries at an athletic clinic in Japan, there were only 28 peripheral nerve problems among 9,550 athletes. Over an 18-year period, the authors found that 5.7% of 1,167 peripheral nerve injuries were related to sports, with most injuries involving the upper extremity.

Pathophysiology

When a nerve is injured, a series of events take place that lead to various degrees of dysfunction, depending on the extent of the inciting cause. In 1943, Seddon described three different types of nerve injury and helped to form the foundation of our understanding and treatment of these challenging problems.

The least severe injury type is termed "neurapraxia," and is described as a minor injury to the nerve, typically resulting from blunt trauma, traction, or local compression. The pathologic process consists of local demyelinization of the Schwann cell, without disruption of the axon, leading to a conduction block. The effect of this injury is a temporary loss of motor strength of the muscles and occasionally sensory function of the dermatomes of the involved nerve. There is no atrophy, or loss of normal reflexes, and spontaneous recovery generally occurs within 3 to 4 weeks. The prognosis for complete recovery is excellent.

The next level of injury is "axonotmesis," referring to disruption of the myelin sheath of the Schwann cell and the axon, but with the outer epineurium remaining intact. In this scenario, there is complete loss of motor and sensory function distal to the injury, with atrophy, and absence of the muscle reflex. A process called "Wallerian degeneration" takes place distal to the injury, involving loss of the functional integrity of the nerve, whereas the structural integrity remains intact. Because the epineurium remains in continuity, the nerve has the innate ability to regenerate within the epineurial sheath. This process has been measured to occur at the rate of 1 mm/day, or 1 inch/month, ultimately leading to return of normal, or near-normal function.

The most severe type of injury is "neurotmesis," in which there is complete disruption of the myelin sheath, axon, and epineurium. Patients with this injury will have no motor or sensory function, with muscle atrophy, and loss of reflexes. Wallerian degeneration occurs distal to the injury; however, because the epineurial sheath is transected, there is little chance of nerve regeneration and, consequently, little chance of functional recovery.

When evaluating athletes with nerve injuries, the classification scheme noted previously can help in the diagnosis and treatment of the patient, as well as offer an assessment of the prognosis for recovery.

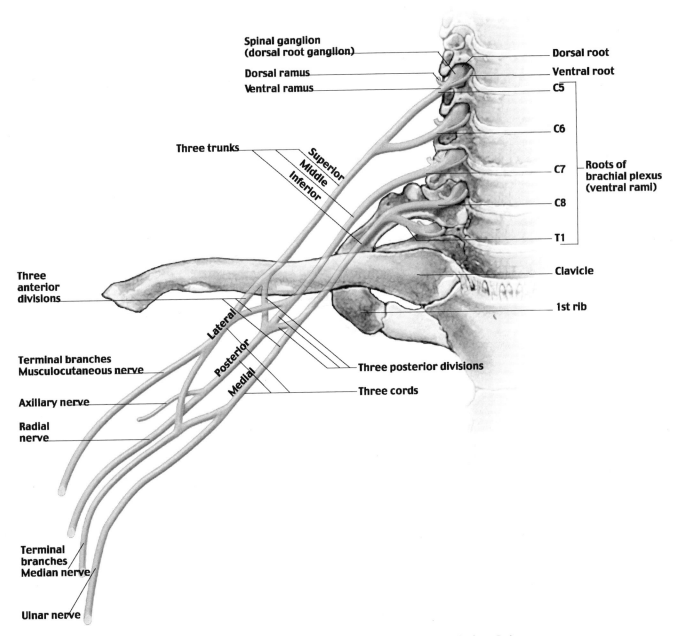

Figure 21-2 Brachial plexus anatomy. (Courtesy of Anatomical Chart Co.)

Classification

In this chapter, we will focus our attention on the sports-related neurologic injuries that impact the function of the shoulder and upper arm. To enhance our understanding and evaluation of these injuries, it is necessary to have a thorough knowledge of the local anatomy. As discussed earlier, the brachial plexus is the origin of the neurologic structures of the upper extremity. The peripheral nerves supplying the muscles and sensory dermatomes of the shoulder and arm arise from the brachial plexus as it courses distally from its cervical and thoracic nerve root origins. Although any of the individual nerves can be affected, we will concen-

trate on the more common injuries that can occur during athletic activities, including the brachial plexus, axillary nerve, musculocutaneous nerve, suprascapular nerve, and long thoracic nerve.

For our purposes in this chapter, we will address the neurologic dysfunction of the upper extremity that evolves from sports injuries, but it is important to remember that there are numerous other causes of neurologic abnormalities that must be considered when evaluating patients, such as closed-head injury, stroke, multiple sclerosis, muscular dystrophy, and a variety of other neurologic diseases. A thorough discussion of these conditions is beyond the scope of this chapter, and you are encouraged to review the appropriate literature.

DIAGNOSIS

History

The specific components of the history and physical examination will depend on the initial presentation. The evaluation of an unconscious athlete in the trauma room of an emergency room will obviously be different from the evaluation of an athlete in your office. The basic principles of a thorough exam should be followed whenever possible, acknowledging the challenges and limitations encountered in the emergency room setting.

- The evaluation of a neurologic injury to the upper extremity may begin on the playing field or sidelines during a sports event, in the emergency room, or in a more controlled environment, such as the office.
  - A physician who provides coverage for sporting events may witness a tackle, collision, or fall of sufficient force to cause a neurologic injury.
  - An injured athlete may be transferred from the playing field to an emergency room for evaluation of a more severe injury, or the athlete may present to your office with complaints of pain, weakness, and possibly numbness of the upper extremity without any inciting event.
- In the treatment of an athlete, just as with any patient, the history will often give clues to the underlying problem.
  - Inquire as to whether there was a traumatic event, and the specifics of the event, or whether the symptoms developed insidiously.
- Depending on the injury, the patient may present with a variety of complaints, including pain, paresthesias, numbness, weakness, fatigue, aching discomfort, and diminished athletic ability.
  - Patients may describe tingling, "pins and needles," and burning as they relate their subjective complaints.
  - The symptoms may emanate from the cervical spine and radiate all the way to the hand.
- Distinguish between symptoms that occur with activity and those that occur at rest, as well as with activity.
- A competitive athlete may express frustration with his or her altered performance associated with the problem.
  - In many cases, the patient will be anxious to resume sports participation as soon as possible, and there may be a tendency to minimize symptoms and how they affect performance.
- With pediatric patients, parents, coaches, and trainers may be able to provide additional observations related to the injury and subsequent problems experienced by the patient.

Physical Examination

- A careful physical examination will provide much of the information that will help elucidate the nature of the condition that is causing the patient's symptoms.
- When assessing neurologic abnormalities of the upper extremity, it is important to remember that injuries to the cervical spine can be manifested by dysfunction of the upper extremity.
  - It is imperative to thoroughly examine the cervical spine of any athlete presenting with altered neurologic function of the upper extremity.
  - When possible, begin your examination standing in front of the patient, but also be sure to examine the patient from behind, looking for any muscle atrophy or loss of symmetry that may be present.
  - Look for any obvious bony abnormalities that might suggest a fracture or dislocation.
  - Palpate the cervical spine for any areas of tenderness or spasm, which may suggest an underlying injury.
  - Observe the range of motion of the cervical spine, taking notice of any limitations or pain reproduced during the motion.
  - Specific maneuvers to localize a particular nerve lesion will be discussed in the appropriate section.
- Once the cervical spine evaluation is complete, the focus of the examination shifts to the shoulder and arm.
  - Compare active and passive range of motion of the shoulder, elbow, wrist, and hand between the involved and uninvolved extremity.
  - Determine if any limitations in motion are related to muscle weakness and an inability to move the involved extremity, or if there may be limitations related to a contracture that may suggest a longer time interval between the onset of symptoms and the presentation in your office.
  - Evaluate strength of the muscles of the shoulder and throughout the upper extremity, including the periscapular musculature, rotator cuff, elbow and wrist flexors and extensors, as well as the muscles of the hand.
  - Document any sensory deficits to light touch, pinprick, and 2-point discrimination with a careful examination of the dermatomes throughout the shoulder, and upper extremity, because this may further localize the area of involvement.
  - A check of the reflexes in the upper extremity should complete the basic portion of the examination, noting any discrepancies between the two upper extremities.

Diagnostic Tests

- Although the history and physical examination will provide much of the information necessary to suggest the cause of a particular problem, additional information may be helpful in arriving at a definitive diagnosis.
- If the clinical presentation includes a history of trauma, radiographs may be required to rule out a fracture or dislocation.
- A computed tomography (CT) or magnetic resonance imaging (MRI) scan may be appropriate to provide more detailed information regarding the bony and soft-tissue structures of the cervical spine, shoulder, and throughout the upper extremity.
- A cervical myelogram may be indicated in traumatic injuries of the brachial plexus that could suggest a nerve root avulsion. An arteriogram may be necessary in the

setting of high-energy trauma to assess the integrity of the major arteries of the shoulder girdle.

- The role of nuclear medicine studies is limited to an adjunct tool for assessing bony problems, such as occult fracture, infection, neoplasm, or osteonecrosis, because these conditions are rarely associated with neurologic dysfunction.
- The primary diagnostic tools for evaluating neurologic abnormalities are the electromyogram (EMG) and nerve conduction studies (NCS).
  - The two tests combined allow the examiner to determine:
    - The presence of a nerve injury.
    - The anatomic region of the injury.
    - Whether the injury is acute or chronic.
    - Single or multiple nerve injuries.
    - The return of function after an injury.
    - Typically, it takes approximately 3 weeks before any abnormalities will become measurable with an EMG/NCS, so there is limited utility in the setting of an acute injury.
    - It may be appropriate to obtain an EMG/NCS early after an injury to determine the baseline measures in an athlete with a history of previous neurologic dysfunction.
- An EMG analyzes spontaneous and voluntary electrical activity in a muscle. *Insertional activity* refers to the electrical activity measured when the needle is inserted into a muscle or is moved within the muscle.
  - It is normal for there to be insertional activity.
    - Nerve damage can cause increased insertional activity in cases of mild degeneration (neuropraxia) or decreased insertional activity in cases of severe degeneration (axonotmesis or neurotmesis).
  - Normally, there is no spontaneous activity in a muscle unless it is stimulated.
    - The presence of spontaneous activity in a muscle indicates an abnormal condition.
  - Spontaneous activity consists of *fibrillation potentials* and *positive sharp waves*, and these may be seen in association with chronic denervation (axonotmesis or neurotmesis) and also reinnervation after neurologic injury.
  - *Motor unit potentials* measure the number of muscle fibers stimulated by a particular axon.
    - After an injury—whether it is a neuropraxia with conduction block, axonotmesis, or neurotmesis—there will be diminished or absent motor unit potentials.
    - As reinnervation occurs through regenerated axons or collateral reinnervation, motor unit potentials become larger and polyphasic in nature, allowing an objective measurement of recovery.
  - NCSs measure the velocity, duration, and amplitude response of a peripheral nerve to an electrical stimulus.
- Both motor and sensory components of a nerve can be assessed, with abnormalities being associated with prolonged latency (slower velocity) between the stimulus

BOX 21-1 ELECTROMYOGRAM AND NERVE CONDUCTION STUDY FINDINGS WITH NERVE INJURY

Needle Electrode Examination (EMG)
- Increased insertional activity
- Fibrillation potentials
- Positive sharp waves
- Increased motor unit firing rate
- Decreased number of motor units firing

Nerve Conduction Studies
- Diminished motor nerve amplitude
- Diminished sensory nerve amplitude
- Prolonged latency
- Slowed conduction velocity

EMG, electromyogram.

and a measured response, along with prolonged duration and decreased amplitude of the response.
- A summary of electrodiagnostic studies in peripheral nerve injuries is listed in Box 21-1.

TREATMENT

When considering treatment alternatives for athletes with nerve injuries of the upper extremity, it is important to consider the different options for treating acute versus chronic symptoms. There are several scenarios that may necessitate emergent operative treatment, including open fractures or dislocations, unreducible dislocations, compartment syndromes, and injuries with neurovascular compromise. Traumatic lacerations with neurologic symptoms may require exploration and nerve repair. Alternatively, the majority of patients who present with neurologic dysfunction of the upper extremity related to sports may be managed nonoperatively, with a period of relative rest, physical therapy, and if symptoms do not improve, surgery may be appropriate. A more thorough discussion of the surgical alternatives will follow the specific injuries discussed in the next section.

SPECIFIC INJURIES

Brachial Plexus

Anatomy
The brachial plexus (Fig. 21-2) arises from the nerve roots C5 to T1 as they exit from the spinal cord and travel distally in the neck, under the clavicle, and into the upper arm. The nerve roots combine to form the upper, middle, and lower trunks, then each trunk sends off an anterior and posterior division to form the lateral, posterior, and medial cords. At various levels, peripheral nerves branch off and continue to become motor and sensory nerves of the shoulder, trunk, and upper extremity.

Etiology

Injuries to the brachial plexus can occur through blunt or penetrating trauma, traction from fractures or dislocations, and laceration from fracture fragments. Be aware of the possibility of vascular injuries in the setting of penetrating trauma or comminuted fractures with significant displacement.

Most commonly, brachial plexus injuries can occur in athletes participating in contact sports such as football, wrestling, and hockey. These patients may suffer what is frequently referred to as a "burner." They will relate a history of striking another player, or the ground, with their shoulder, often, as their head is pushed to the contralateral side. Most frequently, a burner results from traction on the upper roots of the plexus, C5 and C6, as the shoulder is pushed downward, and the head is pushed to the opposite side (Fig. 21-3A). Other mechanisms include a compression-type injury in which the head is pushed to the same side as the symptomatic extremity (Fig. 21-3B), or a direct blow to the plexus from a helmet, a hockey stick, or lacrosse stick (Fig. 21-3C). It has been estimated that 20% to 65% of college football players experience a "burner" during their careers.

As athletes pursue "extreme" sports such as motocross, skateboarding, snowboarding, and mountain biking, the possibility of high-energy trauma increases. Severe injuries are rare but can occur, including scapulothoracic dissociation, in which the bony and soft-tissue structures attaching the scapula to the trunk are disrupted. This can include cervical root avulsions and vascular injury. Clinical suspicion is warranted to rule out this devastating injury.

Be aware of other diagnoses that can cause neck pain, weakness, and numbness of the upper extremity, including herniated disc, cervical spine fracture or instability, and spinal cord contusion.

Diagnosis

History

- Patients with a brachial plexus injury can present with a variety of symptoms, depending on the nature of the injury and the anatomic level of the injury.
- Patients who suffer burners report a confluence of symptoms ranging from burning, "pins and needles," weakness, tingling, and numbness, all the way to temporary paralysis of the upper extremity.
- The symptoms can last for a few seconds to several minutes, and occasionally beyond that, and may radiate from the shoulder to the hand and fingers.
- Patients with severe traumatic injuries of the brachial plexus may present with pain, strength, and sensory deficits related to the specific structures damaged by the injury.

Physical Examination

- The evaluation of patients with a brachial plexus injury should begin with the cervical spine to make sure there is no underlying damage that could result in a catastrophic event if undetected.
- When assessing patients on the playing field, spine precautions should be enacted for any athlete with a suspected cervical spine injury.
- When a high-speed injury occurs, patients should be treated following Advanced Trauma Life Support guidelines, including controlling the airway, providing CPR when indicated, and instituting spine precautions.
- Generally, a "burner" is not associated with neck pain or restricted motion of the cervical spine.
- Brachial plexus injuries can be divided into supraclavicular and infraclavicular injuries.

Figure 21-3   Burner mechanism of injury.

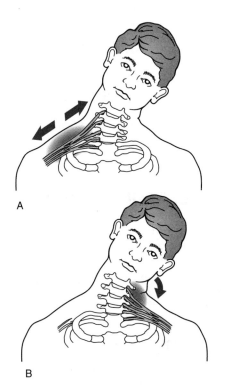

A

B

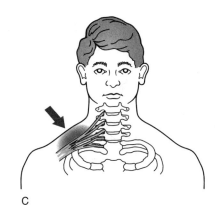

C

- Those injuries that occur above the clavicle, are supraclavicular, and are frequently associated with Horner's syndrome (ptosis, miosis, and anhydrosis).
  - These are generally more severe injuries and suggest the possibility of a cervical root avulsion, with loss of autonomic function.
- Passive and active range of motion should be assessed throughout the shoulder and upper extremity, along with careful evaluation of the motor strength, sensation and reflexes, in an effort to localize the level of injury.
- If possible, examine the patient from behind, looking for muscle atrophy or scapular winging.
- Peripheral pulses should be checked, because these may be altered in more severe injuries such as scapulothoracic dissociation or compartment syndrome.
- When there is no evidence of a traumatic neck injury, the physician can perform Spurling's test to differentiate between cervical disc disease and a brachial plexus problem.
  - Standing behind the patient, the examiner hyperextends the patient's cervical spine, flexes the head laterally toward the involved side, and applies a downward force on top of the head to axially load the spine.
  - If the patient experiences symptoms radiating into the arm, the result is positive, suggesting a cervical nerve root impingement related to disc disease or foraminal narrowing and not a brachial plexus problem.

Diagnostic Tests

- Athletes with neck pain in association with a burner should be evaluated with x-rays of the cervical spine to rule out a fracture or other bony injury.
- If radiographs are nondiagnostic, then further evaluation with an MRI or CT scan may be indicated if neck pain persists.
- Radiographs may be indicated to rule out fractures or dislocations of the upper extremity.
- In the setting of high-energy trauma, the diagnostic workup should follow Advanced Trauma Life Support protocols.
  - Radiographs and CT scans will provide initial data regarding the injured structures.
  - If scapulothoracic dissociation is suspected, an arteriogram should be considered to rule out vascular injury.
  - After the life-threatening injuries have been treated, additional information can be obtained with an MRI of the cervical spine, the brachial plexus, and the shoulder if indicated.
- There is little indication for an EMG/NCS in the acute setting, except as discussed previously.
- Patients with symptoms that persist beyond 3 weeks should be referred for further evaluation.
- Abnormalities may help to localize the level of involvement.
  - Patients will have normal sensory responses and abnormal spontaneous activity in the paraspinal muscles when the injury involves the cervical roots.

- Abnormal spontaneous activity in the upper extremity muscles with normal activity in the paraspinal muscles suggests a brachial plexus injury.

Treatment

- Most patients recover spontaneously from burners with little sequelae.
- In some athletes, the symptoms can occur repeatedly with future contact episodes.
- The treatment of a burner should include keeping the athlete out of sports until the symptoms resolve and the physical examination returns to normal.
- Encourage the patient to work on regaining full range of motion of the cervical spine and the upper extremity.
- Any strength deficits should be addressed through a focused rehab program.
- The athlete should be instructed on proper technique to avoid recurrent injury.
- For football players, protective collars on the shoulder pads may lessen the likelihood of recurrence.
- Patients need to be evaluated on a daily basis for the first few days after injury and then weekly until the symptoms have resolved.
- The treatment of a traumatic brachial plexus lesion depends on the mechanism of injury, the associated injuries, and the level of involvement.
  - After the life-threatening injuries have been stabilized, the orthopaedic injuries can be addressed, including reduction of dislocations and fractures, and internal fixation when appropriate.
  - In severely injured patients, the secondary survey may delineate the extent of neurologic deficits, whereas additional diagnostic studies will provide information to aid in planning the treatment.
  - Initially, in the setting of a closed injury without radiographic or electrophysiologic evidence of a nerve root avulsion or nerve disruption, a shoulder sling may be appropriate for comfort, along with physical therapy to help restore motion and strength of the extremity.
  - If functional deficits persist after 3 to 6 months, surgical alternatives include neurolysis, nerve repair, nerve grafting, neurotization, nerve transfer, and muscle transfer.

IDIOPATHIC BRACHIAL NEURITIS

A rare cause of brachial plexus dysfunction can be idiopathic brachial neuritis—also known as acute brachial neuropathy, neuralgic amyotrophy, brachial plexus neuropathy, and Parsonage-Turner syndrome—which was named after two physicians who reported on 136 soldiers treated during World War II.

Etiology

In one population study, the incidence of Parsonage-Turner syndrome was 1 to 2 cases per 100,000 citizens. The typical patient with this condition is between 30 and 70 years of age, with men being affected twice as frequently as women. There is a belief that the syndrome may be a sequela of a viral infection, although other possible etiologies include heavy exertion, autoimmune disease, and recent immunizations.

Diagnosis

History and Physical Examination

- Patients can present with gradual or occasional sudden onset of pain in the shoulder and upper arm, along with varying degrees of muscle weakness and occasional sensory deficits.
- The symptoms can manifest with activity, as well as at rest.
- Typically, the shoulder and upper arm muscles are affected; but in severe cases, the entire extremity can be involved.
- The symptoms can mimic other conditions such as rotator cuff disease, cervical spine disorders, and compressive neuropathy.
- Athletes with this condition may demonstrate weakness and atrophy of several muscles of the shoulder girdle and upper extremity, including muscles of the hand and wrist.
- Reflex and sensory deficits may be present.

Diagnostic Tests

- The diagnosis of idiopathic brachial neuritis is based on the exclusion of other more common conditions.
- Routine radiographs will generally provide little information.
- An MRI scan of the shoulder should be obtained to rule out rotator cuff disease, ganglion cysts that may cause nerve compression, and to assess the presence of muscle atrophy.
- It may be appropriate to obtain an MRI of the cervical spine to evaluate any cervical disc disease.

- The essential diagnostic tool is an EMG, typically showing changes 3 weeks after symptoms develop.
  - The findings of fibrillation potentials and positive sharp waves indicate muscle denervation in association with axonal neuropathy.
  - Increased latencies and decreased active potentials are also noted.

Treatment

- Treatment of brachial neuritis consists of analgesics, physical therapy to prevent arthrofibrosis, and work on strengthening exercises to restore function.
- Spontaneous recovery generally occurs over several months, although occasionally the process may take several years.
- Athletes can return to participation as their functional recovery allows.

SUPRASCAPULAR NERVE

As our understanding of shoulder problems has evolved, physicians have recognized the subtleties of dysfunction that can occur as a result of injuries other than rotator cuff disease and glenohumeral ligament laxity. Although there is a long list of differential diagnoses that need to be considered when evaluating patients with shoulder problems, no list would be complete without considering injury to the suprascapular nerve.

Anatomy

Arising from the C5 and C6 nerve roots, the suprascapular nerve branches off of the superior trunk of the brachial plexus (Fig. 21-4). The nerve supplies motor innervation to the supraspinatus and infraspinatus muscles, along with

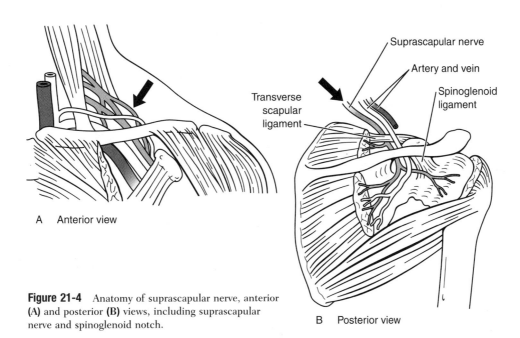

A   Anterior view

Suprascapular nerve

Artery and vein

Spinoglenoid ligament

Transverse scapular ligament

B   Posterior view

Figure 21-4   Anatomy of suprascapular nerve, anterior **(A)** and posterior **(B)** views, including suprascapular nerve and spinoglenoid notch.

sensory innervation to the subacromial bursa, acromioclavicular joint, and glenohumeral joint. The nerve traverses posteriorly, deep to the trapezius, where it passes under the superior transverse scapular ligament, through the suprascapular notch, before giving off a motor branch to the supraspinatus muscle and sensory branches to the subacromial bursa and acromioclavicular joint. The nerve continues posteriorly and winds around the spine of the scapula as it enters the spinoglenoid notch, under the spinoglenoid ligament. From there, the nerve gives off a sensory branch to the posterior glenohumeral joint and then terminates in motor branches to the infraspinatus muscle.

Etiology

The suprascapular nerve can be injured through several mechanisms such as fractures of the scapula and clavicle or penetrating trauma. The nerve can become entrapped in either the suprascapular or spinoglenoid notch, typically by a thickened superior transverse scapular or spinoglenoid ligament, respectively (see Fig. 21-4). The nerve may be compressed by a ganglion cyst in either notch or other soft-tissue mass along its course. With athletes who participate in repetitive overhead activities, the nerve is at risk for traction injury associated with these sports. There have been several reports in the literature noting the occurrence of suprascapular neuropathy in volleyball players. As with many peripheral nerves, there is also a risk of damage to the suprascapular nerve during shoulder surgery. In a cadaver dissection, Warner et al. found that the nerve could be injured if the supraspinatus and infraspinatus were mobilized more than 3 cm. However, the occurrence of such injuries has not been documented in the literature.

Diagnosis

History and Physical Examination

- Typically, there is no specific injury that precedes the development of symptoms with suprascapular nerve problems.
- Patients will usually complain of aching pain in the posterior aspect of the shoulder, often exacerbated by overhead activities.
- Some patients may seek treatment because of weakness of the shoulder girdle.
- With overhead athletes, diminished performance may be the impetus to seek medical consultation.
- Occasionally, patients can be asymptomatic, and the only manifestation of the injury may be muscle atrophy.
- A routine part of the physical examination of any athlete with shoulder pathology is an assessment from behind the patient, looking for atrophy of the muscles of the shoulder girdle.
- With suprascapular nerve palsy, the physical findings will depend on the level of involvement.
- If the nerve is entrapped in the suprascapular notch, there may be atrophy of the supraspinatus and infraspinatus, along with weakness of the external rotators, and a positive supraspinatus test (see Fig. 15-3 in Chapter 15).
- Additionally, pain may be exacerbated with crossed adduction because this places the nerve under additional tension.
- If the site of injury is the spinoglenoid notch, the supraspinatus will be spared, and the patient may have atrophy of the infraspinatus and weakness of the external rotators.
- Some patients, however, may not have any weakness, as the teres minor can help to maintain strength against resisted external rotation, and, in that situation, they may be asymptomatic.
- Generally, patients will have normal range of motion of the shoulder unless limited by muscle weakness.

Diagnostic Tests

- When considering suprascapular nerve palsy in the differential diagnosis of posterior shoulder pain, an EMG/NCS will provide diagnostic information, including the presence of a nerve palsy, as well as the location of the lesion.
  - It is important to localize the site of the nerve injury, because that will determine the surgical approach if necessary.
- Routine x-rays of the shoulder will generally offer little information for patients with suprascapular nerve palsy, unless there is a clavicle or scapula fracture as an underlying cause.
  - If there is a question of a cervical radiculopathy, x-rays of the c-spine should be obtained to evaluate any abnormalities.
- MRI (Fig. 21-5) may be helpful in patients with suprascapular nerve palsy, looking for a ganglion cyst in the suprascapular or spinoglenoid notch.
  - These cysts can frequently be seen in association with a labral tear.
  - A routine MRI scan will delineate the cyst, but an MRI arthrogram may be better at detecting labral pathology associated with the cyst. MRI scans will also reveal the presence of any other soft-tissue mass that may be a source of compression of the nerve.
- If the EMG or NCS is abnormal and the MRI scan fails to show any abnormalities, the patient is most likely suffering from entrapment of the suprascapular nerve in the suprascapular or spinoglenoid notch, depending on the EMG/NCS findings.

Treatment

Nonsurgical

- The initial treatment of patients with suprascapular nerve palsy includes avoidance of the activities that produce symptoms, along with a physical therapy program to improve flexibility and strength of the rotator cuff and scapular stabilizers.
- Anti-inflammatory medication and analgesics may be appropriate.
- Several small studies have shown that most patients can anticipate gradual relief of symptoms and improvement in strength and muscle bulk over a period of 6 to 12 months.
- Nonoperative treatment is less likely to be successful in patients with a ganglion cyst.

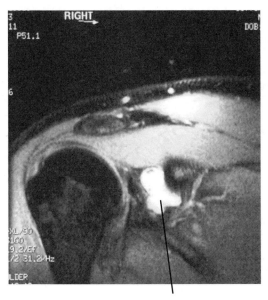

Ganglion cyst

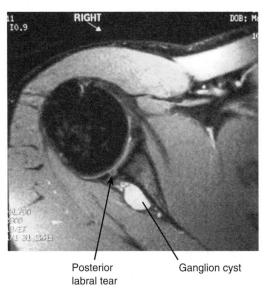

Posterior   Ganglion cyst
labral tear

Figure 21-5 MRI scans of cyst in spinoglenoid notch.

- A review of the literature revealed less than 25% success with nonoperative treatment of these patients.
- Mixed results have been reported with ultrasound- and CT-guided aspiration of ganglion cysts associated with suprascapular nerve palsy.

Surgical Treatment
- Surgical intervention should be considered when pain symptoms and weakness persist despite nonoperative management for 3 to 6 months.
- The surgical approach to treat suprascapular nerve palsy is determined by the underlying pathology as evaluated with EMG/NCS and MRI scan.
  - When the MRI scan fails to reveal a cyst or other soft-tissue mass, and the EMG/NCS show abnormalities of the supraspinatus and infraspinatus—the site of involvement is the suprascapular notch.
- Surgical treatment is to release the superior transverse scapular ligament through a posterior approach to the shoulder.
  - The patient is placed on a beanbag in a lateral decubitus position, with the affected arm draped free.
  - The skin incision runs along the spine of the scapula, with the trapezius being elevated superiorly, and the underlying supraspinatus being reflected inferiorly to expose the suprascapular notch.
  - While protecting the underlying nerve and adjacent vascular structures, the ligament is released.
  - Numerous reports have demonstrated relief of pain and gradual return of muscle strength with this intervention.
- The decision to operate when the EMG/NCS localizes the lesion to the spinoglenoid notch is based on pain symptoms that occur with atrophy of the infraspinatus.
  - Ferretti noted that, despite atrophy of the infraspinatus muscle, a majority of volleyball players were able to function without impairment.

- The surgical approach varies by exposing the nerve on both sides of the spinoglenoid notch.
- The trapezius and supraspinatus are retracted superiorly, and the deltoid and infraspinatus are reflected inferiorly.
- The spinoglenoid ligament is released under direct visualization while protecting the nerve.
- On occasion, the spinoglenoid notch may need to be deepened to alleviate traction on the nerve.
- If the MRI scan reveals a ganglion cyst, arthroscopic examination of the glenohumeral joint is indicated to look for and repair a labral tear, or other intra-articular abnormality that may have led to the development of the cyst.
  - It may be possible to decompress and debride the cyst arthroscopically through the labral defect; however, in some patients, the cyst may need to be excised through an open approach.
- Postoperatively, patients are placed in a sling for 1 to 3 weeks, with early range of motion, depending on the intra-articular findings at the time of surgery.
- The rehabilitation program includes active and passive range-of-motion exercises, along with scapular stabilization and rotator cuff strengthening.
- Most athletes return to sports within 2 to 4 months.
- Even with successful resolution of symptoms after surgical decompression of the suprascapular nerve, nearly half of patients may have persistent atrophy.

AXILLARY NERVE

Injuries of the axillary nerve are the most common nerve injury of the shoulder. Considerable dysfunction of the upper extremity can occur as a sequela of axillary nerve damage.

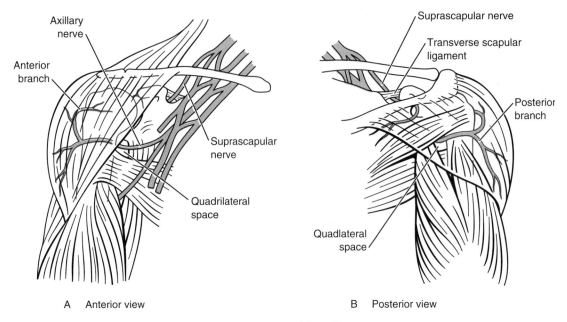

Figure 21-6   Anatomy of the axillary nerve.

Anatomy

The C5 and C6 nerve roots contribute to the posterior cord of the brachial plexus (Fig. 21-2), from which the axillary nerve continues distally, as it runs along the anterior surface of the subscapularis muscle (Fig. 21-6A). As the axillary nerve reaches the inferior surface of the subscapularis, it curves posteriorly and inferiorly under the glenohumeral joint. The nerve passes through the quadrilateral space (Fig. 21-6B), where it divides into anterior and posterior branches. The posterior branch supplies motor innervation to the teres minor and posterior deltoid, and sensory innervation to the lateral aspect of the shoulder via the superior lateral cutaneous nerve. The anterior branch curves anteriorly and superiorly around the humerus, where it innervates the middle and anterior deltoids. Anatomic studies have shown the axillary nerve enters the middle deltoid approximately 5 cm below the lateral edge of the acromion, a point to remember when performing surgery through a deltoid-splitting approach.

Etiology

As with other peripheral nerve problems, axillary nerve injuries can occur through a variety of mechanisms, including traction, blunt trauma, entrapment, and iatrogenic causes. The nerve is most commonly injured after anterior dislocation of the glenohumeral joint, with resultant traction and compression from the dislocated humeral head. Several studies have shown the incidence of axillary nerve injury after glenohumeral dislocation to range from 5% to 54%, with older patients and shoulders left unreduced for several hours being more susceptible. Displaced fractures of the shoulder may also damage the nerve through traction or, in rare cases, laceration of the nerve from fracture fragments. The axillary nerve can be damaged from blunt trauma during contact sports such as football, and hockey, although this is a less frequent scenario.

A rare cause of axillary nerve dysfunction has been termed "quadrilateral space syndrome," a condition in which the nerve becomes entrapped by fibrous bands and hypertrophied muscle in the quadrilateral space (teres minor, long head of triceps, teres major, and humeral shaft).

The axillary nerve is also at risk of injury during various surgical procedures to correct shoulder pathology, including anterior stabilization, arthroplasty, fracture fixation, rotator cuff repairs, and arthroscopy. Surgeons need to identify and protect the nerve from injury during open surgical techniques, and maintain an awareness of proximity to the axillary nerve during arthroscopic and open procedures. The nerve is more likely to be injured in revision shoulder surgery, because the anatomy is frequently abnormal and scar tissue may inhibit adequate visualization.

Diagnosis

History and Physical Examination
- Manifestations of axillary nerve palsy can include sensory and motor components, depending on the nature and location of the injury, as well as the presence of any associated involvement of the brachial plexus.
- Patients may present with weakness of the shoulder, typically in flexion and abduction, along with numbness of the lateral aspect of the shoulder.
- With quadrilateral space syndrome, the athlete may complain of aching pain in the posterior shoulder, and paresthesias of the lateral shoulder, without significant weakness.
- After surgical procedures of the shoulder, diminished sensation over the lateral aspect of the shoulder may be the earliest sign of axillary nerve injury because deltoid function after surgery may be impaired by pain.
- Physical findings associated with axillary nerve palsy are related to the degree of injury, ranging from normal appearance and strength of shoulder flexion and abduction to severe deltoid atrophy and weakness (Fig. 21-7).

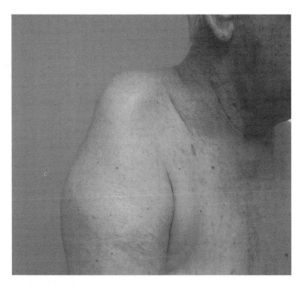

Figure 21-7 Atrophy associated with axillary nerve palsy.

- Patients will typically demonstrate altered sensation over the lateral aspect of the shoulder.
- With any shoulder injury, it is important to document sensory deficits that may suggest axillary or other nerve dysfunction.
- Range of motion of the shoulder may be impaired, depending on the underlying cause of the nerve injury.
- Unless there is an associated brachial plexus injury, reflexes will be normal.
- Patients with quadrilateral space syndrome may present with no significant findings on exam, other than tenderness of the posterior shoulder.

Diagnostic Tests
- Routine x-rays of the shoulder are indicated to reveal any fractures or dislocations that may be associated with axillary nerve palsy.
  - If the patient complains of neck pain, cervical spine films should be obtained.
- The diagnostic test of most value will be an EMG/NCS, looking for alterations of the deltoid and teres minor function, along with the sensory changes that are common with axillary nerve palsy.
  - The electrophysiologic studies will also elucidate any abnormalities of the brachial plexus that may suggest a more significant problem.
  - Because most axillary nerve palsies are related to traumatic or iatrogenic causes, the test will be of little benefit until 3 weeks or more after the injury.
  - Abnormal findings are summarized in Box 21-1.
- In evaluating quadrilateral space syndrome, an arteriogram may provide additional information with altered flow through the posterior circumflex artery as the arm is brought into abduction and external rotation.

Treatment
- When an axillary nerve injury is diagnosed, the treatment is influenced by a variety of factors.

- With closed injuries such as dislocations or fractures, a prompt reduction is indicated to alleviate traction on the nerve and lessen the risk of injury from a fracture fragment.
- A careful physical examination before treatment is necessary to document any baseline neurologic abnormalities.
  - The examination should be repeated after the reduction maneuver, and any changes should be noted.
- If symptoms persist for more than 3 weeks, an EMG/NCS should be performed to assess any electrophysiologic abnormalities, including the axillary nerve and the brachial plexus.
- Most injuries of the axillary nerve can be managed nonoperatively with sling immobilization for a short period of time, depending on the underlying injury, and a rehabilitation program focusing on range-of-motion and strengthening exercises.
  - The recovery of nerve function may take 3 to 6 months, depending on the initial injury, and a repeat EMG/NCS may be indicated to provide objective evidence of recovery if an athlete has ongoing symptoms and functional limitations.
- If there is no clinical or electrophysiological evidence of recovery by 3 to 6 months after a closed injury, surgical exploration may be indicated.
  - When an axillary nerve palsy occurs in the setting of penetrating trauma, early exploration of the wound and nerve repair within a few weeks of the injury may be indicated if the EMG/NCS shows severe changes.
- Patients who develop axillary nerve dysfunction after a surgical procedure can be managed with careful observation.
  - Frequently, the nerve can suffer a neurapraxia, resulting from traction during surgery.
  - An EMG/NCS should be obtained if no improvement is noted after 3 weeks.
  - If the results of the study suggest disruption of the nerve, exploration is indicated.
- Surgical options depend on the findings at the time of surgery and include primary nerve repair, neurolysis, and sural nerve grafting.
  - Patients are generally placed in a lateral decubitus position because anterior and posterior approaches may be necessary to perform a successful repair, frequently with sural nerve grafting.
  - There are a few studies in the literature reporting successful results in 50% to 100% of patients.
  - The best results were noted in patients who underwent surgery within 6 months of the injury.
- For some patients, salvage procedures may be indicated to treat severe deltoid atrophy and weakness that does not resolve with nerve grafting and repair.
  - In those patients, if the posterior deltoid function is preserved, it may be possible to rotate the posterior deltoid anteriorly on the acromion.
  - Alternatively, a shoulder fusion can be considered to provide a stable fulcrum for the upper extremity during activities of daily living.

■ Athletes with quadrilateral space syndrome can be treated using a rehab program that focuses on stretching and strengthening as a part of anticipated recovery.

■ Rarely, surgical decompression through a posterior approach to the shoulder is indicated for patients who remain symptomatic after nonoperative treatment.

■ Cahill and Palmer achieved good or excellent results in 16 of 18 patients treated with decompression.

MUSCULOCUTANEOUS NERVE

Isolated injury of the musculocutaneous nerve rarely occurs with athletic activities. The nerve is more frequently injured after trauma to the shoulder or surgical procedures around the shoulder and has been reported to account for less than 2% of 14,000 nerve injuries treated in World War II.

Anatomy

The musculocutaneous nerve arises from the C5 and C6 nerve roots as they contribute to the lateral cord of the brachial plexus (Fig. 21-2). The nerve sends motor branches that enter the undersurface of the coracobrachialis and brachialis muscles approximately 5 cm distal to the coracoid process, as well as a motor branch to the biceps brachii muscle (Fig. 21-8). The nerve courses distally beyond the elbow, where it provides sensory innervation to the radial aspect of the forearm via the lateral antebrachial cutaneous nerve.

Etiology

In sports activities, the musculocutaneous nerve can be injured as a result of traction from an anterior glenohumeral

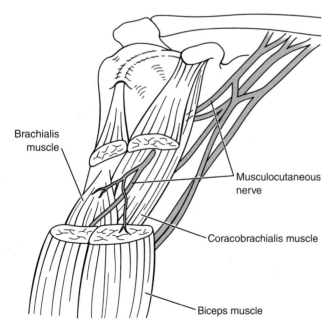

Brachialis muscle

Musculocutaneous nerve

Coracobrachialis muscle

Biceps muscle

Figure 21-8   Anatomy of the musculocutaneous nerve.

dislocation. Rarely, patients can develop musculocutaneous nerve palsy as a result of weight lifting, either from entrapment of the nerve associated with hypertrophy of the biceps musculature or stretching and compression of the nerve during repetitive biceps strengthening exercises. More commonly, the musculocutaneous nerve can be injured during shoulder surgery via a deltopectoral incision because retractors are placed under the conjoined tendon to visualize the anterior aspect of the glenohumeral joint. The nerve's proximity puts it at risk for injury. Entrapment of the lateral antebrachial cutaneous nerve resulting in isolated sensory deficits has been reported in association with racquet sports.

Diagnosis

History and Physical Examination

■ Patients with musculocutaneous nerve dysfunction may present with weakness of elbow flexion and supination, along with numbness of the radial aspect of the forearm.

■ It is important to consider a biceps tendon rupture, C5 to C6 cervical radiculopathy, or brachial plexus injury in the differential diagnosis when evaluating patients with symptoms suggesting injury to the musculocutaneous nerve.

■ After an acute event such as a shoulder dislocation or anterior shoulder surgery, a patient with damage to the musculocutaneous nerve may have weak elbow flexion and supination.

■ It is possible that elbow flexion strength deficits may be subtle, however, because of an intact brachioradialis, which acts as a synergist, and that weakness of supination may be the more predominant finding.

■ Typically, there will be an absent biceps (C6) reflex and diminished sensation over the radial aspect of the forearm.

■ It is important to assess for diminished sensation, altered reflexes, and weakness of other muscles around the shoulder girdle and upper extremity that might suggest a broader injury to the brachial plexus.

■ In some patients, spontaneous recovery of normal function can occur within hours after a musculocutaneous palsy related to strenuous overuse.

Diagnostic Tests

■ Radiographs are indicated to assess for fractures or dislocations in the setting of traumatic injuries.

■ If dysfunction persists after 3 weeks of symptoms, the primary diagnostic tool for evaluating musculocutaneous nerve damage is the EMG/NCS, looking for fibrillation potentials in the biceps, positive waves, decreased voluntary motor unit action potentials, and prolonged latency on nerve stimulation.

Treatment

■ The treatment of musculocutaneous nerve injury related to sports participation includes relative rest, with gradual resumption of activities as symptoms resolve.

- Recovery may take several months, with most patients regaining full function, although some atrophy and sensory deficits may persist.
- For patients who show persistent weakness and EMG/NCS deficits after 3 months, surgical treatment should be considered.
- Surgical options include neurolysis, primary nerve repair, and nerve grafting.
- In the cases of injury related to trauma or surgical procedures, surgical exploration led to 67% good results after early nerve repair in a series of 85 patients.

LONG THORACIC NERVE

Injury of the long thoracic nerve is rare but can occur in a variety of sports, including volleyball, gymnastics, weight lifting, hockey, and tennis.

Anatomy

Branches from cervical roots C5 to C7 combine immediately after they exit the intervertebral neuroforamina to form the long thoracic nerve before it travels distally and laterally under the clavicle and first rib. The nerve becomes more superficial as it travels along the chest wall, where it innervates the serratus anterior muscle. The serratus anterior arises from ribs 2 through 9, and inserts on the medial (vertebral) border of the scapula (Fig. 21-9). The muscle helps to stabilize, protract, and elevate the scapula during shoulder motions.

Etiology

Patients may develop palsy of the long thoracic nerve from traumatic or nontraumatic causes. Because of the nerve's subcutaneous location, it is at risk of injury from a direct blow during contact sports, or less commonly from direct pressure that can occur when a patient lies on his or her side for a prolonged period of time during a surgical procedure. Long thoracic nerve injury can occur during various surgical procedures, including first rib resection for thoracic outlet syndrome and axillary node dissection for breast cancer. The nerve can also suffer repetitive microtrauma during activities that cause traction on the nerve with overhead activities such as volleyball, tennis, and baseball. The nontraumatic causes of long thoracic nerve palsy include compression from adjacent bony and soft-tissue structures as the nerve courses from the cervical spine to the serratus anterior muscle. As discussed earlier in this chapter, nerve compression can lead to ischemia of the microcirculation and subsequent dysfunction. There have also been cases of long thoracic nerve palsy after a viral illness and brachial neuritis.

Diagnosis

History and Physical Examination

- Patients with long thoracic nerve palsy may present with diffuse complaints of aching pain in the shoulder, neck, and scapular region, typically brought on by various overhead activities.
- There may be some degree of weakness that can affect athletic performance such as throwing or tennis.
- The athlete may notice deformity of the shoulder and back with efforts to lift the arm.
- Patients typically do not complain of numbness unless there is a more extensive process involved, such as brachial neuritis, because the long thoracic nerve has no sensory components
- The most obvious physical finding for patients with injury of the long thoracic nerve is scapular winging.
  - As the athlete attempts to forward flex the arm, the winging will typically become more pronounced (Fig. 21-10).
  - A wall push-up is a provocative maneuver that may exacerbate scapular winging.
- Frequently, the patient may have loss of motion related to weakness of forward flexion and abduction of the shoulder.

Diagnostic Tests

- As with many of the nerve injuries in this chapter, the most useful diagnostic test is an EMG/NCS, which can show the level and severity of the injury, as well as any recovery of function.
- The test may also help differentiate between other neurologic conditions, such as brachial neuritis or spinal accessory nerve injury, which can also cause scapular winging.
- It may be reasonable to get plain radiographs to look for any unusual bony abnormalities, such as a cervical rib, which can cause compression of the nerve.
- More advanced imaging techniques such as MRI and CT are rarely indicated for this condition.

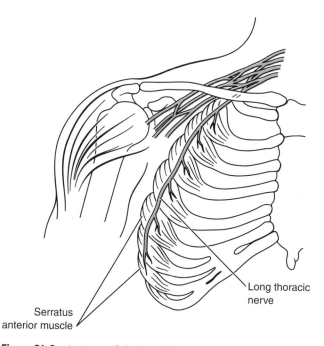

Figure 21-9 Anatomy of the long thoracic nerve and the serratus anterior muscle.

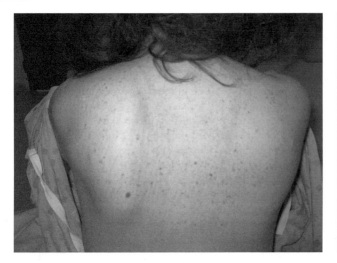 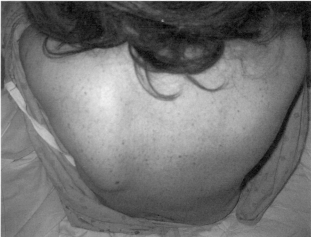

Figure 21-10   Scapular winging.

Treatment

Nonsurgical Treatment

- In general, most patients with dysfunction of the long thoracic nerve can be treated nonoperatively because spontaneous recovery tends to occur over a period of 12 months after the onset of symptoms.
- Patients should be restricted from the causative sport and be referred for physical therapy to maintain range of motion of the shoulder, along with strengthening exercises for the scapular stabilizers and surrounding muscles that are trying to compensate for the weakened serratus anterior.
- Some authors have attempted to stabilize the scapula with a special brace worn around the torso with limited success.

Surgical Treatment

- For patients whose symptoms or EMG results do not improve after 1 to 2 years of nonoperative treatment, surgery may be appropriate.
- The surgical options include pectoralis major transfer, pectoralis minor transfer, rhomboid transfer, teres minor transfer, scapulothoracic fusion, or scapular stabilization without fusion.
- Several reports in the recent literature present data on transfer of the sternal head of the pectoralis major, augmented with autograft hamstrings, fascia lata, or allograft.
  - The technique involves detaching the sternal head portion of the pectoralis major from the humerus, creating a longer construct by weaving an autograft hamstring, fascia lata or allograft, and then passing the tendon through a hole created in the inferior aspect of the scapula.
  - Noerdlinger et al. reported that 75% of 15 patients in their study would undergo the procedure again.
  - Warner and Navarro reported satisfactory results in 7 of 8 patients using autogenous semitendinosus or gracilis augmentation.
  - In a series of 11 patients published by Connor et

al., 91% of the patients were improved at an average follow-up of 41 months.
- There have also been several articles reporting successful treatment of scapular winging in a small series of patients with neurolysis of the long thoracic nerve, or with nerve transfer of the thoracodorsal or medial pectoral nerve to the long thoracic nerve with favorable results.

SPINAL ACCESSORY NERVE

Thus far in this chapter, we have focused on peripheral nerve injuries around the shoulder associated with sports participation. The spinal accessory nerve, cranial nerve 11, can also affect function of the shoulder and upper extremity.

Anatomy

The spinal accessory nerve provides motor innervation to the trapezius and the sternocleidomastoid muscles (Fig. 21-11). The nerve exits the base of the skull via the jugular foramen and travels through the sternocleidomastoid muscle where it continues subcutaneously along the floor of the posterior cervical triangle until it reaches the trapezius. The trapezius is a large, broad muscle that arises from the spinous processes of the neck, the upper and middle back, and inserts along the spine of the scapula, the medial acromion and the lateral clavicle. The muscle has three functional components: (1) the upper portion elevates and laterally rotates the scapula, (2) the middle portion stabilizes and retracts the scapula medially, and (3) the lower portion depresses and downwardly rotates the scapula. As the muscle facilitates scapular stabilization, elevation, and depression, it is vital to the normal function of the shoulder and upper extremity.

Etiology

Injuries to the spinal accessory nerve during sports are rare and can be caused by a direct blow from a helmet, hockey

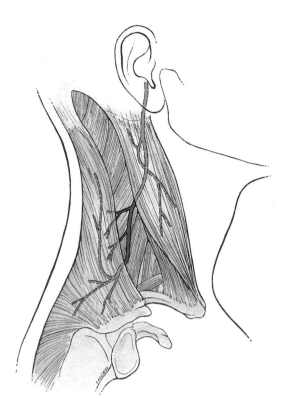

Figure 21-11   Anatomy of the spinal accessory nerve. (From Agur AM, Dalley AF II. Grant's Atlas of Anatomy, 11th ed. Philadelphia: Lippincott Williams & Wilkins, 2004.)

stick, or lacrosse stick. There have also been cases of spinal accessory nerve palsy in patients wearing a shoulder sling for prolonged periods of time. More commonly, injury occurs from penetrating trauma, or during surgical procedures in the neck, including lymph node biopsy, carotid endarterectomy, and tumor resections. Weakness and scapular winging in the absence of trauma or surgical intervention may suggest an underlying neurologic disease or other process.

Diagnosis

History and Physical Examination
- An athlete suffering an injury to the spinal accessory nerve during sports may not experience any symptoms at first.
  - Subsequently, the patient may notice aching pain, along with weakness and difficulty lifting and abducting the arm.
  - Over time, the patient may notice drooping of the shoulder and loss of normal muscular contour.
- Patients can develop pain secondary to impingement of the rotator cuff, as well as pain from muscle spasm of the levator scapula or rhomboids, which are working to compensate for the trapezius dysfunction.
- As the shoulder droops, traction on the brachial plexus may cause discomfort.
- Overhead athletes will generally experience diminished

performance as a result of these previously described symptoms.
- A patient with injury to the spinal accessory nerve will typically have an abnormal contour of the shoulder and neck related to atrophy of the trapezius muscle, the sternocleidomastoid muscle, and associated drooping of the shoulder.
- When the athlete attempts to forward flex the shoulder, winging of the scapula may occur.
- Typically, there will be weakness with abduction and shrugging of the shoulder although, in some patients, a strong levator scapulae can compensate somewhat.
- Shoulder range of motion should be assessed because patients can develop adhesive capsulitis.
- The examination should conclude with a thorough neurologic assessment of the entire extremity to rule out a more involved process such as a brachial plexopathy or some other neurologic condition.

Diagnostic Tests
- As with most orthopaedic conditions, routine x-rays may be part of the patient evaluation.
  - Radiographs of the cervical spine, shoulder, and chest can be considered, with low expectation of any significant abnormalities.
- Similarly, CT and MRI scans may offer minimal information unless there is suspicion of cervical disc disease or a neoplastic process.
- EMG/NCS will provide the most useful information regarding the level of injury, the degree of involvement, and any neurologic recovery that may occur.

Treatment

Nonsurgical Treatment
- Athletes suffering spinal accessory nerve palsy related to sports participation can generally be managed nonoperatively.
  - It may be appropriate to offer a sling initially for comfort, along with mild analgesics for pain.
  - A referral for physical therapy is important to allow the patient to maintain shoulder range of motion, as well as a strengthening program to focus on the surrounding musculature to minimize drooping of the shoulder.
  - Patients may benefit from modalities and transcutaneous nerve stimulation in an effort to alleviate pain symptoms.
  - There may also be a role for electrical muscle stimulation to help lessen muscle atrophy.
  - EMG/NCS should be repeated after several months to assess functional recovery.
  - If symptoms and strength do not improve after 1 year, it is unlikely that continued nonoperative treatment will offer any benefit.
  - At that point, surgery should be considered in active patients.

Surgical Treatment
- In the setting of spinal accessory nerve palsy resulting from a penetrating injury, early exploration with nerve

repair or nerve grafting is recommended to offer the best chance for recovery.

- Surgical treatment of spinal accessory nerve palsy consists of static or dynamic procedures to restore function.
  - Static procedures such as scapulothoracic fusion or fasciodesis are designed to stabilize the scapula to the chest wall or spinous processes, respectively.
  - In a review article, Bigliani states that the results of static procedures for spinal accessory palsy tend to deteriorate with time as grafts stretch out.
- Alternatively, several authors recommend dynamic procedures using local muscle transfers to mimic the function of the trapezius.
  - The "Eden-Lange procedure" involves lateral transfer of the levator scapula, rhomboid minor, and rhomboid major muscles, with each muscle substituting for various portions of the dysfunctional trapezius.
    - The Eden-Lange procedure originally involved transfer of the levator scapula through the trapezius to the lateral spine of the scapula, along with transfer of the rhomboid minor and major to the infraspinatus fossa.
    - The levator scapula mimics the upper trapezius, the rhomboid minor, the middle trapezius, and the rhomboid major the lower trapezius.
  - Bigliani has modified the procedure by transferring the rhomboid minor to the supraspinatus fossa in an effort to more closely reproduce the function of the middle trapezius.
    - Together, the three muscles help to restore mobility and the appearance of the shoulder girdle, although return to sports is less predictable.
    - As described by Bigliani, the technique involves placing the patient in a lateral decubitus position, with an incision between the spinous processes and the medial border of the scapula.
    - The trapezius is elevated off the scapula, and the levator and two rhomboids are identified and detached from the medial scapula border with a sliver of bone using an osteotome.
    - The muscles are then mobilized toward the spinous processes to allow for advancement.
    - The next step in the procedure involves elevating the supraspinatus and infraspinatus from medial to lateral.
    - Drill holes are made in the supraspinatus and infraspinatus fossas 4 or 5 cm lateral to the medial border of the scapula.
    - The rhomboid minor is transferred to the supraspinatus fossa, and the rhomboid minor is transferred to the infraspinatus fossa, where they are sutured to the drill holes with nonabsorbable sutures while maintaining the shoulder in 90 degrees of abduction and the scapula in a reduced position.

- A second incision is then made along the spine of the scapula, medial to the posterolateral corner of the acromion.
- The deltoid, trapezius, and supraspinatus are elevated off the spine of the scapula, while protecting the suprascapular nerve from injury.
- Drill holes are made in the scapular spine 5 to 7 cm medial to the posterolateral corner of the acromion, and the levator scapula is passed through the trapezius and sutured in to place.
- Postoperatively, the patient is placed in an abduction brace for 4 weeks while undergoing rehabilitation.

SUGGESTED READING

Beghi E, Kurland LT, Mulder DW, et al. Brachial plexus neuropathy in the population of Rochester, Minnesota, 1970–1981. Ann Neurol 1985;18:320–323.

Bigliani LU, Compit CA, Duralde XA, et al. Transfer of the levator scapulae, rhomboid major, and rhomboid minor for paralysis of the trapezius. J Bone Joint Surg Am 1996;78:1534–1540.

Cahill BR, Palmer RE. Quadrilateral space syndrome. J Hand Surg 1983;8:65–69.

Connor PM, Yamaguchi K, Manifold SG, et al. Split pectoralis major transfer for serratus anterior palsy. Clin Orthop Relat Res 1997; 341:134–142.

Cummins CA, Messer TM, Nuber GW. Suprascapular nerve entrapment. J Bone Joint Surg Am 2000;82:415–424.

Ferretti A, De Carli A, Fontana M. Injury of the suprascapular nerve at the spinoglenoid notch. Am J Sports Med 1998;26:759–763.

Hirasawa Y, Sakakida K. Sports and peripheral nerve injury. Am J Sports Med 1983;11:420–426.

Krivickas LS, Wilbourn AJ. Peripheral nerve injuries in athletes. Semin Neurol 2000;20:225–232.

Long RR. Nerve anatomy and diagnostic principles. In: Pappas AM, ed. Upper Extremity Injuries in the Athlete. New York: Churchill Livingstone, 1995:43–75.

Magee KR, DeJong RN. Paralytic brachial neuritis. JAMA 1960;174: 1258–1262.

Noerdlinger MA, Cole BJ, Stewart M, et al. Results of pectoralis major transfer with fascia lata autograft augmentation for scapula winging. J Shoulder Elbow Surg 2002;345–350.

Osborne AWH, Birch RM, Munshi GB. The musculocutaneous nerve. J Bone Joint Surg Br 2000;82:1140–1142.

Safran MR. Nerve injury about the shoulder in athletes. Part 1: suprascapular and axillary nerve. Am J Sports Med 2004;32:3:803–819.

Safran MR. Nerve injury about the shoulder in athletes. Part 2: long thoracic nerve, spinal accessory nerve, burners/stingers, thoracic outlet syndrome. Am J Sports Med 2004;32:1063–1076.

Seddon HJ. Three types of nerve injury. Brain 1953;66:237.

Steinmann SP, Moran EA. Axillary nerve injury: diagnosis and treatment. J Am Acad Orthop Surg 2001;9:328–335.

Steinmann SP, Spinner RJ. Nerve problems about the shoulder. In: Rockwood CA, Matsen FA, Wirth MA, et al., eds. The Shoulder. Philadelphia: WB Saunders: 2004:1009–1031.

Warner JJP, Navarro RA. Serratus anterior dysfunction: recognition and treatment. Clin Orthop Relat Res 1998;349:139–148.

Warner JP, Krushell RJ, Masquelet A, et al. Anatomy and relationships of the suprascapular nerve: anatomical constraints to mobilization of the supraspinatus and infraspinatus muscles in the management of massive rotator cuff tears. J Bone Joint Surg Am 1992;74:36–45.

Wiater JM, Bigliani LU. Spinal accessory nerve injury. Clin Orthop 1999;368:5–16.

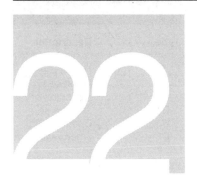

ELBOW INJURIES

ANTHONY SCHENA
ILYA VOLOSHIN

Although not the most common type of elbow injury sustained by athletes, fractures still occur and must be treated appropriately to allow the athlete to return to sport. Given the current explosion of extreme sports, all types of fractures are now being seen in the athletic population. The ultimate goal for the treating physician is to identify the fracture and follow through with proper care. Management of both the fracture and the soft-tissue envelope is critical in the final outcome for injuries about the elbow.

General principles established in fracture and trauma texts hold true for the athlete with an elbow fracture. In general, all athletes who are skeletally mature (closed physes—females aged 14 years or older, males aged 15 years or older) can be treated with standard rigid fixation. Rigid fixation supports osseous healing while allowing for early passive and active assisted range of motion, which will influence the overall outcome for athletes, especially throwing athletes.

The following text is not meant to replace the treatment algorithms established in fracture texts, but rather to augment this treatment by focusing on the athletic elbow.

BIOMECHANICS

The elbow consists of two distinct diarthrodial joints: the ulnohumeral and the radiocapitellar joints. The ulnohumeral provides flexion and extension, while the radiocapitellar provides supination and pronation. There also exists a third joint, between the ulna and radius, which allows the radius to rotate around the ulna with pronation and supination. Activities of daily living require a flexion-extension arc of 30 to 130 degrees and 50 degrees of supination and pronation. Anteroposterior (AP) stability of the elbow relies heavily on the constrained ulnohumeral joint for static control. Dynamic control is provided by the brachialis and biceps anteriorly and the triceps posteriorly. The articular surfaces, as well as the radial and ulnar ligamentous structures, also lend AP support. Valgus stressors are resisted primarily through a combination the anterior portion of the medial collateral ligament (MCL), the radial head, and the anterior capsule. Varus stressors are primarily resisted by the combination of the anconeus muscle and the lateral collateral ligament.

OLECRANON FRACTURES

ANATOMY AND PATHOPHYSIOLOGY

The olecranon makes up the proximal end of the ulna and is the primary articular contact for the distal humerus. This articular surface extends from the tip of the olecranon to the coronoid with one significant interruption, a "bare area" that exists approximately halfway between the tip and the

TABLE 22-1 CLASSIFICATION OF OLECRANON FRACTURES

Type	Description
I	Nondisplaced
II	Displaced
A	Avulsion
B	Transverse
C	Comminuted
D	Fracture/dislocation

(Adapted from Colton CL. Fractures of the olecranon in adults: classification and management. Injury 1973;5:121–129.)

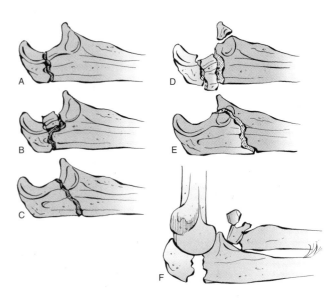

Figure 22-1   Schatzker classification of olecranon fractures. **A:** Transverse. **B:** Transverse impacted. **C:** Oblique. **D:** Comminuted. **E:** Oblique distal. **F:** Fracture dislocation. (From Court-Brown C, McQueen M, Tornetta P III. Orthopaedic Surgery Essentials: Trauma. Philadelphia, Lippincott Williams & Wilkins, 2006.)

coronoid. Along with the coronoid process, it makes up the greater sigmoid notch. When in extension, the olecranon sits within the olecranon fossa of the distal humerus and confers bony stability for the elbow. The olecranon articulates with the trochlea of the humerus throughout the elbow arc of motion. As the elbow moves into flexion, the bony stability decreases, and the soft-tissue envelope of the elbow becomes the primary dynamic and static stabilizing force for the elbow. The olecranon serves as the insertion point for the triceps brachii and anconeus muscles and the origin for ulnar aspect of the flexor carpi ulnaris muscle.

Olecranon fractures are usually the result of a direct blow to the olecranon or the indirect result of falling on an out stretched arm. If the force is significant enough, the proximal aspect of the olecranon will be displaced proximally with the triceps tendon. The remainder of the ulna can move anteriorly with the radius, resulting in a fracture dislocation of the elbow.

CLASSIFICATION

There are multiple classification schemes for the olecranon, none of which is universally accepted by orthopaedists. The simplest one, created by Colton (1973), focuses on fracture displacement and type (Table 22-1). Schatzker's (1987) classification is relatively simple and may be the most useful to the orthopaedist because it allows one to assess different treatment options (Table 22-2 and Fig. 22-1). Whichever

scheme is chosen, the important aspect of the assessment is fracture stability and overall condition of the articular surface.

DIAGNOSIS

- Fractures of the olecranon tend to have a concomitant effusion due to intra-articular extension.
- There can be a large amount of soft-tissue edema, which may make palpation of a step-off difficult.
- When assessing the function of the elbow, the ability to actively extend the elbow is the most important test to conduct.
  - Failure of the extension mechanism usually results in the decision for surgical repair.
- As with any fracture, a careful neuralgic examination should be performed, as well as a thorough inspection of the skin.

Radiologic Examination

- AP and true lateral views are needed.
- Oblique lateral views can obscure the true extent of the intra-articular fracture.
- Most olecranon fractures do not need more than clinical and radiographic workups.

TABLE 22-2 CLASSIFICATION OF OLECRANON FRACTURES

Type	Description
A	Transverse
B	Transverse impacted
C	Oblique
D	Comminuted
E	Oblique distal
F	Fracture dislocation

(Adapted from Schatzker J. Fractures of the olecranon. In: Schatzker J, Tile M, eds. The Rationale of Operative Fracture Care, 2nd ed. Berlin: Springer-Verlag, 1996;113–119.)

TREATMENT

Nondisplaced Fractures

- Nondisplaced fractures can be treated in a long arm cast flexed between 45 and 90 degrees for 3 weeks.
- This period of immobilization is then followed by a protected range of motion (0 to 90 degrees) in a hinged elbow brace until the fracture has united.

- Bony union takes approximately 6 to 8 weeks.
- Once bony union is achieved, physical therapy should focus on obtaining full flexion.
- For older patients, it is advisable to start range of motion before 3 weeks because they are more prone to stiffness.
    - These patients can be protected in the hinged brace or a sling to encourage earlier motion.

Displaced Fractures

- There are four established goals for operative fixation of displaced fractures:
    - Maintain power of the extensor mechanism
    - Avoid incongruity of the articular surface
    - Restore stability of the elbow
    - Prevent stiffness of the joint
- How the surgeon achieves these goal depends on the fracture pattern and the surgeon's experience.

Avulsion Fractures

- Avulsion fractures can be treated with Kirschner (K) wire and tension band fixation.
- The goal of tension band fixation is to convert the tensile forces found along the dorsum of the olecranon into dynamic compressive force across the articular surface.
- The approach for this and most other olecranon fractures is posterior, with the incision slightly lateral to the olecranon.
    - This helps to avoid a painful scar over the tip of the olecranon and keeps the approach away from the ulnar nerve.
    - The ulnar nerve does not need to be isolated or transposed, but its location should be palpated and noted throughout surgery.
- Once through the soft tissue, the avulsed olecranon is usually readily identifiable.
- The hematoma is evacuated and the joint copiously irrigated.
- A trial reduction is conducted and held with reduction clamps.
- K-wires are then passed antegrade through the avulsed tip and into the shaft of the olecranon.
    - The target point is the volar cortex just distal to the coronoid.
    - The position of the K-wires is checked with fluoroscopy.
- Once satisfied with the reduction, the drill hole in the ulna shaft is made for the tension band. It is placed in the dorsal half of the shaft of the ulna distal to the fracture site.
- Next, 16- or 18-gauge wire is then passed through the drill hole and passed dorsally over the ulna. A loop is created on the radial side.
- A 14-gauge angiocatheter is passed between the triceps and tip of the olecranon from ulnar to radial.
    - This allows safe passage of the wire and protects the ulnar nerve.
- Once passed, the ends are twisted together, and tension is placed on the wire by tightening the loop and the twisted ends simultaneously, which will result in increased tension.

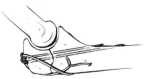

Figure 22-2   Example of tension band wiring of elbow. (From Court-Brown C, McQueen M, Tornetta P III. Orthopaedic Surgery Essentials: Trauma. Philadelphia, Lippincott Williams & Wilkins, 2006.)

- The wire knots are then cut to 3 to 4 mm after being bent distally so that they lie along the radial and ulnar sides of the olecranon (Fig. 22-2).
- Once completed, the fixation is tested by bringing the elbow through a range of motion.
- Final position of the hardware is checked with plain films.
- The wound is copiously irrigated and then closed.
- The arm is placed in a posterior splint.

Simple Transverse Fractures

- These fractures are treated in the same manner as the avulsion fractures.
- A 6.5 cancellous screw with a washer can be used in place of the K-wires (Fig. 22-3).
    - After the reduction, the triceps tendon is split in line with its fibers.
    - The olecranon and ulnar shaft are then drilled and tapped for a 6.5 (4.5 can be used for a small ulna) partially threaded cancellous screw.
    - The cancellous screw needs to engage the cortex of the ulna shaft, usually requiring an 80 to 120 mm screw.
    - Before fully seating the screw, the pilot hole for the

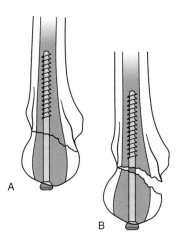

Figure 22-3   **A:** Proper placement of an intramedullary screw. **B:** Placement of the screw slightly off the intramedullary axis results in fracture malreduction. (After Hak D, Golladay G. Olecranon fractures: treatment options. J Am Acad Orthop Surg 2000;8: 266–275. © 2000 American Academy of Orthopaedic Surgeons.)

tension band should be made and the wire passed as described previously.

- ■ The tension is set and the screw tightened.
- ■ Care must be taken not to overseat the screw because this can translate the fracture.
- ■ Proponents of this technique cite application of static and dynamic compression, security of the screw, and strength of the construct as reasons to use the screw.
- ■ Opponents believe that prominent hardware and potential overreduction and translation are reasons to avoid screw fixation.

Transverse Fractures with Comminution

- ■ Fractures with minimal comminution are amenable to fixation with K-wires and tension band, but great care must be taken to avoid compressing the comminution and disrupting the arc of motion between the trochlea and olecranon.
- ■ In cases with extensive comminution, it is best to treat the fracture with plates and screws.
  - ■ These fractures usually require bone graft to support the articular surface.
    - ■ Reconstruction plates, low-contact dynamic compression (LCDC) plates, or preformed olecranon plates can be helpful in dealing with these fractures (Fig. 22-4).
  - ■ Once initial reduction is achieved, K-wires are used to hold the fragments in place.
  - ■ Bone graft is added as necessary to support the articular surface.
  - ■ The plates are then applied using AO technique.
  - ■ Once again, care must be taken to avoid placing too much compression across the fracture.

Oblique Fractures without Comminution

- ■ These fractures are amenable to fixation with a lag screw and plate.
- ■ The lag screw is placed through a plate, from the tip of the olecranon to a point just distal to the coronoid process.
- ■ Screws are then placed, using AO technique, into the proximal aspect of the prebent plate.
- ■ The distal screws are then placed using AO compression techniques.

Oblique Fractures with Comminution

- ■ These fractures are fixed as noted previously, but great care must be taken to avoid excess compression when the lag screw and plate are being placed.

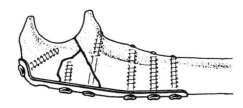

Figure 22-4 Plate fixation of the comminuted fracture.

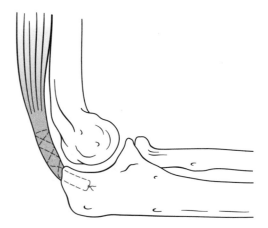

Figure 22-5 When excision and triceps advancement are performed, the triceps should be attached adjacent to the articular surface. (After Cabanela ME, Morrey BF. Fractures of the proximal ulna and olecranon. In: Morrey BF, ed. The Elbow and Its Disorders, 2nd ed. Philadelphia: WB Saunders, 1993:416. Modified with permission from the Mayo Foundation for Medical Education and Research. All rights reserved.)

- ■ In some instances, the lag screw or the compression through the plate may not be used to protect a severely comminuted fracture.

Severe Comminution or Osteopenic Bone

- ■ In some cases, adequate reduction is not achievable.
- ■ It is then advisable to excise the proximal end of the olecranon and repair the extensor mechanism.
- ■ When conducted, the triceps should be reattached adjacent to the articular surface (Fig. 22-5).

POSTOPERATIVE CARE

- ■ As described previously, all of these surgical cases will be placed in a long posterior splint after surgery.
- ■ After an early rest period (1 to 7 days), early motion is begun.
- ■ The extent and start time for early motion will depend on the fracture type and fixation used.
- ■ Fractures treated with tension banding are usually amenable to movement by day 7.
  - ■ Hinged elbow braces or cast braces help to protect the repair.
- ■ More complicated fractures, those fixed with neutralization plates, or patients who are unreliable should be protected in a cast for 2 to 3 weeks.
- ■ This period of immobilization is followed by passive and active assisted range of motion, as well as protection in a brace.
- ■ Once the patient demonstrates radiographic and clinical union, active range of motion is started.

RESULTS

- ■ About 76% to 98% of patients achieve good to excellent results.

- Most experience a loss of extension (~10 degrees), flexion (~5 degrees), some pronation and supination (~5 degrees each), and loss of strength when compared with the contralateral side.
- Poorer results have occurred with elderly patients, delayed surgery, malreduction, and extensive comminution.

COMPLICATIONS

- The most significant complications occur due to painful hardware.
    - 20% to 80% of patients will complain of hardware issues
    - 30% to 70% of patients will require hardware removal
    - 1% to 5% of all hardware will break
- Other complications include infection (0% to 6%), ulnar neuritis (2% to 12%), and heterotopic ossification (2% to 13%).

RADIAL HEAD FRACTURES

PATHOPHYSIOLOGY

The radial head is the proximal, intra-articular portion of the radius. It is involved in both the flexion/extension and pronation/supination arcs of motion. It forms articular joints with both the capitellum, as well as the ulna via the sigmoid notch. The highest level of force is exerted across the radiocapitellar joint at full extension and across the radioulnar joint during pronation. The radial head also provides stability to the elbow when a valgus force is exerted.

Radial head fractures are the result of direct loading of the radius, usually after a fall onto an outstretched arm. Fractures also occur during an elbow dislocation or a direct blow to the posterior aspect of a flexed elbow.

CLASSIFICATION

The Hotchkiss modification of the Mason classification is given in Table 22-3.

DIAGNOSIS

History and Physical Examination

- Most patients complain of pain along the lateral side of the elbow with motion along the flexion/extension plane or pronation/supination plane.

TABLE 22-3 CLASSIFICATION OF RADIAL HEAD FRACTURES

Type	Description
I	Nondisplaced/minimally displaced head or neck fracture Forearm rotation limited by acute pain only Intra-articular displacement <2 mm
II	Displaced (>2 mm) Mechanically limited/incongruous Minimal comminution/more than marginal lip of articular surface
III	Severe comminution Requires excision

(Adapted from Hotchkiss RN. Fractures and dislocations of the elbow. In: Rockwood CA Jr, Green D, Bucholz R, et al., eds. Fractures in Adults, 4th ed. Philadelphia: Lippincott-Raven, 1996.)

- With more severe injuries, there will be a mechanical block to motion, although pain with motion may mimic a mechanical block.
- With higher-grade injuries, there is often gross edema around the elbow.
- With type I injuries, pain may be the only pertinent physical finding.

Radiologic Examination

- As with any suspected fracture, plain films are the first line of a diagnostic workup. AP, lateral, and oblique views of the elbow are obtained to diagnose the fracture.
- A radiocapitellar view, achieved by angling the x-ray tube 45 degrees cephalad with the forearm in neutral, may also be helpful.
- If the patient complains of wrist or forearm pain, then films of the wrist and forearm should also be obtained.
- If the fracture appears amenable to a surgical procedure, it is often helpful to obtain a computed tomography (CT) scan of the elbow as well.

TREATMENT

Type I Fractures

- Type I fractures are treated without surgical intervention.
- The patient is placed in a sling for several days to recover from the acute trauma.
- Aspirating the hematoma and injecting a local anesthetic can provide significant analgesia (Fig. 22-6).
- Most patients will recover functional range of motion within 2 to 3 months.
- Some may have a residual loss of extension, pain, or stiffness, even with a nondisplaced fracture.

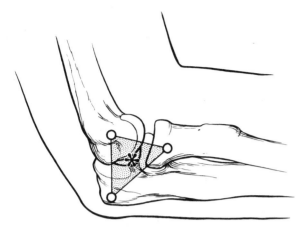

Figure 22-6 The landmarks for aspiration of the elbow joint are the radial head, lateral epicondyle, and tip of the olecranon. A needle inserted into the center of the triangle (*asterisk*) penetrates only the anconeus muscle and capsule before entering the joint. (From Mezera K, Hotchkiss RN. Fractures and dislocations of the elbow. In: Bucholz RW, Heckman JD, eds. Rockwood and Green's Fractures in Adults, 5th ed. Philadelphia: Lippincott Williams & Wilkins, 2002:943.)

Type II Fractures

- All type II fractures should be considered for open reduction with internal fixation (ORIF), especially when the patient is less than 55 years old.
- Fractures associated with instability should be fixed at any age.
- The best indication for fixation are type II fractures that consists of <30% of the radial head or a "slice" fracture that is displaced more than 3 mm.
- Some type II fractures will not have a mechanical block and may be treated similarly to type I.
- Surgery to fix a type II radial head fracture is conducted through the classic Kocher approach to the lateral elbow.
    - Once the fracture is identified, the hematoma is removed and care is taken not to strip any soft-tissue attachments from the fracture fragments.
    - The articular surface is then reconstructed and the reduction held with a 0.425 K-wire.
    - A 2.7 screw is inserted using AO technique.
        - The screw should be placed through the bare area on the radial head (located on the lateral aspect of the radial head when the forearm is held in neutral) (Fig. 22-7).
    - A second screw should be placed if necessary.
    - On some occasions, a small T-plate can be used if the fracture fragment is large enough.
    - When associated with an Essex-Lopresti lesion, ORIF of the radial head fracture is especially helpful.

Type III Fractures

- In the presence of severe comminution of the radial head, the only option is often excision.

- When considering excision of the radial head, it is imperative to be sure that there is not a concomitant Essex-Lopresti lesion.
- Without the radial head present, the radius will migrate proximally due to the incompetent interosseous ligament.
    - Because of this phenomenon, the space once occupied by the radial head must be accounted for.
- Some success has been reported with delayed excision of the radial head, as well as with silicone implants.
    - Silicone implants have caused soft-tissue reaction and have other problems associated with them.
    - Titanium implants allow for maintenance of the radial length when the radial head needs to be excised; however, there has been some documented failure even with these prostheses.
    - Indications for use of a metallic radial head are given in Box 22-1.
    - Because of the questionable outcomes with prosthetic replacement, every effort should be made to save the radial head, especially in the young athlete.

POSTOPERATIVE CARE

- For patients who undergo ORIF of the radial head, a posterior splint is used for 3 to 4 days and a passive motion machine for 2 to 3 weeks.
- At 3 weeks, the patient is allowed to start active assisted and gentle active range of motion.
- This range of motion should be along the extension and supination planes.
- Flexion and pronation are avoided.
- At 6 weeks, with evidence of healing, physical therapy is begun in all planes.
- Complete healing usually occurs by 3 months, and motion is usually achieved by 12 months.
- For patients who undergo a radial head replacement, motion is allowed on postoperative day 2.
- Active assisted and passive range of motion are initiated at first, followed by active range of motion. Similar postoperative management is used for pure excisions of the radial head.

COMPLICATIONS

- Early complications include forearm motion loss, poor fixation, loss of fixation, and injury to the posterior interosseous nerve.
- Early fixation failure should be treated with delayed radial head excision (3 to 4 weeks later).
- Late complications include nonunion, painful hardware, and elbow stiffness.
- The plate, if used, may be removed safely after 6 months.
- Heterotopic bone may form, especially in cases associated with head trauma and other associated elbow injuries.
    - The heterotopic bone can be dealt with once it has matured.

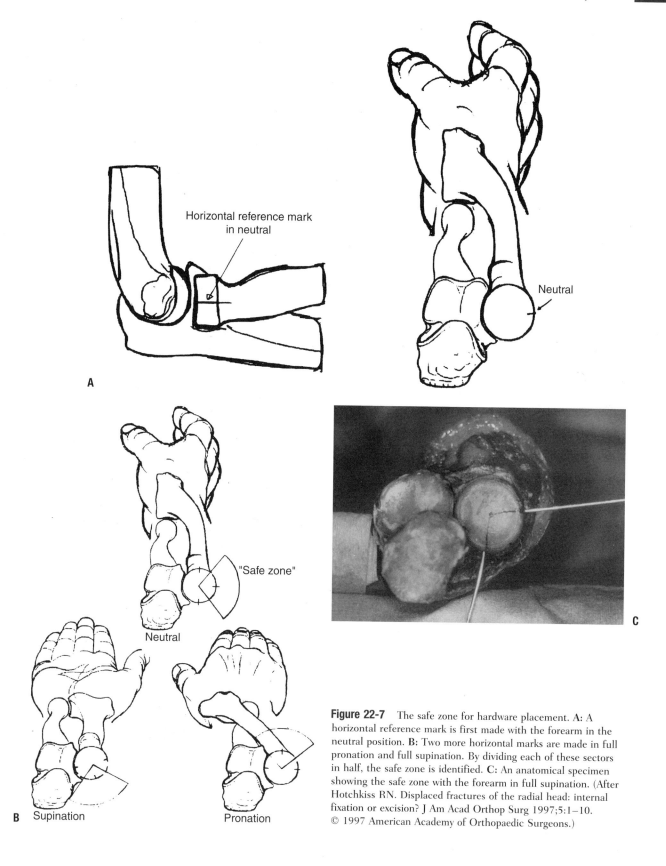

Horizontal reference mark
in neutral

Neutral

A

"Safe zone"

Neutral

C

B   Supination   Pronation

Figure 22-7   The safe zone for hardware placement. A: A
horizontal reference mark is first made with the forearm in the
neutral position. B: Two more horizontal marks are made in full
pronation and full supination. By dividing each of these sectors
in half, the safe zone is identified. C: An anatomical specimen
showing the safe zone with the forearm in full supination. (After
Hotchkiss RN. Displaced fractures of the radial head: internal
fixation or excision? J Am Acad Orthop Surg 1997;5:1–10.
© 1997 American Academy of Orthopaedic Surgeons.)

BOX 22-1 INDICATIONS AND CONTRAINDICATIONS FOR USE OF A METALLIC RADIAL HEAD

Indications
Acute trauma
   Type III radial head fracture associated with:
      Elbow dislocation or Essex-Lopresti injury
      Coronoid type II/III fx or olecranon type III fracture
      After radial head excision with continued elbow instability

Reconstruction
   With interposition arthroplasty if radial head removed and evidence of continued instability
   Stabilization of the forearm and elbow after an Essex-Lopresti injury
   Failed silicone radial head replacement if needed for stability

Contraindications
Acute trauma
   Older patient (>65) with type III fracture without elbow instability or other associated injury
   Open fracture of the radial head, olecranon, or open dislocation with a high risk of infection
   Mason type I or II
   Mason type III without elbow or forearm instability

Reconstruction
   Poor radiocapitellar alignment
   Proximal radial shaft fractures with comminution into the head
   Disease or injury to the capitellum

Absolute Contraindications
   Prior sepsis or question of wound contamination
   Known sensitivity to makeup of prosthesis
   Skeletal immaturity
   Insufficient tissue to provide stability
   Resected radius is malaligned with the capitellum

(Adapted from Morrey B. Radial head fractures. In: Morrey B, ed. The Elbow, 2nd ed. Philadelphia: Lippincot Williams & Wilkins, 2002.)

CORONOID FRACTURES

PATHOPHYSIOLOGY

Once underappreciated, the coronoid fracture has now become an important factor in determining and treating injuries to the elbow. In general, at least 50% of the coronoid is required to maintain elbow stability. Usually, overall elbow stability must take into account ligamentous stability, radial head involvement, as well as the coronoid. Injury to all three of these components, known as the "terrible triad," will be discussed later in the chapter. This section will focus on the lower-grade injuries to the elbow that involve a coronoid fracture.

TABLE 22-4 CLASSIFICATION OF CORONOID FRACTURES

Type	Description	Management
I	Shear or avulsion fracture as a result of the pull of the anterior capsule Involves up to 50% of the coronoid and represents a significant injury to the coronoid and the elbow	Usually marks the occurrence of an elbow dislocation and requires no further treatment than the standard care for an elbow dislocation
II	Involves greater than 50% and is unstable	Elbow is considered to be unstable until proven otherwise
III	When the fracture is caused by a varus force on an extended elbow, the medial collateral ligament is attached to the fragment	Elbow is unstable and needs to be treated aggressively

(Adapted from Morrey B. Fractures of the coronoid and complex instability of the elbow. In: Morrey B, ed. The Elbow, 2nd ed. Philadelphia: Lippincott Williams & Wilkins, 2002.)

Coronoid fractures tend to result from a varus moment on and extended elbow or direct impact of the coronoid against the trochlea. The most widely accepted classification concerning the coronoid is given in Table 22-4 and Figure 22-8.

DIAGNOSIS

■ Initial workup consists of x-rays. In most cases of coronoid injuries, there will be pre- and postreduction film (due to the elbow dislocation).

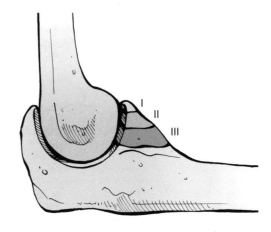

Figure 22-8 Regan-Morrey classification of coronoid fractures. (From Court-Brown C, McQueen M, Tornetta P III. Orthopaedic Surgery Essentials: Trauma. Philadelphia: Lippincott Williams & Wilkins, 2006.)

- After the reduction, it is important to document the stability of the elbow, as well as the arc of motion in which the elbow is stable.
- For patients in whom a more severe injury is suspected, a magnetic resonance imaging (MRI) is usually helpful in determining the extent of the ligamentous damage.

TREATMENT

Indications and contraindications for fixation of coronoid fractures are given in Box 22-2.

Type I Injuries

- Type I injuries essential represent an elbow dislocation.
- Once the ulnohumeral joint has been reduced, this fracture does not need to be addressed acutely.
- Occasionally, the small avulsion can cause anterior elbow discomfort or represent a loose body in the elbow and can be dealt with arthroscopically.

Type II and III Fractures

- This type of fracture can be approached from the posterior side.
  - The patient is placed supine and the operative arm is draped across the chest and over a bolster.
  - A posterior incision is made just medial to the tip of the olecranon.
    - This allows access to the fracture and ulnar nerve.
  - Once the subcutaneous flap is made, the ulnar nerve is identified.
    - The nerve can be left in place or released and transposed anteriorly.
- If transposed, the intermuscular septum is released.
- The soft tissues are elevated off the anterior septum, and the brachialis is elevated off the anterior surface of the humerus.
- The pronator is elevated, but the flexor carpi ulnaris (FCU) is left for closure.
- The MCL is identified and protected.
- The muscle flap is elevated off the capsule and the brachialis is swept radially, exposing the capsule.
- The capsule is split longitudinally, exposing the anterior joint and the coronoid fracture.
- The fracture is reduced with bone-holding forceps and the fragment held with a 0.045 or 0.062 K-wire.
- It is then stabilized with a 2.7 screw (Fig. 22-9).
- In some cases, the fracture involves a more extensive medial piece of the ulna.
  - Screw fixation alone is not adequate and a contoured buttress plate should be added.
- In cases in which the fracture fragments are very small or comminuted, suture fixation may be the only available means for fixation (Fig. 22-10).
  - Drill holes are made in the fragments if possible, and no. 2 or no. 5 sutures are passed through the drill holes and the capsule.
  - If possible, the insertion of the brachialis should be incorporated into the repair.
  - Retrograde drill holes are then made from the subcutaneous border of the ulna to the base of the fracture near the articular surface.
  - The sutures are passed through and tied over the dorsal aspect of the ulna.
  - During the reduction, care should be taken to align the fragments as best as possible close to the joint surface.

BOX 22-2 INDICATIONS AND CONTRAINDICATIONS FOR FIXATION OF CORONOID FRACTURES

Indications
- Type II fractures with intact radial head and a grossly unstable ulnohumeral joint when flexed less than 50 to 60 degrees
- Type II coronoid fractures associated with a radial head fracture and elbow dislocation (terrible triad)
- Isolated anteromedial coronoid fracture

Contraindication
- Patients who are more than 5 to 6 days postinjury with a reduced ulnohumeral joint (to avoid heterotopic calcification)

(Adapted from Morrey BF, O'Driscoll SW. Fractures of the coronoid and complex instability of the elbow. In: Morrey BF, ed. The Elbow. 2nd ed. Philadelphia: Lippincott Williams & Wilkins, 2002.)

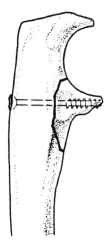

Figure 22-9 Lag screw fixation of the coronoid may be crucial to stability if the fracture is associated with dislocation. (After Heim U, Pfeiffer KM. Internal Fixation of Small Fractures, 3rd ed. Berlin, Springer-Verlag, 1988.)

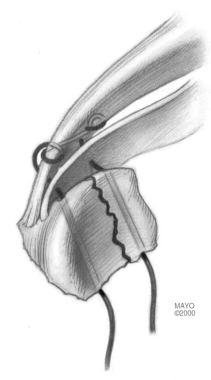

MAYO
©2000

Figure 22-10   Krachow suture technique. The stitch is used to secure the brachialis muscle, capsule, and fractured fragments. (From Morrey BF, O'Driscoll SW. Fractures of the coronoid and complex instability of the elbow. In: Morrey BF, ed. The Elbow, 2nd ed. Philadelphia: Lippincott Williams & Wilkins, 2002:134.)

ELBOW DISLOCATION/ TERRIBLE TRIAD

PATHOPHYSIOLOGY

Elbow dislocations account for 10% to 25% of all elbow injuries. The mechanism of injury is usually a fall onto an outstretched arm. The median age for injury is 30 years old, and the occurrence is spread between sports (40%) and high-energy accidents (50%). Ninety percent are either posterolateral or straight posterior and, if present, the most common associated fractures involve the radial head and coronoid process.

CLASSIFICATION

Although traditional classification schemes have dealt with direction, Morrey (2003) found classifying the dislocation as perched or complete much more clinically relevant (Fig. 22-11). O'Driscoll et al. (1992) found a significant difference in stability between a perched and complete dislocation but could not find much significance between a complete dislocation that was posterior, posterolateral, or anterior. When a varus extension force is placed on an elbow, the lateral ulnar collateral ligament (ULCL) is dis-

rupted as the olecranon rotates and moves posteriorly out of the fossa. If the force ends at this point, the elbow is perched but still has some intrinsic stability due to the intact MCL and the anterior capsule. When the force continues, the olecranon completely dislocates, tearing the remaining soft-tissue restraints. This creates a "ring of instability" and results in a much more unstable elbow. A complete dislocation may also have other associated injuries with it. Concomitant injury to the brachial artery, ulnar and median nerves, radial head, and coronoid process have all been reported.

DIAGNOSIS

History and Physical Examination

- As with other injuries about the elbow, the patient usually presents with pain, edema, and loss of motion.
- A gross step-off posteriorly may be appreciated with complete dislocation.
- Along with the elbow examination, a thorough neurovascular examination should be conducted.
- The ipsilateral shoulder and wrist should be examined because there is a 10% to 15% chance of an associated injury to these joints.

Radiologic Examination

- AP, lateral, and oblique views of the elbow, along with proper films of other suspected sites of injury, should be obtained.
- Postreduction films are essential.
- If other fractures are noted after reduction, proper imaging of these injuries should be performed.

TREATMENT

Nonsurgical Treatment

- The first priority in treating an elbow dislocation is reduction.
- For perched dislocation, the reduction can often be conducted with an intra-articular injection of a local anesthetic.
  - Once the joint has been anesthetized, longitudinal traction is placed on the affected arm at 45 degrees.
  - Pressure is then applied to the olecranon to guide it back into the fossa.
- For a complete dislocation, the same maneuver is used, but it is usually necessary to use either full-blown conscious sedation or general anesthesia.
- Once reduced, x-ray confirmation needs to be made by obtaining an AP and true lateral views of the elbow.
  - These films need to be scrutinized for widening of the joint and possible fractures.
- If adequately reduced, the next step is to determine the stable range of motion.
- The elbow is then splinted in the appropriate position to confer stability.

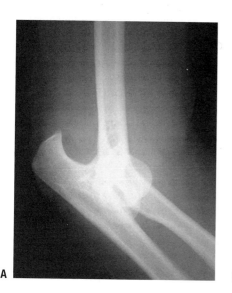
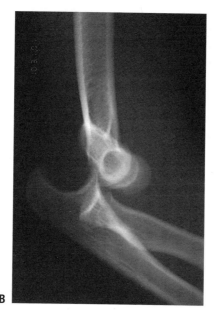

Figure 22-11 A: Complete dislocation. B: Perched dislocation. (From Court-Brown C, McQueen M, Tornetta P III. Orthopaedic Surgery Essentials: Trauma. Philadelphia: Lippincott Williams & Wilkins, 2006.)

- For perched dislocations, the elbow is splinted at 90 degrees for 2 to 3 days and then range of motion is started.
- For complete dislocations, the elbow is protected for 5 to 10 days before starting therapy.
- Immobilization for greater than 3 weeks results in loss of motion.
- X-rays should be checked at least at weeks 1 and 3.
  - Dislocations that were thought to be unstable should be checked more often.
- Perched dislocations usually achieve normal range of motion by 6 to 8 weeks.
- Complete dislocations usually attain 80% to 90% of their motion by 3 months.
- Any patient who displays a contracture of 50 degrees or more after 3 weeks should be placed in an extension brace.
- Strengthening begins in earnest by 8 to 10 weeks.

Surgical Treatment

- Surgical intervention is reserved for patients who require an extreme amount of flexion to remain reduced, who fail to have a congruous reduction, or who have unstable fractures associated with the dislocation.
- The most common fracture/instability pattern is the "terrible triad," which consists of an elbow dislocation, as well as a radial head and coronoid fracture.
- Once the elbow dislocation is reduced, the radial head and coronoid fractures need to be addressed as described previously in this chapter.
- When dealing with these fractures, both the MCL and ULCL should be repaired to achieve the best possible outcome.
- Multiple studies have looked into the repair of the ULCL, the MCL, and both ligaments.
  - Both ligaments play important roles in elbow stability, with the MCL providing stabilization of the ulno-

humeral joint and the ULCL stabilizing the radiocapitellar joint.
  - In instances of simple elbow dislocations, there is no merit in repairing the ligaments acutely.
- For a completely dislocated elbow that remains unstable despite the repair of the collateral ligaments, a hinged external fixator may be the best option.

COMPLICATIONS AND RESULTS

- Stiffness and loss of motion are the most common outcomes following reduction and treatment for an elbow dislocation.
- Most report a loss of up to 30 degrees of extension at 10 weeks and a final loss of 5 to 15 degrees.
- Associated fractures of the radial head and coronoid adversely affect this result. On rare occasions, the primary concern is instability and not stiffness.
- Morrey (2003) reported that posterolateral rotatory instability was the most common pattern among his patients and that this diagnosis is not an easy one to make.
  - In this instance, the ULCL needs to be reconstructed.
- Many patients report general pain with activity.
  - This is most likely due to the trauma that the cartilage undergoes with the initial dislocation.
  - All complete elbow dislocations may have some osteochondral damage.
  - Patients may also lose up to 15% of their strength and feel that their injured side is inferior to the contralateral elbow.
- Heterotopic ossification (HO) has also been documented after an elbow dislocation.
  - The best prevention of HO is to perform an early and definitive reduction.
  - Delayed treatment or multiple reduction attempts have been linked to the development of HO.

- To help prevent postsurgical HO, indomethacin SR 75 mg daily for 3 weeks, or a single postoperative dose of radiation (700 cGy) can be used.
- When it does occur, it is best to remove the ossification once it has matured.

STRESS FRACTURES

OLECRANON

Pathophysiology

Although not quite as common as in children and adolescents, adults can have olecranon stress fractures. The typical patient is an overhead-throwing athlete with pain during the acceleration and follow-through phases of throwing. This pain is usually located directly posterior on the olecranon, although it can also be found along the lateral border of the olecranon. Unlike throwers with MCL laxity and pain, these athletes tend to have negative valgus stress tests and pinpoint pain over the sites described.

Diagnosis

- Although x-rays may show the stress fracture, they are often negative.
- If a fracture is suspected, MRI is currently the best study to evaluate the bone.
- Both bone scans and CT have been used in the past, but neither have the same specificity and sensitivity as MRI.
- MRI is helpful not only with initial diagnosis but also for following the healing of the fracture.
  - In general, MRI results depict poorly defined, patchy areas of low signal intensity continuous with the cortex on T_1-weighted images and high signal intensity on STIR images.
  - In one study, all of the irregularity was noted in the posteromedial aspect of the olecranon.

Treatment
Nonsurgical Treatment
- Treatment for olecranon stress fractures is similar to stress fractures at other sites.
- Initial treatment is to rest the arm and avoid throwing activities for 6 weeks.
- Protecting the elbow in a hinged brace set between 20 degrees to full flexion for the first 4 weeks has been suggested.
- Once the acute pain and discomfort resolves, the patient will begin on a physical therapy regimen.
- This regimen is similar to that used for throwers with other injuries.
- It focuses on rehabilitating the shoulder as well as the elbow.
- If the athlete is able to work through the program without pain, then a graduated throwing program is initiated at 8 to 10 weeks.

Surgical Treatment
- For those athletes who have recurrent pain or who fail rehabilitation, then surgical options can be considered.
- The treatment of choice is fixation with a 6.5 or 4.5 cannulated screw.
- The screw can be placed through a small posterior incision at the tip of the olecranon.
- The triceps is split, and a guidewire is passed antegrade down the shaft of the ulna.
- The ulna is drilled and tapped, and the screw is placed in the standard fashion.
- Once the acute surgical pain has resolved, the patient starts regaining range of motion.
- Once healing is observed, the athlete enters the same program described for nonoperative treatment.
- Occasionally, the hardware is painful and needs to be removed before the thrower is able to fully recover.

CORONOID

Morrey (2003) reported on the case of a coronoid stress fracture in a juvenile gymnast. The diagnosis was made by three-dimensional CT reconstruction of the coronoid. Treatment consisted of withdrawing from athletic participation until the symptoms resolved. Activities of daily living were allowed and splints were not used.

OLECRANON BURSITIS

PATHOPHYSIOLOGY

Olecranon bursitis is a common injury in both the athletic and nonathletic population. Due to the superficial nature of the bursa, it can become quite inflamed, even after a minor injury to the elbow. It can be either acute or chronic, septic or nonseptic.

There are three different bursa in the elbow: the subcutaneous, the intratendinous, and the subtendinous (Fig. 22-12). The subcutaneous bursa is the one that plays the most prominent role in olecranon bursitis.

DIAGNOSIS

Acute Bursitis

Acute olecranon bursitis usually presents with warmth, swelling, and erythema over the olecranon.
  - Symptoms are usually initiated by trauma to the posterior elbow, although a specific history of trauma is not always evident.
  - The amount of swelling can be quite dramatic and can be limited to a small area, causing an egg-like appearance over the olecranon.
- It is usually not painful, although in the process of flexing the elbow, the patient may feel discomfort due to stretching of the skin.

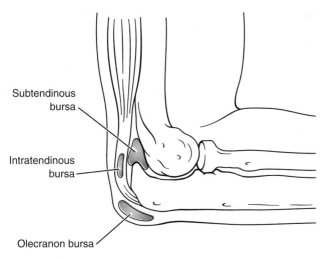

Subtendinous bursa

Intratendinous bursa

Olecranon bursa

Figure 22-12 Bursae of the elbow joint: the superficial olecranon bursa; the intratendinous bursa, which is found in the substance of the tendon; and the subtendinous bursa, which lies between the tip of the olecranon and the triceps tendon.

- The elbow range of motion is maintained.
- Differential diagnosis includes tendonitis, arthritic flare, and pseudogout.
- X-rays are usually done as a matter of course.
- Soft-tissue swelling is usually evident.
- There should be no sign of an effusion or fracture.
- An aspiration can be conducted if the swelling is so severe that it limits motion or if, in the elderly, there is a question of pseudogout as the cause.
  - In this case, the aspirate should be sent for culture, Gram stain, cell count, and crystals.
  - Bursal fluid should have a low white cell count with 80% monocytes.

Chronic Bursitis

- After several bouts of bursitis, the bursal lining can become quite thickened.
- The thickened bursal tissue consists of villi that represent granulation tissue.
- Early in the course, the chronic bursitis presents as soft, thickened tissue over the olecranon.
- Eventually, the bursa becomes quite thickened and can contain multiple solid loose bodies.

Septic Bursitis

- Patients with septic bursitis can present in many ways.
  - Often, the patient will have had several days of insidious pain over the posterior aspect of the elbow.
  - He or she may recall trauma to the site; however, usually the trauma was so minor that they never registered it.
  - There may be a small abrasion over the bursa that served as the entry point for the bacteria.
  - He or she may have a history of fever, chills, and other signs of a systemic infection, but most of the symptoms are related to the local infection.

- Cellulitis can travel both up the arm and down the forearm and can be accompanied by edema.
- The posterior aspect of the elbow is very painful, and range of motion can be limited because of discomfort.
- Every case of suspected septic bursitis should have an aspiration done.
  - Once again, the fluid should be sent for culture, Gram stain, crystals, and cell count.
  - The most common pathogen is *Staphylococcus aureus*.

TREATMENT

Acute Bursitis

- Most acute bursitis can be treated conservatively.
- Usually, ice packs and anti-inflammatory medication are enough to relieve the acute symptoms associated with the bursitis.
- After 24 hours, warm packs can be used to help resorb the bursal fluid.
- Some patients will need aspiration.
- The bursal sac does not need to be openly drained, and a drain should not be placed after aspiration.
  - The bursal cells can line the tract of the drain and create a fistula.
- After aspiration, a compressive dressing needs to be applied for 48 to 72 hours.
- The patient should be advised that there is a greater risk for recurrent bursitis after the first event, and protective padding may be needed if the elbow is at risk of repetitive trauma.

Chronic Bursitis

- In most cases, patients have exhausted the conservative treatment regimen described for acute bursitis. Many present with an acute case superimposed on a chronic case of bursitis.
  - In this instance, conservative treatment will not solve the problem.
- The goal of operative treatment is to remove the entire bursal sac, as well as the loose bodies.
- A posterior approach made slightly lateral to the olecranon is used.
  - An attempt is made to remove the entire bursal sac without disrupting the contents.
  - If there is an olecranon spur, it is removed.
  - Once removed, suturing the subdermal tissue to the underlying fascia obliterates the dead space.
- An alternate approach is to close the wound and then obliterate the dead space by passing mattress sutures on either side of the incision.
  - The skin is closed with suture, a compressive dressing applied, and the elbow protected from flexion greater than 45 degrees for 2 weeks.

Septic Bursitis

- Treatment usually consists of intravenous antibiotics, elevation, and analgesia.

- Until the pathogen and its sensitivities return, the antibiotic coverage is usually broad.
- Once the sensitivities return, it can be tailored to the specific pathogen.
- Most patients require 1 to 3 weeks of intravenous antibiotics, followed by several weeks of oral antibiotics.
- In some cases, especially immunocompromised hosts, surgical treatment is warranted.
- For those who get worse or fail to show clinical improvement, surgical debridement similar to that described earlier is conducted.
  - A drain may be necessary for the first 24 hours for particularly aggressive infections.
  - The patient is placed in a compressive dressing and splint as outlined previously.
- Morrey and Regan (2003) outlined a treatment plan that avoids the operating room in most cases.
  - The septic bursa is aspirated, and if the aspirate is purulent or cloudy or if the patient is febrile, then the bursa is lavaged, and 0.5 g of methicillin mixed in 10 cc of saline is injected.
  - The patient is then placed on proper oral antibiotics to treat *Staphylococcus aureus*.
  - If the fluid reaccumulates, a second aspiration is performed.
  - The elbow is splinted at 45 degrees.
  - If the patient has several bouts of the septic bursitis, he or she is taken to the operating room for a formal incision and drainage of the bursa.

LITTLE LEAGUE ELBOW

MEDIAL TENSION INJURIES

Pathophysiology

"Little League elbow" is a term originally introduced to describe the lesions around the medial aspect of the elbow. Medial elbow injuries are quite common in a young patient population and are related to increased tensile forces across the medial elbow in late cocking and early acceleration phases of throwing. Year-round training, breaking pitch, requiring more forceful flexion and pronation of the wrist compared with standard straight pitch, and improper throwing mechanics contribute to the development of medial-sided elbow injuries. The affected patients are usually less than 10 years of age.

The pathophysiology of this condition is related to the increased tensile stress on the medial epicondyle transmitted through flexor pronator mass and MCL. This ultimately results in stress fracture and separation of the medial epicondylar apophysis.

Medial elbow pain of gradual onset is the primary complaint in medial epicondylar apophysitis. It is also associated with decrease in throwing velocity and the effectiveness of pitching. The medial pain is generally worse with throwing but eventually can occur with other activities.

Diagnosis

- On physical examination, characteristic findings include medial tenderness over the epicondyle, swelling, and occasionally flexion contracture.
- Early radiographic findings include irregular ossification of the medial epicondylar apophysis.
- Later findings exhibit apophyseal enlargement, separation, and eventual fragmentation (Fig. 22-13).

Treatment

- Nonoperative treatment consists of rest and nonsteroidal anti-inflammatory drugs (NSAIDs) for 2 to 4 weeks, followed by stretching and range-of-motion exercises.
- Once motion is restored, strengthening is initiated with return to overhead activities at 6 weeks if pain-free.
- Occasionally, pain persists secondary to inadequate period of rest.
  - In such cases, brief periods of immobilization are appropriate to control inflammation and pain before resumption of rehabilitation.
- Shoulder rehabilitation is important to start at the same time to optimize the conditioning of the kinetic chain in throwers.
  - Throwing mechanics are examined and corrected if improper technique is used.
  - Number of pitches thrown and innings pitched must be monitored to avoid exacerbations of this condition.
- In cases of acute avulsions of the medial epicondyle, which usually result from extreme valgus loads during throwing, treatment is guided based on fracture displacement.

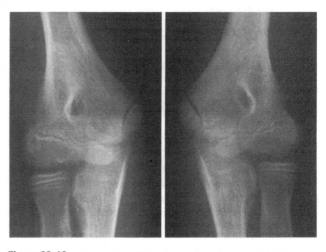

Figure 22-13 Comparison AP radiographs demonstrating left elbow medial epicondyle apophysitis with subtle widening in the throwing arm of a 10-year-old boy. (From Rudzki JR, Paletta GA Jr. Juvenile and adolescent elbow injuries in sports. Clin Sports Med 2004;23:581–608.)

- Minimally displaced fractures are treated by immobilization at 90 degrees for 2 to 3 weeks followed by range-of-motion exercises.
- If the fragment is displaced greater than 5 mm, valgus stability is tested.
- If instability is present, open reduction and internal fixation is performed with smooth K-wires.
- In chronic medial apophysitis, nonoperative management is successful in returning patients back to sport.
  - Occasionally symptoms are recurrent, and the athlete has to miss a season.
  - In acute injuries, nonunions rarely occur from inadequate immobilization.
  - Late surgical excision may be indicated for pain.
  - Open reduction and internal fixation are generally successful at restoring stability and prevention of future radiocapitellar arthrosis.

LATERAL COMPRESSION INJURIES

Pathophysiology

Although reported in adults, osteochondritis dissecans (OCD) of the elbow is much more common in the immature athlete. The capitellum is the most common aspect of the elbow to be involved. In the immature population, there are two entities that can involve the capitellum. The first, Panner's disease, is a self-limiting process that involves general fragmentation and sclerosis of the capitellum. It usually resolves without any long-term sequelae and is not associated with overuse or repetitive elbow activity. It generally involves children between the ages of 7 and 12 years old. The second, OCD, usually presents itself between ages 11 and 15 years and is associated with repetitive trauma. The area of the capitellum involved is well defined. Unlike in Panner's disease, the capitellum does not recover. Instead, the area undergoes progressive flattening and fragmentation. Fifty percent of the involved elbows will eventually develop osteoarthritis.

The cause of OCD of the capitellum is multifactorial. Repetitive trauma clearly plays a role in its development. Multiple studies have linked OCD with the trauma that occurs to the dominant arm of male Little League pitchers. Studies have also linked the constant stress of gymnastics on the immature elbow as a source of OCD in the female athlete. Genetic predisposition may play a role in the development of OCD. The nature of the vascular supply to the capitellum may also play a role. The capitellum is supplied primarily by one or two vessels traveling from posterior to anterior. There is no metaphyseal collateral flow. The repetitive microtrauma experienced by the elbow during pitching may be enough to disrupt the blood flow to the capitellum and cause Panner's disease or OCD (Fig. 22-14).

Diagnosis

History and Physical Examination

- As described, the typical patient with Panner's disease is 7 to 12 years old, whereas OCD affects children 11 to 15 years old.

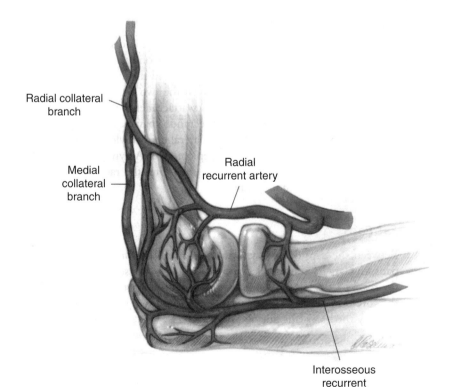

Figure 22-14 Lateral view of the right elbow showing the radial and interosseous recurrent arteries and the medial and radial collateral branches. (After Yamaguchi K, Sweet FA, Bindra R, et al. The extraosseous and intraosseous arterial anatomy of the adult elbow. J Bone Joint Surg Am 1997;79: 1653–1662.)

- With Panner's disease, the child usually complains of stiffness and pain in the dominant elbow after activity.
  - The discomfort is relieved with rest.
- With OCD, the patient may also experience pain and stiffness in the elbow.
  - As the fragmentation progresses, however, the child will start to demonstrate catching and locking of the elbow.
  - These symptoms are due to loose bodies within the joint.
- Physical examination of the elbow usually reveals lateral elbow pain.
  - Although some may have pain specifically over the capitellum, most usually have poorly localized pain over the radiocapitellar joint.
- Range of motion is limited, with a loss of extension more common than a loss of flexion.
- Pain can be evoked with the active radiocapitellar compression test, which involves pronation and supination of the forearm while in full extension.

Radiologic Examination

- Diagnostic evaluation of an immature patient with elbow pain usually begins with radiographs.
- AP and lateral x-rays are standard.
  - Early on in the disease process, these films may be negative.
- Comparative views of the opposite elbow should be obtained.
- AP radiographs at 45 degrees of flexion have been recommended to identify capitellar OCD lesions.
- As the disease progresses, flattening and sclerosis are seen on the radiographs.
  - The classic lesion involves the anterolateral aspect of the capitellum.
- Although radiographs can be quite helpful with the diagnosis of an OCD, MRI is now the best method to detect and define an OCD of the capitellum.
  - MRI has the ability to detect the subtle bone marrow changes that occur early on in the disease process.
  - With progression, the MRI is also able to define the separation of OCD from the underlying subchondral bone and damage to the articular cartilage.
- The diagnostic ability of the MRI can be enhanced with the addition of intra-articular contrast.
  - The contrast can show the separation between the lesion and the subchondral bone, denoting an unstable lesion.
  - Not all unstable fragments can be identified through this method, however.
- MRI can allow for the misdiagnosis of a pseudodefect, which occurs in the posteroinferior aspect of the capitellum as opposed to an OCD, which usually occurs in the anterolateral aspect of the capitellum.
- Classification in Table 22-5 is based primarily on MRI finding.
- OCD lesions of the elbow can also be staged arthroscopically (Table 22-6).

Treatment

- Management of Panner's disease is focused on relieving the symptoms.

TABLE 22-5 CLASSIFICATION OF OSTEOCHONDRITIS DISSECANS OF THE ELBOW BASED ON MRI FINDINGS

Type	Description
IA	Normal or near-normal x-rays/ T1 signal in superficial capitellum and normal T2
IB	Radiographic findings/signal in both T1 and T2
II	MRI with contrast shows margin around lesion
III	Chronic lesions with loose bodies
IV	Associated radial head OCD

MRI, magnetic resonance imaging; OCD, osteochondritis dissecans. (Adapted from Petrie R, Bradley J. Osteochondritis dissecans of the humeral capitellum. In: DeLee J, Drez D, Miller M, eds. Orthopaedic Sports Medicine: Principles and Practice. Philadelphia: W. B. Saunders, 2003.)

- By decreasing physical activity, especially activities that load the lateral aspect of the elbow (throwing, hand springs), the pain will usually resolve.
- For more intense cases, immobilization for 3 to 4 weeks may be necessary.
  - Long-term reports show excellent results for these patients.
- Treating a young athlete with an OCD of the capitellum requires a review of both the clinical and radiographic evidence:
  - How old is the patient?
  - How long has the patient had lateral elbow pain?
  - Has the patient failed conservative treatment?
  - Does the patient demonstrate mechanical symptoms?
  - Is there evidence of an unstable lesion or loose body?

TABLE 22-6 CLASSIFICATION OF OSTEOCHONDRITIS DISSECANS OF THE CAPITELLUM

Type	Description	Definition
IA	Intact/stable	Intact articular cartilage/no loss of subchondral stability
IB	Intact/unstable	Intact articular cartilage/unstable subchondral bone with impending collapse
II	Open/unstable	Cartilage fracture/collapse or partial displacement of subchondral bone
III	Detached	Loose fragments with joint

(Adapted from Defelice GS, Meunier MJ, Paletta GA Jr. Elbow injury in the adolescent athlete. In: Altchek DW, Andrews JR, eds. The Athlete's Elbow. Philadelphia: Lippincott Williams & Wilkins, 2001.)

Type Ia Lesion

- Whether viewed arthroscopically or established radiographically, type Ia lesions can be treated conservatively.
- Cessation of all physical activity involving the affected arm is warranted.
    - Some advocate 3 to 6 weeks of protection in a hinged elbow brace with an anticipated return to activity by 3 to 6 months.
    - Others will allow strengthening of the affected arm once the symptoms have resolved but will not return the athlete to sports for at least 6 months.
- Follow-up radiographs are obtained at 3 and 6 months.
- In general, return to sports is based on a clinical response rather than a radiographic response because the radiographic changes may remain for months or years.
- If the symptoms return after the allotted period, the athlete is kept from athletics for additional time.
- Pitchers may be changed to positional players, whereas competitive gymnasts may have to change to a different sport altogether.

Type Ib Lesion

- Initial treatment of a type Ib lesion is the same as for a type Ia lesion.
- For patients who fail conservative treatment, have persistent pain, or who have developed an unstable lesion, surgical intervention is warranted.
- An arthroscopic or possibly an open procedure through an anterolateral approach is conducted.
- Bradley and Dandy (1989) described subchondral drilling for lesions consisting of less than 55% of the capitellum with less than a 60-degree angle.
- For larger, acute lesions, an attempt should be made to fix the lesion in situ with metallic or bioabsorbable implants.
    - Large lesions (greater than 70% with greater than 90 degrees on the lateral) have a poor outcome.
- Chronic lesions with fragmentation should be debrided and drilled.
- If the lesion is not completely detached, an attempt to fix it internally is made.
    - The subchondral bone is debrided, and autograft from the ulna is used before fixing the lesion with a metallic compression screw, which can be removed at 3 to 5 months.
- For chronic, fragmented lesions, the area is debrided.
    - One must then consider use of an autograft or allograft osteochondral reconstruction.

Type II Lesion

- Most patients with unstable type II lesions by radiographs, MRI, or arthroscopy will bypass the conservative treatment stage.
- Surgical treatment is similar to that described for type Ib.

Type III Lesion

- Chronic loose bodies are removed and the donor bed debrided.
- Acute loose bodies may be fixed if the patient had a previously documented OCD, and the displacement of the fragment is clearly documented.
- For most patients, this is a salvage procedure, and they will be unable to return to sports.

Type IV Lesion

- This lesion is not usually encountered in the athletic population.
- It represents damage to both the capitellum and radial head.
- Treatment of the capitellar lesion, as described previously, can be undertaken when the radial lesion is small (<30%).
- Debridement, drilling, or microfracture may all be useful in treating a radial lesion that is larger than 30%.
- In the adult population, a radial head resection may be the best treatment option.

Postoperative Care

- Most surgical patients were protected for 2 to 3 weeks in either a long arm cast or hinged brace. Passive and active assisted range of motion was started at 3 weeks.
- For those with bony fragments reattached, active motion was not started until union was noted on radiographs.
- For those with debridement only, active range of motion was started once the patient had achieved full and pain-free passive range of motion.
- Return to sport was allowed 6 months after surgery.

Results

- The outcome for patients with OCD of the capitellum depends on the type of lesion and the age of the patient.
- Those diagnosed at an early stage and treated with an adequate rest period can do well.
- Most patients, however, are diagnosed at the type Ib or II stage.
    - When followed out over the long term, these patients have a less favorable outcome.
- For the youngest of our athletes, prevention is the still the best medicine.
- Young throwers with good mechanics may be most at risk.
    - These athletes placed similar stresses on their shoulder and elbow as their professional counterparts.
    - Of all pitches, the fastball generates the most stress on the shoulder and elbow.
- Box 22-3 contains recommendations for the young thrower with open physes.
- For those with closed physes, the goal is still prevention.
    - Throwing athletes need to be well conditioned and should cross train to maintain conditioning.
    - Pitch counts should be monitored and controlled.
    - When discomfort is felt, the athlete should rest.
    - Medication can be used but should be used to help recover from and not cover up an injury.
    - During rehabilitation, it is important to incorporate elbow, shoulder, and scapular therapy on the throwing arm.

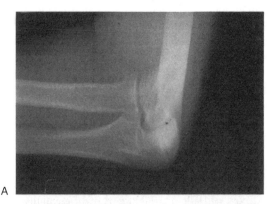

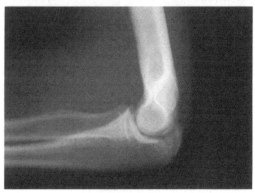

Figure 22-15   Radiocapitellar **(A)** and lateral **(B)** radiographs of persistent olecranon apophysis. (From Rudzki JR, Paletta GA Jr. Juvenile and adolescent elbow injuries in sports. Clin Sports Med 2004;23:581–608.)

OLECRANON APOPHYSITIS AND EPIPHYSEAL FRACTURE

PATHOPHYSIOLOGY

Injury to olecranon apophysis is similar to medial apophysitis. During the acceleration phase of throwing, triceps contractions put tensile forces on the olecranon. In childhood, olecranon apophysitis usually occurs, whereas in adolescents, stress fractures and avulsion of the olecranon apophysis may be seen.

DIAGNOSIS

History and Physical Examination

- Patients can present with acute (more common) or chronic pain and swelling over the posterior elbow.
- Loss of terminal extension can also occur.
- Athletes report decreased level athletic performance.
- Symptoms are worse during physical activity, specifically during the acceleration and follow-through phases of throwing.
- Physical examination findings include tenderness over the olecranon and pain with resisted extension.
- It is important to assess valgus stability of the elbow and palpate ulnohumeral articulation and radiocapitellar articulation for tenderness.
  - Overhead throwers may develop valgus instability with resultant degenerative changes in the posterior compartment and radiocapitellar articulation.

Radiologic Examination

- Radiographs characteristically demonstrate widening or fragmentation of the olecranon physis and sclerosis (Fig. 22-15).
  - Comparison to the contralateral side is useful in this age group to judge significant changes in the bone.
- Absence of radiographic signs does not rule out this condition.
- A technetium bone scan should be ordered when the level of suspicion is high to look for subtle stress fractures.

TREATMENT

- Treatment is determined by severity of the injury.
- Initial treatment includes rest, NSAIDs, cryotherapy, and activity modification.
  - Aggravating activities are avoided.
- Once the symptoms are controlled, rehabilitation is initiated, focusing on range of motion and gradual strengthening.
- Return to sport can usually occur in 6 weeks.
- Occasionally, symptoms rebound and the athlete has to be shut down from aggravating activity for longer period of time and miss a season.
- In cases of chronic olecranon apophysitis, physeal stress fractures, partial tears of the triceps, and persistence of the apophysis into adulthood may occur.
  - Persistent symptoms secondary to these conditions may require operative treatment.
- In general, failure of apophyseal closure after 3 to 6 months of conservative treatment is an indication for internal fixation.

- Usually, this is conducted through a minimal posterior incision with placement of a cancellous screw. This treatment is generally successful in achieving union.

POSTOPERATIVE CARE

- Postoperatively, patients are immobilized for 7 to 10 days with subsequent gradual active flexion and passive extension exercises.
- At 6 weeks, active extension is allowed.
- At 8 weeks, gradual strengthening begins and range-of-motion exercises are continued.
- Return to athletic activity usually occurs in 3 months.

OSTEOARTHRITIS

Epidemiology

Primary osteoarthritis of the elbow is a very rare diagnosis, constituting only 1% to 2% of elbow arthritis. The diagnosis is often a result of chronic overuse associated with repetitive motion. Male to female ratio is 4:1, and the dominant extremity is affected 80% to 90%, with bilateral involvement in 25% to 60% of cases. Common age at the time of presentation is 50 years old, with variation from 20 to 65 years. Typical presentation in an athlete is a 35- to 45-year-old male participating in a sport with intense repetitive motion of the upper extremity.

DIAGNOSIS

History and Physical Examination

- The clinical presentation often consists of a mildly limited range of motion (30 to 120 degrees), which may compromise athletic performance (loss of extension in boxing), and pain in terminal extension.
- It is important to ask the patient to actively flex and extend elbows through arc of motion and determine at which position symptoms occur.
  - If pain occurs in the mid-arc of motion, as well as end-arc of motion, this may influence treatment options.
  - Forearm rotation is usually unaffected.
- Ulnar nerve symptoms may be present and must be sought to make appropriate treatment plan.
  - The ulnar nerve must be palpated and checked for subluxation.
  - Tinel's sign should be assessed.

Radiologic Examination

- Radiographic workup consists mainly of AP and lateral views.
  - These views usually demonstrate osteophyte formation at the coronoid and olecranon processes and in their respective fossae.
  - Loose bodies can also be seen around ulnar-humeral and radiocapitellar articulations.
  - Radial head involvement is evident in about 50% of cases.
- Occasionally, cubital tunnel view may be useful if the ulnar nerve is involved based on physical examination findings.
- Regular x-rays are usually all that is needed to establish diagnosis.
- CT is useful as a preoperative tool to understand the exact location of osteophytes and plan surgical address.

TREATMENT

Nonsurgical Treatment

- Nonoperative treatment must be instituted first, since the symptoms may be minimal and adjustment of technique or activity may yield a satisfactory result.
- A course of anti-inflammatory medications may be helpful.
- In athletic populations, activity modification is usually not a realistic option, and recalcitrant symptoms preventing sport participation justify surgical intervention.
- Several surgical options to treat primary osteoarthritis of the elbow exist.
- Treatment depends on the ulnar nerve symptoms and the extent of the disease in the elbow joint.

Surgical Treatment

- Elbow arthroscopy is an option in experienced hands in patients who do not have ulnar nerve symptoms.
  - This technique allows removal of loose bodies and osteophytes, as well as capsulectomy in patients with limited motion.
  - Recent reports generally report quick recovery period and pain relief at the end-arc of motion is relieved in most cases.
  - Modest improvement of motion is also achieved but must be maintained with proper postoperative rehabilitation protocol.
  - Complications are rare but can be serious, involving surrounding neurovascular structures.
- When motion is the dominating symptom, extensive capsulectomy must be performed, as well as osteophyte and loose body removal.
  - The posterior band of the MCL must be released to gain full flexion.
  - This can be performed safely when the ulnar nerve is protected through medial incision.
  - The ulnar nerve is identified and protected first.
  - After this crucial step, the elbow joint is entered from the medial side, and posterior and anterior capsulectomy are performed.
  - Osteophytes and loose bodies are removed.
  - The ulnar nerve is transposed or left in situ, depending on the preoperative symptoms.
- Lateral column procedure accomplishes similar goals through the lateral approach.

- The ulnar nerve cannot be protected during this approach.
- The joint is entered laterally and anterior and posterior capsulectomy, and osteophyte and loose body removal are performed in a similar manner.
- In cases with extensive radiographic disease, ulnohumeral arthroplasty allows access to the ulnar nerve and circumferential removal of osteophytes and loose bodies.
  - A posterior approach is used, and the ulnar nerve is identified and protected.
  - The medial edge of the triceps is reflected and posterior capsulectomy, as well as removal of osteophytes and loose bodies, is performed.
  - Olecranon fossa is debrided with a trephine.
  - The resultant smooth curvature allows access to the prominent coronoid process, osteophytes, and loose bodies in the anterior compartment of the joint.
- Interposition arthroplasty and total elbow replacement are potential options for patients with extensive disease and pain throughout the arc of motion.
  - After these procedures, the patients are advised not to return to activities that put any significant stresses on the elbow joint.

RESULTS AND COMPLICATIONS

- The results of both the medial and lateral open approaches, as well as the arthroscopic approach, are similar and achieve reliable pain relief and improvement in range of motion between 30 and 60 degrees.
  - Recurrence of motion loss may occur and must be addressed by a judicious postoperative rehabilitation program.
  - Other reported complications include intra-articular bleeding and nerve palsy. Fortunately, these complications are rare but serious and usually can be prevented by meticulous surgical technique.
- With ulnohumeral arthroplasty, pain relief is achieved in about 90% of patients, and modest improvement in motion can be achieved.
  - This motion can be lost in the postoperative period, as with other procedures described previously.
  - Recurrence of symptoms and radiographic changes occur in 20% of patients at 10 years after surgery.
  - Ulnar nerve symptoms occur in 10% of patients postoperatively.

LOOSE BODIES

- Loose bodies within the elbow joint can occur in two distinct populations.
  - In the athletic population, overhead-throwing athletes can develop loose bodies as the result of the repetitive overhead motion and the stress that it places on the elbow.
  - Other patients can develop loose bodies as the result of trauma or degenerative arthritis in the elbow.
- In the overhead-throwing athlete, persistent valgus extension overload can cause impingement between the

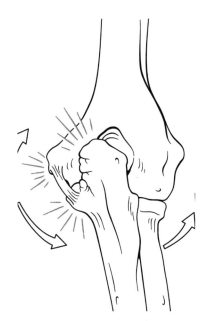

Figure 22-16   Medial tension overload secondary to repetitive valgus stress at the elbow, resulting in attenuation of the UCL complex medially, lateral radiocapitellar compression, and extension overload within the posterior compartment. (After Kvitne RS, Jobe FW. Ligamentous and posterior compartment injuries. In: Jobe FW, ed. Techniques in Upper Extremity Sports Injuries. Philadelphia: Mosby-Year Book, 1996:414.)

posteromedial olecranon and the medial aspect of the olecranon fossa (Figs. 22-16 and 22-17).

- As in other parts of the body, the repetitive stress can result in the development of osteophytes along the posteromedial olecranon.
- Some patients can have concomitant MCL pain, which can cloud the diagnosis.

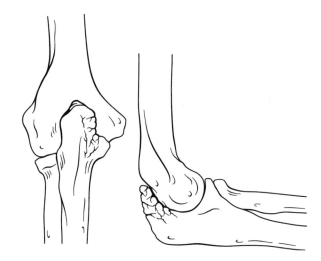

Figure 22-17   Valgus-extension overload of the posterior compartment results in posteromedial osteophytes within the olecranon fossa. (After Miller CD, Savoie FH III. Valgus extension injuries of the elbow in the throwing athlete. J Am Acad Orthop Surg 1994;2:261–269. © 1994 American Academy of Orthopaedic Surgeons.)

- Throwing athletes with MCL pain generally have discomfort at the medial epicondyle, whereas patients with valgus extension overload will experience pain more proximally near the tip of the olecranon.
- Both can experience pain during the early acceleration phase of throwing and both can experience pain with a valgus stress in the office.

Diagnosis

Physical Examination

- In the valgus extension overload test, the examiner repeatedly forces the slightly flexed elbow rapidly into full extension while applying a valgus stress (see Fig. 15-28 in Chapter 15).
  - A positive test points to the presence of posteromedial osteophytes.

Radiologic Examination

- Standard AP, lateral, and oblique films should be obtained.
- Up to 30% of loose bodies can be missed on standard films.
- When considering the possibility of an MCL tear, an MRI is usually obtained. This will also help to delineate the loose bodies.

Treatment

Nonsurgical Treatment

- When an overhead thrower is diagnosed with valgus extension overload and osteophytic changes, the first line of treatment is conservative.
- Rest, ice, and anti-inflammatory medication may reduce the discomfort.

Surgical Treatment

- If a loose body accompanies the osteophytic changes, arthroscopy is the treatment of choice.

BOX 22-4 BASIC PRINCIPLES OF ELBOW ARTHROSCOPY

- Avoid penetrating the subcutaneous tissue with the scalpel blade when making a portal
- Flex the elbow 90 degrees to insert an arthroscopic sheath
- Outline bony landmarks before capsular distention
- Measure precisely the portal placement from the appropriate landmarks
- Direct the arthroscopic sheath and trocar directly toward the center of the joint during insertion
- Local anesthesia is not recommended
- Postoperative neurovascular examination is mandatory

(Adapted from Lynch GJ, Meyers JF, Whipple TL, et al. Neurovascular anatomy and elbow arthroscopy: inherent risks. Arthroscopy 1986;2 : 191–197.)

- Elbow arthroscopy can be conducted with the patient supine, lateral, or prone.
- The most important factor for elbow arthroscopy is placement of the portals.
  - Unlike other major joints, the elbow has several neurovascular structures that lie very close to all possible portal sites.
  - Because of the possible injury to these structures, some basic principles for elbow arthroscopy should be followed (Box 22-4).
  - The anteromedial portal has the highest risk as a result of the proximity of the ulnar nerve (Fig. 22-18).
    - The most important aspect of placement of this portal is to stay anterior to the intermuscular septum.
    - A portal 2 cm above and 1 to 2 cm anterior to the medial epicondyle has been described, but this places the ulnar nerve at risk.

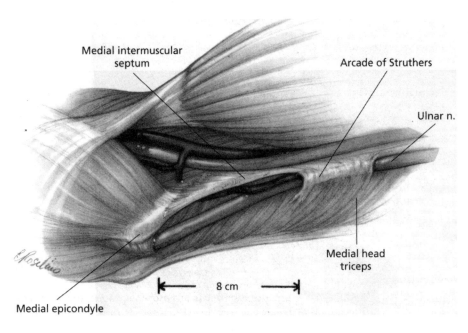

Figure 22-18 The ulnar nerve courses around the medial aspect of the elbow. Proximally, the nerve passes beneath the arcade of Struthers, runs along the medial intermuscular septum, enters the cubital tunnel around the medial epicondyle, and passes through the two heads of the FCU. (From Doyle JR, Botte MJ. Elbow. In: Hand and Upper Extremity Surgery. Philadelphia, Lippincott Williams & Wilkins, 2003: 389.)

- The standard anteromedial portal is made 2 cm distal and 2 cm anterior to the medial condyle. This portal places the brachial artery, ulnar nerve, and median nerve at risk.
  - Laterally, four portal sites have been described.
    - The standard site is located 1 cm distal and 3 cm anterior to the lateral epicondyle.
    - The midanterolateral portal, the proximal antero-lateral portal, and the straight lateral portal have all been described.
    - The straight lateral, or soft spot, can also be used to distend the joint before the start of arthros-copy.
  - Three posterior portals exist for inspection of the posterior elbow.
    - The posterocentral portal is 3 cm above the tip of the olecranon.
      - Both medial and lateral gutters, as well as the olecranon fossa, can be observed through this portal.
    - The proximal posterolateral portal is located along the lateral gutter anywhere from the ole-cranon tip to 3 cm proximal.
    - The inferior posterolateral portal is created at the level of the radiocapitellar joint within the lateral gutter.
- After the removal of the loose bodies, the spurs along the medial aspect of the olecranon and within the fossa can be addressed.
  - Usually, the central and proximal posterolateral por-tals are used for this purpose.
- Care must be taken to protect the ulnar nerve and the triceps tendon.
  - In this instance, suction should never be used when the shaver or other instrument is within the medial gutter.

Postoperative Care

- All patients are started on immediate range of motion.
- After return of full range of motion, strengthening of the upper extremity is started.
  - For overhead athletes, this includes incorporation of shoulder and scapular rehabilitation into the re-covery phase.
- Most throwing athletes can begin rehabilitative throw-ing by 6 to 8 weeks.
- Anticipated return to sport is 3 to 4 months.

Results

- Arthroscopic removal of loose bodies has up to a 90% success rate.
- Even more favorable results have been reported when loose body removal is accompanied by ulnohumeral arthroplasty.

Complications

- The most common complications are as follows: Persistent drainage from the arthroscopy portals

- Deep infection
- Minor contractures
- Transient palsies
  - Permanent nerve damage
- Permanent nerve damage has been reported for each of the three nerves around the elbow.

BICEPS TENDON RUPTURE

PATHOPHYSIOLOGY

Biceps tendon rupture can occur in several locations: mus-culoskeletal junction, incontinuity tendon tear, and at the tendon insertion to the radial tuberosity. Avulsion from the radial tuberosity is the most common location of injury. This injury occurs routinely in male patients with dominant extremity involvement in 80% of the cases.

The mechanism of injury is usually traumatic insult with resistance to elbow flexion at around 90-degree position. Anabolic steroids and chronic degenerative changes in the tendon are common predisposing factors. Radiographic findings of radial tuberosity spurring are the result of degen-erative process at the tendon–bone junction (Fig. 22-19). Previous history of pain in antecubital fossa may represent pre-existing partial rupture. Systemic conditions, such as hyperparathyroidism and lupus erythematosus associated with tendon disorders elsewhere, may predispose to biceps tendon rupture.

DIAGNOSIS

History and Physical Examination

- Clinical presentation usually consists of acute sudden pain in antecubital fossa followed by a dull ache that can persist for several weeks.
- The usual patient is a young or middle-aged male, healthy and physically fit.

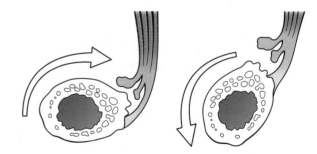

Figure 22-19 Pathophysiology of the distal biceps rupture. Hypertrophic changes at the radial tuberosity cause irritation of the tendon, predisposing it to degenerative changes and rupture during pronation and supination. (After Davis WM, Yassine Z. An etiologic factor in the tear of the distal tendon of the biceps brachii. J Bone Joint Surg Am 1956;38:1368.)

- On physical examination, ecchymosis and obvious characteristic biceps deformity with attempted contraction are noted.
- Diminution of strength must be determined and compared with the contralateral side.
  - Supination strength is mostly affected by flexion strength.
  - Grip strength diminution is also common.
- If the deformity is not present, partial rupture may have occurred, and crepitus is usually present with pronation and supination of the forearm.

Radiologic Examination

- Radiographic evaluation usually will demonstrate edema in soft tissues and degenerative changes of radial tuberosity.
- Routine MRI is not necessary but is occasionally helpful in cases with vague previous traumatic episodes when the injury may not be acute, resulting in tendon contraction and disappearance into the muscular substance.

TREATMENT

- In cases of acute disruption, operative repair is clearly superior to the nonoperative management.
- Partial ruptures can be treated nonoperatively initially; however, if chronic pain develops, surgical approach may be necessary.
- The two-incision approach popularized by Morrey and the single incision anterior approach using various devices securing soft tissue to bone are the two most common techniques of distal biceps repair.
- In the two-incision technique, the tendon is identified, secured with stitches, and passed with a hemostat along the biceps tendon tract right next to the radius without exposure of the ulna.
  - The second incision is made over the hemostat, radial tuberosity is prepared, and repair is performed through the bone tunnels.
  - Exposure of the ulna is associated with increased incidence of heterotopic ossification.
- The anterior single-incision approach has become more popular since the advent of suture anchors.
  - The anterior approach is used, and usually two suture anchors are secured in the radial tuberosity.
  - The suture limbs from the anchors are passed through the tendon using various techniques, and the tendon is repaired back to the radial tuberosity.
- After repair of the tendon in the more common insertion avulsion injuries, the arm is usually immobilized for 5 to 7 days at 90 degrees of flexion and then passive and active gradual motion is begun. Strengthening is started at 3 months postoperatively.
- For tendon tears in continuity and for tears at the musculotendinous junction imbricating repair, graft augmentation is usually necessary.
  - These tears are very rare, and no reports on the results of treatment have been published.

- The repair is usually protected for 3 weeks, and then gradual motion is begun over next 3 months.
- In chronic injuries when the tendon has retracted into the muscle belly, allograft reconstruction with repair to the radial tuberosity is an option for patients who require restoration of strength.
  - Various graft tissues have been described, including fascia lata, semitendinosus tendon, and Achilles tendon allograft.
  - Rehabilitation focuses on protection of the graft and restoration of motion in the first 3 months.
  - Gradual strengthening is started after 3 months.
  - If the needs of the patient are satisfied with decreased supination strength, simple repair to the brachialis may be sufficient.
  - Rehabilitation is much simpler with no restriction on pronation and supination postoperatively.

RESULTS AND COMPLICATIONS

- The repair of the tendon in avulsion injuries, regardless of the technique, results generally in restoration of normal flexion and supination.
- Complications include radial nerve, posterior interosseous nerve, and musculocutaneous nerve injury, which are more associated with anterior approach.
- Heterotopic ossification is more common after the two-incision technique.
- Meticulous passage of the tendon without exposure of the ulna prevents the occurrence of heterotopic ossification.
- If the osseous bridge develops, successful resection can be performed 8 to 9 months after the repair. Recurrence of the tendon avulsion is very rare.

TRICEPS TENDON RUPTURE

PATHOPHYSIOLOGY

Triceps tendon rupture is among the rarest of tendon ruptures. This injury occurs in both men and women, with a male/female ratio of 3:2. This injury can occur in a wide spectrum of ages, with a mean of 33 years. The three sites of injury are muscle belly, musculotendinous junction, and boney avulsion of the tendon, which is the most common.

Mechanism of injury can be traumatic, spontaneous, or secondary to previous surgical release and repair. Traumatic rupture most often occurs due to excentric contraction of the triceps of a flexing elbow as it commonly happens during a fall. Uncoordinated contraction of the triceps during physical activity may also cause this injury. Direct blows to the distal triceps have also been reported to result in tendon rupture. This is a much more rare mechanism of traumatic injury. Spontaneous ruptures are usually secondary to other inflammatory or systemic conditions affecting the strength of the tendon and its insertion to bone. Local inflammatory conditions—such as olecranon bursitis and rheumatoid arthritis and systemic conditions like secondary hyperparathyroidism, lupus erythematosus, osteogenesis imperfecta, and renal osteodystrophy—have been implicated in association with tendon ruptures. Triceps deficiency after triceps detachment and repair as part of another procedure (e.g., total elbow arthroplasty) occurs rarely and its incidence depends on the repair technique, which is beyond the scope of this chapter.

DIAGNOSIS

History and Physical Examination

- Patients usually present with acute onset of pain at the posterior elbow and variable weakness of extension.
- Some residual extension may be preserved secondary to the anconeus confluence with triceps.
- Extension against gravity, however, is usually absent in complete tendon ruptures.
- Palpable defect can be palpated depending on the amount of retraction of the tendon.
- Swelling and ecchymosis are common findings.
- Neurovascular examination is usually normal, although subluxation of the ulnar nerve with triceps tendon rupture has been previously reported.
- Partial ruptures can be more difficult to diagnose because of preservation of extension and less pain, compared with complete ruptures.
  - These patients can also present late because of delayed weakness, compared with the contralateral side.

Radiologic Examination

- Radiographic examination—including AP, lateral, and oblique views—is useful for several reasons.
  - Olecranon bony avulsions can often be noted and assist in establishing diagnosis.
  - Concomitant fractures, especially the radial head, have been reported.
- MRI, although not routinely performed, can provide information about the extent of partial tears.

TREATMENT

- Surgical repair is the treatment of choice for complete tendon ruptures.
  - A common finding is the preservation of the lateral tendinous portion in continuity with anconeus.
  - Nonabsorbable sutures through drill holes provides strong repair.
  - Care must be taken medially to avoid injury to the ulnar nerve.
- Partial ruptures can be treated nonoperatively.
  - One must make sure that most of the tendon is still in continuity because later reconstructive options are not as reliable in achieving good results.

- Delayed reconstructive options include various fascial flaps and V-Y lengthening techniques.
  - We generally use anconeus slide alone or in conjunction with allograft tissue.
  - For significant tendon retraction, Achilles tendon is an ideal choice.
  - It provides secure fascial attachment proximally to the triceps and distally allows boney fixation to the olecranon with a screw.

POSTOPERATIVE CARE

- Postoperatively, the arm is protected at 90 degrees of flexion for 3 weeks, and gentle active motion is allowed subsequently.
- Strengthening is begun at 3 months.
- Strength is often slow to gain, with 80% recovery at 6 months even for acute repairs.

RESULTS

- Results have been generally good with repair or reconstruction up to 1 year after injury.
- Strength is restored even though its recovery may take up to 6 to 8 months.
- Terminal 5-degree loss of extension strength is a common finding.
- Complications are not frequent and include olecranon bursitis, loss of terminal extension strength, and delayed recovery of strength.

ADULT LATERAL ELBOW

LATERAL EPICONDYLITIS

Pathophysiology

Lateral epicondylitis is a much more common condition than its medial counterpart. The peak incidence is in the fourth and fifth decades of life. The prevalence rates are similar in males and females. Seventy-five percent of cases occur in the dominant extremity. The condition has been named "tennis elbow" because of the initial implication of racket sports as the primary cause of the lateral epicondylitis. Ten to 50% of tennis players experience this condition at some point in their career. Many other sports and occupational activities have been found to cause lateral epicondylitis. The common etiologic factor is repetitive forearm activity and wrist motion, especially forced extension. The pathologic lesion is located at the origin of the common extensor tendon of the forearm consisting of extensor carpi radialis longus, extensor carpi radialis brevis, extensor digitorum communis, and the extensor carpi ulnaris. Specifically, extensor carpi radialis brevis is the most commonly involved tendon in this disorder. It originates off the lateral epicondyle, lateral collateral ligament, annular ligament, the investing fascia, and the intermuscular septum. Electromyographic studies have shown increased activity in the extensor muscles of the forearm in professional and collegiate tennis players during ground strokes. These muscles stabilize the wrist in acceleration and follow-through phases. The greatest activity was noted in extensor carpi radialis brevis. In athletes, improper technique and equipment have been implicated as potential causative factors. In tennis, leading with the elbow, hitting the ball late and off-center on the racket, has been associated with increased incidence of lateral epicondylitis. Improper grip size, racket weight, and racket stringing can also generate higher loads on the extensor muscle origin.

The pathologic process responsible for lateral epicondylitis seems to be tendinosis. The initial trauma to the tendon causes intrasubstance microtear, which fails to heal secondary to continued repetitive aggravating activity. The result is the formation of the reparative vascular granulation tissue in the tendon. Nirschl has described this tissue as "angiofibroblastic dysplasia" and proposed a classification system for this process (Table 22-7).

Diagnosis

History and Physical Examination

- Typical presentation consists of insidious onset of lateral elbow pain often associated with repetitive activity.
  - The pain often radiates distally through the forearm.
  - Patients often report weakness and difficulty carrying items in their hand.
  - Rarely is there a history of acute traumatic event associated with symptoms.
- Physical examination must include the entire upper extremity and cervical spine.
- The shoulder must be thoroughly examined because degenerative disorders in the elbow are often associated with overuse conditions in the shoulder.
- Range of motion of the elbow is usually normal.
- Patients have tenderness to palpation, with the greatest tenderness 2 to 5 mm distal to the lateral epicondyle over the extensor carpi radialis brevis.
  - Pain is increased with resisted wrist extension and maximal wrist flexion while the elbow is extended.

TABLE 22-7 STAGES OF THE DEVELOPMENT OF LATERAL EPICONDYLITIS

Stage	Description
1	Initial inflammatory response
2	Formation of angiofibroblastic tissue
3	Structural failure
4	Recurrence of the process described in stages 2 and 3 accompanied by fibrosis or calcification; normal parallel orientation of fibers is lost and vascular fibroblastic tissue without any acute or inflammatory component fill the area in the tendon

- Resisted wrist extension creates tension in the diseased tendon, and maximal flexion puts the tendon on stretch.
- Grip strength is often diminished, compared with the contralateral side.
- The radiocapitellar joint must be palpated to evaluate for plica and potential chondral damage with loose body formation.
  - Tenderness over radiocapitellar joint is generally more distal than lateral epicondylitis tenderness.
- Posterior interosseous nerve entrapment often presents with similar symptoms and has been reported to actually coincide with lateral epicondylitis in 5% of the cases.
  - Patients with posterior interosseous nerve entrapment usually demonstrate pain with resisted supination when a nerve is entrapped in the supinator, or resisted long finger extension when a nerve is entrapped in the extensor digitorum communis.
  - Differentiating these diagnoses from lateral epicondylitis is a difficult task.

Radiologic Examination

- Radiologic workup occasionally reveals calcification in the extensor origin.
  - The presence of calcification does not alter the treatment and has no reported influence on prognosis.
- MRI has limited value, although some reports indicate that the size of the tear and degeneration of the tendon can be reliably determined on MRI.

Treatment

Nonsurgical Treatment

- Nonoperative approach is the mainstay of treatment for lateral epicondylitis and is usually divided into three phases.
- The *first phase* focuses on control of associated synovitis and pain.
  - Rest, activity modification, cryotherapy, NSAIDs, and cortisone injections can be used to control symptoms.
  - Physical therapy modalities such as friction massage, manipulation, phonophoresis, and iontophoresis may also control symptoms.
  - Counterforce bracing decreases the force on the tendon origin by controlling the musculotendinous unit expansion.
- The *second phase* is focused on rehabilitation, including stretching, range-of-motion exercises, and strengthening.
  - It is important to include shoulder rehabilitation, especially in athletes to avoid disuse atrophy and preserve healthy kinetic chain.
- The *third phase* focuses on functional rehabilitation, sports-specific exercises, correction of improper technique and equipment, and interval program of activity to return an athlete to competition.

Surgical Treatment

- Operative treatment is offered for those rare patients who fail nonoperative treatment.

- The goal of surgical treatment is to remove the diseased portion of the tendon and preserve lateral collateral ligament.
- Multiple techniques have been described over the years. Currently, open, arthroscopic, and percutaneous techniques are used to address the lateral epicondylitis surgically.
- Open technique uses a lateral approach over the lateral epicondyle.
    - The interval between extensor carpi radialis longus (ECRL) and extensor carpi radialis brevis (ECRB) is identified, and ECRL is elevated to reveal the ECRB tendon.
    - The degenerative tissue is often located on the undersurface of the ECRB tendon.
    - The tendon is split, and the degenerative tissue is excised.
    - Surgical address of concurrent posterior interosseous nerve (PIN) entrapment can be performed at the same time if indicated.
    - Different subsequent steps can be used, and multiple reports have shown successful results with different techniques.
        - The origin of the tendon can be reattached to the epicondyle. The epicondyle can be drilled and rongeured to increase the vascular supply, the tendon can be lengthened, synovial fringe can be excised, and the tendon can be released without reattachment.
        - All these techniques have shown similar outcomes and depend on the surgeon's preference.
- Arthroscopic lateral release is another surgical approach that has become available with the advent of arthroscopic techniques.
    - The advantage of arthroscopic technique is that concomitant intra-articular pathology can be addressed at the same time.
    - The patient is placed in either a supine, lateral decubitus, or prone position.
    - Proximal medial portal is created after the elbow is distended.
    - Diagnostic arthroscopy of the anterior compartment is performed.
    - Three types of lateral capsular lesion associated with lateral epicondylitis have been described.
        - Type 1 has intact lateral capsule.
        - Type 2 demonstrates a linear rent in the capsule.
        - In type 3, the entire lateral capsular origin is peeled off and reflected distally with ECRB visible behind it (Fig. 22-20).
    - The proximal lateral portal is created with an outside-in technique. Shaver and bipolar or monopolar radiofrequency probes can be used to debride the lateral capsule and the origin of the ECRB until the ECRL is visible.
    - Care must be taken to stay over the anterior 50% of the radial head to avoid injury to the lateral collateral ligament.
    - The posterior compartment can be inspected through various posterior portals.
- Percutaneous release have also been reported, with similar results as open procedures.
    - The procedure can be performed in the office.
    - The patient is given local anesthetic injection. One-centimeter incision is made transversely just distal to the lateral epicondyle.
    - Common extensor origin is incised with a scalpel just distal to the lateral epicondyle.
    - Hemostasis is controlled and the wound is closed.

Postoperative Care

- The postoperative rehabilitation after open approach includes early immobilization for 7 to 10 days, with subsequent range-of-motion and isometrics exercises for 3 to 4 weeks.
- Gradual strengthening starts at that point.
- After arthroscopic approach, range of motion and isometrics are started immediately.
- Progressive strengthening starts at 4 weeks.
- Patients often return to work in 2 to 4 weeks, depending on their vocation. Rehabilitation after percutaneous release is similar.

Results

- The results of the nonoperative treatment are successful in up to 90% of the patients.
- Regardless of the nonoperative approach, most patients seem to improve with time up to 1 year.
- Surgical treatment, regardless of the technique, has

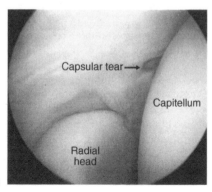
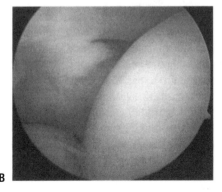

Figure 22-20 A: Arthroscopic view of the lesion associated with lateral epicondylitis. The arthroscope is in the proximal port looking laterally into the anterior chamber of the elbow joint. **B:** A type 3 lesion. (From Whaley AL, Baker CL. Lateral epicondylitis. Clin Sports Med 2004;23:677–691.)

A   B

been successful in more than 90% of the patients who failed nonoperative treatment.

- Arthroscopic and percutaneous approaches seem to be associated with faster recovery and return to occupational activities.

POSTEROLATERAL ROTATORY INSTABILITY

Pathophysiology

- Posterolateral rotatory instability is a fairly recently described condition.
- In this condition, the ulna and the radial head rotate externally on the distal humerus when the forearm is in maximal supination and the elbow is in slight flexion (see Fig. 15-31 in Chapter 15).
    - This occurs when static and dynamic stabilizers of the lateral elbow are deficient.
- The static stabilizer on the lateral side of the elbow is the LCL complex.
    - The complex consists of lateral ulnar collateral ligament (LUCL), radial collateral ligament (RCL), annular ligament, and accessory lateral collateral ligament (Fig. 22-21).
    - The LUCL and RCL originate at the lateral epicondyle and are indistinguishable at this location.
    - The LUCL inserts on the crista supinatoris on the ulna, where distinct broad attachment of the ligament can be identified.
        - O'Driscoll described the LUCL as the "essential lesion" in posterolateral rotatory instability (PLRI).

- The pathoanatomy of injury is a continuum of soft-tissue disruption that occurs in elbow dislocation.
    - In stage 1, LUCL is disrupted creating PLRI.
    - Stage 2 involves further disruption of the anterior and posterior capsule.
    - In stage 3A, the posterior band of the ulnar collateral ligament (UCL) is torn and the elbow dislocates, pivoting on the anterior band of the UCL.
    - The anterior band is disrupted in stage 3B.
- There is controversy as to what static stabilizers must be deficient for PLRI to occur.
    - Several studies pointed out that the proximal origin of the LCL complex (LUCL and RCL) must be detached for the PLRI to occur.
    - It seems that proximal detachment is much more significant in creation of instability as opposed to distal injury.
- The dynamic stabilizers preventing PLRI are also not very clear.
    - The structures that have been implicated in providing dynamic stability include lateral triceps, anconeus, extensor muscles of the forearm, brachialis, intermuscular septum between extensor digitorum communis and extensor digitorum quinti, and deep fascial bands of extensor carpi ulnaris.
- Disruption of the static and dynamic stabilizers can occur in three different scenarios: elbow dislocation, acute varus injury to the elbow, and iatrogenic causes.
    - Elbow dislocation is the most common cause of PLRI.
    - Acute varus injury of the elbow can occur in elderly patients during falls.

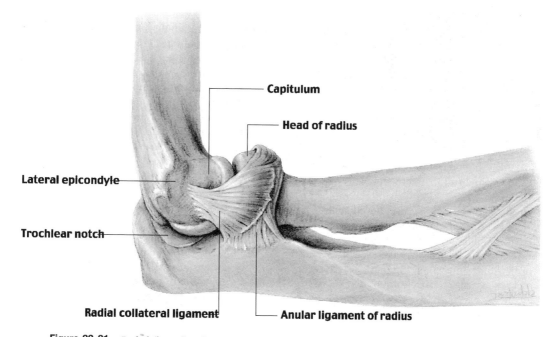

Figure 22-21   Radial (lateral) collateral ligament. The fan-shaped lateral ligament is attached to the anular ligament of the radius, but its superficial fibers continue on to the ulna. (From Moore KL, Dalley AF II. Clinical Oriented Anatomy, 4th ed. Baltimore: Lippincott Williams & Wilkins, 1999.)

Labels in figure: Capitulum; Head of radius; Lateral epicondyle; Trochlear notch; Radial collateral ligament; Anular ligament of radius

- Repetitive stretching of the LCL rarely occurs, as it does to its medial counterpart, the UCL.
- However, congenital or traumatic conditions of the elbow, leading to cubitus varus, can cause gradual stretching of the LCL resulting in PLRI.
- Iatrogenic causes of LCL injury include surgical procedures for lateral epicondylitis and radial head excision or replacement when the LCL is inadequately repaired back to the lateral epicondyle.

Diagnosis

History and Physical Examination

- Clinical presentation of patients with PLRI is highly variable.
- Presenting symptoms can be anywhere from pain to frank recurrent elbow dislocations.
- Most of the time, patients present with pain when loading the elbow.
- This is especially noted when the forearm is supinated and elbow slightly flexed, such as when pushing off with arms while getting up out of a chair.
- Symptoms of snapping, popping, and giving way can also be present.
- It is important to ask about previous injuries and surgical procedures on the involved elbow.
- A high index of suspicion and awareness about possibility of PLRI is important to avoid missing this diagnosis.
- Physical examination may appear remarkably normal.
  - The range of motion is usually normal.
  - Tenderness is likely to be absent of traumatic event to the elbow, which occurred a long time before presentation.
  - Routine varus and valgus stress usually does not show any abnormal laxity.
- Specific provocative tests have been shown to be helpful in making diagnosis.
  - These are difficult to perform in an awake individual.
  - The most sensitive test is the lateral pivot shift test of the elbow (see Fig. 15-31 in Chapter 15).
    - The patient's shoulder is flexed and maximally externally rotated with the examiner standing above the patient's head. The forearm is maximally supinated with valgus stress on the elbow flexed at 90 degrees. Axial load is provided by the other arm of the examiner, and the elbow is extended and apprehension response or frank radial head subluxation may occur. This may create a dimple in the skin overlying the radiocapitellar joint. When the elbow is flexed again past 40 degrees, the radial head reduces and may produce an audible and palpable clunk.
    - The test is considered positive, even if the maneuver elicits pain, since the patient's guarding may prevent actual subluxation of the radial head.
  - The posterolateral drawer test is another test for PLRI (Fig. 22-22).
    - The elbow is flexed to 30 or 90 degrees, and the forearm is translated in anterior and posterior directions relative to the distal humerus to create

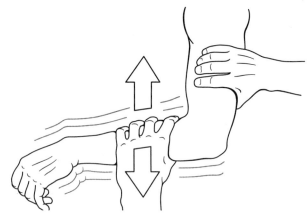

Figure 22-22 Lateral translation, which consists of superior and inferior stress to the lateral aspect of the flexed elbow while the forearm is fully supinated. (After Morrey B, O'Driscoll S. Lateral collateral ligament injury. In: Morrey BF, ed. The Elbow and Its Disorders, 3rd ed. Philadelphia: WB Saunders, 2000:556–562. Modified with permission from the Mayo Foundation for Medical Education and Research. All rights reserved.)

subluxation of the ulnohumeral joint. Pivoting of the lateral forearm around intact medial structures will occur in PLRI.
- The test is positive if instability is felt by both the examiner and the patient.
- Another two tests consist of the patient pushing up from either a prone position or from a chair with palms supinated. The same maneuvers are performed with forearms pronated.
  - If maneuvers are painful when the forearms are supinated and nonpainful when they are pronated, the tests are positive.

Radiologic Examination

- Radiographic studies usually do not show any abnormalities unless there is cubitus varus secondary to previous fracture or congenital deformity.
- Stress views while applying varus stress or posterolateral pivot shift can demonstrate LCL complex laxity and radial head subluxation.
- MRI is rarely useful, although special sequences may demonstrate LCL pathology.

Treatment

- There is no successful nonoperative treatment for deficient LCL complex and PLRI.
- Less active patients who modify their activity may adapt and accept the limitations of function.
- In active patients, treatment of PLRI is surgical.
- Examination under anesthesia is important because this is the only time when a physician can truly assess the extent of instability without the patient's guarding.
- Repair of the LCL complex is indicated in children, adolescents, and adults, with adequate ligamentous tissue for repair back to the lateral epicondyle.
  - The patient is positioned in a supine position with

arm adducted over the chest or extended on a hand table.

- A lateral 8- to 10-cm incision is made along the supracondylar ridge proximally and anterior to the anconeus distally.
- The Kocher approach provides excellent exposure to the LCL complex and radiocapitellar joint.
- If the tissue of the LUCL and RCL is adequate, two nonabsorbable no. 2 or no. 5 sutures are placed in the tissue in locked fashion.
- Three bone tunnels are created starting on the lateral epicondyle and exiting over the posterolateral supracondylar ridge.
- Sutures are passed through the bone tunnels and tied over the bone bridge, whereas the elbow is held in valgus and 40 degrees of flexion, with the forearm in pronation.
- Anterior and posterior capsules are plicated, and the extensor muscles, anconeus, and lateral triceps are repaired back to the lateral epicondyle and lateral supracondylar ridge.
- Most of the patients have attenuated ligamentous structures and require reconstruction of the LUCL.
  - Graft choices include ipsilateral palmaris longus, contralateral palmaris longus, gracilis tendon, semitendinosus tendon, fourth toe extensor tendon, plantaris tendon, or a 3-mm-wide strip of the Achilles tendon.
  - The approach is similar to the approach described for the repair.
  - The LUCL is split longitudinally along its fibers to identify the origin of the lateral epicondyle.
  - Ulnar tunnel and two lateral epicondylar tunnels are created.
  - The graft is passed through the tunnels.
  - The elbow is held at 40 degrees of flexion and full pronation, and the graft is sutured to itself.
  - Muscles and skin are repaired in the same manner as described for LCL repair.

Postoperative Care

- Postoperative care after repair or reconstruction initially consists of immobilization with elbow at 90 degrees of flexion and forearm in full pronation for 2 weeks.
- A brace is placed after 2 weeks; and motion is allowed with block of extension at 60 degrees, 45 degrees, and 30 degrees at 2-week intervals over a 6-week period.
- At 8 weeks, the brace is removed, but supination, extension, and varus forces are avoided.
- Generally, patients return to activity at 9 months.

Results

- Long-term data on LUCL reconstruction are limited.
- Repair of the ligaments when the tissue is adequate, and reconstruction restored stability in 89% of the patients in one report.
- About 73% of the patients in this report achieved good or excellent results.
- The results were better in patients with a history of

trauma, subjective complaints of instability, and reconstruction with autograft tissue.

ADULT MEDIAL ELBOW

Repetitive overhead motion, specifically throwing, is associated with medial-side tension injuries in adults. The spectrum of the pathology includes tendonitis of the volar-pronator mass, medial epicondylitis, ulnar nerve traction injuries, hyperextension valgus overload, and UCL injuries. These conditions become more prevalent with age and often interfere with athletes' performance. Just as most of overuse conditions, the medial-sided elbow disorders in athletes often respond to rest, NSAIDs, and physical therapy. About 50% of athletes undergo operative intervention to return to sports, however.

MEDIAL EPICONDYLITIS

Anatomy and Pathophysiology

Medial epicondylitis is a much more rare diagnosis than its counterpart, lateral epicondylitis. Consequently, much less literature has been written about medial epicondylitis. The underlying pathologic process seems to be similar; however, the anatomy in the region of the medial elbow, specifically in close proximity of the anterior oblique band of the UCL and the ulnar nerve, make medial epicondylitis unique in terms of diagnostic workup and treatment.

The peak incidence is in the fourth and fifth decades of life, with equal rates in males and females. Dominant extremity is involved 75% of the time. Just as others overuse diagnosis, medial epicondylitis is associated with repetitive stress over the medial side of the elbow. Throwing athletes put tremendous strain over the medial side of the elbow as described previously. The volar flexor-pronator mass absorbs significant amount of the forces placed across the elbow leading to degenerative changes at the musculotendinous region and the tendon–bone junction at the medial epicondyle. This disorder has also been associated with other sports, such as golf, tennis, bowling, racquetball, football, weight lifting, and javelin throwing. Certain occupations such as carpentry and plumbing have increased incidence of medial epicondylitis most likely secondary to repetitive forearm pronation and wrist flexion.

The unique anatomy around the medial epicondyle includes the tendinous origin of the flexor-pronator muscles, the ulnar nerve, and the anterior band of the UCL. One must be aware of intimate association of this structures and concomitant pathology that can occur. The pronator teres and flexor carpi radialis are the most lateral muscles of the flexor pronator mass and originate from the anterior aspect of the medial epicondyle. These tendons are most commonly involved in the pathologic process of the medial epicondylitis. Proximity of the ulnar nerve often creates concomitant pathology of ulnar nerve irritation and entrapment. The distal portion of the cubital tunnel, between the two heads of the flexor carpi ulnaris, is the most common location of nerve compression. The proximity of the UCL and the common mechanism of increased valgus strain responsible for medial epicondylitis and degeneration of the UCL make valgus instability an important part of differential diagnosis.

The histologic nature of medial epicondylitis is similar to the lateral epicondylitis. The three stages described for the lateral epicondylitis most likely take place on the medial side.

Diagnosis

History and Physical Examination
- Patients usually present with insidious pain over the medial elbow.
  - Pain is worse with forceful flexion and pronation of the wrist.
  - In athletes, pain is associated with repetitive activity such as throwing and can be associated with other pathologic processes such as ulnar neuritis and UCL insufficiency.
- Range of motion is usually normal initially, but with time, flexion contracture can develop and is very common in overhead athletes.
- On physical examination, patients can have swelling and warmth over medial epicondyle.
- Tenderness is usually present about 8 to 10 mm distal and anterior to the medial epicondyle over the pronator teres and flexor carpi radialis tendons.
  - Pain is exacerbated with resisted flexion and pronation.
- Ulnar nerve neuritis and UCL deficiency may present in similar fashion or coexist in athletic population.
  - Thorough examination of the ulnar nerve—including Tinel's, elbow flexion test, and palpation of the nerve—is an important part of the examination. UCL should be examined by palpation along its course and using provocative tests: the valgus stress test, the milking maneuver, and the Mayo valgus stress test, described earlier.

Radiologic Examination
- Radiographic workup is usually negative but may reveal calcifications and traction spurs.
- EMG testing is useful in patients with concomitant ulnar nerve symptoms.
- MRI or magnetic resonance arthrography is useful in athletes to assess the status of the UCL and evaluate the origin of the volar-pronator muscle mass when acute rupture is suspected.

Treatment

Nonoperative Treatment
- Nonoperative approach to medial epicondylitis is the mainstay treatment for this condition. It is divided in three phases, similar to the lateral epicondylitis.
  - The goal of the first phase is to control the inflammation and alleviate pain.
    - The patient is to stay away from offending activities.

- Complete rest is discouraged to avoid atrophy.
- The medial elbow is iced 3 to 4 times a day for 15 to 20 minutes.
- A short course of NSAIDs and cortisone injection into the subaponeurotic fatty recess may also be helpful to alleviate pain from concomitant synovitis.
- Ultrasound and high-voltage galvanic stimulation have been used to relieve pain; however, these modalities have not undergone the scrutiny of prospective, randomized studies to determine their efficacy.
- Counterforce bracing is also helpful to decrease the intrasubstance tension in the tendon by limiting the contractile expansion of the musculotendinous unit.
  - The brace is worn during daily activities and may also be helpful in returning to athletic activity.
- The second phase of the nonoperative treatment is focused on rehabilitation.
  - This phase is initiated as soon as the pain is controlled.
  - The first goal is to establish painless full range of motion.
  - Stretching and isometrics are instituted at this time.
  - As the strength and flexibility are restored, concentric and excentric strengthening exercises are begun.
  - The goal is to achieve greater strength than at the time of preinjury when tendinous injury occurred.
  - Shoulder and elbow rehabilitation is also very important, especially in athletes before sport-specific and vocational activities.
- The third phase is focused on a safe return of an athlete back to competition.
  - Equipment and proper technique must be monitored to ensure prevention of recurrent symptoms.
  - Various equipment factors related to increased incidence of lateral and medial epicondylitis have been identified in different sports.
  - The main goal is to decrease the vibration transmission and valgus stress to the medial elbow.
  - Experienced coaches, trainers, and physicians can ensure safe return to the sport by using a structured interval program focusing on flexibility, strength, and endurance.

Surgical Treatment
- Surgical treatment is offered when 3 to 6 months of nonoperative treatment fails.
- In high-level athletes with tendon origin avulsion, the operative treatment is offered sooner because return to sport with such injury, especially throwing, is most likely incompatible with conservative treatment.
- The goal of the surgical approach is to excise the degenerative tissue, enhance the vascular environment of the

area, reattach the healthy tendon, and address concurrent ulnar nerve and UCL pathology.

- The medial approach is used, and care must be taken to avoid injury to the medial antebrachial cutaneous nerve.
- The degenerative tissue is excised through the longitudinal muscle-splitting approach or transverse approach, leaving tendon origin on the medial epicondyle.
- The bone bed can be rongeured and drilled to enhance the vascular supply to the area.
- The defect is closed, and the tendon is reattached to the epicondyle through bone tunnels or to the stump of the tendon tissue that was left intact during the approach.
- Ulnar nerve and UCL pathology is addressed through the same approach if warranted.
- Layered closure is performed, and the elbow is splinted at 90 degrees of flexion in neutral forearm rotation.

Postoperative Care

- Postoperative rehabilitation includes immobilization for 7 to 10 days until wound heals.
- Passive and active range of motion is started at this point.
- Isometrics are initiated at 3 to 4 weeks, and resistive strengthening started at 6 to 8 weeks.
- Athletes generally return to their sport in 3 to 6 months.

Results

- Results of nonoperative treatment are variable.
  - Older reports have shown a success rate of 85% to 90%, but others have reported recurrence of symptoms in 26% to 40% of the patients.
- Surgical treatment after failed nonoperative management results in 88% to 96% of successful treatment.
  - Most athletes are able to return to their previous level of competition.
  - Results are better in patients without concurrent ulnar nerve pathology.
  - Objective strength deficits may occur but do not seem to result in functional compromise.

HYPEREXTENSION VALGUS OVERLOAD

Pathophysiology

Ulnar-humeral articulation plays an important role in stability of the elbow. In extension, olecranon articulation with olecranon fossa contributes to stability of the joint in the coronal plane. Extensive valgus forces combined with hyperextension, which occurs in throwing athletes, result in increased pressure between the medial olecranon and the medial half of the olecranon fossa. This process results in formation of osteophytes and loose bodies in olecranon fossa and on the medial surface of the olecranon. Medial ligamentous laxity exacerbates this condition.

Diagnosis

History and Physical Examination

- Clinical presentation usually constitutes pain medially and posteriorly, especially during acceleration and deceleration phases of throwing.
- Patients may report catching, locking, and sharp painful episodes in terminal extension.
- Terminal extension is often limited secondary to osteophytes and loose bodies.
- Pain radiating down the ulnar side of the forearm and tingling may represent ulnar nerve irritation secondary to olecranon osteophytes.
- Physical examination usually demonstrates tenderness along the medial ulnohumeral articulation.
- Crepitus and locking can be observed with active motion of the elbow.
- Range of motion is often limited in extension due to impinging osteophytes.
- Valgus testing and milking maneuver are important to assess anterior band of medial collateral ligament.
- Testing for Tinel's sign should be performed to check for ulnar nerve irritation.
- Ulnar nerve instability must be checked for, especially prior to any surgical intervention.
- Palpation of the radiocapitellar joint, secondary stabilizer to valgus stress, is also important because increased pressure in this articulation can cause articular damage and loose body formation.

Radiologic Findings

- Radiographic workup includes AP, lateral, and axillary views.
- Loose bodies and osteophytes can often be identified with these routine views.
- MRI is often useful to further identify loose bodies and osteophytes, as well as provide information about surrounding soft-tissue structures.

Treatment

Nonsurgical Treatment

- Initially, treatment consists of rest, NSAIDs, physical therapy focusing on excentric elbow flexors contractions, modalities, supervised pitching mechanics, and gradual throwing program as symptoms allow.
- Increased valgus stress at the elbow during pitching was correlated with shoulder abduction angle at stride foot contact and elbow angle at the peak of the elbow valgus stress.
- Modification of pitching mechanics may decrease the valgus stress seen at the elbow.

Surgical Treatment

- Operative options include open removal of osteophytes and loose bodies through posterior incision and arthroscopic approach.
- The arthroscopic option results in less morbidity, faster recovery, and offers the advantage of inspection of the entire joint to address any additional pathology.
- The portals used for posterior compartment include the

posterolateral portal, located 3 cm proximal to olecranon tip along the lateral border of the triceps, and the direct posterior portal, located 3 cm proximal to the olecranon tip through the middle of the triceps tendon.

- The posterolateral portal is usually used as a viewing portal, and the direct posterior portal is used as a working portal.
- Care is taken to remove only osteophytes and preserve native olecranon.
- When working medially, special attention should be paid to avoid injury to the ulnar nerve traveling in the cubital tunnel close to the medial osteophytes.

Postoperative Care

- Postoperative rehabilitation consists of immediate active flexion and extension exercises.
- Care is taken to gain full extension to prevent build of scar in the space created after resection.
- At 6 weeks, the gentle throwing program is initiated, with return to competition allowed around 3 to 4 months postoperatively.

Results and Complications

- Open and arthroscopic treatments showed successful results in about 90% of patients.
- In general, patients with posterior impingement alone do better than patients who developed degenerative changes in the joint.
- One of the concerning findings is that in professional baseball players, resection of the medial olecranon may unmask valgus instability secondary to incompetent medial collateral ligament.
  - In one of the reports, 25% of players required subsequent MCL reconstruction.
- Medial olecranon osteophytes may provide increased valgus stability in patients with incompetent MCL.
  - Resection of these osteophytes leads to further damage of the MCL secondary to increased demand during throwing.
  - Increased sequential resection of the olecranon places increased strain on the MCL.
  - These results further stress the importance of careful medial resection of osteophytes, leaving only the native olecranon intact.
    - The exact amount of safe resection is currently unknown.

ULNAR COLLATERAL LIGAMENT INJURY

PATHOPHYSIOLOGY

The UCL consists of anterior, posterior, and transverse bundles (Fig. 22-23). The anterior bundle is the primary stabilizer of elbow to valgus stress. Throwing athletes with injury to the anterior bundle of the ligament have pain and decreased athletic performance.

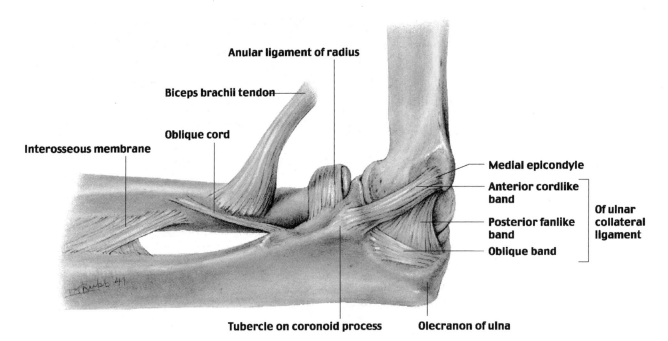

Figure 22-23   Ulnar (medial) collateral ligament. The anterior band (part)—a strong, round cord—is taut when the elbow joint is extended. The posterior band is a weak, fan-like ligament that is taut in flexion of the joint. The oblique fibers merely deepen the socket for the trochlea of the humerus. (From Moore KL, Dalley AF II. Clinical Oriented Anatomy, 4th ed. Baltimore: Lippincott Williams & Wilkins, 1999.)

Throwing athletes place tremendous stresses on the anterior band of the UCL during throwing. The greatest stresses occur during late cocking and early acceleration phases of throwing. During the acceleration phase, the elbow flexes from 90 to 120 degrees and rapidly extends at 40 msec to the ball release. The angular velocity of the elbow during this interval of time is 4,500 deg/sec. The forces placed on the UCL often exceed its tensile strength. Improper throwing mechanics, poor flexibility, and inadequate conditioning may result in additional cumulative stress transmitted to UCL complex. This mechanism of throwing puts repeated stress on the anterior band of UCL, resulting in stretching, attenuation, and sometimes frank failure of the ligament.

DIAGNOSIS

History and Physical Examination

- Two types of presentations can occur in athletes with UCL injury.
  - The more common presentation consists of gradual onset of medial pain during the late cocking and early acceleration phases of throwing.
  - Sometimes athletes can experience first-time medial pain after a particularly intense and prolonged period of throwing, after which they continue having medial pain and can subsequently throw at only 50% to 75% of their normal level.
  - Occasionally, an athlete experiences acute pain and pop after a throw and is unable to continue throwing.
- It is important to collect as detailed a history as possible including time of onset of symptoms and phase of throwing when symptoms are most bothersome.
  - Changes in training regimen, accuracy, velocity, stamina, and strength, as well as prior injuries, are important information.
  - About 85% of athletes experience symptoms during the acceleration phase of throwing.
- Any neurologic and vascular symptoms must be sought.
  - Ulnar neuritis is commonly associated with UCL insufficiency and it is important to assess the symptoms, especially motor abnormalities, because it may influence treatment.

Physical Examination

- If there is an effusion of the elbow, the joint is held at 70 to 80 degrees of flexion corresponding to the greatest capsular volume.
- Carrying angle formed by the axial line of the humerus and the forearm is assessed.
  - Increased carrying angle may be secondary to previous trauma, congenital abnormalities, as well as adaptive changes in throwers secondary to the stretching of the medial structures.
- Range of motion is assessed both actively and passively, taking note of any contractures, crepitus, and pain.
  - Flexion contractures are present in 50% professional throwers and are considered normal adaptations.

- Palpation on bony anatomy and soft tissue is also an important part of the examination.
  - Tenderness of the volar-pronator mass is common in throwing athletes and should alert the physician to the possibility of valgus instability.
- Palpation of the UCL is performed with the elbow flexed 50 to 70 degrees, allowing the volar-pronator mass to move anteriorly.
  - Palpation is performed along the entire course of the ligament.
  - Pain on palpation may indicate a spectrum of pathology from intrasubstance tearing to frank rupture.
  - Some athletes may have rupture of the flexor-pronator muscle origin associated with UCL injury.
    - These patients will have pain on palpation at the medial epicondyle and pain with resisted wrist flexion, as well as weakness of wrist flexion.
- The ulnar nerve should also be palpated along its course from the raphe of Struthers to the flexor ulnaris muscle mass.
  - Ulnar nerve instability is checked by palpation while moving the elbow from extension to flexion.
- Stability of the elbow is assessed with the valgus stress test performed at 20 to 30 degrees of flexion to unlock the olecranon from the olecranon fossa (see Fig. 15-28 in Chapter 15).
  - Opening of greater than 1 mm or pain may indicate abnormality in UCL.
    - This opening medially is difficult to detect on manual testing, which may explain why studies by experienced clinicians have noted the ability on physical examination to detect valgus elbow laxity preoperatively of 26% to 82% of patients.
- The milking maneuver produces a valgus stress to the joint in flexion and is helpful in assessment of UCL (see Fig. 15-29 in Chapter 15).
  - The affected elbow is flexed beyond 90 degrees, and the opposite hand of the patient is placed under the elbow being tested to grasp the thumb of the affected hand, thereby exerting a valgus stress on the affected elbow.
  - The UCL is palpated by the examiner for tenderness and joint space opening during this maneuver.
  - This technique of examination is thought to be more sensitive at 90 degrees of flexion, based on the increased valgus rotation of the elbow at this position, as compared with the 30-degree position.
- Another test for UCL insufficiency is the Mayo valgus stress test (Fig. 22-24).
  - The athlete's shoulder is placed in an abducted and externally rotated position.
  - The elbow is then taken through its flexion-extension arc of motion while imparting a valgus force to the elbow.
  - During this maneuver, pain is usually felt at a specific and reproducible point within the flexion arc of 80 to 120 degrees.
  - This reproduces the pain of throwing in the athlete because of close replication of forces.

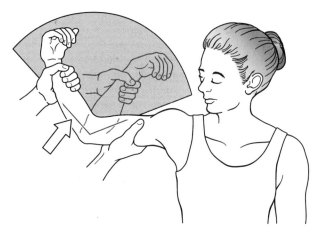

Figure 22-24   Mayo valgus stress test for UCL instability. A positive result is pain between 80 and 120 degrees. (After Safran MR. Injury to the ulnar collateral ligament: diagnosis and treatment. Sports Med Arthrosc Rev 2003;11:20.)

Radiologic Examination

■ Radiographic workup includes AP, lateral, axial, and two oblique views of the elbow.
■ Stress radiographs may be helpful to assess medial joint line opening, compared with the uninjured side.
■ Radiographs are evaluated for olecranon osteophytes, loose bodies, and calcification within the ligament (indicating potential previous injury).
■ Diagnostic imaging for evaluation of soft tissue around the elbow, specifically UCL, continues to be a controversial topic.
   ■ The options include nonenhanced MRI, and CT and magnetic resonance arthrograms.
■ CT and magnetic resonance arthrograms showed similar sensitivity and specificity in diagnosis of complete and partial tears.
■ Nonenhanced MRI seems to be less accurate for partial tears, although some reports demonstrated good sensitivity and specificity using special sequences.

TREATMENT

Nonsurgical Treatment

■ Nonoperative treatment of UCL injuries leads to satisfactory results in nonthrowing athletes.
■ In general, high-demand professional throwing athletes do not do well with nonoperative approach.
■ The nonoperative treatment begins with a period of "active rest" (2 to 6 weeks) when the athlete stays away from throwing and modalities focusing on control of inflammation and range-of-motion exercises are instituted.
■ Shoulder rehabilitation is an important part of elbow recovery because any weakness or soreness at the shoulder level places increased demand at the elbow during throwing.

■ After pain in the elbow is resolved, strengthening of the flexor-pronator muscles is initiated.
■ Progressive strengthening of all muscle groups in the upper extremity is initiated after pain is controlled.
■ Plyometrics and functional exercises are started with an interval-throwing program initiated at 3 months.
■ Return to competition is allowed when the entire rehabilitation program is completed without pain.

Surgical Treatment

■ Operative treatment of UCL injuries is indicated in patients with complete rupture of UCL based on history, physical examination, and imaging studies who want to return to active throwing sports.
■ The operative approach is also offered to throwing athletes with partial tears who failed a comprehensive nonoperative treatment described previously.
■ Occasionally, nonthrowing athletes continue having symptoms of valgus instability despite nonoperative treatment.
■ Operative treatment constitutes reconstruction of the anterior band of the UCL.
■ Based on multiple reports, reconstruction allows higher return to throwing and better overall results compared with ligament repair.
■ Jobe et al. (1986) were the first to report on reconstruction of the anterior band of UCL using graft tissue in the figure-of-eight fashion placed through bone tunnels in the medial epicondyle of the humerus and the proximal ulnar and suturing the graft to itself.
   ■ This procedure allowed 10 of 16 athletes to return to the previous level of competition.
   ■ Several concerns with the approach described in this chapter included detachment of the flexor-pronator mass and routine submuscular ulnar nerve transposition.
■ Subsequently, several authors reported various modifications of the original surgical technique.
   ■ Modifications included a muscle-slitting approach through the flexor-pronator mass with subcutaneous ulnar nerve transposition or without ulnar nerve transposition, and utilization of the Krakow stitch in the graft with fixation in the medial epicondyle through the single bone tunnel (docking procedure).
■ Arthroscopic evaluation can be useful before the open approach to confirm valgus instability and check for concomitant pathology (e.g., olecranon osteophytes, loose bodies).
■ Positioning of the patient for the arthroscopic portion is a matter of preference of the surgeon.
   ■ The anterior compartment is examined either from one of the medial or lateral portals.
   ■ Valgus stress is applied, and medial joint opening is confirmed.
   ■ The posterior compartment can be evaluated after that through the posterolateral portal.
   ■ The posterior portal can be established if osteophytes or loose bodies need to be removed.
■ After the arthroscopic portion of the procedure is finished, a medial approach to the elbow is used.

- Care must be taken to avoid injury to the medial antebrachial cutaneous nerve.
- Depending on the surgeon's preference, the ulnar nerve can be dissected and protected throughout the procedure for subsequent transposition.
- A muscle-splitting approach is less traumatic and allows adequate visualization of the anterior band of the UCL.
- The anterior band is identified and split along its length.
- Valgus stress is applied, and the opening of the medial joint space is confirmed.
- Ulnar tunnels are made 3 to 4 mm distal to the sublime tubercle.
- The ulnar nerve must be meticulously protected during placement of the inferior drill hole.
- Proximally, the surgeon has a choice to use either two tunnels and passing the graft in the figure-of-eight as described in the original technique by Jobe or using a single tunnel and fixing graft tissue over a bone bridge (docking procedure).
- Ulnar nerve transposition is performed if significant ulnar nerve symptoms were present preoperatively.
- Subcutaneous transposition seems to cause less postoperative ulnar nerve symptoms, compared with submuscular transposition.

POSTOPERATIVE CARE

- Postoperatively, the elbow is immobilized for 7 to 10 days, with subsequent institution of active shoulder, elbow, and wrist range-of-motion exercises.
- Progressive strengthening is initiated at 4 to 6 weeks.
- The elbow is protected from valgus stress for 4 months.
- It is important to include shoulder rehabilitation exercises early and continue them throughout the rehabilitation program.
- Rotator cuff strengthening is initiated at 2 months postoperatively.
- Progressive interval-throwing program is started at 4 months.
- Return to competition occurs usually around 12 to 18 months.

RESULTS AND COMPLICATIONS

- Before the UCL reconstruction described by Jobe, rupture of the anterior band of the UCL in a throwing athlete was a career-terminating event.
- Several reports have documented the results of the anterior band of the UCL reconstruction using Jobe's technique with or without modifications.
- The reconstruction allows return to a previous level of activity in 63% to 97% of throwing athletes.

- Postoperative complications most commonly involve injury to the medial antebrachial cutaneous nerve and ulnar nerve irritation.
- Recurrent instability due to stretching or rupture of the graft is uncommon.

SUGGESTED READING

Benjamin HJ, Briner WW Jr. Little League elbow. Clin J Sport Med 2005;15:37–40.

Cain EL Jr, Dugas JR, Wolf RS, et al. Elbow injuries in throwing athletes: A current concepts review. Am J Sports Med 2003;31:621–635.

Chen FS, Rokito AS, Jobe FW. Medial elbow problems in the overhead-throwing athlete. J Am Acad Orthop Surg 2001;9:99–113.

Ciccotti MC, Schwartz MA, Ciccotti MG. Diagnosis and treatment of medial epicondylitis of the elbow. Clin Sports Med 2004;23:693–705.

Colton CL. Fractures of the olecranon in adults: classification and management. Injury 1973;5:121–129.

DeLee J, Drez D, Miller M, eds. Orthopedic Sports Medicine, 2nd ed. Philadelphia: WB Saunders, 2003:1311–1318.

Hak D, Golladay G. Olecranon fractures: treatment and options. J Am Acad Orthop Surg 2000;8:226–275.

Hotchkiss RN. Displaced fractures of the radial head: internal fixation or excision? J Am Acad Orthop Surg 1997;5:1–10.

Jobe FW, Stark H, Lombardo SJ. Reconstruction of the ulnar collateral ligament in athletes. J Bone Joint Surg Am 1986;68:1158–1163.

Kobayashi K, Burton K, Rodner C, et al. Lateral compression injuries in the pediatric elbow: Panner's disease and osteochondritis dissecans of the capitellum. J Am Acad Orthop 2004;12:246–254.

Lynch GJ, Meyers JF, Whipple TL, et al. Neurovascular anatomy and elbow arthroscopy: inherent risks. Arthroscopy 1986;2:191–197.

Mehta JA, Bain GI. Posterolateral rotatory instability of the elbow. J Am Acad Orthop Surg 2004;12:405–415.

Morrey B, ed. The Elbow and Its Disorders. Philadelphia: WB Saunders, 2000.

Morrey BF. Acute and chronic instability of the elbow. J Am Acad Orthop Surg 1996;4:117–128.

Morrey BF, ed. The Elbow, 2nd ed. Philadelphia: Lippincott Williams & Wilkins, 2002.

Morrey BF, Askew LJ, An KN, et al. Biomechanical study of the normal elbow motion. J Bone Joint Surg Am 1981;63:872–877.

Nirschl RP, Ashman ES. Tennis elbow tendinosis (epicondylitis). Instr Course Lect 2004;53:587–598.

Nirschl RP. Prevention and treatment of elbow and shoulder injuries in tennis players. Clin Sports Med 1988;7:289–294.

O'Driscoll SW, Bell DF, Morrey BF. Posterolateral rotatory instability of the elbow. J Bone Joint Surg Am 1991;73:440–446.

O'Driscoll SW, Morrey BF, An KN. Elbow dislocation and subluxation: a spectrum of instability. Clin Orthop 1992;280:186–197.

Ramsey ML. Distal biceps tendon injuries: diagnosis and management. J Am Acad Orthop Surg 1999;7:199–207.

Sanchez-Sotelo J, Morrey BF, O'Driscoll SW. Ligamentous repair and reconstruction for posterolateral rotatory instability of the elbow. J Bone Joint Surg Br 2005;87:54–61.

Schatzker J. Fractures of the olecranon. In: Schatzker J, Tile M, eds. The Rationale of Operative Fracture Care. Berlin: Springer-Verlag, 1987.

van Riet RP, Morrey BF, Ho E, et al. Surgical treatment of distal triceps ruptures. J Bone Joint Surg Am 2003;85-A:1961–1967.

Whaley AL, Baker CL. Lateral epicondylitis. Clin Sports Med 2004;23:677–691.

Williams RJ III, Urquhart ER, Altchek DW. Medial collateral ligament tears in the throwing athlete. Instr Course Lect 2004;53:579–586.

Zarins B, Andres J, Carson W, eds. Injuries to the Throwing Arm. Philadelphia: WB Saunders, 1985.

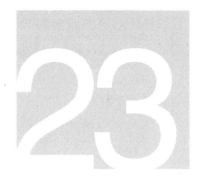

SPORTS-SPECIFIC INJURIES OF THE PELVIS, HIP, AND THIGH

BRETT D. OWENS
BRIAN D. BUSCONI

ANATOMY

The pelvis is formed from the fusion of three separate centers of ossification: the pubis, ischium, and ilium. All fuse into a single bone by early adolescence (Fig. 23-1). The site of convergence and fusion of all three centers of ossification is the triradiate cartilage, which eventually fuses and forms the mature acetabulum. In addition to these primary centers of ossification, the adolescent has seven other centers of secondary ossification, which includes the iliac crest, ischial apophysis, anterior inferior iliac spine, pubic tubercle, angle of pubis, ischial spine, and the lateral wing of the sacrum. These secondary centers of ossification must be recognized on x-ray, and knowledge of fusion is mandatory for a diagnosis of fracture or avulsion to be made.

Proximal femoral development occurs as a result of fusion of three separate centers of ossification: the femoral head, the greater tuberosity, and the lesser tuberosity. The neck-

shaft angle averages 130 degrees, and the anteversion of the femoral neck averages 10 degrees in the adult. Similar to the glenoid cavity of the shoulder, the acetabulum has a fibrocartilaginous labrum attached to its margins. Contrary to the shoulder, the acetabular labrum increases the depth of the joint rather than increasing its diameter. The labrum does not form a complete circle and is continued inferolaterally as the transverse ligament across the acetabular notch. The acetabular fossa lies in the inferomedial portion of the acetabulum and is filled with the triangular-shaped ligamentum teres and the pulvinar (fat and connective tissue). The fovea capitus (bare area) is a small depression on the medial femoral head, which is the insertion site for the ligamentum teres.

The fibrous capsule of the hip joint is reinforced by three prominent thickenings of the joint capsule: the iliofemoral, the pubofemoral, and the ischiofemoral ligaments. The iliofemoral ligament (ligament of Bigelow) is the thickest and strongest of these. This ligament inserts on the intertrochanteric line resulting in more than 95% of the femoral neck being intracapsular. The zona orbicularis (the name

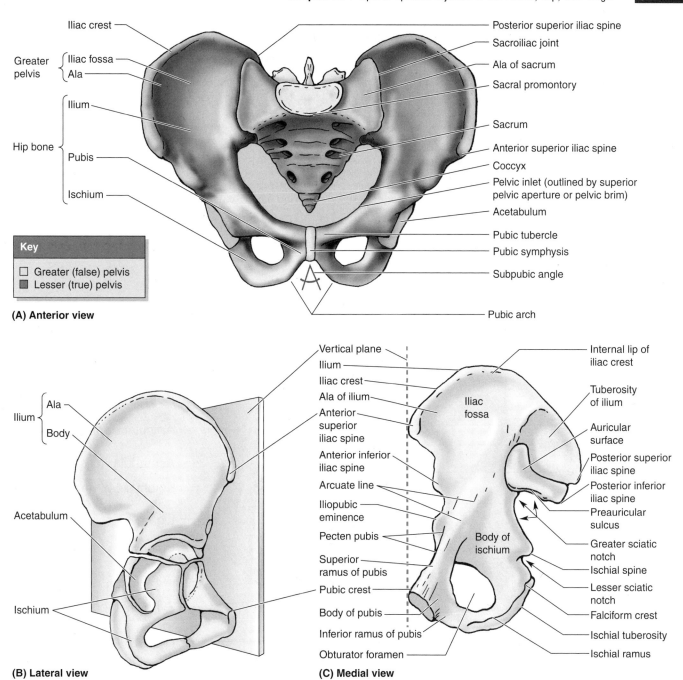

Iliac crest

Greater pelvis { Iliac fossa / Ala }

Hip bone { Ilium / Pubis / Ischium }

Posterior superior iliac spine
Sacroiliac joint
Ala of sacrum
Sacral promontory
Sacrum
Anterior superior iliac spine
Coccyx
Pelvic inlet (outlined by superior pelvic aperture or pelvic brim)
Acetabulum
Pubic tubercle
Pubic symphysis
Subpubic angle
Pubic arch

Key
☐ Greater (false) pelvis
■ Lesser (true) pelvis

(A) Anterior view

Ilium { Ala / Body }
Acetabulum
Ischium

(B) Lateral view

Vertical plane
Ilium
Iliac crest
Ala of ilium
Anterior superior iliac spine
Anterior inferior iliac spine
Arcuate line
Iliopubic eminence
Pecten pubis
Superior ramus of pubis
Pubic crest
Body of pubis
Inferior ramus of pubis
Obturator foramen

Iliac fossa
Body of ischium

Internal lip of iliac crest
Tuberosity of ilium
Auricular surface
Posterior superior iliac spine
Posterior inferior iliac spine
Preauricular sulcus
Greater sciatic notch
Ischial spine
Lesser sciatic notch
Falciform crest
Ischial tuberosity
Ischial ramus

(C) Medial view

Figure 23-1   **A:** Bones of the pelvis. The skeleton of the pelvis is formed by the two hip bones anteriorly and laterally, and the sacrum and coccyx posteriorly. **B:** Lateral view of a child's hip bone. In the anatomical position, the anterior superior iliac spine and the anterior aspect of the pubis lie in the same vertical plane. The hip bone is composed of three bones—the ilium, ischium, and pubis—that meet in the cup-shaped acetabulum. The bones are not fused at this age and unite by a triradiate cartilage along a Y-shaped line. Fusion is usually complete by age 23. **C:** Medial view of the right hip bone in the anatomical position. (From Moore KL, Dalley AF II. Clinical Oriented Anatomy, 4th ed. Baltimore, Lippincott Williams & Wilkins, 1999.)

given to the deep circular fibers of the iliofemoral ligament) may be mistaken for the acetabular labrum arthroscopically. The iliopsoas bursa, directly anterior to the hip joint, communicates with the joint in 15% of normal anatomic specimens. It is not often shown arthrographically, but it may be seen in chronic joint distention with synovitis.

Because of its ball-and-socket configuration, the hip joint has a unique degree of internal stability (Fig. 23-2). Despite this, there is a great mobility between the femoral head and the acetabulum. The motion in the hip joint is in three planes: sagittal, frontal, and transverse, with the greatest motion in the sagittal plane. To perform activities of daily living, a flexion of a least 120 degrees, an abduction of 20 degrees, and a rotation of 20 degrees are preferred, but to participate in sporting events, a significantly greater range of motion is often necessary. During slow walking, the maximum force that is transmitted across the hip joint is about 1.6 times body weight. In running, the force increases to 5 times body weight during the stance phase.

The blood supply to the hip joint is profuse, but the blood supply to the femoral head itself is more tenuous. Until physeal closure (14 to 17 years of age), metaphyseal and epiphyseal blood supplies are separate. Throughout childhood and into adolescence, femoral blood supply is primarily provided by the terminal branches of the medial femoral circumflex artery. These terminal branches form two retinacular vascular systems: posterior-superior and posterior-inferior. The lateral circumflex system is significant until 5 or 6 years of age and supplies blood only to the anterior half of the femoral head. This specific arrangement of me-

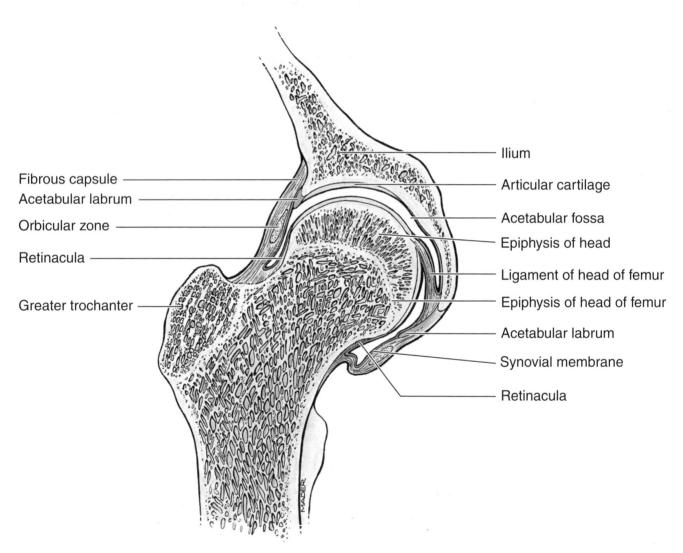

Fibrous capsule

Acetabular labrum

Orbicular zone

Retinacula

Greater trochanter

Ilium

Articular cartilage

Acetabular fossa

Epiphysis of head

Ligament of head of femur

Epiphysis of head of femur

Acetabular labrum

Synovial membrane

Retinacula

Figure 23-2   Coronal section of the hip joint. Observe that the acetabular labrum extends the acetabular rim so that a complete socket is formed, engulfing the head of the femur (thigh bone). Great force must be applied to dislocate the head from the socket, often involving fracture of the acetabular rim and/or avulsion of the labrum. The epiphysis of the femoral head is entirely within the articular capsule of the joint. Observe also that the ligament of the head is surrounded by a tube of synovial membrane. It transmits medial epiphyseal vessels to the femur, which may or may not persist in adults. (From Moore KL, Dalley AF II. Clinical Oriented Anatomy, 4th ed. Baltimore, Lippincott Williams & Wilkins, 1999.)

dial blood supply and poor anastomosis makes the femoral head highly susceptible to avascular necrosis (AVN) from injury to the physis or femoral neck.

Numerous short and long muscles control the hip joint. The main function of the musculature is to meet the requirements of efficient walking by maintaining stability of the weight-bearing leg despite continued change in limb and body position and moving the body forward. Stability is gained by muscle action to resist the force of gravity that acts to pull the body downward. Because the human frame is top-heavy with much of its mass above the pelvis, large muscular forces are required to maintain stability. Also, because the center of gravity must move from behind the supporting stance phase foot to ahead of the stance phase foot to move the body forward, the demands on the muscles are constantly changing. The force to propel the body forward is derived from accelerating the swing phase limb during the gait cycle and positioning the stance phase limb to allow the body to fall forward. Hip muscles participate in both these functions. The gait cycle presents complex and progressively changing demands on the hip musculature. Abnormalities of these muscles, which cause weakness or pain, distort the gait cycle, producing a limp. It is convenient to think of the muscles in functional groups when describing muscular control; however, an individual muscle may contribute to more than one functional movement. These groups are described as the abductors, flexors, adductors, extensors, and rotators. The innervation of these muscles will be noted so that the physician can interpret the effect of neurologic disorder on hip function.

The tensor fascia lata extends its tendinous fibers with the fibers of the gluteus maximus to form the iliotibial tract on the lateral aspect of the thigh. Muscles of this group are innervated by the superior gluteal nerve, which is composed mainly of fibers from the fourth and fifth lumbar nerve roots. The muscles of this group are required to maintain pelvic stability during the stance phase of gait. During stance phase, body weight forces the bearing hip into adduction. Unless the abductors contract with normal strength, there is an excessive pelvic tilt. With deficient abductor function, the individual will compensate by leaning the trunk over the stance phase limb. This compensatory gait pattern is called an abductor lurch and reduces forces across the hip.

The primary flexors of the hip are the iliopsoas, rectus femoris, and sartorius. The pectineus and tensor fascia lata also function as flexors. The strongest flexor is the double-bellied iliopsoas muscle. The iliopsoas is innervated by the femoral nerve, which is composed of fibers originating from the second through fourth lumbar segments. The sartorius and rectus femoris muscles are less powerful flexors and are innervated by the femoral nerve. During gait, hip flexors are important as swing phase is initiated. These muscles contract to accelerate the leg forward. A patient with weak hip flexors circumducts the leg and compensates further by pivoting the body about the opposite stance phase foot, giving the characteristic circumduction limp. The hip flexors are also important in elevating the limb during stair climbing and in such activities as kicking. With kicking, the rectus femoris contracts strongly, and its origin through an apophy-

sis at the anterior inferior iliac spine may be avulsed in adolescents.

The adductor group is composed of five muscles: the adductors longus, brevis, and magnus; the gracilis; and the pectineus. The adductors longus and brevis, the gracilis, and much of the adductor magnus are innervated by the obturator nerve. The posterior portion of the adductor magnus, which is predominantly an extensor of the hip, is innervated by the sciatic nerve, whereas the pectineus is innervated mainly by the femoral nerve. Like the hip flexors, these muscles are largely controlled by the second through fourth lumbar segments. The adductor group has a varied role during gait. At the beginning of stance phase, the adductor magnus is important in assisting the hip extensors to resist flexion of the hip. The adductor longus acts as a hip flexor at the end of the stance phase and as an extensor at the end of the swing phase.

The extensors consist of the gluteus maximus and hamstring muscles, including the long head of the biceps femoris, the semitendinosus, and the semimembranosus. Another extensor is the posterior portion of the adductor magnus. The gluteus maximus is innervated by the inferior gluteal nerve, which is predominantly composed of fibers from the fifth lumbar and first sacral segments. The hamstrings are all innervated by the sciatic nerve, with fibers originating from the fifth lumbar through second sacral segments. Primarily, the hip extensors are responsible for preventing hip and trunk flexion during gait, especially during the early stance phase of gait. The extensors are also responsible for slowing down the accelerating swing phase leg at the end of swing phase. If these muscles fail to function properly, gait becomes unsteady. The gluteus maximus, along with the adductor magnus, is also responsible for climbing and rising from a sitting posture.

Extending across the posterior aspect of the hip are the short external rotators, including the piriformis, superior and inferior gemelli, obturator externus and internus, and the quadratus femoris. Except for the obturator externus, which is innervated by the obturator nerve, the short rotators are innervated by a branch of the sacral plexus. There are no pure internal rotators of the hip. A number of muscles provide internal rotation as well as other functions. For example, the anterior fibers of the gluteus minimus may internally rotate the hip.

Branches of the lumbar and sacral plexus innervate the hip joint. These nerves derive from the second through the fifth lumbar segments. Several of the branches originate from the obturator nerve. The other branches of the obturator nerve innervate the anterior portion of the knee joint, which helps explain why patients with hip disorders may have anterior knee pain in the absence of significant pain about the hip. Occasionally, knee pain may be referred to the hip.

The sciatic nerve emerges from the sacral plexus through the greater sciatic notch between the piriformis and the obturator internus. In the sciatic notch, the sciatic nerve is vulnerable to injury from pelvis fractures and, distal to the notch, vulnerable to injury from posterior dislocation of the femoral head. The femoral artery, vein, and nerve enter the thigh lying on the iliopsoas and pectineus muscles. They are cushioned by these muscles and are not likely to be injured by hip dislocation or pelvic fractures.

DIAGNOSIS

Physical Examination

- A thorough physical examination, including a baseline temperature and vital signs, should be performed.
- Patients who complain of hip pain and are febrile need to be aggressively worked up to rule out hip pyarthrosis or infection.
  - Although hip infections are rare in skeletally mature individuals without a history of hip surgery, one must always consider this diagnosis, especially with the growing number of immunocompromised patients.
  - Usually, pyarthrosis can be ruled out with a careful history and exam, though radiographs and laboratory studies are sometimes needed. Rarely, a hip aspirate is required to eliminate the possibility of pyarthrosis.
  - Other rare causes of hip discomfort and fever include a psoas abscess, prostatitis, pelvic inflammatory disease, and a urinary tract infection.
- The examination begins as the patient walks into the office, with assessment of gait pattern.
  - Intra-articular hip disorders will be manifested by a Trendelenburg gait, but unfortunately some extra-articular causes can present with a similar gait pattern.
- The patient must be adequately undressed for proper examination.
- Inspection normally reveals a level pelvis.
  - Pelvic obliquity suggests leg-length discrepancy or scoliosis, which may or may not be associated with hip disease.
- A thorough spine and neurologic examination should be performed.
  - An upper level lumbar herniated disc (L2–L3 or L3–L4) can produce pain radiating to the groin, thus mimicking hip pain.
- Contracture of the hip may cause a compensatory obliquity of the pelvis.
  - If inspection of the pelvis is difficult because of the patient's size, palpation should be performed at the body prominences to determine position and symmetry.
- Observe the resting posture of the hip.
  - The ligaments of the hip are so oriented that pressure in the joint space is least when the hip is slightly flexed, abducted, and externally rotated. Therefore, patients with an acute synovitis or effusion tend to maintain the hip in this position.
- The Trendelenburg test is performed after inspection.
  - The patient is asked to stand on one leg and lift the other leg with the hip and knee flexed.
  - Normal patients will lift the pelvis contralateral to the stance limb.
  - Patients with deficient abductor muscles or a hip disorder that causes pain on contraction of the mus-

cles have an impairment of this normal mechanism. Consequently, these patients will allow the pelvis to drop contralateral to the stance phase side or may shift the upper body over the stance phase leg to reduce muscular demand.

- The groin should also be examined for inguinal and femoral hernias.
  - The pubis should be palpated to assess for tenderness, which may indicate a condition such as osteitis pubis or athletic pubalgia.
  - Tenderness in the medial proximal thigh may indicate an adductor tendonitis that can also mimic true hip pain.
- The hip examination consists of range-of-motion testing and provocative tests for intra-articular pathology.
  - Patients with intra-articular and certain extra-articular hip disorders will have limitations in range of motion in comparison with the unaffected hip.
  - Provocative tests for labral tears include moving the hip from a flexed, externally rotated and abducted position to an extended, internally rotated and adducted position to test for anterior pathology, and moving from a flexed, internally rotated and adducted position to an extended, abducted and externally rotated position to test for posterior pathology. These tests are positive if they produce a painful click.
- The body landmarks of the pelvis and femur should be palpated.
  - Lateral pain most commonly occurs with trochanteric bursitis, but one must beware of attributing all lateral pain to bursitis as an occult femoral neck fracture can have a similar presentation, especially in an elderly patient.
- Intra-articular hip pathology such as labral tears, loose bodies, and chondral defects can still escape diagnosis on history and physical examination alone. Radiographic evaluation is necessary in all cases of hip pain because it will aid in diagnosis for most common hip disorders.

Radiologic Examination

- Imaging is essential to the complete assessment of the hip.
  - The primary study of choice is plain radiography.
  - An AP pelvis and an AP and lateral view (frog-leg or cross-table) of the symptomatic hip can help rule out pathology of the bone architecture (fracture or bone tumor).
  - If pelvic fracture is found or suspected, pelvic inlet and outlet views are often beneficial.
  - Acetabular fractures are best assessed with Judet views, as well as with computed tomography (CT) with fine cuts through the hip joint.
  - It is imperative to rule out an occult femoral neck fracture in patients with persistent hip pain who cannot bear weight on the extremity.
  - The study of choice to detect occult hip fractures is magnetic resonance (MR), which is superior to scintigraphy.

- MR imaging (MRI) is needed to assess the soft tissues about the hip and pelvis, as well as the marrow elements.
  - Marrow edema is best shown as high signal intensity on T_2 STIR images.
- Assessment of intra-articular pathology can be enhanced with MR arthrography. However, many studies have shown a significant false-negative rate for detecting labral pathology.

Differential Diagnosis

Hip and pelvis injuries encompass a wide spectrum of pathology, resulting from repetitive microtraumatic stresses or acute microtraumatic forces. Fortunately, the majority of these injuries heal without permanent sequelae; however, accurate recognition and prompt appropriate treatment are required to minimize complications. Injuries to the hip and pelvis account for approximately 5% of all injuries sustained by adult athletes. Runners and soccer players may also be somewhat more prone to injuries of the hip and groin. Soft-tissue injuries include muscular, tendinous, or ligamentous inflammation, contusion or strain, rupture or avulsion. Skeletal injuries involve the epiphysis, physis, apophysis, metaphysis, or diaphysis, and skeletal pathology includes incomplete or complete fractures, stress reactions, dislocations, avulsions, infections, inflammations, and acquired or pathologic conditions.

Hip pain typically regarded as nontraumatic—e.g., inflammatory conditions such as rheumatoid arthritis, juvenile arthritis and ankylosing spondylitis, infections, tumors (benign and malignant), and metabolic bone disease—may be induced by physical activity and consequently presented to the sports physician. Nerve entrapment syndromes of the ilioinguinal, genitofemoral, and the lateral cutaneous nerves of the thigh can manifest as pain or paresthesiae in their respective distributions. It is essential that systemic illness manifesting as hip pain be considered when the severity of course of the injury is not in keeping with the presumed diagnosis.

In addition, the differential diagnosis of hip pain must include structures distant to the joint and periarticular tissues. It is important to consider referred pain from the lumbar spine, abdominal and pelvic viscera, genitourinary problems, sacroiliac problems, hernias, and other pelvic conditions. Similarly, pain from the knee and thigh may be referred proximally to the hip and vice versa.

Persistent hip pain can also originate from intra-articular pathology such as synovitis, loose bodies, AVN, acetabular labral tears, or infection. Pain is usually the chief complaint of patients with hip problems. These patients may present with pain over the anterior or lateral aspects of the hip, in the groin, or more medially in the region of the adductors (corresponding to the obturator nerve distribution). Pain may radiate distally to the knee. Pain referred to the hip may be secondary to spinal problems, which must be considered in the differential diagnosis of patients with "hip" pain.

Patients with chronic progressive disease such as osteoarthritis report progressively severe pain. They often report prior problems (e.g., injury or childhood disease, including developmental dysplasia, AVN, or slipped capital femoral epiphysis). Adults with AVN may describe the onset of pain

months or years after cortisone use. Excessive alcohol ingestion may be a contributing cause of AVN.

Patients will complain of stiffness, which may be worst in the morning or may be a more constant problem affecting many activities of daily living. To obtain an accurate analysis, patients should be questioned to determine their impairment in the activities of walking, dressing, stair-climbing, and foot hygiene.

BONY INJURIES

Fracture and Dislocation

Pelvis and Femur

Pelvic and femoral diaphyseal fractures are rare in sports but can have devastating consequences. These injuries require great amounts of energy imparted to occur, although lower-energy mechanisms can be seen in pathologic bone. Most pelvic fractures in athletes are stable injuries of the pelvic ring and require symptomatic treatment with an initial course of protected weight-bearing.

- The determination of pelvic ring stability should be confirmed by inlet/outlet radiographs, in addition to CT.
- The treatment of choice for diaphyseal femur fractures is reduction followed by intramedullary nailing.

Hip

Hip dislocations and fracture dislocations are seen more commonly but are still rare injuries (Fig. 23-3).

- Intertrochanteric hip fractures require surgical reduction and internal fixation.
- Femoral neck fractures in athletes are a true orthopedic emergency.
  - Anatomic reduction and internal fixation are required in a timely fashion because AVN is associated with delays in treatment.
- Another injury that has the devastating risk of AVN is

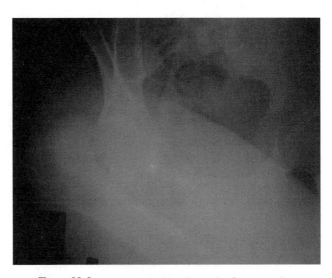

Figure 23-3   Anteroposterior radiograph of posterior hip dislocation.

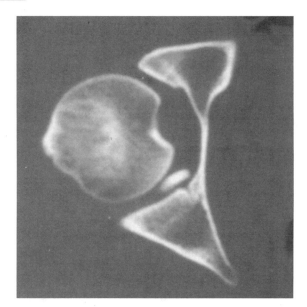

Figure 23-4   CT scan showing intra-articular loose body after hip dislocation.

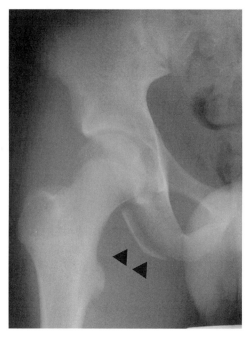

Figure 23-5   This adolescent soccer player had sudden onset of pain while accelerating during a game. He indicated his buttock as the source of his pain, a rather unusual location, and had increasing hip/buttock pain with palpation of his hamstring muscles in the popliteal space or knee flexion. His radiograph shows an avulsion fracture (*arrowheads*) of his ischial tuberosity (the origin of the hamstrings). (From Fleisher GR, Ludwig S, Baskin MN. Atlas of Pediatric Emergency Medicine. Philadelphia: Lippincott Williams & Wilkins, 2004.)

hip dislocation, which may also have associated femoral head or acetabular fractures.

- These require emergent closed (or open if necessary) reduction followed by CT to assess a fracture if present or to rule out an osseous loose body (Fig. 23-4).
- Even in the absence of fracture, the presence of chondral loose bodies and labral pathology can cause persistent symptoms.
    - Hip arthroscopy can be useful in this scenario.

Avulsion Fractures and Apophyseal Injuries

Avulsion fractures about the hip and pelvis are the result of failure of the bone at the tendinous insertion rather than the tendon itself. These injuries are more common in skeletally immature athletes with open apophyses, which are more susceptible to failure than the tendinous insertion. These are usually the result of a sudden, forceful concentric or eccentric contracture or rapid, excessive passive lengthening. Common sites of these avulsions about the pelvis are the insertion of the sartorius into the anterior-superior iliac spine, the rectus femoris superior head insertion into the anterior-inferior iliac spine, and the insertion of the hamstrings into the ischial tuberosity. These injuries are also seen in the proximal femur with the insertion of the hip abductors into the greater trochanter and the insertion of the iliopsoas into the lesser trochanter (Fig. 23-5).

Treatment
- Nonsurgical management has been associated with good to excellent results.
- In the case of severe displacement of the avulsed fragment (especially noted in avulsions of the ischial tuberosity or the greater trochanter), surgical intervention has been recommended but indications remain unclear.
- A rehabilitation protocol for these injuries is given in Box 23-1.

- Skeletally immature patients are also susceptible to chronic traction injuries at these apophyses, and this is referred to as apophysitis.
    - Apophysitis is treated conservatively with rest, followed by functional rehabilitation of the involved muscle group.

Slipped Capital Femoral Epiphysis

- Slipped capital femoral epiphysis (SCFE) is the most common hip disorder in adolescents. It is more common

---

BOX 23-1 REHABILITATION PROTOCOL FOR AVULSION FRACTURES AND APOPHYSEAL INJURIES OF THE HIP AND PELVIS

- Rest, using proper positioning to unload the injured apophysis, and ice/analgesics
- Gentle active and passive range-of-motion exercises
- Progressive resistance beginning when 75% of motion is achieved and ending when 50% of strength is returned
- Integration of stretching and strengthening exercises with functional activity
- Return to competitive sport at 8 to 10 weeks

(Adapted from Metzmaker JN, Pappas AM. Avulsion fractures of the pelvis. Am J Sports Med 1985;13:349–358.)

in overweight males and has an increased incidence in blacks.

■ Bilateral involvement is seen in 20% to 40% of patients.

■ The femoral head remains in the acetabulum while failure at the physis allows the femoral neck to slip anteriorly.

■ SCFE is a poorly diagnosed condition and should be suspected in a skeletally immature patient with hip or knee pain or limp.

■ Anteroposterior and frog-leg lateral radiographs are diagnostic. SCFE is classified based on the ability to bear weight, with "stable" slips allowing weight-bearing.

■ Although unstable slips are associated with a higher incidence of AVN, all slips need to be stabilized with in situ pinning.

Stress Fractures

Pelvis

■ Pelvic stress fractures should be suspected in athletes such as long-distance runners and military recruits.

■ The most common site is the junction between the ischium and inferior pubic ramus.

■ Tenderness to palpation directly over the fractured bone can be helpful in locating the lesion.

■ A positive standing sign has been described in which a patient develops discomfort in the groin while standing unsupported on the ipsilateral leg.

■ Plain radiographic signs, such as periosteal reaction or fracture line, can lag behind the clinical presentation by as long as 3 weeks.

■ MRI and bone scan can provide an earlier diagnosis.

■ Tumors should at least be considered in the differential diagnosis.

■ Treatment consists of rest, with emphasis on protected weight-bearing, flexibility, and aerobic nonimpact exercises such as swimming or cycling. Return to sport can be delayed up to 6 months.

Femoral Neck

■ Although femoral neck stress fractures are not as common as pelvic stress fractures, if treated incorrectly, the results can be disastrous.

■ Similar to pelvic stress fractures, these present with groin pain and an antalgic gait. Pain will be worsened by flexion and internal rotation of the hip.

■ Radiographic evidence may lag behind by 3 to 4 weeks.

■ MRI (Fig. 23-6) and bone scan may be helpful in earlier diagnosis.

■ Two types of femoral neck stress fractures exist.

   ■ The first type is a compression side femoral neck stress fracture. These occur in the inferior medial aspect of the neck and usually respond to restriction to non–weight-bearing status until radiographic evidence of healing has occurred.

   ■ The more worrisome type is the tension side femoral neck stress fracture. This is a transverse fracture along the superior margin of the neck.

■ Because of the high risk of displacement, internal fixation is recommended for nondisplaced fractures.

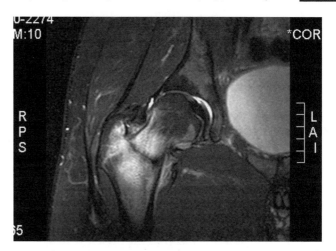

Figure 23-6   MRI of femoral neck stress fracture in an 18-year-old male military recruit.

■ Immediate closed or open reduction and internal fixation are recommended for displaced fractures.

■ Fracture displacement can lead to AVN of the femoral head.

Osteitis Pubis

■ Primary osteitis pubis is caused by repetitive microtrauma and is difficult to treat.

■ Most cases of osteitis pubis are secondary. Retained sutures from hernia or urogynecological repair may cause osteitis pubis.

■ Traumatic osteitis pubis is a fatigue fracture involving the bony origin of the gracilis muscle at the pubic symphysis.

■ When the bony lesion is located at the lower margin of the symphysis, it is referred to as gracilis syndrome.

■ Endometriosis, pelvic inflammatory disease, and tumor must also be considered in the differential, often necessitating a biopsy.

■ On physical examination, patients will have tenderness to palpation directly on the pubis.

■ Although activity may aggravate the symptoms, patients with primary osteitis may get some relief.

■ Although diagnosis is usually confirmed by MRI or bone scan, the distinction between primary and secondary osteitis is usually made on physical examination.

■ Initial treatment consists of rest, range-of-motion exercises, oral nonsteroidal anti-inflammatory drugs, and sometimes corticosteroid injection. Secondary osteitis will respond to treatment of the underlying condition.

■ Surgical intervention can be required in recalcitrant cases but has unpredictable results.

SOFT-TISSUE INJURIES

Intra-articular Pathology

■ The torn acetabular labrum (Fig. 23-7) has been identified as a cause for hip discomfort in athletics.

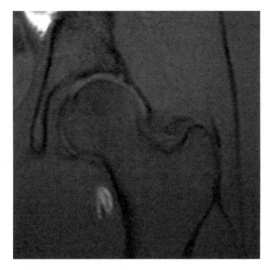

Figure 23-7 A 19-year-old female lacrosse player with a superior labral tear on MRI.

- Its clinical features include a painful click in the inguinal area that radiates toward the gluteus, catching, or giving-way symptoms.
- In general, athletes will remember an antecedent traumatic event, which often involves sports requiring forceful hip flexion, abduction, and forceful knee extension, such as karate.
- On physical examination, the painful click can be reproduced by a Thomas flexion-extension maneuver.
- Radiographic measures have been unreliable and have low diagnostic yields.
- It is this group of patients with refractory hip pain, reproducible physical findings, and equivocal or negative radiographic studies in who hip arthroscopy has been successful in diagnosis and treatment.
- Excellent results have been reported when arthroscopic debridement of the lesions is performed.
- Return to sports can be as early as 6 to 8 weeks after debridement.
- Chondral lesions can be elusive causes of hip symptoms.
  - Patients usually complain of mechanical symptoms.
  - Physical examination can demonstrate clicking.
  - MR arthrography can help with the diagnosis, as well as arthroscopy, which can be both diagnostic and therapeutic.
  - Fibrillated articular cartilage can be removed, whereas full-thickness lesions can be addressed with marrow-stimulating techniques for fibrocartilage ingrowth.
  - Byrd described the "lateral impact injury" in which a blow to the greater trochanter allows transfer of this force, damaging the articular cartilage of the femoral head. This mechanism should be considered in contact athletes.
  - Femoroacetabular impingement is another entity that can present in athletes and can be addressed via either open debridement or arthroscopy.
- Ligamentum teres injuries can also be seen in athletes.

- Although the blood supply provided by the ligamentum in adults is negligible, the exact role of the ligamentum has not been defined.
- Dynamic arthroscopy has shown tightening of the ligamentum during external rotation, suggesting a possible role as a hip stabilizer. Injuries to the ligamentum teres can be isolated or as part of a larger traumatic spectrum (hip dislocation).
- Patients with isolated injuries often report mechanical symptoms and have a clicking noted on physical examination.
- CT can sometimes show a small bony avulsion, which can suggest the diagnosis; however, MR arthrography is usually more helpful.
- Arthroscopic debridement is the usual treatment of ligamentum teres pathology with good results reported.

Muscle Strains

Soft-tissue injuries to the periarticular structures surrounding the hip and pelvis are the most common injuries seen in athletes. In general, the great majority of soft-tissue injuries about the hip and pelvis are musculotendinous strains. The type of injury sustained is highly dependent on skeletal age of the athlete, physical condition, and biomechanical forces involved in both the sport and nature of the trauma. The degree of injury can range from repetitive microinjury associated with each performance to a more significant single macroinjury caused by an abnormal biomechanical force. A certain degree of microtrauma occurs with every major exertional performance immediately manifested by swelling, sensitivity, and a recovery interval. If additional moderate or severe micro- or macroinjury occurs, there may not be a normal healing response, which may lead to more significant changes in tissue structure and a negative effect on future athletic performance.

A strain is an injury to a musculotendinous structure caused by an indirectly applied force. The most common mechanism of injury is a result of eccentric contraction or stretching of an activated muscle. The site of injury is influenced by the rate of loading, mechanism of injury, and local anatomic factors. Low rates of loading will result in a failure at the tendon bone junction by bone avulsion or disruption at its insertion. High rates of loading result in intratendinous or myotendinous juncture injuries.

These injuries can be graded on a three-scale clinical grading system (Table 23-1). Complete disruptions can ben-

TABLE 23-1 GRADING OF MUSCLE STRAINS

Grade	Description
1	Simple stretching of soft-tissue fibers
2	Partial tearing of the musculotendinous unit
3	Secondary to extreme violent forces causing complete disruptions (unusual)

efit from surgical repair, as in the case of proximal hamstring tendon tears (Fig. 23-8).

Contusions

Among the most frequently experienced hip and pelvic injuries sustained by athletes are soft-tissue contusions. Contusions usually result from direct blows to a specific soft-tissue area usually overlying a bony prominence. Contusions are most common in contact sports, especially football, but are also seen in other sports. In contact sports, the blow is usually caused by contact with another athlete. In noncontact sports, athletes usually sustain blows from contact with equipment (e.g., gymnastics), contact with high-velocity projectiles (e.g., a lacrosse ball), or contact from the playing surface.

Contusions are often found over areas of bony prominences of the pelvis, which include the iliac crest (hip pointer), greater trochanter, ischial tuberosity, and pubic rami. Because of the varied anatomy of the pelvis, contusions can be superficial, especially when they overlie a relatively subcutaneous bone or lie deep within a large muscle mass. It is important to determine possible presence and extent of muscular hemorrhage because an increase in muscular hemorrhage often results in more severe symptoms and longer time before returning to sport.

Hip Pointer

- Pain and hemorrhage over the iliac crest has been referred to as a hip pointer.
- These injuries include contusions, avulsion of the iliac apophysis, periostitis, or avulsion of the muscles that insert onto the iliac crest.
- On physical examination, the patient will have superficial or muscular hemorrhage, which will be painful on palpation.
- It is important to note by touch a defect, which would indicate an avulsion injury.
- Patients will have difficulty with rotation and side bending of the trunk.

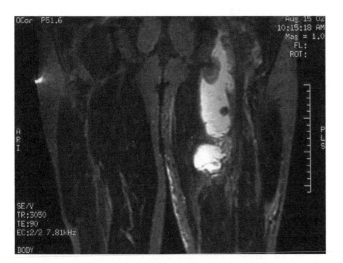

Figure 23-8   MRI showing proximal hamstring tendon avulsion.

- Anterior-posterior and oblique x-rays of the pelvis will rule out an avulsion fracture, periostitis, or an acute fracture of the iliac wing.

Thigh Contusions

- Thigh contusions are common athletic injuries most often encountered in football from direct trauma.
- These injuries can involve significant muscular damage, hematoma formation, and swelling, so the athlete can be extremely uncomfortable.
- Initial treatment is rest, ice, and compression to minimize hematoma formation.
- Immobilization in flexion and initiation of early flexion exercises has been recommended to decrease myositis ossificans formation and improve functional outcome.

Myositis Ossificans

- Myositis ossificans is the ossification of contused muscle hematoma.
- Although this reflects on the severity of the injury, it usually does not limit the function of the athlete.
- In the presence of an ossified mass anterior to the femur, however, osteosarcoma must be ruled out by radiographic and CT imaging.
- Symptomatic myositis ossificans lesions that are refractory to conservative management may be treated with excision once it has matured (usually 6 months); however, this can be associated with recurrence.

Bursitis

Bursitis about the hip is a common condition secondary to inflammation of one of the three major bursae about the hip: the trochanteric bursa, the iliopsoas bursa, and the ischiogluteal bursa (Fig. 23-9). These bursae facilitate the gliding of musculotendinous or ligamentous structures. Bursitis may be secondary to direct injury or overuse of the adjacent musculotendinous structures or degenerative changes in these structures. Because bursae are lined by true synovial tissue, bursitis also can occur with systemic disease, causing synovitis.

The trochanteric bursa is a large bursa that lies between the greater trochanter and the overlying junction of the gluteus maximus and tensor fascia lata, as these merge to form the fascia lata and iliotibial tract. This is the most common bursitis in athletes and is common in runners. Ischiogluteal bursitis, inflammation of the bursa between the ischial tuberosity and the overlying gluteus maximus, is usually associated with injury or with occupations requiring long periods of sitting. The patient complains of pain over the ischial tuberosity that is aggravated by sitting, and the pain may radiate into the posterior thigh. Iliopsoas bursitis is another relatively common bursitis in athletes. This bursa is located between the iliopsoas muscle and the pelvis proximally and the hip capsule and psoas tendon distally. Communication between the hip joint and psoas bursa is common.

- Bursitis at any of these sites is treated conservatively with rest, stretching, and nonsteroidal anti-inflammatory drugs.

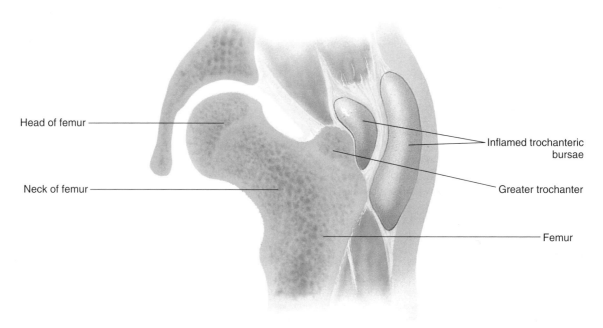

Head of femur

Neck of femur

Inflamed trochanteric bursae

Greater trochanter

Femur

Figure 23-9 Bursitis of the hip. (Asset provided by Anatomical Chart Co.).

■ Corticosteroid injections may provide temporary symptomatic relief.

■ Use of local anesthetics can also provide diagnostic confirmation.

■ Rarely, surgical release of the involved tendon may be necessary in chronic, recalcitrant cases.

Snapping Hip Syndrome

Snapping hip syndrome is a collection of extra-articular and intra-articular pathologies that can be painful and disabling to the athlete. Extra-articular snapping of the hip joint can be caused by (1) the iliopsoas tendon as it passes over the iliopectineal eminence or the lesser trochanter of the femur, (2) the iliofemoral ligaments over the femoral head, (3) the long head of the biceps femoris over the ischial tuberosity, or (4) the iliotibial band over the greater trochanter of the femur. The intra-articular causes include tears of the anterior labrum, synovitis, and loose bodies that can also create a snapping or clicking sensation in the hip. It can be difficult to distinguish the extra-articular lesions from the more disconcerting intra-articular lesions but CT and MRI can assist with the diagnosis. Hip arthroscopy can be both diagnostic and therapeutic for intra-articular lesions.

The most common cause of snapping hip syndrome is irritation of the greater trochanter by the iliotibial band. The iliotibial band is a large, flat tendinous structure that originates on the anterior-superior portion of the iliac crest, crosses over the greater trochanter of the femur, and inserts onto the lateral condyle of the tibia. Iliotibial band syndrome is seen in athletes who undergo repetitive knee flexion such as runners and cyclists.

■ Athletes will have pain over the greater trochanter of the femur, the lateral thigh, or radiating pain down to the knee.

■ Patients often report hip instability symptoms.

■ If severe enough, the snapping sensation will occur during normal ambulation. Once this area becomes inflamed, running or rising from a seated position may hurt continuously.

■ The mainstay of treatment is conservative, with bursal excision with iliotibial band partial release/lengthening reserved for refractory cases.

Nerve Entrapment Syndromes

Nerve entrapment syndromes are rare findings in athletes but need to be considered in patients with pain that does not have an identifiable cause or with diagnosed injuries that do not follow the expected time course for healing.

■ Obturator nerve entrapment can occur when the nerve is tethered by a fascial band as it exits the obturator foramen.

　■ Athletes complaining of burning pain in the medial thigh and can have weakness of the adductor muscles, as well as paresthesias in the medial thigh.

　■ Local anesthetic infiltration around the nerve can be diagnostic.

　■ Conservative treatment is indicated if no electromyographic changes are present.

　■ If evidence of denervation exists, surgical release can be successful.

■ The lateral femoral cutaneous nerve is a purely sensory nerve that supplies the anterolateral thigh. Entrapment of this nerve is called "meralgia paresthetica."

　■ Direct trauma to the region of the anterior superior iliac spine can be the cause of nerve injury, but most cases do not have an identifiable cause.

　■ Local anesthetic injection can be diagnostic.

　■ Conservative treatment is usually successful.

- Surgical exploration and release is reserved for refractory cases.
- Ilioinguinal nerve entrapment can also be seen in athletes, who typically present with inguinal pain that radiates to the scrotum or labia.
  - This entrapment can often be caused by hypertrophy of the abdominal musculature and usually responds to changes in training regimen.
  - Surgical release is reserved for cases that do not respond to conservative management.
- Piriformis syndrome is the compression of the sciatic nerve by the piriformis muscle. The compression of the nerve occurs as it exits deep to the piriformis muscle (Fig. 23-10).
  - Patients will complain of pain and symptoms in the sciatic nerve distribution.
  - A history of acute trauma to the buttock is often present.
  - Patients will have difficulty sitting or participating in activities that cause hip flexion and internal rotation (ice skating).
  - On physical examination, tenderness can be present over the piriformis tendon in the gluteal area.
  - Pain is elicited by forced internal rotation on an extended thigh, or pain and weakness on resisted abduction and external rotation of the thigh (Pace's sign).
  - Rectal or vaginal examination may produce pain in the piriformis area.
  - MRI can be helpful to demonstrate sciatic nerve inflammation in the area of the piriformis tendon.
  - Nonoperative modalities are often successful in achieving some symptomatic relief.
  - Sciatic neurolysis with piriformis tendon release can be necessary in refractory cases.

Hamstring Syndrome

- Hamstring syndrome, described in track athletes, involves severe pain in and around the ischial tuberosity that radiates down the posterior aspect of the thigh to the popliteal area.
- Any activity that puts the hamstring on stretch can create this radiating pain. Sprinting, hurdling, and even sitting for long periods will cause pain.
- Physical examination elicits exquisite tenderness at the ischial tuberosity and, at times, reproduction of sciatic pain with percussion of the nerve at the ischial tuberosity.
- Resisted leg extension will reproduce the pain.
- The sciatic nerve is thought to be entrapped between the semitendinosus and the biceps femoris by a fibrous band that constricts the two muscles.

Athletic Pubalgia

The term "athletic pubalgia" refers to a chronic inguinal or pubic area pain in athletes, which is noted with exertion. The pattern of symptoms in these patients, operative findings, and results of studies all suggest that the lower abdominal or inguinal pain is not due to occult hernia. Only a

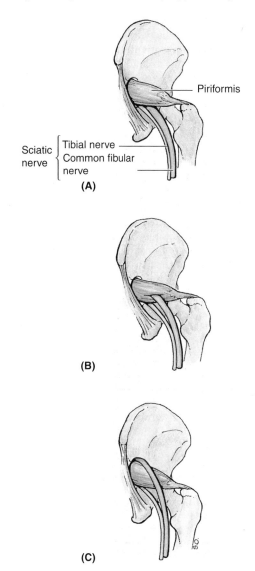

Figure 23-10   Relationship of sciatic nerve to the piriformis. **A:** Usually, as the sciatic nerve emerges from the greater sciatic foramen, it passes inferior to the piriformis. **B:** In 12.2% of 640 limbs studied, the sciatic nerve divided before it entered the gluteal region, and the common fibular division (yellow) passed through the piriformis. **C:** In 0.5% of cases, the common fibular division passed superior to the muscle, where it is especially vulnerable to injury during intragluteal injections. (From Moore KL, Dalley AF IID. Clinical Oriented Anatomy, 4th ed. Baltimore, Lippincott Williams & Wilkins, 1999.)

small percentage of patients are found to have occult hernia at the time of surgery. When this does occur, the occult hernia is usually found on the side opposite the principal symptoms.

The rectus tendon insertion on the pubis seems to be the primary site of pathology. Most patients describe a hyperextension injury in association with hyperabduction of the thigh. The location of pain suggests that the injury involves both the rectus abdominis and adductor longus muscles. Other tendinous insertion sites on the pubic bone may also be involved.

Diagnosis

- The athletes have lower abdominal pain with exertion.
  - A minority of patients have pure adductor related pain that is disabling.
  - Most of the patients remember a distinct injury during exertions.
  - Usually, the abdominal pain involves the inguinal canal near the insertion of the rectus abdominis muscle on the pubis.
  - The pain often causes a majority of patients to stop competing in sports.
- MRI findings in athletic pubalgia are often nonspecific. Conversely, 12% of patients have an MRI finding that clearly indicates a problem at the rectus insertion site.
  - The relatively small incidence of a specific diagnosis by imaging studies suggests that the problem may be an attenuation of the muscle or tendon due to repeated microtrauma.
  - The finding on MRI of adductor longus inflammation is consistent with athletic pubalgia.

Treatment

- Generally, the acute management of groin pain suspected to be athletic pubalgia is conservative, including rest, ice, compression, anti-inflammatory medications, and massage.
- When the process continues over several months and the athlete cannot return to previously expected activity because of pain, operative intervention should be considered.
- Surgical treatment of athletic pubalgia requires a broad surgical reattachment at the inferolateral edge of the rectus muscle with its fascial investments to the pubis and adjacent anterior ligaments.
  - Also performed is an anterior and lateral release of the epimysium of the adductor fascia to expand this compartment. The epimysium is the layer of connective tissue that encloses the entire muscle.
  - This kind of fascial release is often successful in relieving the adductor symptoms in athletic pubalgia.

SUGGESTED READING

Bradshaw C, McCrory P, Brukner P. Obturator nerve entrapment: a cause of groin pain in athletes. Am J Sports Med 1997;25:402–408.

Busconi B, McCarthy J. Hip and pelvic injuries in the skeletally immature athlete. Sports Med Arthrosc Rev 1996;4:132–158.

Byrd JW. Lateral impact injury: a source of occult hip pathology. Clin Sports Med 2001;20:801–815.

Byrd JW, Jones KS. Traumatic rupture of the ligamentum teres as a source of hip pain. Arthroscopy 2004;20:385–391.

Kelly BT, Williams RJ, Philippon MJ. Hip arthroscopy: current indications, treatment options, and management issues. Am J Sports Med 2003;31:1020–1037.

Klingele KE, Sallay PI. Surgical repair of complete proximal hamstring tendon rupture. Am J Sports Med 2002;30:742–747.

McCarthy JC, Day B, Busconi B. Hip arthroscopy: applications and technique. J Am Acad Orthop Surg 1995;3:115–122.

Metzmaker JN, Pappas AM. Avulsion fractures of the pelvis. Am J Sports Med 1985;13:349–358.

Meyers WC, Ricciardi R, Busconi BD, et al. Athletic pubalgia and groin pain. In: Garrett WE, Speer KP, Kirkendall DT, eds. Principles and Practice of Orthopaedic Sports Medicine. Philadelphia: Lippincott Williams & Wilkins, 2000:223–230.

Newberg AH, Newman JS. Imaging of a painful hip. In: McCarthy JC, ed. Early Hip Disease: Advances in Detection and Minimally Invasive Treatment. New York: Springer-Verlag, 2003: 17–43.

Owens BD, Busconi BD. Trauma. In: McCarthy JC, ed. Early Hip Disease: Advances in Detection and Minimally Invasive Treatment. New York: Springer-Verlag, 2003.

Ryan JB, Wheeler JH, Hopkinson WJ, et al. Quadriceps contusions: West Point update. Am J Sports Med 1991;19:299–304.

Sampson TG. Hip morphology and its relationship to pathology: dysplasia to impingement. Op Tech Sports Med 2005;13;37–45.

Shin AY, Gillingham BL. Fatigue fracture of the femoral neck in athletes. J Am Acad Orthop Surg 1997;5:293–302.

ANTERIOR CRUCIATE LIGAMENT INJURIES

VINCENT W. CHEN
ROBERT E. HUNTER
JOHN WOOLF

Anterior cruciate ligament (ACL) injuries and their treatment constitute perhaps the largest segment of orthopaedic sports medicine. Over the past 20 to 30 years, recognition of the devastating effects ACL injury can have on athletes has prompted an enormous amount of research and development into the best methods of treating this entity.

ANATOMY

The ACL first begins to form from mesenchyme in the sixth week of gestation. It initially forms in a ventral location and eventually migrates posteriorly to its final location, remaining extrasynovial throughout development.

The femoral attachment arises from the inner surface of the lateral femoral condyle, with a semicircular footprint (Fig. 24-1). On a notch view of the knee joint, the ACL attachment is completely lateral to a line drawn down from the middle of the intercondylar notch and occupies the superior 66% of the notch. The tibial attachment is located anterior and lateral to the medial intercondylar tubercle, with fibers that fan out onto an attachment site that mea-

sures approximately 11 mm in width and 17 mm in anteroposterior (A/P) length (Fig. 24-2).

The average length of the ACL measures 32 to 33 mm, with a range from 22 to 41 mm. There are two main "bundles" or "segments": the anteromedial and the posterolateral, named for the position in which each bundle inserts onto the tibia.

Pertinent anatomic facts include the following:

- Vascular supply—middle genicular artery.
- Nerve supply—primarily the posterior articular nerve.
- Mechanoreceptors—Ruffini end-organ receptors (stretch) and free nerve endings (mostly subsynovial near the ACL insertion).

BIOMECHANICS

The knee cannot be described as a simple hinge joint. The unique arrangement of ligaments allows for 6 degrees of freedom, with the ability to translate into three planes: medial to lateral, proximal to distal, and anterior to posterior,

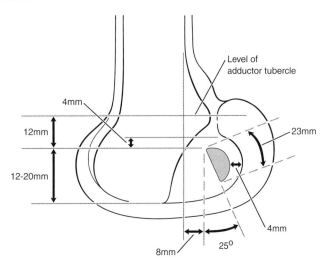

Figure 24-1 Medial aspect of the lateral femoral condyle showing the semicircular shape of the femoral attachment of the ACL. (After Girgis FG, Marshall JL, Monajem A. The cruciate ligaments of the knee joint. Anatomical, functional, and experimental analysis. Clin Orthop 1975;106:216–231.)

as well as rotate in three planes: flexion-extension, internal-external, and abduction-adduction (Fig. 24-3). The biomechanical properties of the ACL are difficult to discuss in isolation and are best considered in conjunction with the posterior cruciate ligament (PCL). The "crossed four-bar linkage" model most easily breaks down the complexity of the ACL/PCL interaction in the sagittal plane by reducing the degrees of freedom to one plane, as well as by utilizing two dimensions as opposed to three. The ligaments form a linked system in which the changing center of knee rotation and the combination of roll and glide of the femur on the tibia are predicted by this linkage of the PCL and ACL (Fig. 24-4).

As with other ligaments, the ACL is viscoelastic; therefore, it exhibits stress-strain behavior that is time rate-dependent, such that the amount of deformation depends

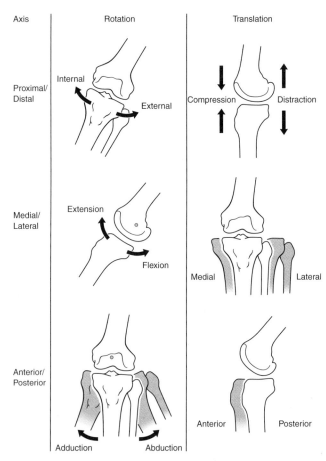

Figure 24-3 Translation and rotation around each of the three axes provide the six degrees of freedom needed for knee motion. (After Larson RL, Taillon M. Anterior cruciate ligament insufficiency: principles of treatment. J Am Acad Orthop Surg 1994; 2:26–35.)

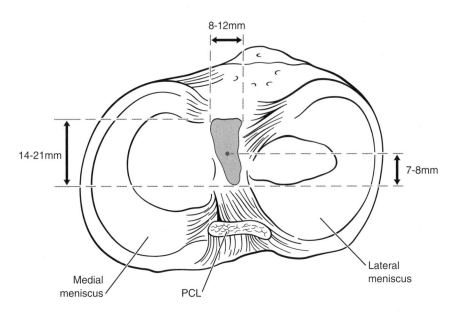

Figure 24-2 Tibial attachment for the anterior cruciate ligament. (After Girgis FG, Marshall JL, Monajem A. The cruciate ligaments of the knee joint. Anatomical, functional, and experimental analysis. Clin Orthop 1975;106:216–231.)

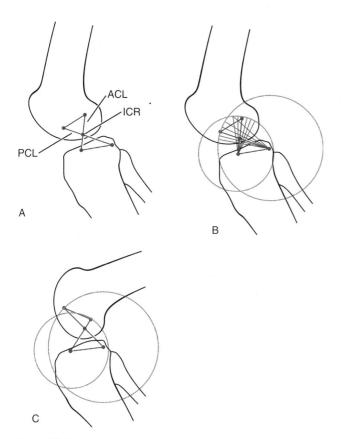

Figure 24-4 Crossed four-bar linkage schematic, demonstrating the changing center of knee rotation during knee range of motion. **A:** Full extension of the knee. **B:** Note posterior migration of the tibiofemoral contact point with knee flexion. **C:** Model of the knee joint in flexion. ACL, anterior cruciate ligament; ICR, instant center of joint rotation; PCL, posterior cruciate ligament.

on the load and the rate of application. The faster a load is applied, the more elastic the ligament behaves.

The ACL serves as the primary restraint to anterior translation of the tibia on the femur. Studies have shown that this effect is best isolated at 15 to 30 degrees of flexion. The ACL also serves as a secondary restraint to internal rotation, especially near full extension. Finally, it may be a minor secondary restraint to external rotation and varus-valgus angulation under weight bearing conditions.

PATHOGENESIS

Etiology

ACL injury occurs most commonly via a noncontact mechanism, with no direct blow to the knee. Multiple studies estimate the percentage of noncontact ACL injuries to be in the range of 70% to 78% of total ACL injuries. Football, basketball, and soccer are the most common sports in which participants suffer an ACL injury.

The classic mechanism has been described as a valgus external rotation twisting injury during deceleration that usually occurs when the athlete lands on the leg and quickly pivots in the opposite direction. However, several other mechanisms may also cause ACL injury, including varus internal rotation, hyperextension, or a pure deceleration. From this data, it is clear there is no one way to damage an ACL and that the mechanism of injury is more sports-dependent than twisting, cutting, or any one specific loading event.

Epidemiology

- There are approximately 150,000 new ACL injuries per year in the United States.
- Between 64,000 and 100,000 ACL reconstructions are performed yearly in the United States, with numbers increasing each year.
- Overall incidence is approximately 1 in 3,000 persons (all ages).
- For ages 15 to 45, the incidence is approximately 1 per 1,750 persons.

Although no specific numbers have been reported concerning the percentage of female versus male ACL injuries per year, there has been a definite increase in the number of females suffering ACL injury. The recent increase of sports participation for females cannot fully explain the increasing numbers. As will be discussed later in this chapter, numerous hypotheses have arisen to attempt to explain why females participating in jumping and pivoting sports have from 4 to 8 times more likely chance of sustaining an ACL injury than their male counterparts.

Pathophysiology

Risk factors can be classified into four categories: environmental, anatomical, hormonal, and biomechanical.

Environmental Risk Factors

Knee bracing first arose in the 1970s, and early reports showed a decrease in the number of ACL injuries in college and high school athletes. However, subsequent studies showed that braces were ineffective and may even increase the incidence of ACL injury. Despite these findings, many athletes continue to use prophylactic knee bracing, for supposed psychological and proprioceptive benefits.

Researchers have investigated the playing surface, as well as type of shoe wear as primary contributors to injury. A study of National Football League ACL injuries found that most noncontact injuries occur on dry playing surfaces, and a Norwegian study noted that a high friction level between shoes and surface was a major risk factor for ACL injury in team handball. A study of football cleat design found that cleats with a predominance of grip on the periphery of the shoe generate the highest friction on turf and seem to result in a higher incidence of ACL tears. Issues of performance versus safety must be balanced because higher friction between surface and shoe generally improves performance but carries higher risk of injury.

Anatomic Risk Factors

Females have an up to eight times greater chance of suffering an ACL tear than males competing in the same sport.

They tend to have increased femoral anteversion, Q-angle, tibial torsion, and foot pronation (see Fig. 4-1 in Chapter 4).

In general, it has been postulated that ligamentous laxity (in either gender) may increase the predisposition to ACL injury. However, studies have found conflicting results. One article found a mild increase in both anterior and posterior knee laxity after playing basketball and jogging for greater than 30 minutes, which returns to normal after 60 minutes. Perhaps this exercise-associated laxity may increase susceptibility to injury.

Femoral notch size has been extensively studied and, as of yet, no conclusive statement can be made that notch size increases the chance of an ACL tear, since studies have found conflicting results.

One study found that there was a significant difference in the cross-sectional area of the ACL between men and women, in which a larger area was found for males. Their results, however, could not correlate this with notch width, nor specifically with ACL injury.

Hormonal Risk Factors

Numerous recent studies have attempted to define the role of estrogen and progesterone in the etiology of female ACL injury. Estrogen has been found to reduce tensile properties in the rabbit ACL and estrogen, as well as progesterone target cells, has been detected in the human ACL. The direct effect of these hormones has yet to be established.

Studies that have investigated the timing of ACL injuries during the menstrual cycle have reported conflicting results due to differences in patient population with regard to usage of oral contraceptives (which in themselves have been linked to lower general sports injury rates in women). A study of 128 female athletes found that high-risk intervals were associated with the follicular phase of the menstrual cycle, regardless of oral contraceptive use. Other studies, however, did not find any hormonal impact.

Biomechanical Risk Factors

Neuromuscular control refers to the unconscious activation of the dynamic restraints surrounding a joint in response to sensory stimuli. Researchers have tried to determine if there is any association between differing neuromuscular patterns between men and women to explain the increased incidence of ACL injury in females. A dynamic electromyographic study compared knee motion patterns between male and female recreational athletes in running, cutting, and jumping tasks. It was found that women tended to have a decreased knee flexion angle and increased knee valgus angle compared with men in all tasks. It also showed that women had increased quadriceps muscle activation and decreased hamstring muscle activation in every task. Interestingly, these knee positional differences were apparent before landing, suggesting that neuromuscular control may be occurring via different mechanisms for men versus women.

Another study examined knee flexion-extension moment, varus-valgus moment, and proximal tibial anterior shear force during stop-jump tasks. Women had a significantly higher anterior tibial shear force, greater knee extension moment, greater knee valgus moment, and smaller knee flexion angle. This also supports the hypothesis that differing patterns in knee motion may be associated with differences in lower extremity neuromuscular control.

Histopathology

The normal healing response of an injured ligament is to form a local hematoma. In extra-articular ligaments, the hematoma is organized into a fibrinogen mesh, in which invading cells such as macrophages, monocytes, and other inflammatory cells can settle. These inflammatory cells secrete cytokines and growth factors that can mediate inflammation and attract fibroblasts and stem cells to the injured ligament, eventually leading to scar or fibrous tissue formation. However, the ACL differs in that it is intra-articular and has only a thin synovial lining that is almost always torn along with the ACL. Therefore, a local hematoma cannot form, thus impairing the healing response.

Besides loss of synovial integrity, cytokine proportions change in the knee joint, with marked increases in the proinflammatory cytokines interleukin-1 and tumor necrosis factor-α. This aggressive environment may also inhibit healing response.

CLASSIFICATION

The objective description of ACL laxity requires assessment of the degree of displacement, as well as the character of the end point. Laxity can be judged by clinical "feel," measured using specific instruments designed to measure amount of bony translation between the femur and tibia. As with other ligaments, ACL laxity can be classified by the number of millimeters of anterior translation (Table 24-1).

Use of instrumented laxity measurement has both its proponents and opponents, yet the KT-1000 and its newer versions do provide a quantitative measurement of knee laxity for use in clinical studies. A side-to-side measurement difference of more than 3 mm is indicative of a complete ACL tear.

Partial tears may be difficult to distinguish from a complete tear on clinical examination. In a partial tear, plastic deformation of the ligament has occurred without reaching the ultimate failure point. This can result in increased A/P translation but with a firmer endpoint. Partial tears are very rare.

TABLE 24-1 ACL LAXITY CLASSIFICATION

Grade[a]	Amount of Excess Motion
I	Up to 5 mm of motion
II	6 to 10 mm of motion
III	11 to 15 mm of motion
IV	More than 15 mm of motion

ACL, anterior cruciate ligament.
[a] Subclassification: A, firm end point; B, soft end point.

DIAGNOSIS

History

- ACL injury is most commonly due to a twisting type of mechanism.
- Injury usually occurs during deceleration, cutting, or jumping.
- The patient may hear a pop.
- Skiers often have "giving way" with distraction and rotation.
- Patients often cannot ambulate immediately after the injury due to pain.
- Immediate effusion (within a few hours) is common.

Physical Examination

- Physical examination should include assessment of the following:
  - Effusion
  - Joint line tenderness
  - Range of motion
  - Gait (if possible)
- Ligamentous and ACL-specific testing is required, and arthrometry is optional.
- Examination under anesthesia may be required (although clinical examination should exceed 90% accuracy).
- The Lachman examination is the most sensitive test to detect acute ACL injury.
- Table 24-2 summarizes the primary diagnostic knee tests.

Radiologic Examination

- Plain radiographs
  - Standing AP, lateral, and merchant (patellofemoral) views are recommended.
  - The Segond sign, a small avulsion fracture of the posterolateral tibial plateau, is pathognomonic for ACL rupture.
  - Radiographs may show a tibial spine avulsion.
- Magnetic resonance imaging
  - MRI has high sensitivity and specificity for ACL tears.
  - Its overall accuracy is around 95%.
  - It is not cost efficient in the initial evaluation and is not mandatory for proceeding with surgical reconstruction.
  - MRI can be useful to document associated pathology (damage to other soft-tissue structures, bone bruises).
  - Characteristics that may be noted on MRI include a noncontinuous ACL ligament, best seen on sagittal views (Fig. 24-5), an irregular wavy anterior margin, increased signal in the ligament on T_2-weighted images, and the presence of a sharply buckled PCL, indicative of an anteriorly positioned tibia and therefore an ACL tear.

TREATMENT

Surgical Indications

- A patient with an acute ACL tear in the cruciate dominant knee (genu varum and hyperlaxity) requires ACL

TABLE 24-2 DIAGNOSTIC KNEE TESTS

Test	Anatomic Structure	Technique
ACL tests		
Lachman	ACL	Flex knee to 20–30 degrees, pull tibia forward on the femur
Anterior drawer	ACL	Flex knee to 90 degrees, pull tibia forward on femur
Pivot shift	ACL	Place valgus stress while internally rotating tibia, then flex and extend knee
Associated knee tests		
Posterior drawer	PCL	Push tibia posteriorly on femur at 90 degrees knee flexion
Reverse pivot shift	PCL	Opposite of pivot shift
McMurray	Meniscus	Twist knee from flexion to extension, feel for joint line click
Dial	Posterolateral corner	Externally rotate foot with knee flexed 30 degrees
Varus stress	LCL	Apply at 30 degrees of knee flexion
Valgus stress	MCL	Apply at 30 degrees of knee flexion

ACL, anterior cruciate ligament; LCL, lateral cruciate ligament; MCL, medial cruciate ligament; PCL, posterior cruciate ligament.

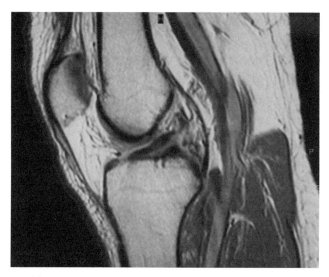

Figure 24-5   Sagittal MRI demonstrating detachment of the femoral origin of the ACL ligament.

reconstruction due to anatomic alignment that predisposes the knee to further injury.

- With severe varus deformity, consideration should be made for concurrent high tibial osteotomy.
- Patients who are unwilling to give up high-demand sports activities (Table 24-3):
  - Level III activities can usually be performed without difficulty with ACL deficiency.
  - Level II activities can also often be performed, as long extreme laxity does not exist and the patient possesses good coordination. A brace is often quite beneficial.
  - Level I activities are difficult to perform with an ACL-deficient knee.
- Patients with significant associated pathology, such as meniscal lesions or other ligamentous injuries, and patients experiencing instability (giving way of the knee) with daily activities.

TABLE 24-3 ACTIVITY LEVEL CLASSIFICATION

Level	Description
I	Jumping, pivoting, or hard cutting (e.g., football, soccer)
II	Heavy manual work or side-to-side sports (e.g., skiing, tennis)
III	Light manual work or noncutting sports (e.g., jogging, running)
IV	Sedentary activity without sports

(From Christel P, Dijan P, Darman Z, et al. [Results of Marshall-MacIntosh reconstruction according to 3 scoring systems (ARPEGE, Lysholm, IKDC). 90 cases reviewed with at least a one-year follow-up]. Rev Chir Orthop Reparatrice Appear Mot 1993;79:473–483.)

Contraindications

Partial tears involving less than 50% of the ACL with a negative pivot shift do not need reconstruction. Another group of patients who may not require surgery includes those over the age of 30 who are not involved in high-demand activities or who are willing to modify activities, do not have recurrent instability, and have an arthrometric side-to-side difference of less than 5 mm.

Age alone is not a contraindication to surgery, but should be factored in with activity level. Most surgeons would consider ACL reconstruction in a patient approaching middle age if they are extremely fit and active, with no evidence of arthritic change. For those older, less active patients, a well-supervised rehabilitation program and activity modification provide excellent results.

Nonsurgical Treatment

- The primary options if surgery is to be delayed or not performed at all consist of rehabilitation programs, activity modification, and bracing.
  - Some patients will have minimal functional problems with no treatment at all.
- Physical therapy to strengthen the surrounding muscles (especially the hamstrings) can significantly benefit patients, especially those who are older and more sedentary.
  - Other goals of physical therapy are to regain range of motion and help proprioceptive function.
- Activity modification is perhaps the main option for nonoperative treatment because ACL-deficient knees are most susceptible to an acute subluxation episode with twisting and cutting type activities. A typical scenario may be the weekend warrior who does not have much time for sports, who decides to give up basketball after suffering an ACL rupture, and who instead takes up biking or hiking.
- Bracing has been studied extensively in the literature, yet there is no clear answer whether bracing can either prevent ACL injuries or reduce instability episodes and further knee damage in the ACL-deficient knee.
  - The proposed mechanisms of protection are mechanical constraint of joint motion and improvement of joint proprioception.
  - Despite the fact that brace use does not have concrete support in the literature, the majority of surgeons do use braces in certain cases.
  - The older patient may do very well with bracing, and bracing is the primary option for an in-season athlete who is attempting to delay surgery until after the season.
  - Bracing can be used for the skeletally immature athlete until growth plates approach closure to avoid performing growth plate violating procedures.
  - Some patients feel more secure wearing the brace and feel they have a subjectively better idea of the position of their leg due to the brace.

Surgical Goals

Once the decision has been made to proceed with surgery, certain goals become important. The purpose of surgery is to provide a stable knee, which will enhance performance and at the same time protect the knee from further damage to other structures—in particular, the menisci and the articular cartilage. This cascade of injuries may ultimately lead to arthritis, although long-term outcome studies addressing arthritic changes are lacking. One researcher did find that 11.6% of 225 ACL reconstructions followed 6 to 11 years showed radiographic evidence of progressive arthritic changes. Related to the concept of regaining stability is the goal of returning athletes to an appropriate level of function. Primary ACL reconstruction has been reported to have success rates from 75% to 93%, defined as relief of symptoms of giving way, restoration of functional stability, and return to normal or near-normal activities.

Surgical Principles

Certain principles should guide the surgeon who will perform ACL reconstruction:

- Correct all components of instability.
  - This necessitates a meticulous physical examination, along with detailed arthroscopy.
  - Failing to diagnose and treat posterolateral corner instability, a meniscal tear, or severe genu varum will ultimately cause the surgical reconstruction of the ACL to be unsuccessful.
- Provide secure fixation to allow for early motion.
  - One of the more severe complications of ACL surgery is postoperative stiffness, which is largely preventable.
  - The development of newer methods of secure fixation, especially for soft-tissue grafts, makes aggressive postoperative rehabilitation less dangerous to the graft and ultimate knee stability.
- Place grafts appropriately to provide full range of motion without subjecting the graft to excess stress.

Surgical Techniques

ACL surgery was initially performed as an open procedure. With the advent of arthroscopy, ACL reconstruction progressed to a two-incision endoscopic procedure and finally has evolved into a one-incision endoscopic technique.

BOX 24-1 GRAFT SOURCES

Autograft
- Bone–patellar tendon–bone
- Hamstring tendons (semitendinosus/gracilis)
- Quadriceps tendon
- Iliotibial band

Allograft
- Bone–patellar tendon–bone
- Hamstring tendons
- Tibialis anterior tendon
- Achilles tendon

Graft Sources and Selection Principles

Box 24-1 lists the most common grafts in use today.

Bone–patellar Tendon–bone. The bone–patellar tendon–bone (BTB) graft has been considered the gold standard for primary ACL reconstruction. BTB has initial strength that is comparable with or greater than the native ACL, with four times greater stiffness (Table 24-4). An important advantage is that BTB allows for bone-to-bone healing in both the femoral and tibial tunnels, which is quicker and perhaps more reliable than soft-tissue healing to bone. Bone-to-bone healing was shown to occur (in a dog model) by 6 to 8 weeks.

Ipsilateral central one-third BTB has been the most popular choice, though several surgeons have promoted contralateral BTB harvesting to theoretically accelerate recovery time, by sharing the surgical trauma with the otherwise healthy opposite knee. Medial one-third BTB grafts have been used, although fears of subsequent lateral patellar maltracking have deterred most surgeons. Lateral one-third BTB is another option rarely used, with little reported data in the literature. The primary concerns associated with using BTB are listed in Box 24-2.

Hamstring Tendon. With the recent improvement in fixation devices, reconstruction with hamstring tendon has become increasingly popular. Originally, single-looped semitendinosus or gracilis tendons were used, but failures led

TABLE 24-4 BIOMECHANICAL GRAFT PROPERTIES

Graft	Ultimate Strength (N)	Stiffness (N/mm)	Cross-sectional area (mm²)
Intact ACL	2160	242	44
BTB	2376	812	35
Quadruple hamstring	4108	776	53
Quad tendon	2352	463	62
Anterior tibialis	3412	344	38
Posterior tibialis	3391	302	48

ACL, anterior cruciate ligament; BTB, bone–patellar tendon–bone; N, Newtons.
(Adapted from Miller SL, Gladstone JN. Graft selection in anterior cruciate ligament reconstruction. Orthop Clin North Am 2002;33:675–683.)

BOX 24-2 DRAWBACKS OF BONE–PATELLAR TENDON–BONE GRAFTS

- Patellofemoral/anterior knee pain (5% to 55%)
- Postoperative quadriceps weakness
- Division of the infrapatellar branch of the saphenous nerve, leading to at least transient numbness
- Possible patellar fracture, patellar tendon rupture, and patellar tendonitis
- Discomfort with kneeling

to the current common use of a quadruple-looped semitendinosus/gracilis graft. This quadruple construct possesses stiffness three times greater than the native ACL and ultimate strength twice that of BTB. The ultimate tensile load is almost three times that of the native ACL. The cross-sectional area for hamstrings is greater than BTB and closer to the size of a normal ACL.

One study addressed the issue of harvest site morbidity, as well as quantified hamstring weakness after hamstring reconstruction. They found that donor site morbidity was low, and hamstring strength was abnormal only for 1 month when harvested from the ACL reconstructed knee. They concluded that hamstring grafts are a viable option to reduce donor site morbidity. The primary disadvantages of hamstring grafts are given in Box 24-3.

Quadriceps Tendon. The incision for a quadriceps tendon harvest avoids the infrapatellar branch of the saphenous nerve. In addition, bone can be harvested from the patella to enable bone-to-bone healing on one end of the graft. However, biomechanical studies have shown the quadriceps tendon to be significantly less stiff than the BTB, as well as to possess a much lower ultimate tensile stress value. This graft is used in very few centers currently.

Iliotibial Band. The iliotibial band graft has primarily been used in extra-articular procedures, which alone have been found to be inadequate for an ACL-deficient knee. Techniques have also been described using the iliotibial band as an augment to another graft in an intra-articular procedure.

Allograft Tissues. Common allografts used include hamstring, BTB, tibialis anterior, and Achilles tendon. They play a paramount role in revision surgery, as well as in the multiply injured ligament; now, many surgeons use allografts for primary ACL reconstruction. A January 2001 report issued by the Office of the Inspector General of the U.S. Department of Health and Human Services estimated that tissue banks distributed more than 750,000 allografts for transplantation in all medical fields in 1999 alone. The greatest advantage lies in the elimination of harvest site morbidity. Subsequently, muscle strength is not hindered during the postoperative period. Surgical time is decreased, as is the ability to use a smaller incision. Finally, graft size can be chosen, as well as the option for bone plugs, thus making allografts very attractive for revision surgery.

The disadvantages of allografts are listed in Box 24-4.

Fixation Issues

Successful ACL reconstruction relies on graft healing in the tunnels, which requires fixation that can withstand the forces generated during rehabilitation. Fixation can be categorized as direct and indirect. Direct fixation involves devices that fix the tendon–bone within the bone tunnels. Examples include interference screws and cross-pins. Indirect fixation devices secure the graft at a distance from the graft end. Examples of this include the Endobutton (Smith and Nephew, Memphis, TN) and suture posts. One theoretical advantage of direct fixation is decreased longitudinal graft-tunnel motion ("bungee effect"), as well as decreased sagittal graft-tunnel motion ("windshield wiper effect").

Bone-to-bone Fixation. Metal interference screws have a long track record of success in ACL reconstruction. A classic study found that interference screw fixation was stronger and had greater load to failure for BTB than either staples or sutures tied over a button. Recently, bioabsorbable screws have gained popularity, with similar strength profiles as metal screws, though cyst formation has been reported with their use. Potential problems with interference screws include the possibility of divergence, wherein the screw path deviates from the bone plug (greater than 30 degrees of tunnel divergence places the graft at greater risk of failure), and abrasion of the soft-tissue portion of the graft with either improper interference screw placement

BOX 24-3 DRAWBACKS OF HAMSTRING GRAFTS

- Soft-tissue healing to bone—studies suggest longer time to heal than bone–patellar tendon–bone (12 vs. 8 weeks)
- Residual hamstring weakness, because hamstrings are the primary muscular antagonist to anterior tibial translation
- Risk of amputation of the graft during harvest or inadequate tissue
- Inferior fixation techniques (this has improved in recent years)

BOX 24-4 DRAWBACKS OF ALLOGRAFTS

- Possibility of disease transmission
  - There have been more than 26 reports of bacterial infections associated with a musculoskeletal tissue allograft
  - The estimated risk of human immunodeficiency virus transmission with graft implantation is 1:1,000,000
  - Hepatitis C transmission has occurred in two recipients, even after development of advanced immunoassays and improved screening
- Slower graft healing or incorporation
- Cost

or a screw that is too long. In general, interference screw fixation has supplanted staples and the suture post for bone–tendon–bone fixation.

Tendon-to-bone Fixation. Earlier procedures utilized extra-articular types of fixation, such as screws with washers, staples, and sutures over a post. Initially, the screw and washer construct was found to be the strongest. The Endobutton was then developed to eliminate the need for the second lateral incision. It also provided cortical instead of cancellous bone fixation, along with avoiding graft abrasion. There is also no risk of graft abrasion. The disadvantage of these techniques is that aperture fixation is not achieved, so the graft may be susceptible to the "bungee effect."

Cross-pin fixation systems, such as the TransFix (Arthrex Corp., Naples, FL) and RigidFix (Mitek/Johnson & Johnson, Piscataway, NJ), have been recently developed. In the TransFix technique, a soft-tissue graft is looped around a pin that has been inserted through cancellous bone from the lateral femoral condyle. The RigidFix uses bioabsorbable pins that pierce the graft from across the condyle. Some of the possible complications unique to these types of devices include the risk of avascular necrosis, as well as fracture of the lateral femoral condyle.

Specific Surgical Procedures

ACL Surgical Technique
- Perform an examination under anesthesia before prepping the leg, and document this finding in the operative note.
- Place a tourniquet as high as possible on the leg, and then place the leg in a leg holder.
- Be sure to pad the nonoperative leg and abduct the leg enough to enable access to the posteromedial joint line, in case meniscal repair is needed.
- Diagnostic arthroscopy is performed first, evaluating all knee compartments, paying particular attention to meniscal pathology.
- At this point, perform meniscal repair, partial meniscectomy, and/or chondroplasty as needed.
- Next, graft harvest should be performed, with exsanguination of the limb using an Esmarck bandage.

Bone–patellar–bone Harvest
- Make a longitudinal incision starting at the distal end of the patella and extend distally to the tibial tubercle.
- Expose the patella and patellar tendon, being careful not to violate the peritenon, patellar tendon, or the underlying fat pad.
- The incision can be translated proximally and distally as needed once the subcutaneous tissues have been released.
- Measure the width of the patellar tendon, which will decide the width of central third tendon to harvest.
  - Do not take more than one third of the tendon (e.g., 10 mm if the total tendon width is 30 mm).
- Use a scalpel or double-bladed scalpel to incise the central third of the tendon, being careful to maintain longitudinal alignment with the tendon fibers.

- Outline the patellar and tibial bone plugs using a marking pen.
  - Standard dimensions are approximately 9 to 10 mm width, 20 mm length, and 8 mm depth.
- Use a small saw and outline the plugs, angling the cuts to create a triangular patellar plug and a trapezoidal tibial tubercle plug.
- Gently release the patellar bone plug from the proximal end using osteotomes.
- Carefully release the fat pad from the distal patellar pole to avoid a leak of fluid from the joint.
- Release the tibial tubercle bone plug in a similar fashion.
- The patellar tendon defect can be filled with cancellous bone trimmed from the plugs.
- Repair the patellar tendon and peritenon.
- Place a moist lap in the incision.
- On the back table, use a rongeur to round off the bone plugs, and use sizers to estimate bone tunnel size.
- Measure the length of the whole graft.
- Drill two holes each in the tibial and patellar bone plugs, placing heavy, strong, nonabsorbable sutures through these holes to be used for graft passage.
- Set the graft aside wrapped in a moist sponge until ready for passage.

Hamstring Harvest
- Make a longitudinal incision approximately 3 cm long directly over the insertion of the pes anserinus, starting approximately three fingerbreadths below the joint line, and 1 to 2 cm medial to the tibial tubercle.
  - In thinner patients, the pes anserinus tendons, and in particular the gracilis, can often be palpated directly through the skin.
- Clear away subcutaneous tissue from the tibial crest to the posteromedial edge of the tibia.
- Identify the pes tendons inferior to the sartorius expansion.
  - The gracilis, a smaller, narrower tendon, will lie proximal to the larger semitendinosus tendon.
- Make an incision parallel to the tendons and along the proximal edge of the gracilis.
- By pulling on the gracilis tendon, the pes bursa and the interval between the medial cruciate ligament (MCL) and the overlying pes tendons can be identified.
- Start in the bursa and release the tendons off the tibial crest.
- By turning the tendons over, the interval between the semitendinosus and gracilis can be identified.
- Divide the two and separate them from the overlying sartorius.
- Beware of inferior fascial expansions originating from the semitendinosus. One to two expansions almost always need to be isolated and released.
- As more soft tissue is released, pulling on the tendon will increase its excursion.
- Once comfortable with the soft-tissue release, apply a whipstitch to the released end using no. 2 Ethibond.
- Thread this end through a closed tendon stripper, extend the knee partially, and then slowly push the tendon stripper into the thigh, aiming for the ipsilateral ischial tuberosity.

- Make sure to hold counterpressure on the sutures in line with the tendon.
- Do not torque on the stripper.
- If the stripper will not advance, consider performing more soft-tissue release.
- Once both tendons are harvested, remove all of the residual muscle on the tendon using a scissors.
- Trim away all fascial bands and excess tissue at the ends that may make passage difficult.
- Place no. 2 Ethibond whip stitches in the opposite ends.
- Fold both tendons in half and tension all four limbs equally on a tension board.
- Size the graft to 0.5 mm.
- The method of femoral and tibial fixation will then dictate how to proceed to prepare the tendons for passage and fixation.

Tibialis Anterior Allograft Preparation
- Once it is confirmed that an ACL reconstruction needs to be performed (e.g., after examination under anesthesia), have the circulating nurse defrost the allograft by placing it in a warm saline bath.
- Preferentially, the allograft should be procured from a male under age 40, with a length of at least 20 cm and a folded diameter of 9 mm.
- The graft should then be doubled over on the graft master table and whip-stitched in the same manner as for the hamstring graft.

Notchplasty
- There has been recent controversy about the amount of notchplasty to perform.
  - We perform only enough notchplasty to be able to visualize the posterior cortex of the lateral femoral condyle.
  - This may involve removing some cartilage from the anterior lateral femoral condyle to see around the corner.
- Be sure to clear away the soft tissue at the back of the notch, avoiding the fat around the PCL, which contains many small blood vessels.
- Also, be sure not to leave any sharp edges that may abrade the graft during range of motion.

Tibial Tunnel
- The starting point for the tibial tunnel should be halfway between the tibial crest and the medial border of the tibia.
  - This will result in a 60-degree coronal angle, allowing better rotatory control of the knee.
- The proximal/distal starting point will vary with the amount of angle desired for the tibial tunnel.
  - This can be set with the tibial tunnel drill guide that is used.
- A guide pin should be placed so that the pin enters the knee joint in the posteromedial area of the ACL footprint, or at the free edge of the anterior horn of the lateral meniscus and at the junction of the medial and middle thirds of the interspinous region, about 7 mm anterior to the PCL.

- The tunnel should be drilled with a constant diameter drill based on predetermined graft size.
- When using soft-tissue grafts, it is best to underdrill 1 to 2 mm and dilate the hole to match the graft diameter if interference screw fixation is used to improve pullout values by compaction of tibial bone.

Femoral Tunnel
- An offset guide should be used (sized for the appropriate tunnel) to make the femoral tunnel, with the offset allowing about 2 mm of posterior wall when the socket is created.
- Position the pin at the ten o'clock to 10:30 position on the right knee and at the 1:30 to two o'clock position on the left knee.
- The tunnel should be drilled to the appropriate depth, depending on how far you want the graft to be seated in the femoral tunnel.
- Hyperflex the knee and place a long Beath pin (has distal eyelet for sutures) by hand into the femoral tunnel.
- Tap this into place for purchase, then drill up through the lateral femoral cortex, maintaining hyperflexion, and continue drilling until the pin breaks through the skin.
- Use a screw-on handle or Kocher to hold the Beath pin proximally.
- Alternatively, you can place the Beath pin through the offset guide and drill the femoral tunnel directly over the Beath pin.

Graft Passage
- Take the finished graft and thread sutures that are looped around the proximal end of the graft through the Beath pin eyelet.
- Pull the Beath pin up and out of the knee.
- For Endobutton fixation, a no. 5 and no. 2 Ethibond are threaded through opposite ends of the Endobutton.
  - The no. 5 Ethibond is pulled to clear the Endobutton past the lateral femoral cortex, then the no. 2 Ethibond is firmly pulled to "flip" the Endobutton.
- For interference screw fixation, the graft should be advanced up into the femoral tunnel along with a guide pin for an interference screw that has been placed anterior to the graft.
  - This guide pin can enter the joint either through the anteromedial portal or via a stab incision just medial to the patellar tendon at the level of the tibial plateau to give the best angle to avoid divergence of the screw with the femoral tunnel.
  - While pulling resistance on both ends of the graft, the interference screw is placed with care not to amputate the graft.
  - The screw should not be prominent in the notch and ideally should be anterior to the graft, placing the graft as posterior as possible in the tunnel.
- For distal fixation by interference screw, preposition another guide pin in the anterior aspect of the tibial hole.
  - With BTB grafts, the tibial guide wire can be passed anterior to the bone plug.
  - You can reduce creep of the graft (from tendon elongation) by pulling on the graft 10–20 times after femoral fixation has been performed, or by holding

tension on the graft and cycling the knee multiple times through a full range of motion.

- Extend the knee to approximately 20 degrees of flexion, hold tension on the distal end of the graft using hemostats, and place the interference screw.
- Make sure the screw is not prominent, but do not place the screw in too deep, because cortical fixation will then be lost.
- Use the arthroscope to confirm the screw is not protruding into the joint, then range the knee and perform a gentle Lachman to check for stability.

■ Close all incisions and deep layers as necessary and place the dressing and an unlocked hinge brace on the leg.

■ Cold applying devices and pain pumps also work well to control postoperative swelling and pain.

Revision Surgery

As the number of primary ACL reconstructions increases, the number of revision surgeries will likely increase. With success rates ranging from 75% to 90%, it is obvious there is a population of patients that can be classified as failures for a variety of reasons.

Causes of Failure

Early failure (defined as less than 6 months after surgery) most commonly occurs due to errors in surgical technique. Late failure (after 1 year) is most commonly due to trauma.

Errors in Surgical Technique. Correct tunnel placement is essential for success in ACL surgery. Range of motion and stability are directly affected by tunnel position. The most common error in tunnel placement is femoral tunnel placed too anterior, thus producing a graft too tight in flexion and loose in extension. This is most likely due to inadequate visualization of the posterior notch region. The phrase "resident's ridge" directly references the error of not finding the "over-the-top" position (visualizing the posterior cortex of the notch) with subsequent anterior femoral tunnel placement. This can best be avoided by meticulous soft-tissue removal and by ensuring one can feel and visualize the back of the notch using a probe. The ideal anatomic placement for the femoral tunnel should be as posterior as possible without violating the posterior femoral cortex.

Tibial tunnel placement has more recently been recognized as vital to obtaining good results. Originally, techniques stressed an anteromedial placement of the tunnel in the ACL footprint, whereas current techniques suggest placement in a more posteromedial portion of the footprint. Many surgeons try to place the guide pin in the posterior area of the ACL footprint so that the pin just brushes against the PCL. Others use the free edge of the anterior horn of the lateral meniscus to guide pin placement. The whole tunnel should also lie fairly posterior to avoid graft impingement in the notch. To avoid notch impingement with extension, the entire tibial hole should be posterior to the roof of the intercondylar notch with the knee in full extension (Fig. 24-6). However, placing the tibial tunnel too posterior results in poor biomechanical performance of the graft.

Graft impingement denotes contact of the graft with the

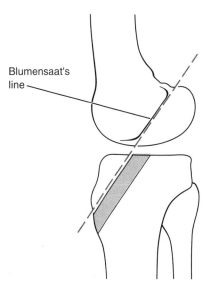

Figure 24-6 The correct position of the tibial tunnel is parallel and posterior to Blumensaat's line. (After Howell SM, Barad JM. Knee extension and its relationship to the slope of the intercondylar roof: implications for positioning the tibial tunnel in anterior cruciate ligament reconstructions. Am J Sports Med 1995;23: 288–294.)

femoral notch with the knee in full extension. This occurs mainly due to improper tunnel placement but can also be due to inadequate notchplasty. A classic postoperative finding also causing impingement is a "cyclops" lesion. This occurs from inadequate removal of soft tissue anterior to the ACL footprint or partial damage to the graft itself, resulting in accumulation of scar tissue causing a block to extension. This soft-tissue lesion may require arthroscopic debridement to regain full extension. Of note, recent trends have favored a less aggressive notchplasty to avoid distortion of femoral tunnel placement, as well as the belief that much of the tissue removed undergoes significant regrowth. Nevertheless, attention should always be paid to the area anterior to the tibial tunnel to avoid cyclops formation.

Graft tensioning is a controversial topic in ACL surgery, with no consensus as to the ideal amount of tension to use during graft fixation or the best flexion angle to apply the tension. Although most surgeons rightly fear inadequate tensioning leading to a nonfunctional graft, several authors have shown that overtensioning can have deleterious effects on motion and graft vascularization, leading to possible graft failure. In addition, overconstraint of the knee joint from overtensioning may lead to heightened joint pressures and subsequent osteoarthritis. Most authors currently recommend tensioning in full to near full extension, with approximately 20 to 40 N of force.

Failure to Recognize Secondary or Associated Injuries. Although isolated ACL injury is perhaps the most common injury pattern, the surgeon must be aware of combined instability patterns such as concomitant injury to the MCL, posterior horn medial meniscus, or posterolateral corner. Missing these injuries at the time of index surgery will place increased loads on the ACL and likely will result in eventual failure of the graft. Likewise, during revision surgery, these problems must be addressed in order for revision surgery to succeed. A chronically lax MCL may require reefing or augmentation. A more aggressive meniscectomy may need to be performed—and even meniscal transplantation considered—if the meniscus is deemed to be nonfunctional.

Posterolateral instability may be the most commonly missed associated injury with ACL tears. The Dial test (as described in Table 24-2) must be used to avoid missing this injury. In a chronic situation, a lateral thrust during walking may be observable. Treatment options may include primary repair versus augmentation or reconstruction of the popliteus tendon, popliteofibular ligament, and lateral collateral ligament.

Failure of Graft Incorporation. Some causes of graft failure can be attributed to insufficient vascularity, immunologic reaction, and stress shielding associated with use of an augmentation device. Other causes include loosening in the tunnel before bony ingrowth and delayed remodeling of allografts. Time to healing in the tunnel varies with the graft choice.

Failure Due to Trauma. Early failure from trauma may occur with overaggressive rehabilitation or a premature return to athletics, causing failure likely due to incomplete incorporation of the graft. Late failure occurs after resumption of full activities, after the graft has matured. The prevalence of traumatic reinjury has been estimated to be around 5% to 10% in the athletic population. It has been shown that graft stiffness and strength are only 30% to 50% of normal the first year after reconstruction, so excessive loads during this time may lead to elongation and plastic deformation of the graft.

Preoperative Planning

A meticulous history and physical examination must be performed in the revision situation. Prior office notes and operative notes are also essential for preoperative planning.

History

- The history should be very specific as to mechanism of injury and any previous symptoms or instability events.
  - For example, a patient may have had a long-standing incompetent ACL that was asymptomatic, but had a new event in which their medial meniscus was torn, thereby making the knee symptomatic.
- A review of previous notes can help determine whether any preexisting laxity was evident, and the operative note contains a great deal of information on the status of the menisci and articular cartilage, as well as graft type, choice of fixation, and any other intraoperative problems.
- Infection should always be considered as a possible reason for graft failure. Although uncommon, the history may provide clues to an indolent infection.
  - This may be particularly pertinent in the case of synthetic grafts.
  - If infection is suspected, a full workup must be performed before surgery, including possible aspiration of the knee, x-rays, and blood work.

Physical Examination

- A meticulous physical examination, besides testing the competency of the ACL graft, should stress the other structures of the knee, such as the posterolateral corner, the menisci, and the MCL.
- The presence of varus alignment may require a valgus producing osteotomy.
- Range of motion must be performed to evaluate for arthrofibrosis.

Radiologic Evaluation

- Radiographs
  - X-rays are essential to preoperative evaluation and should include a standing AP view, lateral, Merchant, and a 45-degree posteroanterior flexed weight-bearing view.
  - If warranted, a standing long leg film will help with measuring alignment.
  - The presence of tunnel expansion and cysts must be addressed, with staged bone grafting, if necessary.
  - The type of fixation (metal/bioabsorbable screws, Endobutton, etc.) can be categorized, as well as tunnel position.
  - The 45-degree flexed weight-bearing view will provide information about the degree of arthrosis, as well as give a view of the notch.
- MRI
  - Just as in primary ACL injury, an MRI is not necessarily needed; however, a new MRI may be helpful to determine the status of the menisci, articular cartilage, and ligamentous structures.
  - Because of its usefulness for surgical planning, we routinely obtain an MRI in the revision situation.

Surgical Plan. Issues such as bone tunnel expansion and arthrofibrosis often require a two-stage approach. Widened bone tunnels may necessitate removal of existing hardware with bone grafting of the tunnels, then waiting approximately 12 to 24 weeks before performing the definitive procedure. Preexisting arthrofibrosis may require extensive physical therapy or manipulation under anesthesia to regain sufficient motion to undertake revision reconstruction.

If only one procedure needs to be performed, some general issues must be addressed. The necessary equipment to perform hardware removal must be in the operating room, as well as other special equipment depending on type of fixation chosen. Previous skin incisions should be used if at all possible, avoiding skin bridges of 7 cm or less if other incisions must be made. Other issues to decide on include graft choice, as well as type of fixation.

Graft Selection. Tissues available for revision surgery can be divided into autograft and allograft categories. Synthetic grafts are no longer in use for any type of ACL surgery, although future research may someday provide a viable synthetic biologic ACL. The results of allograft and autograft revisions are quite similar, and because of tissue availability, allografts are the more common grafts used in revision surgery. Achilles tendon and patellar tendon are the most common allografts used due to the ability to achieve bone-to-bone healing on one or two ends. The bone plug can also be fashioned to fill in gaps from tunnel widening or bone loss after screw removal.

Graft Fixation. The surgeon has many choices for revision fixation; often, several techniques may be successful for a given scenario. On the femoral side, depending on position, metal screws can either be bypassed or removed if they interfere with the new tunnel. If removed, the subsequent bone defect must be filled, either with a bone block, a larger diameter soft-tissue graft, or a larger metal screw. Screws can be stacked side to side as well. Bioabsorbable screws rarely need removal because they can be easily drilled through if in the area of the new tunnel. Two incision techniques can be revised to one-incision endoscopic techniques and, in general, most situations can be revised to either Endobutton or two-incision/over-the-top fixation. Revision of the newer transosseous fixation devices has not been studied in depth due to the recent introduction of these products into the market.

Intraoperative Considerations. Instrumentation to consider having readily available include coring reamers; large 10-mm plastic sheathes; and various sizes of screwdrivers, osteotomes, bone pick, curettes, flexible guide wires of assorted sizes, and pituitary graspers. An ACL revision tray often contains most of these instruments, as well as specially designed devices such as a screw expander, trephine drill, and stripped screw screwdriver.

The most common surgical error that needs to be addressed is a femoral tunnel placed too far anterior. In this case, as long as the previous tunnel is more than one tunnel diameter anterior to where the new tunnel would be placed, a new tunnel can be simply drilled, avoiding the need to address the previous tunnel and its hardware. In the case where the femoral tunnel has been placed properly, re-drilling of the previous tunnel can be performed. Where difficulty arises is when the previous tunnel is just slightly anterior to the anatomic site, causing overlap of the two tunnels, producing an enlarged tunnel diameter. Options in this scenario include trying to fit a smaller diameter graft posteriorly, avoiding tunnel overlap (usually with a soft-tissue graft of 7 to 8 mm), or enlarging the previous tunnel to incorporate the correct tunnel site and using an allograft with a bone block. By positioning the bone plug to fill the previous hole, the tendon can be moved to a more posterior position. In situations in which the previous tunnel is too far posterior, with posterior wall blowout, a two-incision technique or Endobutton fixation provides stable fixation.

In cases in which a greatly enlarged tunnel diameter is encountered (>15 mm wide), staged reconstruction with bone grafting of the tunnel should be considered. Other options include stacking interference screws, using a two-incision technique or filling the defect with a large allograft bone block.

Errors in tibial tunnel placement can be addressed with principles similar to errant femoral tunnel placement. Most commonly, the tibial tunnel has been placed too far anterior. Difficulties also arise from attempting to remove interference screws. Direct visualization by placing the arthroscope up the tibial tunnel often works well; another technique uses fluoroscopy to thread a guidewire inside the cannulated screw. The quality of the tibial bone is generally compromised due to hole size and osteopenia. Because of

that, fixation with interference fit alone is risky, and backup sutures tied over a screw and washer are generally preferred.

COMPLICATIONS

Intraoperative Complications

Intraoperative complications can be subdivided into graft problems and tunnel problems. Meticulous surgical technique must always be performed to prevent infection and guarantee the best chance for success via correct tunnel placement and graft utilization.

Graft Problems

Problems associated with patellar and hamstring tendons are listed in Box 24-5.

A complication that must be avoided is contamination of the graft, most commonly from dropping the graft on the floor. If this occurs, another graft should be considered for implantation, but if the contaminated graft must be used, one should follow this protocol:

- Wash the graft with chlorhexidine gluconate and triple antibiotic solution (gentamicin, clindamycin, polymyxin) for 10 minutes each using pulsed lavage.
- Treat with postoperative antibiotic prophylaxis (an oral cephalosporin) for 5 days.

Tunnel Placement

Incorrect tunnel placement was addressed in an earlier section; however, blowout of the posterior femoral wall merits further discussion. The key in avoiding the consequences of this error is recognition during surgery. An easy solution is to use an Endobutton, which does not require a posterior wall for fixation. If so desired, a two-incision technique may also be used, which changes the angle of femoral tunnel placement away from the errant tunnel.

Postoperative Complications

Postoperative complications include infection, abnormal healing responses, arthrofibrosis, graft rejection, complex regional pain syndrome, and failure of the graft. All of these complications can be detected by early, systematic follow-up examinations. Careful preoperative planning, appropri-

---

BOX 24-5 PROBLEMS ASSOCIATED WITH GRAFTS FROM PARTICULAR TENDONS

Patellar tendon
- Bone plug fracture
- Obtaining an inadequate bone plug circumference
- Acute patellar fracture
- Breaching of the fat pad

Hamstring tendon
- Inadequate length or width
- Transection of a tendon during harvesting

ate patient selection, and meticulous surgical technique can minimize the number of complications.

REHABILITATION

Once surgery has been performed, the impetus is on the patient to rehabilitate their knee to regain full function. Most surgeons permit return to sports after 6 months, although some authors have brought athletes back to sports as early as 3 to 4 months after surgery. At the very least, an early return to sports requires a highly motivated patient with access to skilled physical therapy.

A dedicated rehabilitation program after an anterior ligament reconstruction is a critical step in returning an athlete back to competition (patient back to activity). There has been a full swing of the pendulum over the past 20 years from postoperative casting to the "accelerated" rehabilitation program of recent years. Recent advances in rehabilitation sciences are elucidating the importance of the rehabilitation program and the return-to-sport decision process and

improving our ability to better serve our patients in the long term. The potential consequences of early return to sports are currently being discussed in the literature, as are the factors that define the potential problems. The surgeon must work with an experienced physical therapist or athletic trainer to decide on a rehabilitation program that is specific to each individual patient, protects the knee, and is cost effective.

Successful return to activity, athletic or other, requires optimal function of the neuromuscular system to protect the repair and to protect the joint surface by attenuating shock during activity. Our understanding of motor control, resultant joint forces, and joint kinematics is improving because of research using electromyography, force plates, cineradiography, and the open MRI. Results from this research suggest that neuromuscular function does not fully return until between 18 and 24 months after an anterior cruciate ligament reconstruction. We are rapidly moving from a paradigm that considers only "strength" of the quadriceps and hamstrings as a measure of readiness to return to activity to espousing the importance of other key factors such as

TABLE 24-5 RESULTS OF ACL SURGERY STUDIES

Graft Type	Author	Notes
Retrospective studies		
BTB	Buss (1993) Bach (1994) Aglietti (1993) Howe (1991)	■ 85% to 90% to be stable (≤4 mm difference), with a 2- to 5-year follow-up ■ More than 90% had successful return to function ■ 15% to 40% complications, primarily loss of motion, and patellofemoral pain
STG	Sgaglione (1993) Anderson (1994) Grana (1992)	■ 85% to 90% stable ■ 90% return to function ■ 15% complications ■ The issue with both retrospective groups is that there was no control or comparison group
BTB versus STG	Otero (1993) Holmes (1991)	■ Compared 56 BTB with 36 STG ■ BTB concluded to be better (tighter knee function was the same) ■ Limitation was varied rehabilitation ■ Compared 27 BTB with 48 STG ■ For acute injuries, results were equal ■ BTB was better for chronic cases
Prospective studies		
BTB versus STG	Warren (1994) Aglietti (1994)	■ Function was equal ■ BTB causing more problems with loss of motion, pain, and swelling
Prospective randomized studies		
BTB versus STG	Marder (1991) O'Neill (1998) Corry (1999)	■ No significant differences for laxity, function, or subjective complaints ■ BTB groups had more patellofemoral pain and loss of motion
Meta-analysis		
BTB versus STG	Yunes (2001)	■ The only meta-analysis in the ACL literature ■ Concluded that BTB was a better graft ■ Controversial finding, since by nature meta-analyses have design flaws as a result of differences in grading systems and study design in the compiled studies

ACL, anterior cruciate ligament; BTB, bone–patellar tendon–bone; STG, semitendinosus/gracilis.

proprioception, balance, time to peak torque of key muscles, and compensation patterns used by postsurgical athletes to perform. These variables should be addressed as part of a "neuromuscular" rehabilitation program that incorporates a progression of balance, strength, and power activities to create adaptation of the neuromuscular system. In addition, the exercises should reach beyond the muscles of the knee to integrate specific training of the hip, core abdominal, and ankle muscles.

The decision to allow an athlete to return to full activity must consider the nature of the sport, the condition of the knee (including any evidence of subchondral bruising), and the status of the neuromuscular system. In addition to a predetermined time goal, the results of "functional testing" should be weighted heavily to better understand when the athlete and the knee are ready to return in a manner that is safe for the repair and healthy for the knee in the future.

RESULTS

It is difficult to compare ACL studies because of the tremendous changes in both surgical technique and technology. New fixation devices, the numerous graft choices, and variations in rehabilitation, patient population, and associated injuries make it almost impossible to evaluate studies directly with each other. Table 24-5 summarizes publications based on type (e.g., retrospective, prospective, prospective randomized, and meta-analysis).

SUGGESTED READING

Arnoczky SP. Biology of ACL reconstructions: what happens to the graft? Inst Course Lect 1996;45:229–233.

Chappell JD, Yu B, Kirkendall DT, et al. A comparison of knee kinetics between male and female recreational athletes in stop-jump tasks. Am J Sports Med 2002;30:261–267.

Frank CB, Jackson DW. The science of reconstruction of the anterior cruciate ligament. J Bone Joint Surg Am 1997;79:1556–1576.

Fu FH, Bennett CH, Lattermann C, et al. Current trends in anterior cruciate ligament reconstruction: Biology and biomechanics of reconstruction. Am J Sports Med 1999;27:821–829.

Griffin LY, Agel MA, Albohm MJ, et al. Noncontact anterior cruciate ligament injuries: Risk factors and prevention strategies. J Am Acad Orthop Surg 2000;8:141–150.

Harner CD, Giffin JR, Dunteman RC, et al. Evaluation and treatment of recurrent instability after anterior cruciate ligament reconstruction. Instr Course Lect 2001;50:463–474.

Hunter RE, Grana WA, Blessey PB, et al. Anterior cruciate ligament injury. Online Tutorial. Orthopaedic Knowledge Online. Available at: www.aaos.org/oko.

Martin SD, Martin TL, Brown CH. Anterior cruciate ligament graft fixation. Orthop Clin N Am 2002;33:685–696.

Rodeo S, Arnoczky S, Torzilli PA, et al. Tendon-healing in a bone tunnel. A biomechanical and histological study in the dog. J Bone Joint Surg Am 1993;75:1795–1803.

Simonian PTM, Larson RV. Anterior cruciate ligament injuries in the skeletally immature patient. Am J Orthop 1999;28:624–628.

Yu B, Kirkendall DT, Taft TN, Garrett WE. Lower extremity motor control-related and other risk factors for noncontact anterior cruciate ligament injuries. Inst Course Lect 2002;51:315–324.

Yunes M, Richmond JC, Engels EA, et al. Patellar tendon versus hamstring tendons in anterior cruciate ligament reconstruction: a meta-analysis. Arthroscopy 2001;17:248–257.

COLLATERAL LIGAMENT INJURIES OF THE KNEE

ANDREW F. ARTHUR
ROBERT F. LAPRADE

MEDIAL COLLATERAL LIGAMENT COMPLEX

The medial collateral ligament (MCL) complex of the knee is the primary restraint to preventing valgus opening and external rotation of the tibia. The MCL complex has also been demonstrated to play an important secondary role in preventing anterior translation of the tibia in knees with anterior cruciate ligament (ACL) deficiency. A thorough understanding of the MCL complex is essential for accurate history-taking, clinical examination, radiographic imaging, diagnosis, and subsequent treatment of ligamentous injuries of the knee.

Pathogenesis

Epidemiology
The MCL complex is the most commonly injured ligament of the knee. Many grade I injuries are often never seen by physicians, making the true incidence of MCL complex injuries likely higher than reported. As such, physicians should have a high clinical suspicion for these injuries. In addition, understanding the pathogenesis of injured anatomic structures will help determine the appropriate course of treatment, including rehabilitation and surgical repairs or reconstructions when indicated.

MCL complex injuries can occur in isolation or with other concomitant ligamentous or meniscal injuries. As expected, more severe injuries are more likely to have additional ligamentous injuries: 20% of grade I, 52% of grade II, and 78% of grade III MCL complex injuries will have concomitant ligamentous injuries. The ACL is the most commonly injured ligament in combined injuries, accounting for 95% of the mixed lesions in grade III MCL complex injuries in one study. Concurrent meniscal injuries are found to occur in only 0% to 5% of isolated MCL complex injuries, but may approach 50% in knees with combined MCL complex and ACL tears.

Etiology
The majority of MCL complex injuries are caused by valgus stresses to a slightly flexed knee. These injuries can occur as a result of noncontact injuries, such as skiing or pivoting maneuvers (which tend to produce less severe injuries), or contact injuries, such as a lateral blow to the knee during

TABLE 25-1 AMA GUIDELINES FOR GRADING MCL OR LCL COMPLEX INJURIES

Grade	Description
I	0 to 5 mm joint line opening
II	5 to 10 mm joint line opening
III	>10 mm opening; no firm end point (complete tear)

AMA, American Medical Association; LCL, lateral collateral ligament; MCL, medial collateral ligament.

American football. Contact injuries usually produce more severe injuries and account for the majority of grade III MCL complex lesions.

Other structures that may be injured include the vastus medialis obliquus (VMO) muscle, the ACL, menisci, and the medial patellofemoral ligament, which may be disrupted as a result of a concomitant lateral patellar subluxation or dislocation.

Classification

MCL complex injuries are graded according to the amount of medial joint line opening to valgus stress with the knee in 30 degrees of flexion. It is important to compare this measurement to the contralateral side to assess for any side-to-side differences.

The American Medical Association (AMA) guidelines for quantitating the degree of ligamentous injury are given in Table 25-1.

Anatomy

The MCL complex consists of one large ligament and a series of capsular thickenings and tendinous attachments that function together to provide dynamic and static stability to the medial aspect of the knee. The important static stabilizers are the superficial MCL, the deep MCL, and the posterior oblique ligament. The dynamic stabilizers include the semimembranosus complex with its multiple heads of insertion, the adductor magnus tendon, the VMO muscle, and the medial gastrocnemius tendon (Fig. 25-1).

Superficial Medial Collateral Ligament

The superficial MCL (also called the tibial collateral ligament) is the largest structure in the MCL complex. It attaches on the femur just distal and posterior to the medial epicondyle and has two attachments on the tibia. The more proximal tibial attachment is 2 cm distal to the joint line and is just anterior to the posteromedial border of the tibia. The second tibial attachment passes deep to the pes anserine tendons, attaching to the anteromedial aspect of the tibia 5 to 7 cm distal to the joint line.

Deep Medial Collateral Ligament

The deep MCL consists of medial capsular thickenings on either side of the medial meniscus that are designated as the meniscofemoral and meniscotibial portions of the deep MCL. These ligaments are in continuation with the medial capsule and have separate attachments to both the femur and tibia, as well as to the middle of the medial meniscus.

Posterior Oblique Ligament

The posterior oblique ligament is a tendinous expansion of the semimembranosus muscle. It reinforces the posterior aspect of the meniscofemoral ligament and has widespread fascial attachments to the posteromedial capsule and adductor tubercle. The posterior oblique ligament resists valgus stresses at 0-degree flexion.

Diagnosis

History and Physical Examination

- Diagnosis of MCL complex injuries is often suspected based on the patient's description of the injury, which usually involves either a noncontact valgus and external rotation injury, or a direct lateral blow to the knee.
- Careful palpation of the specific anatomic structures

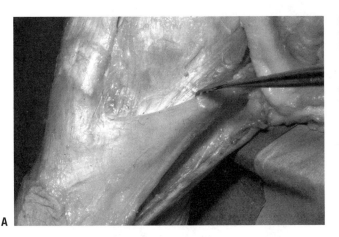
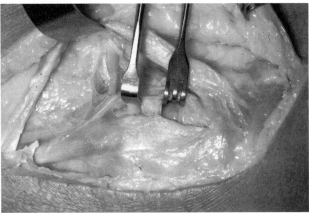

A   B

Figure 25-1   Anatomy of the medial structures of the knee. **A:** Lateral view, left knee, demonstrating the pes anserine tendons overlying the tibial collateral ligament (*pointer*). **B:** Lateral view, left knee, with the meniscofemoral and meniscotibial components of the deep MCL incised and retracted.

before motion testing can often determine which structures are injured.

■ Pain over the meniscofemoral or meniscotibial attachments may indicate a specific portion of the MCL complex that is injured.

■ This distinction is important as treatment parameters and prognosis differ according to the type and location of MCL complex injuries.

■ Associated injuries, such as medial meniscus tears or patella dislocations, may be elucidated from medial joint line tenderness or medial patellofemoral pain, respectively.

■ The clinical examination should also include assessment of range of motion and ligamentous stress testing for both injured and uninjured knees.

■ Side-to-side differences are essential to determining the overall significance of any objective laxity.

■ The main clinical maneuver is the valgus stress test performed with the knee flexed to 30 degrees over the side of the examination table.

■ The examiner's fingers are placed over the joint line to stabilize the knee and assess the degree of subsequent laxity as a valgus stress is applied with the other hand placing the force over the foot/ankle to control for rotation (Fig. 25-2).

■ Medial joint line crepitation, or a palpable "clunk," felt during the valgus stress test may also indicate a medial meniscus tear, a chondral injury, or baseline medial compartment arthritis.

■ Valgus stress to the knee at 0-degree flexion can also be assessed.

■ Increased laxity in this position indicates a severe amount of underlying ligamentous injury, usually in-

volving the ACL, posterior cruciate ligament (PCL), or both ligaments.

■ In these instances, there is a significant injury to the MCL complex as well.

■ The anterior drawer test in external rotation is another test used to determine the extent of MCL complex injury. It assesses the amount of anteromedial translation of the tibia on the femur.

■ With the patient supine, the knee is flexed to 80 degrees with the foot externally rotated as an anterior drawer maneuver is performed.

■ Increased laxity, compared with the uninvolved knee, may indicate a concurrent ACL tear or may be useful in quantitating the degree of laxity in the chronic MCL complex injury.

■ It is important to differentiate this test from the posterolateral drawer test (discussed later) because both can contribute to a perceived increased amount of external rotation.

■ Injury to the posterior oblique ligament may occur in association with combined ACL and MCL complex injuries.

■ In this setting, increased valgus laxity at 0-degree flexion may occur despite an intact PCL.

■ Avoiding knee hyperextension during the rehabilitation period may be warranted to allow for appropriate healing of these posteromedial knee structures.

Radiologic Examination

Radiographs

■ Anteroposterior, lateral, and patellofemoral radiographs should be obtained to inspect for fractures, lateral capsular avulsions, ligamentous avulsions, loose bodies,

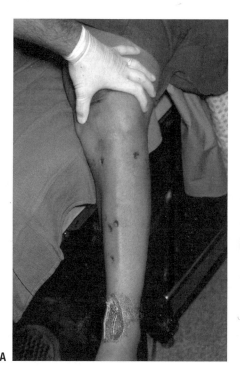
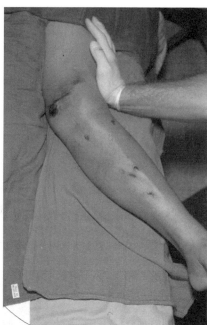

Figure 25-2   Valgus stress test of a left knee with a grade III MCL tear **(A)** reduced; **(B)** valgus stress applied.

Magnetic Resonance Imaging

- When the diagnosis is in doubt, or if other ligamentous injuries are suspected, an MRI of the knee can be useful.
- The coronal MRI views provide the best visualization of the MCL complex and are most useful in determining the severity, extent, and specific anatomic location of MCL complex injuries.
- In acute injuries, MRI scans can differentiate between meniscofemoral, midsubstance, or meniscotibial lesions, which ultimately may affect the prognosis and treatment parameters.
- MRI scans may also be useful in differentiating acute injuries from chronic MCL complex injuries.
- Chronically injured ligaments are significantly thickened at the site of previous injury and may have increased signal on MRI images (Fig. 25-4).

Treatment

Isolated MCL Complex Injuries

Nonsurgical Treatment

- Isolated grade I and II injuries are treated nonoperatively.
  - The patient should be allowed full weight-bearing as tolerated, and crutches can be discontinued once the patient is able to walk without a limp.
  - Range of motion is encouraged within the first 24 to 48 hours after the injury, and attempts are made to achieve a full range of motion as soon as possible.
  - Icing and elevation are used to control pain from swelling and edema.
  - Quadriceps strengthening exercises (straight-leg raises, quadriceps setting exercises, leg presses, lightweight squats to a maximum of 70 degrees of knee flexion), and an exercise bike are implemented as soon as tolerated.

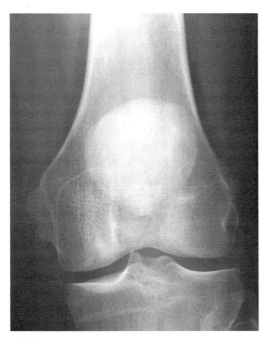

Figure 25-3 Pellegrini-Stieda lesion. Anteroposterior x-ray left knee.

calcification of the MCL complex (Pellegrini-Stieda lesion), or evidence of a patellar dislocation (Fig. 25-3).
- Skeletally immature patients should have varus and valgus stress radiographs to verify that the injury is not a Salter-Harris physeal fracture.
- Stress radiographs may also be valuable in the chronically injured MCL complex to quantitate the degree of injury and whether an MCL complex injury has healed or not.

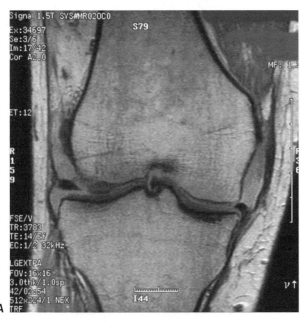
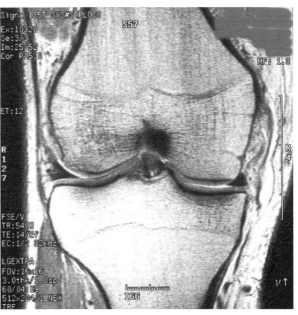

Figure 25-4 Coronal MRI images of acute meniscofemoral-based (A) and chronic meniscotibial-based (B) MCL injuries.

- Emphasis on full functional recovery to include full range of motion, no laxity, and adequate strength within 4 to 6 weeks is stressed to the patient.
- Isolated grade III MCL complex injuries are also initially treated nonoperatively.
    - It is important to distinguish between tibial-sided lesions and femoral-sided lesions because treatment and prognosis may differ.
    - Meniscotibial lesions are more problematic, with a higher incidence of rotational instability and subsequent development of chronic grade III instability.
    - The use of a knee brace to prevent varus/valgus stresses through the knee, although not proven, may be beneficial to patients with grade III instability and a meniscotibial lesion.
    - Regardless, this population of MCL complex injuries should be followed closely throughout the rehabilitation program.
    - In general, patients who have completed the functional rehabilitation program should have a grade I or less valgus stress test by the fourth week after injury.
    - Continued grade III instability may indicate a need for surgical intervention and warrants close clinical monitoring.
    - Grade III injuries are allowed return to activities with demonstration of normal knee motion, grade I or less instability, and adequate functional strength.
- Functional testing is recommended for in-season athletic participation to make sure that patients do not have instability with twisting and pivoting activities.
    - Athletes who return to full participation within the first 4 to 6 weeks after a grade III MCL complex tear are encouraged to wear a functional hinged knee brace to protect against reinjury during contact sports.
- Casting or immobilization has not proved beneficial and may, in fact, be detrimental to the healing and restoration of normal ligament function.
    - It may lead to arthrofibrosis and an extended period of rehabilitation to restore normal range of motion.
    - Although unproven, use of a brace that still allows full range of motion may be beneficial for meniscotibial lesions. Further clinical outcome studies are needed to confirm this practice.

Surgical Treatment

- Operative treatment of isolated MCL complex injuries should be undertaken only after completion of the functional rehabilitation program and symptomatic grade II or III instability persists.
    - It is becoming increasingly recognized that chronic, symptomatic injuries are more common than traditionally thought.
- Chronic grade III MCL complex injuries will not heal and should ultimately be repaired or reconstructed if they cause functional limitations.
- The goal of a surgical reconstruction is to restore normal stability and allow early range of motion and rehabilitation.
- Reconstructions should be performed anatomically to restore normal MCL complex anatomy.

- Reconstruction is performed with either a pes anserine tendon autograft (gracilis and/or semitendinosus tendons) or an Achilles tendon allograft.
    - The choice to use autograft versus allograft is dependent on allograft availability, the status of the gracilis and semitendinosus tendons, and patient and surgeon preference.
- MCL complex reconstruction is performed with concurrent plication of the middle third medial capsular ligaments (deep MCL ligament) and the posterior oblique ligament, especially in patients with concurrent anteromedial rotatory instability.
- As previously noted, restoration of normal ligamentous anatomy is crucial to prevent stretching out of the graft over time, thereby preserving the long-term stability of the reconstruction.

Combined Medial Cruciate Ligament Complex Injuries with Other Ligament Injuries

- More severe knee injuries may result in MCL complex injury with concomitant injury to additional structures about the knee.
- The ACL is the most commonly concurrently torn ligament.
    - Grade III MCL complex injuries have been shown to have a 78% incidence of concomitant ligament injury, and greater than 95% of these multiligament-injured knees have ACL tears.
- Injury to the medial meniscus is rare in isolated MCL complex injuries (less than 5% incidence).
    - With concomitant injury to the ACL, however, the medial meniscus is more easily injured, resulting in the classic O'Donoghue triad of an ACL, MCL, and medal meniscus tear.
- Appropriate diagnosis and subsequent repair or gentle debridement of medial and/or lateral meniscus tears should be carefully considered in knees with combined ACL and MCL complex injuries.
- Combined injuries of the ACL and MCL complex should be managed with the goal of restoring normal functional anatomy to provide a stable and completely rehabilitated knee.
- Regardless of the severity of MCL complex injury, initially this should usually be treated nonoperatively.
- Rehabilitation should be performed similarly as previously described, with emphasis on restoration of full range of motion and quadriceps strength.
    - This initial period of rehabilitation allows the MCL complex to heal and also allows the inflammatory phase of injury to subside, thereby optimizing the timing for ACL reconstruction.
- Once full range of motion and normal quadriceps strength have been achieved, the MCL complex can be re-evaluated and the ACL can be reconstructed in appropriately selected patients.
- Patients with continued grade III MCL complex laxity should be carefully evaluated for concurrent MCL complex repair at the time of an ACL reconstruction.
    - Tibial-sided (meniscotibial) injuries with significant rotational instability and femoral-sided (meniscofemoral) "peel-off" injuries with significant instabil-

ity in extension are especially prone to developing chronic symptomatic instability.

■ These patients need careful clinical evaluation.
■ Intraoperatively, before the ACL is reconstructed, a thorough examination under anesthesia—including a valgus stress at 30 degrees of knee flexion—is performed.
  ▨ Residual instability (2+ or greater) to the MCL complex warrants repair and/or reconstruction.
  ▨ Arthroscopic examination of the knee may demonstrate a medial "drive-through sign," indicating significant MCL complex laxity and a need for subsequent repair or reconstruction (Fig. 25-5).
■ Failure to recognize clinically significant MCL laxity before ACL graft fixation could result in the ACL graft overconstraining the knee and masking underlying residual MCL laxity.
  ▨ This overconstraint of the knee could increase the stress on the ACL graft, causing it to stretch out or even fail over time.
■ The individual anatomic structures (posterior oblique ligament, superficial MCL, and deep MCL) are carefully dissected and their integrity assessed.
  ▨ Midsubstance tears can be repaired directly or reconstructed.
  ▨ Femoral or tibial-sided lesions are repaired with suture anchors or a screw and soft-tissue washer to its anatomic insertion sites.
  ▨ Direct repair and/or reefing of the posterior oblique ligament and semimembranosus complex are also performed as needed to eliminate any associated rotational instability.
  ▨ The soft tissues in knees with chronic MCL complex injuries may limit direct repair techniques, and reconstruction with a hamstring tendon autograft or Achilles tendon allograft may be necessary.
■ MCL complex injuries associated with knee dislocations or concomitant posterolateral corner (PLC) injuries

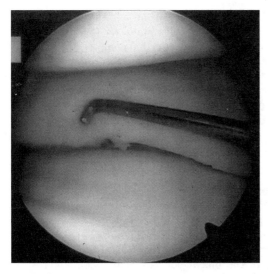

Figure 25-5   Chronic grade III MCL tear with an arthroscopic medial compartment "drive-through" sign (right knee).

should be treated surgically within the first 2 weeks of injury.
  ▨ Individual structures are most easily identified during this early phase of healing before scar formation and loss of normal tissue planes.
  ▨ Surgical goals include anatomic fixation of individual structures and early range of motion postoperatively to limit the complication of arthrofibrosis.

Results and Outcome

Long-term prognosis of isolated MCL complex injuries is dependent on the degree of laxity after the completion of the functional rehabilitation program. Patients with initial grade I and II laxity have been shown to have excellent knee function and sporting ability, despite increased residual valgus laxity on clinical examination at long-term follow-up. Knee joint instability and early osteoarthritis is largely spared in patients with isolated partial MCL complex injuries. In a prospective study of patients with isolated partial ruptures of the MCL, Lundberg et al. showed only 13% of patients developed Fairbank's grade I osteoarthritis changes at 10-year follow-up.

The results of nonoperative treatment for isolated grade III injuries have varied considerably. Indelicato found that by following a rigid protocol to rule out concurrent meniscus and cruciate tears, good and excellent results can be expected in more than 90% of patients. Other authors have reported less favorable results with isolated grade III MCL complex injuries. Kannus found long-term results to be poor and unacceptable in every respect: 63% decrease in physical activity, 22% change in occupation, 22% with continued subjective instability, 63% incidence of radiographic osteoarthritis, and only 11% of patients were asymptomatic with respect to knee stability.

As described previously, we believe that regardless of the degree of MCL complex laxity, combined ACL and MCL injuries should initially be managed nonoperatively within the functional rehabilitation program. If, on completion of 4 to 8 weeks of the rehabilitation program, grade II or III laxity persists, operative repair and/or reconstruction should be performed. Reconstruction of concomitantly injured ligaments (e.g., ACL) should similarly be performed once the initial inflammatory phase has subsided and full range of motion and normal quadriceps strength has been achieved. This treatment protocol has been similarly found to be effective by Hughston who reported excellent long-term results (22 years) for acutely repaired MCL complex injuries (with and without concomitant ACL tears), stressing the importance of precise anatomical repair of the MCL complex.

POSTEROLATERAL CORNER

The posterolateral ligament complex of the knee functions to statically and dynamically resist varus opening and external tibial rotation relative to the femur. The PLC has also been demonstrated to play a secondary role in preventing anterior and posterior tibial translation in the ACL- and PCL-deficient knees, respectively. A thorough understanding of the components of the PLC is essential for accurate history-taking, clinical examination, radiographic imaging, diagnosis, and subsequent treatment of both simple and complex ligamentous injuries to the knee.

Pathogenesis

Epidemiology

The true incidence of injuries to the posterolateral structures of the knee is unknown because many injuries are initially undetected or underreported. Studies in which MRI has been performed after acute knee injuries show a 6% to 8% incidence of PLC injury. Isolated PLC injuries are rare and more commonly occur in combination with ACL or PCL injuries. Studies show that approximately 75% of knees with PLC injuries will have additional ligamentous injuries. In addition, there is also a 15% incidence of peroneal nerve injury after grade III PLC injuries. The presence of numbness of the dorsum of the foot, weakness to dorsiflexion, or a footdrop should alert the clinician to possible injury to the common peroneal nerve.

Persistent knee instability after ACL or PCL reconstruction may be the first recognition of PLC. Failure to recognize concomitant PLC when performing ACL or PCL reconstruction may result in graft failure or residual instability symptoms. For optimal results, a thorough evaluation of the entire knee is essential before undergoing any ligamentous reconstruction of the knee. Perhaps a more thorough understanding of PLC knee injuries by health care providers may prove these injuries to be more common than currently suspected.

Etiology

Injury to the PLC of the knee is most common during sports activities and accounts for 40% of PLC injuries. Historically, the mechanism of injury involves a blow to the anteromedial aspect of the knee. More recent studies have shown the mechanism to involve twisting (30%), noncontact hyperextension (21%), contact hyperextension (16%), and an anterior force to a flexed knee (10%) (Table 25-2). These mechanisms of injury may also produce injury to the cruciate ligaments, and the integrity to these structures must also be considered.

Classification

Varus instability after PLC injuries is graded according to the amount of lateral joint line opening to a varus stress with the knee in 30 degrees of flexion. It is important to

TABLE 25-2 MECHANISM OF POSTEROLATERAL KNEE INJURIES

Mechanism	Incidence (%)
Twisting	30
Noncontact hyperextension	21
Contact hyperextension	16
Anterior blow to flexed knee	10

compare this measurement with the contralateral side to assess for any side-to-side differences.

As with MCL complex injuries, the AMA has established guidelines for quantitating the degree of ligamentous injury to the lateral collateral ligament and PLC (see Table 25-1).

Anatomy

The anatomy of the posterolateral knee is more complex than the medial side. The fibula once articulated with the femur and, through evolutionary changes, the fibula has pulled away from the femur while still maintaining its ligamentous and capsular attachments. The bony anatomy of the lateral knee is also significantly different from the medial side. Although the concavity of the medial tibial plateau provides inherent stability to the medial compartment, the convex surface of the lateral tibial plateau provides no such stability. This inherent bony instability to the lateral structures of the knee provides a teleological explanation for why the ligamentous structures to the posterolateral aspect of the knee are so complex. As such, injury to these structures often produces dramatic functional instability during even simple gait (e.g., varus thrust gait patterns). Such persistent functional instability is the reason why ligamentous injuries to the posterolateral structures heal poorly with nonsurgical treatments.

The normal function of the posterolateral structures of the knee is to provide restraint to varus forces, posterolateral (external) tibial rotation, and posterior tibial translation near full knee extension. Thus, posterolateral knee instability will demonstrate increased varus opening, external tibial rotation, and posterior tibial translation. A thorough understanding of the functional anatomy of the posterolateral knee is essential to guiding the physician to the appropriate timing and technique involved in treating the complex array of injuries that occur to the posterolateral structures of the knee. Restoration of both the dynamic and static stabilizing structures is necessary for achieving good outcomes.

Iliotibial Band

The iliotibial band acts as an accessory anterolateral ligament and is a secondary stabilizer to varus forces. There are four main components that comprise the iliotibial band: the superficial layer (main structure) that attaches to Gerdy's tubercle, the deep layer that attaches to the lateral intermuscular septum of the distal femur, the capsuloosseous layer, and the iliopatellar band. During knee flexion, the iliotibial band becomes tight, exerting a posterior force on the lateral tibia. In knee extension, the iliotibial band moves anteriorly, serving as a secondary restraint to varus and posterolateral rotation forces.

Biceps Femoris

The biceps femoris muscle acts as a powerful dynamic external rotator of the tibia and contributes as a lateral stabilizer of the knee. The muscle consists of a long head and a short head, each with numerous arms and attachments. The long head of the biceps consists of five components: a direct arm, an anterior arm, a reflected arm, and two aponeurotic expansions (anterior and lateral). The main attachments are

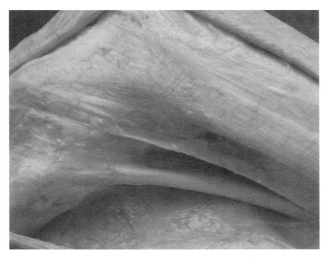

Figure 25-6 Superficial posterolateral anatomic dissection demonstrating the superficial layer of the iliotibial band and the long head of the biceps femoris (lateral view, left knee).

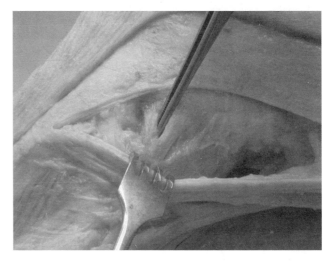

Figure 25-7 Lateral view, left knee, with superficial layer of iliotibial band horizontally split and retracted. The hemostat is between the popliteus (to left/anterior) and FCL femoral attachments.

the direct arm, which inserts on the posterolateral edge of the fibular head, and the anterior arm, that attaches to the lateral edge of the fibular head and lies directly over the fibular collateral ligament (FCL)-biceps bursa (Fig. 25-6).

The short head of the biceps femoris muscle is composed of six attachments: a proximal muscular attachment to the tendon of the long head of the biceps, a capsular arm to the posterolateral joint capsule, two tendinous attachments (the direct arm and anterior arm), a confluence with the capsulo-osseous layer of the iliotibial band, and a final fascial attachment that expands onto the posteromedial aspect of the FCL. The three main attachments of the short head of the biceps are the two tendinous attachments (the direct and anterior arms) and the capsular arm. The direct arm is a tendinous insertion just posterolateral to the fibular styloid. The anterior arm passes medial to the FCL and inserts on the posterior aspect of the tibial tuberosity. Avulsions of the meniscotibial portion of the middle third lateral capsular ligament (Segond fracture) may tear this anterior arm due to its close proximity. The final major component is the capsular arm, which attaches to the posterolateral joint capsule, as well as distally onto the lateral gastrocnemius tendon and fabella. This distal edge of the capsular arm is known as the fabellofibular ligament which originates at the fabella, or cartilaginous fabella-analog, and inserts onto the tip of the fibular styloid. The fabellofibular ligament is tight in extension and relaxed in flexion.

Popliteus Tendon and Ligament Complex

The popliteus tendon and popliteofibular ligament (PFL) play a major role in both dynamic and static stabilization of the lateral tibia on the femur. Together, the popliteus complex restricts posterior tibial translation and external tibial rotation, provides secondary resistance to varus forces, and acts as a dynamic internal rotator of the tibia.

The popliteus tendon originates on the femur in the popliteal sulcus, passes distally and posteroinferiorly through the popliteal hiatus, and inserts on the posterior aspect of the tibia (Fig. 25-7). At the hiatus, the tendon has three popliteomeniscal fascicles that insert into the posterior joint capsule and posterior horn of the lateral meniscus. These provide dynamic stability to the lateral meniscus.

The PFL is a static stabilizer to the lateral and posterolateral knee, which provides resistance to varus forces and posterolateral (external) tibial rotation. The PFL is composed of two divisions (anterior and posterior) and attaches the popliteus tendon to the fibular styloid. This is also known as the arcuate ligament in older literature. The PFL is a vital component to any reconstruction procedure of the PLC of the knee.

Fibular Collateral Ligament

The FCL (lateral collateral ligament) is the primary static restraint to varus stress of the knee and also provides additional resistance to external tibial rotation. The FCL is rarely injured in isolation. Ligament sectioning studies of the posterolateral structures have shown that significant varus instability cannot be produced without injury to the FCL. Thus, injury to the FCL—as well as any number of the surrounding structures—is necessary for true varus instability.

The FCL attaches on the femur just posterior and proximal to the lateral epicondyle and inserts on the midportion of the lateral fibular head. Attachments from the long head of the biceps femoris insert onto the FCL and a large biceps-FCL bursa is identifiable at the distal aspect of the FCL insertion (Fig. 25-8). The middle third lateral capsular ligament lies deep to the FCL. Similar to the medial capsular thickenings, the lateral knee capsule exists as meniscofemoral and meniscotibial ligamentous attachments. These ligaments provide secondary restraint to varus stress. Avulsion of the meniscotibial portion of the middle third lateral capsular ligament may produce a characteristic Segond fracture or a soft-tissue avulsion variant.

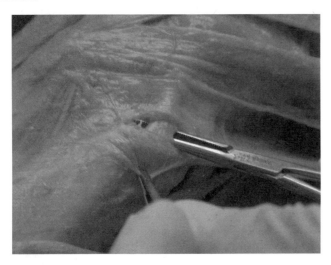

Figure 25-8 Lateral view, left knee, demonstrating a horizontal incision through the anterior arm of the long head of the biceps femoris to expose the biceps bursa. The hemostat is medial to the distal aspect of the FCL.

Diagnosis

History and Physical Examination

- The signs and symptoms of injury to the posterolateral structures depend on various factors that should be considered for each individual case.
  - The extent of injury, the timing of injury (acute vs. chronic), mechanical alignment, gait pattern, presence of knee hyperextension, and patient age and activity level are all important factors to consider when assessing patients with posterolateral instability.
- Patients with knee hyperextension and a varus alignment may present with a varus thrust gait and instability, which is particularly disabling.
  - Patients with minimal knee hyperextension and valgus alignment may have significant objective instability but clinically have relatively few symptoms.
- Patients with posterolateral instability will typically complain of instability that is most noticeable near full extension as a "toggling" instability near extension.
  - The knee may also subjectively "buckle" into hyperextension.
- Patients may also have particular difficulty with stairs and side-to-side activities.
- When examining patients, it is important to remember the normal function of the posterolateral structures: restraint to varus, external tibial rotation, and posterior tibial translation near full extension.
  - Thus, injury to the posterolateral structures will produce laxity to varus stress, external tibial rotation, and posterior tibial stress near extension.
  - All clinical examination tests should be compared with the contralateral unaffected knee to assess side-to-side differences.
  - In addition, a detailed neurovascular exam should be performed because up to 15% of grade III PLC injuries will have a concomitant common peroneal nerve injury.

Testing

Dial Test. The dial test attempts to identify the degree of instability to external tibial rotation. The femur is stabilized while the foot, ankle, and tibia are externally rotated at both 30 and 90 degrees of knee flexion. An increase of external rotation (as noted by the position of the tibial tubercle) of 10 to 15 degrees, compared with the contralateral side, is consistent with an injury to the PLC structures. Greater than 10 degrees of increased external rotation at 90 degrees of knee flexion indicates that the PCL and/or ACL may also be injured. Conversely, isolated PLC injuries usually have less than 5 degrees of increased external rotation at 90 degrees.

Posterior Drawer Test

- The posterior drawer test attempts to identify the degree of posterior tibial translation.
- The position of the anterior tibia relative to the femoral condyles is noted, whereas a posteriorly directed force is applied to the tibia with the knee in 30 and 90 degrees of knee flexion.
- Combined injury to the PCL and PLC will show increased posterior tibial translation at both 30 and 90 degrees of flexion.
- Isolated injury to the PLC will show increased posterior tibial translation at 30 degrees, but not 90 degrees.
- These examination findings confirm that the PCL is the primary restraint to posterior tibial translation at all flexion angles, whereas the PLC resists posterior tibial translation mainly near full extension.

Posterolateral Drawer Test

- The posterolateral drawer test assesses the degree of combined external tibial rotation and posterior tibial translation.
- The patient is supine with the knee flexed to 80 to 90 degrees and the hip flexed to 45 degrees.
- A posterior drawer test is then performed with the foot held in internal rotation, neutral, and external rotation.
- Injury to the PCL will show increased posterior tibial translation with the foot in neutral and internal rotation.
- Injury to the PLC will show increased posterior tibial translation with the foot in external rotation (as compared with the contralateral unaffected knee).
- Combined PCL and PLC injuries will show increased posterior translation in all foot positions.
- The sensitivity of the posterolateral drawer test for injury to the PLC has been shown to be 70% to 75%.

External Rotation Recurvatum Test

- The external rotation recurvatum test assesses the integrity of the posterior structures through the amount of existent knee hyperextension.
- The patient is supine with the knees and hips extended.
- The great toe of each extremity is then lifted off the table sequentially and assessed for the degree of hyperextension and external tibial rotation present.
- Increased hyperextension and external rotation of the affected extremity indicates PLC instability with a concurrent cruciate ligament injury.

- We have rarely found this test to be positive with an isolated PLC injury.

Reverse Pivot Shift Test

- The reverse pivot shift test assesses the amount of posterolateral tibial rotation.
- This test is the opposite maneuver from the pivot shift test used to assess for ACL stability.
- In the reverse pivot shift test, the knee is started at 90 degrees of flexion.
- The foot is then externally rotated, while a valgus force is applied at the knee, thus causing posterolateral tibial subluxation.
- As the leg is brought slowly into extension, the iliotibial band will act to statically reduce the tibia at 30 to 40 degrees of flexion.
- This test has high variability and low specificity, and up to 35% of normal knees will have a positive reverse pivot shift test during an examination under anesthesia.
- Most normal knees with some amount of genu recurvatum will have a positive reverse pivot shift test.

Varus Stress Test at 30 Degrees of Flexion

- The varus stress test is used to assess the primary static stabilizer of the knee, the FCL.
- The patient is supine while the examiner stabilizes the foot with one hand and places the other hand over the lateral joint line (while simultaneously stabilizing the femur) as a varus stress is applied to the knee at 30 degrees flexion.
- Laxity is graded according to the AMA guidelines (Table 25-1).
- We have found this test to be the most important test to assess for a posterolateral knee injury.

Radiologic Examination

Radiographs

- Anteroposterior, lateral, and patella sunrise views should be obtained for all injuries about the knee.
- Most often, plain radiographs are normal but it is important to determine if any fractures or ligamentous avulsion injuries have occurred before planning any treatment.
- Plain radiographs may reveal a proximal fibular tip avulsion fracture, a fibular head or styloid fracture (arcuate fracture), an avulsion of Gerdy's tubercle, a tibial plateau fracture, a tibiofemoral dislocation, or a Segond fracture.
    - As described previously, a Segond fracture is an avulsion of the meniscotibial portion of the midthird lateral capsular ligament and is commonly seen with a concomitant ACL injury.
    - An arcuate fracture refers to a fracture of the fibular head and styloid in which the biceps femoris insertion, fabellofibular ligament, PFL, and FCL are usually attached to the fracture fragment.
        - Open reduction and internal fixation are usually necessary for all displaced or unstable arcuate fractures.

- Stress radiographs may be obtained to help quantitate the amount of lateral joint line opening with a varus stress at 30 degrees of knee flexion.
    - Comparison should be made to the unaffected knee as well. In the skeletally immature patient, stress radiography should be obtained to verify that a Salter-Harris fracture is not responsible for the knee instability.
- Standing, full-length anteroposterior radiographs of the affected lower extremity should be obtained for all patients with chronic PLC injuries to assess the mechanical alignment.
    - An alteration in the mechanical axis through the medial aspect of the knee will usually result in abnormal joint reactive forces with PLC injuries.
    - Most commonly, varus alignment will displace the weight-bearing axis medially, placing the medial compartment in compression and the lateral compartment in tension. Severe clinical instability and varus thrust gait may result.
    - By realigning the mechanical axis through the center of the knee with a proximal tibial opening wedge osteotomy, normal balanced joint reactive forces are reproduced, creating a much more stable knee.
    - Failure to correct the varus malalignment before any ligamentous reconstruction will lead to an unacceptably high rate of failure and recurrent instability.
    - Patients with chronic ligamentous injuries and varus alignment should have a proximal tibial opening wedge osteotomy to correct their malalignment before any ligamentous reconstruction of the knee.
    - A certain subset of these patients will have enough clinical stability after the osteotomy that a subsequent ligamentous reconstruction becomes unnecessary.

Magnetic Resonance Imaging

- MRI has been shown to predictably identify and assess the structures of the PLC of the knee.
- Standard high-resolution imaging sequences—as well as thin-cut coronal oblique views oriented along the course of the popliteus tendon (which include the entire fibular head)—are necessary for accurate diagnosis (Fig. 25-9).
- MRI may be especially useful in the acutely injured and painful knee in which an accurate and comprehensive examination is not possible.
- Most importantly, accurate assessment of the menisci, articular cartilage, and surrounding muscles and ligaments is useful for appropriate surgical planning.

Treatment

Isolated Posterolateral Corner Injuries

Isolated Grade I and II Instabilities

- The treatment of isolated grade I and II PLC instability is almost always nonsurgical.
- Isolated grade I and II injuries typically result from low-energy injuries and often cause little functional impairment, particularly in patients with valgus alignment and no knee hyperextension.

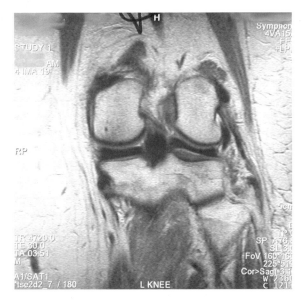

Figure 25-9   Coronal MRI scan, left knee, demonstrating both a tear of the meniscotibial capsule off the tibia and the FCL off the fibular head.

- Treatment consists of immobilization of the knee in full extension for 3 weeks, followed by a functional rehabilitation program.
- Quadriceps strengthening exercises (straight-leg raises, quadriceps setting exercises, and leg presses) and an exercise bike are implemented as soon as tolerated after the immobilization.
- Emphasis on full functional recovery to include full range of motion, no laxity, and adequate strength within the next 4 to 6 weeks is stressed to the patient.
- Patients who do not respond to initial rehabilitation and those with varus alignment and grade II instability should be carefully re-evaluated 4 months after injury.
- A subset of patients who do not respond to the initial rehabilitation may have lateral meniscal hypermobility caused by tearing of the popliteomeniscal fascicles.
  - This may present itself as lateral joint line pain accentuated by placing the affected knee in the figure-4 position.
  - During arthroscopy, a hypermobile meniscus tends to sublux medially with varus stress and laterally with valgus stress. If the lateral meniscus is found to be unstable to arthroscopic probing, patients may benefit from repair of the popliteomeniscal fascicles back to the lateral meniscus to better stabilize the meniscus.
  - In a study by Kannus et al., it was found that isolated grade II injuries generally do favorably, whereas grade III injuries do poorly.

Isolated Grade III Instability
- Grade III PLC injuries do poorly with nonoperative treatment.
  - It is generally believed that the lateral and posterolateral structures do not heal after injury. Sectioning

of the FCL and popliteus tendon in a rabbit model has confirmed that these structures do not heal after rupture.
  - As such, surgical repair or reconstruction becomes necessary for the more severe PLC injuries.
- Anatomic repair of individual structures as soon as possible, usually within the first 1 to 2 weeks after injury, is generally advised.
  - Acute repairs have a more favorable outcome for a number of reasons. Individual structures are more easily identified early after injury.
  - Scar formation after the first 2 weeks complicates the repair, as normal tissue planes are lost and muscles and ligaments have retracted. In addition, it can be very difficult to identify the common peroneal nerve after the onset of scar tissue planes.
  - After the repair, early range of motion is instituted as the integrity of the repair allows.
- Initial arthroscopic evaluation may be performed to assist surgical decision making, or if intra-articular pathology is suspected by clinical examination and MRI.
  - Arthroscopy may help identify tibial versus femoral-sided lesions, may confirm popliteus tendon or popliteomeniscal fascicle injury, and may demonstrate the severity of the injury through a lateral compartment "drive-through sign" (Fig. 25-10).
  - The arthroscopic portion of the procedure should be limited to prevent excessive fluid extravasation, which may interfere with subsequent open surgical exploration.
- The open surgical approach involves a lateral curvilinear incision beginning distally at Gerdy's tubercle and traveling proximally along the posterior third of the iliotibial band.
  - The iliotibial band is split, and a posteriorly based skin flap is used to expose the lateral structures (Fig. 25-11).
  - Peroneal nerve neurolysis is performed to decom-

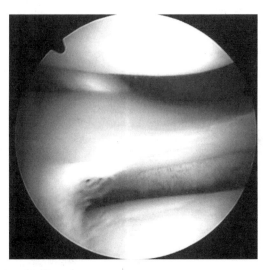

Figure 25-10   Arthroscopic view, lateral component of a knee, demonstrating gapping consistent with a grade III posterolateral knee injury and its "drive-through" sign.

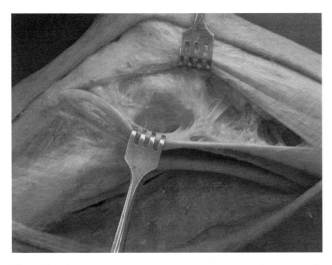

Figure 25-11   Lateral view, left knee, demonstrating the posteriorly based skin flap and split superficial layer of the iliotibial band (retractors). The lateral capsule over the deep femoral structures is exposed.

press the nerve and to gain access to the structures that attach to the fibular head.
  - An arthrotomy incision is made 1 cm anterior to the FCL to assess the popliteus tendon and popliteomeniscal fascicles.
- Many techniques have been described for repair and reconstruction of the posterolateral structures.
  - Suture anchors, recess procedures, direct suture repair, and allograft or autograft reconstructions are all possible surgical options.
  - Irrespective of the technique used, the most important aspect to any surgical approach is to perform an anatomic repair of individual structures to restore normal muscle and ligament anatomy and to attempt early knee motion postoperatively.
- Avulsions of the popliteus tendon or FCL off the femur should be repaired using a recess procedure.
  - The recess procedure is performed using a bone tunnel directed just anterior and proximal to the medial epicondyle to avoid the intercondylar notch.
  - Sutures tied into the avulsed structures are pulled into a small bone tunnel and tied over a button on the medial femur.
- Proximal fibular avulsion fractures, or arcuate fractures, involve the PFL, insertions of the long and short head of the biceps femoris, the FCL, and the fabellofibular ligament.
  - Open reduction and internal fixation using cerclage or tension-band technique with nonabsorbable suture or wire are indicated.
- Ligamentous injuries without bony attachments are repaired using suture anchors or direct suture repair, depending on the proximity to its anatomic bony insertion site.

Postoperative Management
- Early range of motion without compromise of the surgical repair is ideal. This can be guided on an individual basis, depending on the intraoperative assessment and integrity of the repair.
- Patients are non-weight-bearing, with a knee immobilizer in full extension (avoiding hyperextension) for the first 6 weeks.
- Passive range of motion, quadriceps setting exercises, and straight-leg raises (performed in the knee immobilizer) are instituted during this period.
- At 6 weeks, the knee immobilizer is discontinued, weight-bearing is slowly progressed as tolerated, and a stationary bike with low resistance is begun.
- Hamstring strengthening and isotonic exercises are not started until 4 months postoperatively.
- In cases in which the surgical repair is tenuous, 2 to 4 weeks of cast immobilization may be necessary.
  - Patients are placed into a long-leg cast with neutral plantar flexion, 60 degrees of knee flexion, and slight internal rotation of the tibia.
  - External tibial rotation should be avoided because this may adversely stress the repaired posterolateral structures.

Combined PLC Injuries and Other Grade III Ligamentous Injuries
- Concomitant injury to other ligaments of the knee is common with PLC injuries.
- As with isolated PLC injuries, combined ligamentous injuries should be repaired within the first 1 to 2 weeks of injury.
- Primary repair of the posterolateral structures should be performed during the same surgical setting as reconstruction or repair of the other ligaments.
- It is not recommended to stage repairs or reconstructions because they could result in the initial surgical procedure stretching out.
- Failure to repair (or recognize) injury to the posterolateral structures has been shown to compromise the integrity and longevity of reconstructed cruciate ligaments.
  - Markolf used a cadaver model to demonstrate that sectioning of the PLC in varus knees increased the force on the ACL at all flexion angles and on the PCL at flexion angles greater than 45 degrees.
  - LaPrade has similarly shown increased force on ACL grafts at both 0 and 30 degrees of flexion, and PCL grafts at all flexion angles, after sectioning of the posterolateral structures and application of a varus stress.
  - It is therefore recommended to perform anatomic reconstruction of the PLC at the same time as cruciate ligament reconstruction to best restore normal knee mechanics and long-term stability.
- For combined PLC and ACL injuries, it is recommended that the posterolateral structures are repaired first, followed by ACL reconstruction graft fixation.
  - This avoids excessive external rotation during tensioning of the ACL graft.
- For combined PLC and PCL injuries, it is recommended that the PCL is tensioned first at 90 degrees of knee flexion.
  - It makes no difference whether the PCL or PLC is repaired first (as tensioning of the PCL at 90 degrees

of flexion does not cause an increase in external rotation in PLC-deficient knees), so it is recommended to secure the PCL graft in its tunnels first to restore normal anteroposterior position of the tibia on the femur.

■ Postoperative rehabilitation is similar to that described for isolated grade III PLC injuries.

■ Early range of motion, as the repair allows, is stressed to avoid complications of knee arthrofibrosis.

Chronic Grade III PLC Instability

■ Unlike acute injuries, chronic posterolateral instability must first be addressed through the assessment of the mechanical alignment of the affected lower extremity.

■ Failure to correct genu varus alignment and return the mechanical axis to the lateral compartment will frequently result in failure of the PLC repair or reconstruction (as the genu varus and resultant varus thrust gait will place excessive tension on the lateral structures, causing stretching of the reconstructed tissues over time).

■ As such, chronic posterolateral instability with abnormal mechanical alignment will require a corrective osteotomy before any ligamentous reconstruction.

■ An opening wedge medial proximal tibial osteotomy to correct the mechanical axis to the lateral compartment is the preferred approach (Fig. 25-12).

  ▪ An opening wedge osteotomy has the advantage of tightening the posterior capsule and oblique popliteal ligament complex, which ultimately fosters additional posterolateral stability.

  ▪ An external fixator or plate fixation with allograft matrix provides satisfactory fixation.

■ Patients are reassessed for instability at 6 months postoperatively, once the osteotomy has healed and the patients have worked on a lower extremity strengthening program.

  ▪ In some cases, correction of the malalignment into slight valgus will create sufficient subsequent stability to obviate a need for further ligamentous reconstruction.

  ▪ If subjective and objective instabilities persists after the osteotomy, a second-stage PLC reconstruction should be performed.

Surgical Technique

■ Primary repair of the injured ligaments in chronic injuries is usually not possible due to scar formation, loss of tissue planes, and retraction of torn structures.

  ▪ As a result, the integrity of the posterolateral structures is less important than in the acute setting, and MRI may be unnecessary for preoperative assessment.

■ Multiple techniques have been described for the treatment of chronic grade III posterolateral instability.

  ▪ Most current reconstructions function as sling procedures, are not anatomic, and may rely on using remaining local dynamic structures.

  ▪ These methods include FCL reconstruction, femoral bone block advancements, biceps femoris tenodesis, various allograft or autograft reconstruction weave procedures, and popliteal recess procedures.

  ▪ These techniques have only variable success in restoring early knee stability and do not specifically address anatomic reconstruction of the main stabilizing structures of the knee: the FCL, the popliteus tendon, and the PFL.

■ As for acute repairs, anatomic reconstruction of the key ligamentous structures seems the ideal way to best restore normal knee biomechanics, function, and long-term stability.

  ▪ LaPrade et al. have recently described an anatomic reconstruction procedure of the FCL, popliteus tendon, and PFL using an Achilles tendon allograft.

  ▪ The technique involves use of an Achilles tendon allograft split into two grafts.

  ▪ Bone blocks from each graft are placed into the anatomic femoral attachment sites of the popliteus tendon and FCL.

  ▪ Appropriately placed tunnels are made in the fibula and tibia, and the tubularized grafts are passed and secured into place (Fig. 25-13). Results of this technique in a cadaver model demonstrate excellent restoration of static stability to the PLC during varus and external rotation stresses.

  ▪ Through an anatomic reconstruction approach to the key posterolateral structures (which preserves the remaining dynamic supporting elements), we believe this method to be the treatment of choice for

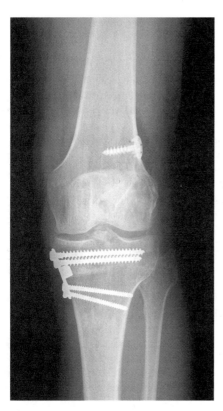

Figure 25-12   Healed left knee, proximal medial opening wedge osteotomy (anteroposterior radiograph).

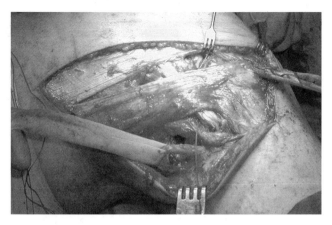

Figure 25-13 Lateral view, right knee, demonstrating the fibular collateral ligament graft in place, the common peroneal nerve (retracted), and the popliteus tendon and popliteofibular ligament grafts exiting anteriorly on the tibia.

the reconstruction of chronic grade III posterolateral instability.

■ Early results of a prospective study (in progress), with more than 100 patients using this technique, are promising.

SUGGESTED READING

Fetto JF, Marshall JL. Medial collateral ligament injuries of the knee: a rationale for treatment. Clin Orthop 1977;132:206–218.

Harner CD, Vogrin TM, Höher J, et al. Biomechanical analysis of a posterior cruciate ligament reconstruction: deficiency of the posterolateral structures as a cause of graft failure. Am J Sports Med 2000;28:32–39.

Hughston JC. The importance of the posterior oblique ligament in repairs of acute tears of the medial ligaments in knees with and without an associated rupture of the anterior cruciate ligament: results of long-term follow-up. J Bone Joint Surg Am 1994;76: 1328–1344.

Hughston JC, Jacobson KE. Chronic posterolateral rotatory instability of the knee. J Bone Joint Surg Am 1985;67:351–359.

Indelicato PA. Non-operative treatment of complete tears of the medial collateral ligament of the knee. J Bone Joint Surg Am 1983;65: 323–329.

Kannus P. Long-term results of conservatively treated medial collateral ligament injuries of the knee joint. Clin Orthop 1988;226: 103–112.

Kannus P. Nonoperative treatment of grade II and III sprains of the lateral ligament compartment of the knee. Am J Sports Med 1989; 17:83–88.

LaPrade RF. Arthroscopic evaluation of the lateral compartment of knees with grade 3 posterolateral knee complex injuries. Am J Sports Med 1997;25:596–602.

LaPrade RF, Johansen S, Wentorf FA, et al. An analysis of an anatomical posterolateral knee reconstruction. Am J Sports Med 2004;32: 1705–1714.

LaPrade RF, Muench C, Wentorf F, et al. The effect of injury to the posterolateral structures of the knee on force in a posterior cruciate ligament graft: a biomechanical study. Am J Sports Med 2002;30: 233–238.

LaPrade RF, Resig S, Wentorf F, et al. The effects of grade III posterolateral knee complex injuries on the anterior cruciate ligament graft force: a biomechanical analysis. Am J Sports Med 1999;27: 469–475.

LaPrade RF, Terry GC. Injuries to the posterolateral aspect of the knee: association of anatomic injury patterns with clinical instability. Am J Sports Med 1997;25:433–438.

Lundberg M, Messner K. Long-term prognosis of isolated partial medial collateral ligament ruptures: a ten-year clinical and radiographic evaluation of a prospectively observed group of patients. Am J Sports Med 1996;24:160–163.

Markolf KL, Wascher DC, Finerman GAM. The effect of section of the posterolateral structures. J Bone Joint Surg Am 1993;75:387–394.

O'Brien SJ, Warren RF, Pavlov H, et al. Reconstruction of the chronically insufficient anterior cruciate ligament with the central third of the patellar ligament. J Bone Joint Surg Am 1991;73:278–286.

Shelbourne D, Patel DV. Management of combined injuries of the anterior cruciate and medial collateral ligaments. J Bone Joint Surg Am 1995;77:800–806.

Terry GC, LaPrade RF. The biceps femoris muscle complex at the knee: its anatomy and injury patterns associated with acute anterolateral-anteromedial rotatory instability. Am J Sports Med 1996;24:2–8.

Terry GC, LaPrade RF. The posterolateral aspect of the knee: anatomy and surgical approach. Am J Sports Med 1996;24:732–739.

Veltri DM, Deng XH, Torzilli PA, et al. The role of the cruciate and posterolateral ligaments in stability of the knee. Am J Sports Med 1995;23:436–443.

POSTERIOR CRUCIATE LIGAMENT INJURIES

JEFFREY A. RIHN
PAUL GAUSE
RICK CUNNINGHAM
CHRISTOPHER D. HARNER

The posterior cruciate ligament (PCL) is one of the main stabilizing structures of the knee. Injuries of the PCL occur between 3% and 38% of all acute knee injuries, with a higher incidence reported in trauma patients who are involved in motor vehicle accidents or who sustain sports-related injuries. Despite a recent increase in PCL research, our understanding of PCL injury and treatment continues to lag behind that of the anterior cruciate ligament (ACL). The overwhelming majority of PCL research is basic science in nature, which has provided a scientific rationale for the current approach to PCL injury. There remains, however, a lack of solid clinical outcomes studies. Much debate exists regarding the natural history of PCL injury, surgical indications for treatment, and optimal technique for PCL reconstruction. This chapter provides a summary of the anatomy and biomechanics of the PCL, an overview of the principles of diagnosis and decision making regarding the treatment of PCL injuries, and a detailed discussion of current PCL reconstruction techniques.

ANATOMY AND FUNCTION

The PCL averages between 32 and 38 mm long. It has a cross-sectional area of 31.2 mm^2 at its midsubstance level, which is 1.5 times that of the ACL. The PCL originates on the lateral border of the medial femoral condyle at the junction of the medial wall and roof of the intercondylar notch. The footprint of femoral attachment is 32 mm in diameter and terminates 3 mm proximal to the articular cartilage margin of the femoral condyle. The tibial insertion is located within a depression between the posterior aspect of the medial and lateral plateaus, approximately 1 cm distal to the joint line (Fig. 26-1). The PCL tibial insertion site lies just anterior to the popliteal neurovascular bundle, necessitating particular consideration when performing PCL reconstruction.

Two PCL bundles—the anterolateral bundle (ALB) and the posteromedial bundle (PMB)—have been defined (Fig. 26-2). The names of the ALB and PMB are based on the

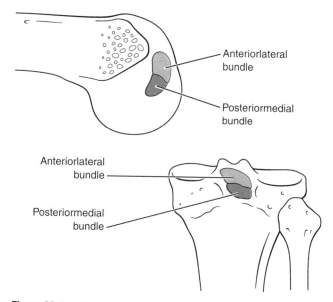

Figure 26-1 Illustration of the femoral and tibial insertion sites of the anterolateral and posteromedial bundles of the posterior cruciate ligament. (From Harner CD, Hoher J. Evaluation and treatment of posterior cruciate ligament injuries. Am J Sports Med 1998;26:471–482.)

femoral origin and tibial insertion for each bundle. The ALB is two times larger in the cross-sectional area than the PMB. Functionally, the two components have different tensioning patterns that depend on the degree of knee flexion. The larger ALB is under greater tension with increasing flexion (making it the important posterior stabilizer with knee flexion), whereas the PMB is under greater tension with increasing extension (making it the important posterior stabilizer with knee extension). Therefore, tension develops in a reciprocal fashion in each bundle during knee flexion and extension, with very few fibers of the PCL exhibiting isometric behavior. The large, ligamentous insertion sites and the lack of isometry complicate the task of replicating PCL function with a single-bundle PCL graft. These characteristics of the PCL support newer surgical techniques involving double-bundle reconstruction and an increased emphasis on optimizing femoral tunnel placement during PCL reconstruction.

Additionally, anterior and posterior meniscofemoral ligaments have been defined. The meniscofemoral ligaments originate from the posterior horn of the lateral meniscus, run adjacent to the PCL, and insert anteriorly (ligament of Humphrey) and posteriorly (ligament of Wrisberg) to the PCL on the medial femoral condyle (Fig. 26-2). The presence of these ligaments is highly variable. Although it has been suggested that theses ligaments contribute to the anterior-posterior and rotatory stability of the knee, the role of the meniscofemoral ligaments has not been fully characterized.

The PCL is the primary restraint to posterior tibial translation. It resists 85% to 100% of a posteriorly directed knee force at 30 and 90 degrees of knee flexion. Because up to 60% of PCL injuries have associated disruption of the posterolateral structures (PLSs), it is important to understand the contribution of these structures to knee stability. The lateral collateral ligament (LCL), popliteus, popliteofibular ligament, posterolateral joint capsule, and the iliotibial band (ITB) are important secondary restraints to posterior translation of the tibia. The amount of posterior tibial translation increases dramatically when both primary and secondary restraints are disrupted, as in the case of a combined ligament injury.

The PLSs are a primary restraint, and the PCL is a secondary restraint to external tibial rotation. Isolated section of the PLS increases external rotation maximally at 30 degrees and has little effect on external rotation at 90 degrees of knee flexion. Combined PCL and PLS sections increase external rotation at both 30 and 90 degrees. This information is particularly helpful during clinical examination. Increased posterior tibial translation and external rotation at 30 degrees—but not at 90 degrees—of knee flexion indicates an isolated PLS injury, whereas increased posterior translation and external rotation at both 30 and 90 degrees indicates a combined PCL and PLS injury. Failure to recognize and address a PLS injury when performing PCL reconstruction may lead to early failure of the PCL graft.

MECHANISM OF INJURY

The most common mechanism of injury to the PCL is an anterior blow to the proximal tibia, which is classically associated with the "dashboard injury" that occurs during a motor vehicle accident. Hyperflexion is the most common cause of PCL injury in sports, often due to a fall on the flexed knee with the foot in plantar flexion. Isolated PCL injuries occur less frequently than combined ligamentous injuries, which most likely result from a posteriorly directed tibial force with an associated rotational component.

DIAGNOSIS

History

Evaluation of knee injury should begin with a thorough history. The mechanism may be indicative of the severity of

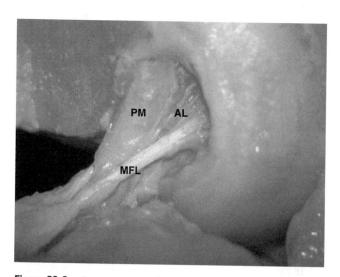

Figure 26-2 Gross specimen demonstrating relationship between the anterolateral (*AL*) and posteromedial (*PM*) bundles of the PCL, and the anterior meniscofemoral ligament (*MFL*) or the ligament of Humphrey.

the injury, whether it is isolated PCL or whether it involves multiple ligaments. In the case of an acute "isolated" PCL injury, the patient may present with only complaints of mild swelling, vague discomfort, and knee stiffness. Patients with isolated PCL injuries do not usually relate a sense of knee instability. A large effusion and substantial loss of motion, instability, and a significant degree of pain should raise concerns for injuries to additional knee structures.

In the setting of trauma, 95% of PCL injuries have associated injuries, including osteochondral, meniscal, and ligamentous injuries. Sixty percent of PCL injuries have associated injury to the PLS. Thus, a thorough examination of all structures of the knee is essential. With any combined ligament injury involving the PCL, knee dislocation and associated neurovascular injuries must be suspected and ruled out. Greater than 50% of knee dislocations spontaneously reduce before presentation. Incidences of associated popliteal artery and peroneal nerve injury ranges are reported to be as high as 45% and 40%, respectively. Mechanism of knee dislocation is not predictive of associated neurovascular injury because injuries to the popliteal artery and peroneal nerve are associated with both high energy (i.e., car accident) and low energy (i.e., twisting during sports activity) injuries. For this reason, a thorough neurovascular examination should promptly be performed in all cases of suspected knee dislocation. Use of an angiogram in evaluation of knee dislocation remains a controversial topic. We currently obtain a popliteal artery angiogram in all cases of suspected knee dislocation, even if palpable pulses are preset in the involved limb. This minimizes the risk of missing a potentially limb-threatening intimal tear in the popliteal artery that may not manifest itself until days after the injury. A more in-depth discussion of the evaluation of knee dislocation is beyond the scope of this chapter.

Physical Examination

The physical examination should begin with an evaluation of the patient's standing, weight-bearing alignment, and gait. Subtle signs of PCL deficiency include tibia vara, external tibial rotation, and genu recurvatum. A slightly bent knee gait may be observed, which allows the patient to avoid terminal extension and excessive external rotation of the tibia on the femur. A varus thrust gait most likely indicates the presence of a combined PCL/PLS injury.

On examination of the injured knee, a mild or moderate effusion may be noted with an isolated PCL injury. Range of motion is usually well preserved and may be symmetric to the noninjured knee. The knee should be examined for signs of collateral ligament and PLS injuries. The LCL and medial collateral ligament (MCL) should be palpated for tenderness, and varus and valgus stress testing should be performed at full extension (stressing PLSs and posteromedial structures) and 30 degrees of flexion (evaluating the integrity of the LCL and MCL). Examination for meniscal injury should include palpation of the medial and lateral joint lines, as well as a flexion McMurray test.

Special care should be undertaken when evaluating the ACL in the setting of PCL disruption. The noninjured knee should be examined first to determine the proper relationship of the tibia to the femur, so that posterior subluxation

of the tibia in the PCL-injured knee can be corrected before assessing anterior laxity. Failure to restore the proper tibial–femoral relationship in a PCL-deficient knee when assessing the ACL may cause the examiner to falsely attribute an increase in anterior-posterior laxity to a torn ACL.

The most sensitive test for PCL deficiency is the posterior drawer test, which is performed with the tibia held in a neutral position and the hip and knee flexed to 45 and 90 degrees, respectively. In performing this test, a posteriorly directed force is applied to the proximal tibia (Fig. 26-3). The extent of posterior translation is determined by assessing the change in the relationship between the medial tibial plateau and the medial femoral condyle. In a normal knee, the medial tibial plateau is usually 1 cm anterior to the medial femoral condyle. A PCL injury should be suspected if this step-off is not present, or if the application of posterior force to the proximal tibia reveals a soft end point.

Severity of PCL injury is graded according to the amount of posterior laxity. A grade I injury is represented by posterior translation of 1 to 5 mm, grade II between 5 and 10 mm (with the anterior border of the tibial plateau lying flush with the femoral condyles), and grade III greater than 10 mm (with the anterior border of the tibial plateau lying posterior to the medial femoral condyle). Grade I and II injuries represent partial PCL tears, whereas grade III injuries represent complete PCL tears and may indicate an associated injury to the PLS.

Additional diagnostic tests for PCL injury have been described. These include Godfrey's test (posterior sag test; Fig. 26-4) and the quadriceps active test. Godfrey's test is performed by flexing the knees and hips of the patient to 90 degrees while the patient is supine. The examiner holds both legs in the air. Gravity causes the tibia of the PCL-deficient leg to rest in a posteriorly subluxated position compared with the intact knee. Posterior tibial translation of the injured leg supports the diagnosis of a PCL injury. The quadriceps active test places the knee at 60 degrees of flexion, with the foot flat on the examination table. The tibia of the PCL-deficient leg is posteriorly subluxated in this position. The patient is asked to fire his or her quadriceps

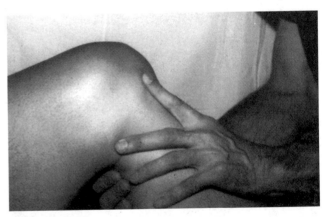

Figure 26-3 Posterior drawer test that is positive for a grade III PCL injury. The knee is held in 90 degrees of flexion. The extent of posterior translation is determined by assessing the step-off between the medial tibial plateau and the medial femoral condyle as a posterior force is applied to the proximal tibia.

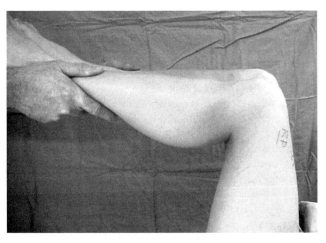

Figure 26-4   Positive posterior sag test. Both knees and hips are held at 90 degrees with the patient supine. Compared with the uninjured knee, the tibia in the PCL-deficient knee subluxes posteriorly.

muscle or extend the knee by sliding the foot on the examination table. When the quadriceps contracts in a PCL-deficient knee, the posteriorly subluxated tibia will visibly translate anteriorly to a reduced position.

Injury to PLS should be ruled out, particularly when the posterior drawer is greater than 10 mm. The tibial external rotation test is used to evaluate the PLS. The test may be performed with the patient supine or prone, with the knee flexed in 30 and then 90 degrees. It is considered positive if the medial border of the foot or the tibial tubercle externally rotates 10 to 15 degrees more than the noninjured side. Increased external rotation at 30 degrees but not 90 degrees is consistent with an isolated PLS injury, whereas increased external rotation at 30 and 90 degrees indicates a combined PLS/PCL injury (Fig. 26-5). The reversed pivot shift test can also be used to assess PLS injury. This test is performed with the patient supine and the knee held in 90 degrees of flexion. The knee is then externally rotated and passively extended. If an injury of the PLS is present, a shift occurs

at 20 to 30 degrees of flexion as the posteriorly subluxated lateral tibia plateau reduces anteriorly. Because of guarding, the reversed pivot shift is often difficult to elicit in the awake patient. It is, however, a useful diagnostic tool during an examination under anesthesia.

Radiographic Examination

Radiographic studies are essential when PCL injury is suspected. These should include a flexion weight-bearing view and a Merchant patellar view, which are helpful in detecting degenerative changes often present in cases of chronic PCL deficiency. Radiographs should be examined closely for evidence of tibial plateau fractures, Gerdy's tubercle avulsions, or fibular head fractures (indicative of a PLS injury). The lateral radiograph is helpful in detecting bony avulsion of the PCL tibial insertion, osteochondral defects, and posterior subluxation of the tibia. Stress radiographs have been shown to be useful in both diagnosing PCL injury and quantifying the associated posterior tibial laxity. The "gravity sag view," a lateral radiograph of the knee flexed to 90 degrees with the hip flexed 45 degrees, has been described in evaluating the tibia-femur step-off in PCL deficiency. In patients with chronic PCL deficiency who complain of pain and instability, a technetium-99 bone scan is helpful in identifying early degenerative changes in the patellofemoral or medial compartment that may not be detected on plain radiographs. These early findings support surgical stabilization to prevent further progression of degenerative joint disease.

Magnetic resonance imaging (MRI) is extremely effective in diagnosing acute PCL injury, with a reported sensitivity and specificity of up to 100%. In addition, MRI is helpful in identifying associated ligamentous, osteochondral, and meniscal injuries. Chronic grade I and II injuries of the PCL have some capacity to heal in an elongated position and may appear normal on MRI. In such cases, an increase in posterior tibial translation on sagittal view may be the only sign of PCL injury. MRI is thus not as sensitive in diagnosing chronic PCL injuries.

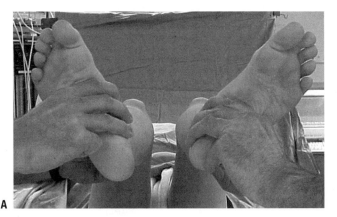
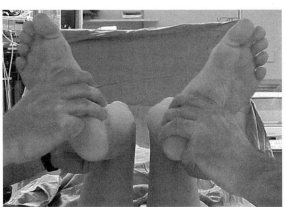

A   B

Figure 26-5   Positive tibial external rotation test. With the patient supine, tibial external rotation of both extremities is tested at both 30 degrees **(A)** and 90 degrees **(B)**. Increased external rotation of the left tibia at both 30 and 90 degrees suggests injuries of both the PLS and PCL.

TREATMENT

The approach to treatment of PCL injuries should take into account the severity of the knee injury, timing, symptoms, patient expectations, and activity level. Although controversy exists regarding the surgical indications for PCL reconstruction, the surgical treatment of certain patterns of PCL injury is agreed on. Most authors agree that avulsion fractures of the PCL should be acutely repaired with sutures through drill holes or screw fixation. This approach to treatment has resulted in a good outcome. Additionally, combined injuries to the PCL and ACL, PCL and PLS, or PCL and MCL should also be surgically reconstructed, preferably within the first 3 weeks after injury. With the exception of these particular scenarios, the treatment decision algorithm for PCL injury should be tailored to the individual patient, with specific attention given to injury severity, timing, and patient expectations. An outline of the treatment protocol for acute and chronic PCL injury can be seen in Algorithms 26-1 and 26-2, respectively.

Nonsurgical Treatment

It is generally accepted that acute, isolated grade I and II PCL injuries can be treated nonoperatively. Conservative treatment involves protected weight-bearing and quadriceps muscle rehabilitation. Patients are usually able to return to sports within 2 to 4 weeks after injury. Treatment of grade III PCL injuries is more controversial. Because of the potential for a subtle injury to the PLS when diagnosis of a grade III PCL injury is made, it is recommended that the knee be splinted in extension for 2 to 4 weeks. Immobilization in extension decreases tension on the ALB of the PCL and the PLS and prevents posterior tibial translation secondary to hamstring contraction and gravity. After 2 to 4 weeks of immobilization, rehabilitation progresses as with grade I and II PCL injuries. Return to sports activity, however, is

delayed for 8 weeks after discontinuation of immobilization (total 10 to 12 weeks). Patients with grade III PCL injuries who develop medial or patellofemoral chondrosis or continued complaints of instability despite adequate physical therapy may require surgical treatment.

Chronic grade I or II PCL tears are treated with physical therapy. Symptomatic patients with recurrent swelling and pain are treated with activity modification because surgical reconstruction of an isolated grade I or II PCL injury does result in a significant improvement in symptoms or function. Chronic grade III PCL injuries are treated surgically if symptoms of pain and/or instability develop or persist despite therapy. Some patients with a symptomatic, chronic grade III PCL injury may in fact have a combined, occult PLS injury. In such combined injuries, reconstruction of the both the PCL and PLS is recommended. Failure to address the injured PLS when performing PCL reconstruction places excessive load on the PCL graft and predisposes the patient to early graft failure.

Surgical Treatment

- When evaluating chronic PCL injuries for surgical intervention, it is important to determine if there is varus malalignment of the knee and to evaluate the patient's gait for the presence of a dynamic varus thrust with ambulation.
    - With these findings, a high tibial osteotomy should be performed before PCL reconstruction.
- A biplanar osteotomy has been used at our institution to correct varus deformity and to reduce dynamic posterior tibial translation (by increasing tibial slope).
- Biomechanical testing has shown that an increase in posterior tibial slope by 5 mm (~4 to 5 degrees) significantly reduces the posterior sag in a PCL-deficient knee.
    - This approach can be used in patients who have

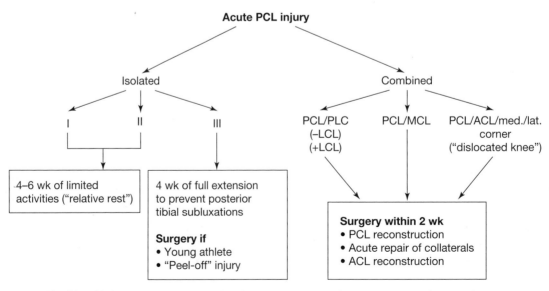

Algorithm 26-1   Treatment algorithm for acute PCL injuries. (After Harner CD, Hoher J. Evaluation and treatment of posterior cruciate ligament injuries. Am J Sports Med 1998;26:471–482.)

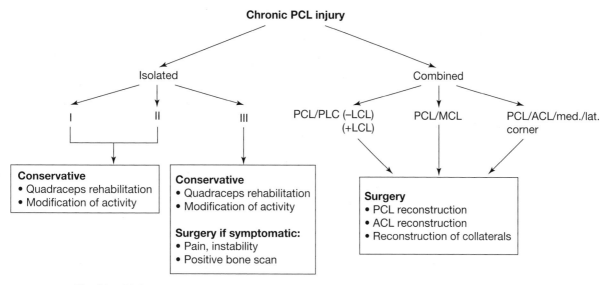

Algorithm 26-2   Treatment algorithm for chronic PCL injuries. (After Harner CD, Hoher J. Evaluation and treatment of posterior cruciate ligament injuries. Am J Sports Med 1998;26:471–482.)

chronic PCL deficiency (or failed PCL surgery) with medial compartment arthritis.
- By combining sagittal slope osteotomy with coronal plane osteotomy (biplanar), the surgeon can reduce the tibia and unload the medial compartment.
- Patients with severe arthrosis should be excluded from consideration for PCL reconstruction.

PCL Repair
- PCL avulsions can be repaired primarily with good results.
- For large bony avulsion, AO screws can be used, whereas smaller fragments can be stabilized by suture repair through drill holes.
- Acute repair of avulsion injuries have superior results when compared with conservative treatment.
- Because the PCL is limited in its healing capacity, primary repair of midsubstance PCL tears is currently not recommended.

PCL Reconstruction
- The two most widely accepted methods of PCL reconstruction are a transtibial technique, using a single- or double-bundled graft and the tibial inlay technique.
- Because of the complexity of tensioning patterns in the two bands of the PCL, it is difficult to reproduce the position and function of the native ligament complex using either technique.

Graft Selection
- Current graft options include both allograft and autograft tissues.
- Considerations in graft selection include length, cross-sectional area, availability, and soft tissue versus bony fixation.
- Autografts commonly used for PCL reconstruction include the patellar tendon, the hamstring tendons, and the quadriceps tendon.

- A patellar tendon autograft is commonly used for PCL reconstruction because it allows for bony fixation at both the femoral and tibial sites of fixation.
- The quadriceps tendon has been popularized due to its large size. The large, cross-sectional area and generous length of the quadriceps tendon graft allow the surgeon to closely approximate size of the native PCL while minimizing problems with graft-tunnel length and size mismatch.
- The disadvantages of autograft tissue include significant donor site morbidity, larger incision size, and increased operative time.
- Allograft tissue is a popular choice for PCL reconstruction, especially in the setting of a combined ligamentous injury.
  - Advantages of the allograft include the avoidance of donor site morbidity, decreased surgical time, and tissue availability in cases of combined ligamentous injury, revision surgery, or double-bundle PCL reconstruction.
  - Disadvantages of the allograft include the increased risk of disease transmission and its considerable cost.
  - Although it has also been shown that allograft tissue exhibits a delay in remodeling and graft incorporation compared with autograft tissue, this difference is not manifested clinically with long-term follow-up.
  - Achilles tendon allograft is a popular graft choice in PCL reconstruction because of its large, cross-sectional area and calcaneal bone plug that allows for bony fixation.

Examination under Anesthesia
- Examination under anesthesia (EUA) is an important component of the evaluation of PCL injury that should be performed before surgical treatment. PCL deficiency

can be confirmed with examination tests discussed previously.

■ Associated injuries are more apparent when the patient is completely relaxed and unable to guard against the examiner.

■ Concomitant PLS injuries that are subtle or even missed on initial clinical examination are often more evident under anesthesia, with asymmetric tibial external rotation and a positive reversed pivot shift test.

■ Contralateral comparison is essential to minimize the risk of falsely diagnosing ligamentous injuries.

Diagnostic Arthroscopy

■ Diagnostic arthroscopy allows for a final confirmation of injury before reconstructing the PCL.

■ A thorough evaluation of all intra-articular structures should be performed and associated injuries should be documented.

■ Presence of associated meniscal and/or osteochondral pathology often affects the surgical treatment plan.

■ Because the PCL is encased in synovium, injury to the ligament can be obscured unless an effort is made to visualize the ligament directly.

■ Several arthroscopic signs can aid in the diagnosing PCL injury.

■ Because of posterior subluxation of the tibia in a PCL-deficient, the intact ACL appears lax (ACL "pseudolaxity").

■ Application of an anterior drawer reduces the tibia and allows for an accurate assessment of the native ACL.

■ Failure to do so may result in misdiagnosis and an unnecessary ACL reconstruction.

■ In the setting of chronic PCL deficiency, chondrosis of the medial and patellofemoral compartments may be noted on arthroscopic examination.

Transtibial Tunnel Reconstruction: Single- and Double-bundle Techniques

■ For both single- and double-bundle transtibial PCL reconstruction, the patient is positioned supine on the operating table, and an examination under anesthesia is performed.

■ The use of a tourniquet is a controversial subject.

■ Although it allows for better hemostasis during surgery, it may increase the risk of venous thrombosis and neurapraxia.

■ At our institution, a well-padded tourniquet is applied to the upper thigh but is not inflated unless necessary during the procedure.

■ A sandbag, on which the foot is rested when the injured knee is flexed, is secured to the operating table at the level of the midthigh.

■ A lateral post is placed at the level of the tourniquet to prevent lateral movement of the flexed leg.

■ The setup should permit the operative knee to be taken trough a full range of motion.

■ The healthy leg is fully extended, supported by the operating table.

■ A Foley catheter is placed, and a Doppler ultrasound is used to confirm the distal pulses at the start and finish of the case.

■ Fluid extravasation and resultant compartment syndrome are also potential problems in arthroscopic reconstruction of the PCL injured knee, especially in the setting of an acute or multiple ligamentous injury.

■ In these cases, we recommend the use of gravity flow through the arthroscope rather than using a fluid pump to reduce this risk.

■ The surgeon should palpate the calf and thigh throughout the case.

■ If there is any concern about excessive fluid extravasation, the arthroscopic procedure should be abandoned and an open reconstruction performed.

■ After the patient is prepared and draped in the usual sterile fashion, standard diagnostic arthroscopy is performed.

■ It is important to document any injury to the PCL and also to address any associated intra-articular pathology.

■ We also carefully assess the meniscofemoral ligaments, as every effort is made to preserve these if one or both of them is intact.

■ Depending on graft selection, the graft is then either harvested or thawed and prepared according to the preferred technique of the surgeon.

■ In cases of midsubstance PCL tears, the remaining ligament is debrided so that tibial and femoral insertion sites are exposed.

■ Visualization of the tibial stump of the torn PCL is accomplished with a 70-degree arthroscope in the AL portal.

■ The scope allows adequate visualization of the tibial insertion site below the slope of the posterior tibial plateau.

■ A posteromedial portal is then established.

■ To avoid injury to the saphenous vein and nerve, the arthroscope is used to transilluminate the posteromedial corner while creating the posteromedial portal.

■ A curette or periosteal elevator is then used to elevate the posterior capsule off the tibia.

■ A shaver is passed through the posteromedial portal and under constant scope visualization, and with the shaver directed anteriorly at all times, the tibial PCL insertion site is debrided.

■ The surgeon must be very careful during this portion of the procedure not to violate the posterior capsule and risk neurovascular injury.

■ A 15-mm offset PCL guide set at 50 to 55 degrees is then introduced through the anteromedial portal and positioned in the distal and lateral aspects of the PCL tibial insertion site under arthroscopic visualization (Fig. 26-6).

■ The starting point for the guidewire on the anterior tibia is 4 cm distal to the joint line and 2 cm medial to the tibial tubercle.

■ In preparation for the drilling of the tibial tunnel, a 2- to 3-cm vertical skin incision is made.

■ A 3/32 Kirchner wire is then advanced under arthroscopic visualization with the knee in 90 degrees of flexion.

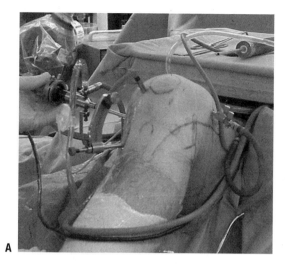
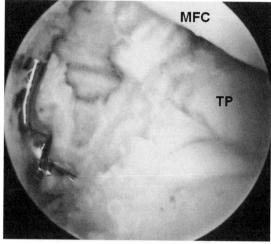

Figure 26-6 **A:** Arthroscopic setup during drilling of the tibial tunnel. The tibial drill guide is introduced through the anteromedial portal. **B:** The tibial drill guide is positioned under arthroscopic visualization in the posterolateral aspect of the tibial PCL insertion site. *TP*, tibial plateau; *MFC*, medial femoral condyle.

- A lateral radiograph or fluoroscopic image is obtained to confirm proper guidewire placement.
  - On the lateral view, the guidewire should be placed at the level of the proximal tibia-fibula joint line and should exit the posterior tibial cortex approximately 10 mm below the tibial plateau (Fig. 26-7).
- If the guidewire is too proximal on the PCL tibial insertion site, a 3-mm or a 5-mm parallel wire guide is used to optimize placement of the guidewire.
- After confirmation of accurate tibial tunnel guidewire placement, the tibial tunnel is drilled.
- A curette is placed directly over the guidewire at the site of tibial PCL insertion to protect the posterior structures during drilling.
- A 10-mm compaction drill bit is passed under direct arthroscopic visualization with a 30-degree arthroscope positioned through the posteromedial portal.
- The drill bit is initially passed using power and is then completed by hand.
  - This allows the surgeon to feel the far cortex and minimizes the risk of overdrilling and perforation of the posterior capsule.
- Using dilators, the PCL tibial tunnel is then expanded to 11 mm in 0.5-mm increments.
- The femoral tunnel is then established.
- The single-bundle PCL reconstruction aims to simulate the larger and stiffer ALB of the PCL.
  - The femoral tunnel is thus positioned at the center of the insertion site of the ALB on the lateral wall of the medial femoral condyle (Fig. 26-8).
  - Several studies have demonstrated that the location of the femoral tunnel in PCL reconstruction significantly affects the resulting knee kinematics.
  - At our institution, we center the femoral tunnel 7 mm off of the articular margin at the 1 o'clock position in the right knee or at the 11 o'clock position in the left knee.
- The femoral guidewire is inserted under arthroscopic visualization through the AL portal (Fig. 26-9).
- The guidewire is then overdrilled with a 10-mm compaction drill to a depth of 30 mm.
- Using dilators, the femoral tunnel is expanded to 11 mm in 0.5-mm increments.
- A 3.2-mm drill bit is use to create a tunnel exit out through the medial femoral condyle to allow graft passage and tensioning during fixation.
- In the single-bundle technique, the method of graft passage is determined by the type of graft utilized.
  - If a patellar tendon graft is used for PCL reconstruc-

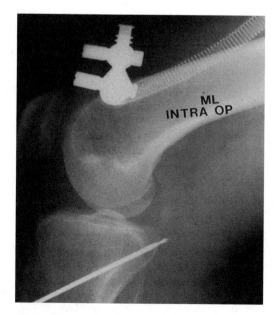

Figure 26-7 Intraoperative lateral x-ray taken to confirm the position of the tibial tunnel guidewire before drilling the tibial tunnel. The guidewire should exit 10 mm distal to the tibial plateau.

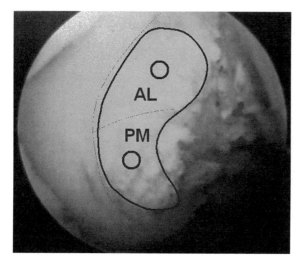

Figure 26-8 Arthroscopic view of the femoral insertion sites of the anterolateral (*AL*) and posteromedial (*PM*) bundles of the posterior cruciate ligament. The femoral tunnel guidewire should be positioned in the center of the insertion site of the AL bundle.

tion, we recommend passing the graft from the tibia to the femur.

■ This will allow easier graft passage around the posterior corner of the tibia.

■ We currently use the Achilles tendon allograft for single-bundle PCL reconstruction.

■ Graft passage is initiated by placing an 18-gauge wire loop up through the tibial tunnel into the knee joint. The wire loop is then pulled out through the AL portal.

■ The whip-stitch sutures from the soft-tissue end of the Achilles allograft are pulled into the knee through the AL portal and out through the tibial tunnel using the wire loop.

■ The soft-tissue end of the graft is then advanced into the tibial tunnel.

■ A Beath needle is placed through the AL portal and advanced into the femoral tunnel and out through the skin of the anteromedial thigh.

■ The AL portal is enlarged to 2 cm.

■ The bone plug sutures of the graft are threaded through the eye of the Beath needle, and the needle and sutures are then pulled out through the femoral tunnel, advancing the bone plug retrograde into the femoral tunnel.

■ The tendinous side of the bone plug is oriented anterior in the femoral tunnel.

■ The double-bundle PCL reconstruction uses two femoral tunnels and a single tibial tunnel in an attempt to recreate the functional anatomy of the ALB and PMB of the native PCL.

■ Double-bundle PCL reconstruction has been shown to more closely restore normal knee biomechanics throughout the entire flexion-extension cycle.

■ Harner et al., in a biomechanical study comparing the single- and double-bundle PCL reconstruction techniques, reported that the double-bundle reconstruction restored posterior tibial laxity to that of the intact knee and restored the in situ force of the PCL more closely to the intact knee than did the single-bundle reconstruction.

■ Two divergent femoral tunnels are required for the double-bundle reconstruction.

■ The femoral tunnel for the AL graft is placed as discussed for the single-bundle technique.

■ For the PM graft, a 7-mm diameter femoral tunnel is placed within the PCL footprint inferior to and slightly deeper in the intercondylar notch than the AL tunnel (3 to 4 mm off the articular margin, at the 2:30 position in the right knee or the 9:30 position in the left knee).

■ A bone bridge of at least 5 mm should be preserved to avoid tunnel bridge collapse (Fig. 26-10).

■ A PCL femoral insertion area of 128 mm² provides enough surface area to accommodate the two tunnels.

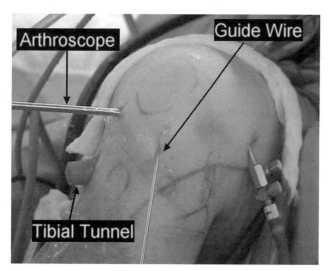

Figure 26-9 Arthroscopic setup during drilling of the femoral tunnel. The femoral tunnel guidewire is placed through the AL portal. Guidewire placement and drilling of the femoral tunnel is visualized arthroscopically through the anteromedial portal.

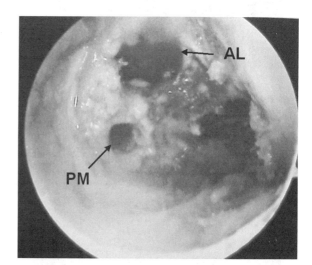

Figure 26-10 Arthroscopic view of the anterolateral (*AL*) and posteromedial (*PM*) femoral tunnels in double-bundle PCL reconstruction. A 5-mm bone bridge is preserved to minimize the risk of bone bridge collapse.

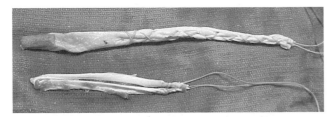

Figure 26-11 Graft selection in double-bundle PCL reconstruction includes an allograft Achilles tendon (top) for reconstruction of the anterolateral bundle and a doubled autograft semitendinosus (bottom) for reconstruction of the PMB. A baseball whip-stitch using no. 5 nonabsorbable suture in the tendinous portion of the Achilles allograft and no. 2 nonabsorbable sutures in each end of the semitendinosus autograft facilitate graft passage.

- At our institution, a 10-mm Achilles allograft and a 7-mm doubled semitendinosus autograft are used to reconstruct the ALB and PMB, respectively (Fig. 26-11).
- These two separate grafts are passed through the tibial tunnel and then fixed in separate femoral tunnels.
- The method of graft fixation for the single- and double-bundle reconstructions will vary greatly depending on graft selection and surgeon preference.
- Rigid bone block fixation can be achieved using an interference screw that is 20 to 25 mm in length with a diameter similar to that of the bone tunnel.
- Several techniques for fixing the soft-tissue end of a graft provide adequate stability, including a screw and spiked washer, an Endobutton, a suture post, or a soft-tissue (bioabsorbable) interference screw.
  - Use of an Endobutton will require modification when drilling the femoral tunnel.
- We achieve initial graft fixation on the femoral side.
- For the single-bundle reconstruction using an Achilles tendon allograft, the calcaneal bone block is fixed within the femoral tunnel using an interference screw.
  - Fixation is achieved from inside to out by placing the interference screw through the AL portal over a guidewire that is positioned adjacent to the bone block, within the femoral tunnel (Fig. 26-12).
- For the double-bundle reconstruction, the calcaneal bone block of the Achilles tendon allograft is fixed using an interference screw, and the doubled semitendinosus graft is fixed using an Endobutton.
- Before tibial fixation, the graft should be preconditioned to minimize graft elongation after fixation.
  - This is accomplished by cycling the knee through the in situ range of motion several times while applying tension (10 lb) to the graft.
- During final fixation of the graft in the single-bundle reconstruction, the knee is held in 70 to 90 degrees of flexion, and an anterior drawer force is applied to recover the normal step-off between the medial femoral condyle and the medial tibial plateau.
  - These fixation conditions have been shown to be optimal in restoring intact knee biomechanics.
- Final fixation is performed using one of the methods discussed previously.

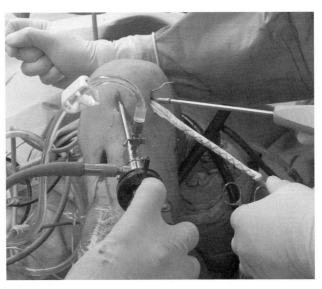

Figure 26-12 Femoral fixation of the Achilles tendon allograft. Fixation is achieved from inside to out by placing the interference screw over a guidewire that is positioned through the anterolateral portal and into the femoral tunnel, adjacent to the calcaneal bone block of the Achilles tendon allograft.

- We prefer a screw and soft tissue washer for fixing the Achilles graft on the tibial side (Fig. 26-13).
- In the double-bundle reconstruction, the AL graft is fixed under the same conditions described previously.
- The PM graft is fixed while an anterior drawer is applied to the tibia near full extension as tension is held on the graft.
- Like the AL graft, the PM graft should be preconditioned to minimize elongation after fixation.
- Fixing the PM graft under these conditions provides increased posterior stability near full extension.
- We prefer to fix the PM graft sutures over a separate post and washer (Fig. 26-14).

Tibial Inlay Technique
- The inlay technique requires a posterior approach to the knee, which allows for placement of the graft's bone block into a trough created at the tibial insertion site of the native PCL.
  - This provides a more anatomic site of tibial fixation and avoids the sharp angle of the graft observed at the proximal margin of tibial tunnel in the traditional transtibial technique ("killer turn").
  - It has been proposed that this "killer turn" generates increased graft stress and friction that may contribute to graft elongation or failure after initial fixation.
  - Despite these theoretical advantages, several biomechanical studies have shown no significant difference in knee kinematics and PCL graft forces when comparing tibial inlay and transtibial tunnel techniques of PCL reconstruction at the time of initial graft fixation.
  - When comparing these techniques of PCL reconstruction under cyclic loading, however, increased graft degradation and thinning has been shown to

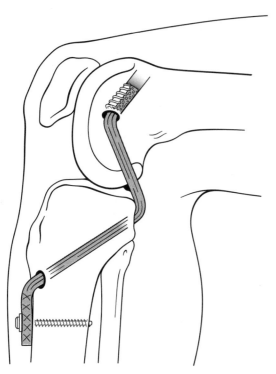

Figure 26-13 Single-bundle PCL reconstruction using an Achilles tendon allograft. (After Margheritini F, Mauro CS, Rihn JA, et al. Biomechanical comparison of tibial inlay versus transtibial techniques for posterior cruciate ligament reconstruction: analysis of knee kinematics and graft in situ forces. Am J Sports Med 2004; 32:587–593.)

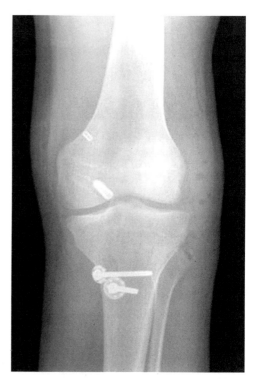

Figure 26-14 Anteroposterior x-ray of the knee obtained postoperatively after double-bundle PCL reconstruction. Fixation of the Achilles tendon allograft is achieved using an interference screw on the femoral side and a screw and soft-tissue washer on the tibial side. Fixation of the double semitendinosus autograft is achieved using an Endobutton on the femoral side and screw and soft-tissue washer on the tibial side.

occur at the site of the "killer turn" in the transtibial tunnel, which may predispose the graft to elongation and failure over time.

■ The clinical implications of these findings remain unknown.

■ Clinical outcome studies are needed to adequately compare the efficacy of the techniques of PCL reconstruction.

■ For the tibial inlay technique, the patient is positioned in the lateral decubitus position with the operative leg up.

■ From this position, a posterior approach to the tibial insertion of the PCL can be made directly.

■ Additionally, the hip can be abducted and externally rotated 45 degrees and the knee flexed to 90 degrees, with the foot on the operating table to perform standard arthroscopy, graft harvest, femoral tunnel placement, and graft passage.

■ This method of positioning avoids having to reposition the patient intraoperatively from a supine to a prone position.

■ Following EUA, the patient is positioned in the lateral decubitus position. The hip is abducted and externally rotated, and the knee is flexed.

■ Arthroscopy is carried out to document injury to the PCL and to address any associated intraarticular pathology.

■ Depending on graft selection, the graft is either harvested or thawed.

■ The inlay technique requires that at least one end of the graft has a bone block for fixation, limiting graft selection to the patellar tendon, quadriceps tendon, or Achilles tendon.

■ Berg originally described this technique using a bone–patellar tendon–bone graft, which remains the most commonly used graft for the inlay procedure.

■ The bone block that will be fixed in the tibial trough is fashioned with a flattened surface and is drilled during graft preparation to accept a 4.5-mm cortical screw.

■ The bone block to be fixed on the femoral side is contoured into a bullet-tipped cylinder shape to facilitate graft passage.

■ After arthroscopic debridement of the PCL stump, a femoral drill guide is positioned in the anterior portion of the PCL footprint at its femoral insertion.

■ The starting point is centered on the medial cortex of the medial femoral condyle.

■ The entry point is more proximal to preserve subchondral bone and reduce the risk of avascular necrosis of the medial femoral condyle.

■ The guide tip should be placed 6 mm from the medial femoral condyle articular surface at the 11 o'clock position (left knee) or 1 o'clock position (right knee) and the tunnel drilled to the appropriate size for the prepared graft.

■ A looped 18-gauge wire or graft passer, which will later

be used to pass the graft, is then placed antegrade through the femoral tunnel into the joint.

■ The injured leg of the patient is then repositioned in preparation for the posterior approach, with the knee extended and the leg abducted.

■ Different posterior approaches used in the tibial inlay procedure are described in the literature.

■ A horizontal incision can be made over the popliteal crease that has an extension over the medial head of the gastrocnemius.

■ The interval between the medial head of the gastrocnemius and semitendinosus is developed bluntly to expose the posterior joint capsule.

■ Lateral retraction of the gastrocnemius provides access to the posterior capsule of the knee and protects the neurovascular structures of the popliteal fossa.

■ The posterior tibial sulcus (PCL insertion site) and wire loop should be palpable, and a vertical capsule incision will then expose the PCL footprint on the tibia.

■ After exposing the tibial sulcus, an osteotome is used to create a unicortical bone trough at the site of tibial PCL insertion large enough to accommodate the tibial side of the graft.

■ Both the size of the bone plug and/or trough can be adjusted to ensure a tight fit.

■ The tibial side of the graft is placed in the trough and fixed to the tibia.

■ Fixation can be achieved using a flat washer and either a 6.5-mm cancellous screw or 4.5-mm cortical screw.

■ The graft is passed retrograde through the notch and into the femoral tunnel using the prepositioned 18-gauge wire.

■ If a bone–patellar tendon–bone graft is used, the femoral bone plug is positioned in the femoral tunnel, and the graft is tensioned and preconditioned by passively cycling the knee through its full range of motion.

　■ Ideally, the bone plug is positioned flush with the articular joint surface.

　■ If the graft is too long, the tibial trough and tibial bone plug can be moved distally.

■ Fixation is achieved using an interference screw in the femoral tunnel.

■ If an Achilles or quadriceps graft is used, the soft-tissue end of the graft is passed retrograde through the femoral tunnel, tensioned, preconditioned, and fixed using a screw and spiked washer (Fig. 26-15).

■ The graft is fixed in a manner similar to that described previously with the transtibial technique.

■ To review, the knee is flexed 70 to 90 degrees, an anterior drawer force is applied to the tibia, and the sutures exiting the graft are fixed over a post and washer.

■ A posterior drawer test after fixation assesses stability of the reconstruction.

Treatment of Associated Injury of the Posterolateral Structures

As stated previously, isolated PCL injuries are much less common than combined injuries. Up to 60% of PCL injuries involve associated injury to the PLS. Appropriate treatment of concomitant PLS injury is crucial. Failure to restore the integrity of the PLS places excessive force on a recon-

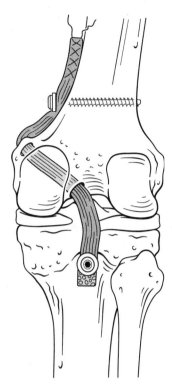

Figure 26-15 Tibial inlay technique for PCL reconstruction using an Achilles tendon allograft. (After Margheritini F, Mauro CS, Rihn JA, et al. Biomechanical comparison of tibial inlay versus transtibial techniques for posterior cruciate ligament reconstruction: analysis of knee kinematics and graft in situ forces. Am J Sports Med 2004; 32:587–593.)

structed PCL graft, predisposes the graft to elongation and early failure, and yields less favorable results than combined treatment of the PCL and PLS injury. Several different techniques for repairing the posterolateral structures have been described in the literature. Surgical options for posterolateral injuries include primary repair, advancement, augmentation, and reconstruction.

■ Acute surgical treatment of posterolateral corner injuries has achieved better clinical results than reconstruction of chronic injuries.

■ Primary anatomic repair of the posterolateral structures in an acute setting (<3 weeks after injury) offers the best surgical outcome.

■ The approach to the PLS involves a 12- to 18-cm curvilinear incision that begins midway between the fibular head and Gerdy's tubercle and then continues proximally over the lateral epicondyle, paralleling the posterior border of the ITB.

■ The peroneal nerve is identified and tagged with a vessel loop.

■ All of the posterolateral structures are then evaluated in a systematic fashion.

■ In acute injuries, there may be significant stripping and detachment of both ligaments and tendons.

■ The interval between the posterior edge of the ITB and the biceps femoris is developed as structures are identified.

- The ITB insertion can also be partially released in subperiosteal fashion from Gerdy's tubercle to increase exposure to the LCL and popliteus insertions.
- Direct suture repair of the injured structures is performed from deep to superficial.
- Severe injuries that are not amenable to primary repair may require augmentation.
- Many options exist for augmenting the structures of the posterolateral corner, including use of the iliotibial tract, the biceps femoris tendon, the hamstrings tendon, or an allograft.
- Excessive scar formation and inadequate tissue usually preclude primary repair of chronic posterolateral corner injuries.
- Reconstruction of the posterolateral structures is preferred in this case.
- The goals of surgical treatment are to restore intact knee kinematics and reduce the likelihood of progressive degenerative arthritis.
  - Numerous techniques for PLS reconstruction have been described in the literature. The current goal is to achieve an anatomic reconstruction of the injured components of the PLS.
- For LCL reconstruction, we prefer to use Achilles tendon allograft, fixing a 7- to 8-mm bone block to the fibular head with a metal interference screw.
  - The Achilles tendon allograft is secured to the lateral femoral epicondyle using suture anchors.
  - The remaining LCL is meticulously dissected to preserve its proximal and distal remnants.
  - These remnants are tensioned and sutured to the Achilles tendon allograft that has been secured to the lateral femoral condyle (Fig. 26-16).
- In chronic injury of the popliteal tendon and/or popliteofibular ligament, we prefer to reconstruct the popliteofibular ligament using either a hamstring autograft or a tibialis anterior allograft.
- A tunnel is created in the proximal fibula.

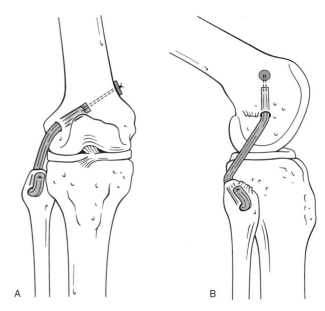

Figure 26-17   Reconstruction of the popliteofibular ligament. (After Cole BJ, Harner CD. The multiple ligament injured knee. Clin Sports Med 1999;18:241–262.)

- The graft is passed deep to the LCL and placed into a closed-end tunnel at the anatomic femoral insertion site of popliteus tendon.
- Its femoral attachment is then tied over a plastic button on the medial femoral cortex.
- The distal end is pulled through the tunnel created in the fibular head and tensioned with the knee in 30 degrees of flexion.
- Fixation is achieved with a bioabsorbable interference screw placed in the fibular head tunnel (Fig. 26-17).
- In cases of combined LCL and popliteofibular ligament reconstruction, the distal end of the popliteofibular graft is brought posterior to anterior through a soft-tissue tunnel created at the insertion of the biceps tendon.

POSTOPERATIVE CARE

- Most postoperative PCL reconstruction protocols brace the knee in extension for 4 weeks, supporting the tibia to prevent posterior translation and excessive stress on the graft.
- Partial weight-bearing as tolerated and quadriceps exercises start on the first postoperative day.
- Mini-squats and closed-chain exercises start at approximately 6 weeks, followed by proprioceptive training at 12 weeks, increasing knee stability.
- Range-of-motion exercises are essential to regaining full knee flexion.
- Patients are progressed slowly through passive flexion exercises in the early postoperative period and, in most cases, regain full flexion in 5 to 7 months.
- Hamstring exercises are delayed for 4 months, as they place excessive posterior loads on the tibia during the early stages of graft healing.

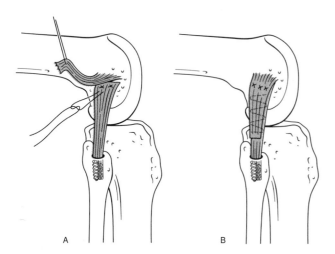

Figure 26-16   Reconstruction of the lateral collateral ligament. (After Cole BJ, Harner CD. The multiple ligament injured knee. Clin Sports Med 1999;18:241–262.)

- Light jogging begins at 6 months.
- The patient is allowed to return to full activities 9 to 12 months after surgery, depending on the individual demands of daily activity and the progression of physical therapy.
- The goal of rehabilitation is to achieve adequate knee stability, full range of motion, and quadriceps strength that is symmetric to that of the contralateral leg.
- A structured physical therapy program is essential to regaining motion, strength, and proprioception.

SUGGESTED READING

Berg EE. Posterior cruciate ligament tibial inlay reconstruction. Arthroscopy 1995;11:69–76.

Fanelli GC, Giannotti BF, Edson CJ. Arthroscopically assisted combined posterior cruciate ligament/posterior lateral complex reconstruction. Arthroscopy 1996;12:521–530.

Grood ES, Stowers SF, Noyes FR. Limits of movement in the human knee. Effect of sectioning the posterior cruciate ligament and posterolateral structures. J Bone Joint Surg Am 1988;70:88–97.

Harner CD, Janaushek MA, Kanamori A, et al. Biomechanical analysis of a double-bundle posterior cruciate ligament reconstruction. Am J Sports Med 2000;28:144–151.

Harner CD, Vogrin TM, Hoher J, et al. Biomechanical analysis of a posterior cruciate ligament reconstruction. Deficiency of the posterolateral structures as a cause of graft failure. Am J Sports Med 2000;28:32–39.

Harner CD, Xerogeanes JW, Livesay GA, et al. The human posterior cruciate ligament complex: an interdisciplinary study. Ligament morphology and biomechanical evaluation. Am J Sports Med 1995; 23:736–745.

Noyes FR, Barber-Westin SD. Surgical reconstruction of severe chronic posterolateral complex injuries of the knee using allograft tissues. Am J Sports Med 1995;23:2–12.

Shelbourne KD, Davis TJ, Patel DV. The natural history of acute, isolated, nonoperatively treated posterior cruciate ligament injuries. A prospective study. Am J Sports Med 1999;27:276–283.

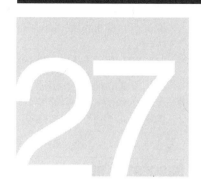

MULTIPLE LIGAMENT INJURIES OF THE KNEE

GREGORY C. FANELLI
DANIEL R. ORCUTT
JUSTIN D. HARRIS
DAVID ZIJERDI
CRAIG J. EDSON

A multiple ligament–injured knee most often occurs after a significant force is applied to the knee resulting in a knee dislocation. The knee may have spontaneously reduced and may not demonstrate radiographic evidence of a dislocation at initial presentation. Because these injuries typically involve a high-energy mechanism, the physician evaluating the patient must have a high index of suspicion for additional trauma, especially involving the contralateral lower extremity. Neurovascular injuries commonly occur in the multiple ligament–injured knee, and a detailed assessment of these structures is imperative.

Knee dislocations may be easily missed, especially if one has spontaneously reduced. Estimates indicate that approximately 0.01% or less of all hospital admissions are attributable to knee dislocations.

Evaluation beyond the initial trauma workup commonly includes examination under anesthesia, magnetic resonance imaging, and arthroscopy. These tools in conjunction with one another can give valuable information on the injury complex, as well as assisting in formulating a treatment plan.

ANATOMY AND BIOMECHANICS

Several anatomic features, both static and dynamic, contribute to knee stability. Static stabilizers include the bony articulations, menisci, and ligaments. Dynamic stabilizers include the musculature that crosses the knee joint. The articulation of the tibiofemoral joint is maintained in part by the bony anatomy of the femoral condyles and tibial plateau, as well as the menisci, which increase contact area between the tibia and femur (Fig. 27-1). The most significant ligamentous stabilizers are the anterior cruciate ligament (ACL) and the posterior cruciate ligament (PCL), the medial collateral ligament (MCL) and the lateral collateral ligament (LCL), and the posteromedial and posterolateral corners. The capsular ligaments of the knee are aponeurotic

Anterolateral view

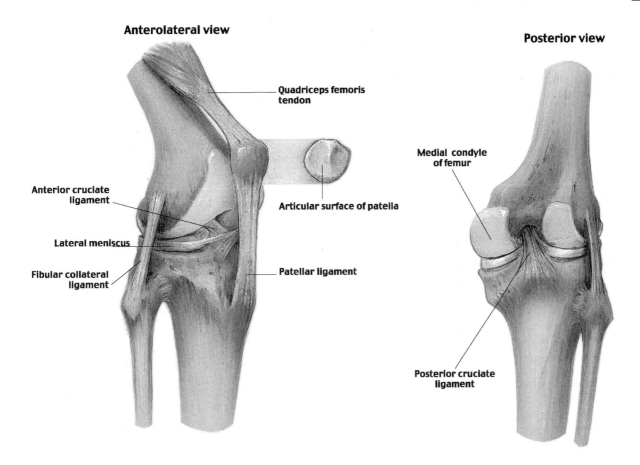

Quadriceps femoris
tendon

Anterior cruciate
ligament

Lateral meniscus

Fibular collateral
ligament

Articular surface of patella

Patellar ligament

Posterior view

Medial condyle
of femur

Posterior cruciate
ligament

Posteromedial view

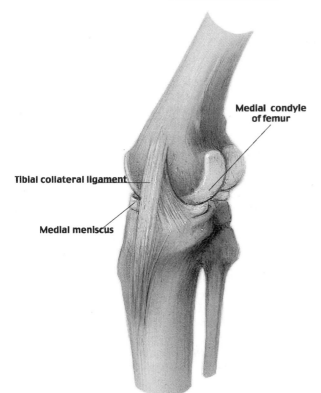

Medial condyle
of femur

Tibial collateral ligament

Medial meniscus

Figure 27-1   Knee ligaments. Asset provided by Anatomical Chart Co.

extensions of the thigh and leg musculature that terminate on the menisci. They function to activate motion of the joint and impart stability as ligament tension is modulated by the attached musculature.

The medial aspect of the knee can be conceptualized in terms of three layers and three longitudinal divisions. The first and most superficial layer is the sartorius and its fascia. Next is the tibial collateral ligament. The third and deepest layer consists of the medial capsular ligament. The gracilis and semitendinosus muscles run between the two superficial layers. The medial aspect of the knee is divided longitudinally into thirds. The anterior third consists of the medial retinacular ligament of the extensor aponeurosis, which has only meniscal and tibial attachments. The middle third contains the medial middle third capsular ligament and the tibial collateral ligament superficially. The posterior third contains the termination of the semimembranosus tendon, which consists of the posterior oblique ligament and the origin of the oblique popliteal ligament. Each ligament can be divided into meniscofemoral and meniscotibial components in the coronal plane.

The lateral aspect of the knee can also be divided into layers. The deepest layer is the lateral capsule, which divides into two laminae just posterior to the overlying iliotibial tract. The laminae encompass the LCL, fabellofibular, and arcuate ligaments. The second layer consists of the quadriceps retinaculum and the two patellofemoral ligaments posteriorly. The most superficial layer consists of the iliotibial tract and the superficial portion of the biceps and its expansion. The peroneal nerve lies deep to the iliotibial tract, just posterior to the biceps tendon.

In the popliteal fossa, the popliteal artery and vein are separated from the posterior capsule by a layer of fat. The artery is tethered proximally by the adductor hiatus and distally by the soleus arch, where it bifurcates into anterior and posterior tibial arteries. Genicular arteries give rise to the collateral circulation around the joint. The proximity of the popliteal artery to the joint, as well as its immobility, makes it especially susceptible to injury with dislocations of the knee joint. The tibial and common peroneal nerves run superficial to the artery and are less vulnerable to injury when the knee is dislocated.

To assess the structural integrity of the ligamentous structures, the function of each must be well understood:

■ The ACL functions to prevent anterior translation of the tibia relative to the femur, limit rotation of the tibia when the knee is in extension, and limit varus and valgus stress when the LCL or MCL are injured (Fig. 27-2A).

■ The PCL is located near the center of rotation of the knee. It functions as the primary static stabilizer of the knee and the primary restraint against posterior translation of the tibia (Fig. 27-2B).

■ The MCL and LCL function to prevent valgus and varus stresses, respectively, when the knee is flexed to 30 degrees.

  ■ A secondary function of both is to limit anterior or posterior translation and rotation of the tibia.

■ The posterolateral corner functions to resist posterolateral rotation, as well as posterior tibial translation relative to the femur.

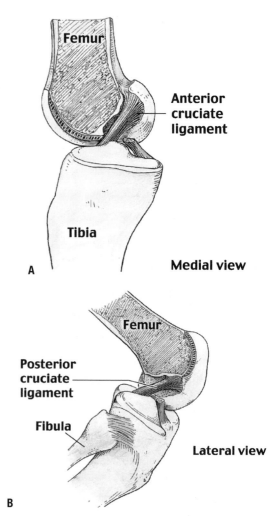

Figure 27-2 **A:** The ACL resists posterior displacement of the femur on the tibial plateau. **B:** The PCL resists anterior displacement of the femur on the tibial plateau. (From Moore KL, Dalley AF. Clinically Oriented Anatomy, 4th ed. Baltimore: Lippincott Williams & Wilkins, 1999.)

■ The posteromedial corner functions to resist posteromedial tibial translation relative to the femur and valgus stress at the knee.

CLASSIFICATION

Each classification system for knee dislocations given here provides valuable information on the type of injury, its risk of neurovascular complication, and its risk of infection. Each knee dislocation needs to be evaluated using a combination of these classification systems.

■ Direction of dislocation of the tibia

  ■ One common way is to describe the direction of displacement of the tibia in relation to the distal femur.

  ■ This gives a combination of possible dislocations, including anterior, posterior, medial, lateral, and rotational.

  ■ Rotational dislocations include anteromedial, anterolateral, posteromedial and posterolateral.

TABLE 27-1 CLASSIFICATION OF KNEE DISLOCATIONS

Type	Description
KDI	Intact posterior cruciate ligament with variable injury to collateral ligaments
KDII	Both cruciate ligaments disrupted completely with collaterals intact
KDIII	Both cruciate ligaments disrupted completely with one collateral ligament disrupted
KDIV	Both cruciate ligaments and collateral ligaments disrupted
KDV	Dislocation with periarticular fracture

(From Schenck RC Jr. The dislocated knee. Instr Course Lect 1994;43:127–136.)

- Presence of an open or closed injury
- Amount of energy required for the dislocation: high-energy versus low-energy
  - Low-energy mechanisms include nonmotorized sports injuries. These injuries have a lower incidence of neurovascular injury.
  - Higher-energy mechanisms include motor vehicle collisions and falls from height.

A classification system was created by Schenck that describes the injury pattern, as well as any associated neurovascular injury (Table 27-1). This classification system may be helpful in planning surgical treatment and for predicting functional outcome.

EPIDEMIOLOGY

Anterior dislocations are thought to be the most common, representing 31% to 70% of all knee dislocations. Posterior dislocations are the next most frequent at 25%. Rotational dislocations occur in 3% to 5%. Many knee dislocations spontaneously reduce. A high index of suspicion must exist if multiple ligaments are injured that a knee dislocation is likely to have occurred.

Open dislocations constitute one fifth to one third of all knee dislocations and have a poorer prognosis. They also limit surgical management because it may make arthroscopic surgery difficult.

The typical mechanism of injury is a violent force on the proximal tibia or knee. The direction that the force is applied will determine the ultimate position of the dislocation, as well as the ligaments injured. Hyperextension results in anterior dislocation. The posterior capsule fails first. The ACL and PCL, as well as the popliteal artery, then fail at approximately 50 degrees of hyperextension.

A posteriorly directed force on the proximal tibia, typical of a dashboard injury, is thought to result in a posterior knee dislocation. Varus and valgus stresses result in lateral and medial dislocations, respectively. A combination of forces in the anterior-posterior plane and in the medial-lateral plane will likely produce a rotational-type dislocation.

The posterolateral dislocation is thought to arise from flexed non-weight-bearing knee with a rapid abduction and internal rotation moment.

ASSOCIATED INJURIES

Several anatomic structures are at risk for injury in the dislocated knee. Patients can present with varying combinations of ligamentous involvement. All four major knee ligaments, as well as the posteromedial and posterolateral corners, can be compromised. Additionally, vascular and neurologic injuries are common. Furthermore, bony avulsion injuries, fractures of the distal femur or tibial plateau, and ipsilateral tibial or femoral shaft fractures are often seen with concomitant knee dislocations.

Numerous reports exist in the literature citing knee dislocations in which less than three of the major knee ligaments were torn, but this appears to be the exception rather than the rule. If a dislocation occurs solely in the sagittal plane, it would not be uncommon to find macroscopic continuity of both collateral ligaments, but several experts propose that frank dislocations invariably result in rupture of at least three of the four major knee ligaments. A meticulous ligamentous examination is essential to evaluate fully the extent of the injury.

Cruciate injuries in knee dislocations typically fall into one of two patterns: either bony avulsions or midsubstance tears. These often exist in multiple combinations with other soft-tissue and ligamentous injuries. Bony avulsion or peel-off injuries are often amenable to surgical reattachment and avoid the need for reconstruction of the involved cruciate. Avulsion injuries are more likely to occur in high-energy knee dislocations. Midsubstance tears of the cruciates occur commonly with knee dislocations. Results of primary repair of midsubstance tears are far inferior to that of surgical reconstruction.

In addition to cruciate rupture, injury to the soft tissues, collateral ligaments, joint capsule, and supporting tendinous structures are common in knee dislocations. These structures also frequently require operative attention. Once again, a careful physical and surgical evaluation is crucial to identify injury to the MCL, LCL, menisci, and tendons of the iliotibial band, the biceps femoris, the popliteus, and the quadriceps mechanism. All open injuries require thorough debridement, pulsatile irrigation, and bony stabilization.

The incidence of vascular compromise in knee dislocation is significant, so there is a need for a complete vascular evaluation. The popliteal artery has very limited mobility secondary to the tethered nature of the vessel at the adductor hiatus and the entrance through the gastrocnemius soleus arch. This tethering makes it extremely vulnerable to injury in cases of blunt trauma to the knee. Two major types of injury mechanisms are described. One involves a stretching of the artery, often seen with hyperextension, which results in extensive intimal damage. This is more common in anterior dislocations. Posterior dislocations, however, typically result in a direct contusion of the vessel by the posterior aspect of the tibial plateau and are more likely to produce complete rupture of the artery. As the popliteal artery is an end-artery to the leg, with minimal collateral circulation provided by the geniculate system, any compromise to the point of prolonged obstruction often leads to ischemia and eventual amputation. Furthermore, the popliteal vein is responsible for the majority of the venous outflow from the knee. Injury to this structure also compromises the viability of the lower limb.

In the case of frank knee dislocations and suspected dislocations, the presence of pulses does not rule out an arterial injury. Serial vascular examinations are essential as intimal flaps may often present as delayed thrombus formation. Additionally, the absence of pulses implies an arterial injury and cannot be attributed to vascular spasm. Failure to recognize an arterial injury can lead to disastrous outcomes.

Nerve injury is also quite common after dislocation of the knee. A reasonable estimate of the documented incidence is anywhere from 20% to 30%. The majority of nerve injuries involve the peroneal nerve, but reports of tibial nerve compromise have been reported. Nerve palsies have been described in all types of knee dislocations, but a common theme is association with injury to the lateral ligamentous complex. The peroneal and tibial nerves are not as tightly tethered as the popliteal artery and are thus less prone to injury. A stretch neurapraxia is the most common mechanism of injury, which often extends well proximal to the fibula. Occasionally, complete nerve transection occurs. Recovery of nerve function is unpredictable, with most series reporting no recovery in more than 50% of injuries. Nerve injury must be differentiated from stocking paresthesias that may be indicative of a developing compartment syndrome as opposed to a simple neurapraxia.

Osseous integrity is also often compromised in knee dislocations. Reports have indicated that the incidence of bony injury may be as high as 60%. Avulsion fractures of ligamentous and tendinous attachments are seen frequently in knee dislocations (Segond fractures, fibular head avulsion fractures, cruciate avulsions) but should be considered ligamentous injuries, unlike major fractures as are seen in true fracture dislocations of the knee.

The term "fracture dislocation" distinguishes between tibial plateau fractures and purely ligamentous knee dislocations because of different treatment protocols. Tibial plateau fractures require bony stabilization, whereas pure knee dislocations necessitate ligamentous reconstruction. Fracture dislocations of the knee are a combination of the two, adding an element of complexity to their treatment. Like pure knee dislocations, these are typically high-energy injuries that can result in marked joint instability and are associated with a high risk of soft-tissue and neurovascular compromise. It is also important to differentiate between these three entities because outcomes correlate directly with the underlying injury. Tibial plateau fractures have the best prognosis, and pure dislocations have the worst prognosis, with fracture dislocations lying somewhere in between.

DIAGNOSIS

History and Physical Examination

- A knee dislocation is the most dramatic example of the multiple ligament–injured knee.

- Obvious deformity may be present, and a grossly dislocated knee is unlikely to escape diagnosis.
- Dislocations that have spontaneously reduced may present more subtly.
  - Complete disruption of two or more knee ligaments should alert the clinician to the possibility of a spontaneously reduced knee dislocation.
  - Without proper evaluation and treatment, considerable adverse sequelae and morbidity may result.
- Perform a thorough history, including mechanism and position of the limb, at the time of injury.
  - Injuries may be classified as low- or high-velocity based on the history.
- Manipulation of the limb before the patient's arrival in the emergency department, and the resting position and alignment of the injured extremity need to be recognized.
- Inspection of the skin for abrasions, ecchymosis, swelling, and open wounds provides clues for possible underlying pathology.
- Gross knee swelling with normal radiographs may indicate a spontaneously reduced knee dislocation.
- Dimpling of the skin may indicate an irreducible posterolateral dislocation.
  - This type of dislocation involves buttonholing of the medial femoral condyle through the medial joint capsule.
  - A high incidence of skin necrosis after attempted closed reduction mandates open reduction.
- The most essential aspect of the initial evaluation of an acutely injured knee is a detailed neurovascular examination.
  - Before any attempted closed reduction, both motor and sensory findings in the superficial peroneal, the deep peroneal, and the tibial nerve distributions must be documented.
  - Check pulses, capillary refill, skin color, and skin temperature.
  - The presence of active hemorrhage, an expanding hematoma, or a bruit over the popliteal artery are all also signs of vascular injury. These must all be carefully evaluated both before and after a closed reduction is performed.
  - Serial neurovascular checks are mandatory in all patients who have or are suspected of having a knee dislocation.
- Laxity testing is often limited in the conscious patient because of significant pain with the examination.
  - A stabilized Lachman test in which the examiner's thigh is placed under the injured knee allows for relatively pain-free evaluation of both anterior and posterior endpoints.
  - Gross laxity in full extension during application of a varus or valgus stress implies disruption of the collateral ligament, one or more of the cruciate ligaments, and associated capsular injury.
  - A more detailed ligamentous examination typically requires conscious sedation or general anesthesia.

Radiologic Examination

- Before any manipulation, anteroposterior (AP) and lateral radiographs of the affected extremity should be ob-

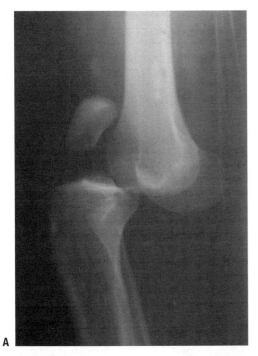

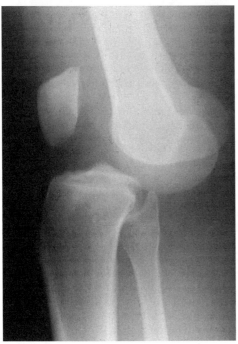

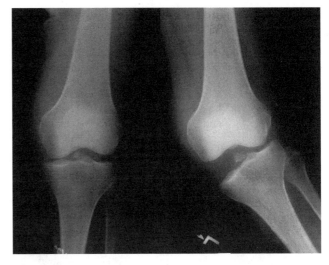

Figure 27-4 Stress radiograph revealing gross medial joint line opening indicating complete tears of the MCL, ACL, and PCL. (From Bucholz RW, Heckman JD. Rockwood & Green's Fractures in Adults, 5th ed. Lippincott Williams & Wilkins, 2001.)

Figure 27-3 Lateral radiographs comparing a posterior cruciate ligament (PCL) intact knee dislocation **(A)** and a complete bicruciate ligament knee dislocation **(B)** in two different patients. Note the parallel alignment of the patellofemoral joint with the femur in the complete bicruciate injury and the close proximity of the femur and tibia in the PCL intact knee dislocation. (From Bucholz RW, Heckman JD. Rockwood & Green's Fractures in Adults, 5th ed. Lippincott Williams & Wilkins, 2001.)

tained to confirm the direction of the dislocation (Figs. 27-3 and 27-4).

- Plain films help determine associated osseous injuries, as well as identify joint surface fractures and bony avulsions.
- Radiographs are also necessary to verify reduction.
- Tibiofemoral widening on AP knee films may be the only radiographic sign of a spontaneously reduced knee dislocation.

- All knee dislocations raise suspicion of potential vascular injury.
  - Any signs of compromised vascularity after a dislocated knee warrant evaluation with an arteriogram.
- After the acute management of the dislocated knee, magnetic resonance imaging (MRI) of the affected knee should be obtained to aid in planning the reconstruction of compromised ligamentous structures.
  - Because of its superior soft-tissue contrast and direct multiplanar acquisition, MRI has become the primary tool used to evaluate the soft tissues of the knee.
  - Improvements in technology now enable a complete examination in less than 20 minutes, inclusive of ligaments, menisci, and articular cartilage.
  - Ligamentous and meniscal lesions, as well as abnormalities of the peroneal nerve, can be evaluated quite accurately on MRI (Fig. 27-5).
- Magnetic resonance angiography (MRA) of the popliteal fossa is now being considered a method to evaluate for possible vascular injury after knee dislocation.
  - At some institutions, it is used in the acute setting, as an alternative to invasive formal arteriography.
  - In addition to being less invasive, it avoids the potential for contrast reactions and arterial punctures.
  - Numerous studies document the utility of MRA in other settings, but its utility in the assessment of

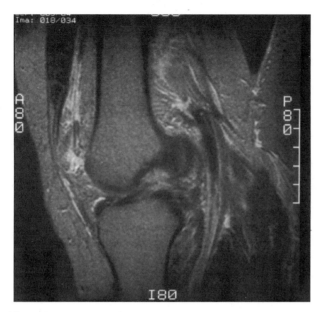

Figure 27-5   Midsubstance ACL and PCL tears on magnetic resonance imaging in a low-velocity knee dislocation. (From Bucholz RW, Heckman JD. Rockwood & Green's Fractures in Adults, 5th ed. Lippincott Williams & Wilkins, 2001.)

vascular injury after knee dislocation has not been cited in the literature.

■ As further studies involving more high-risk patients commence and technology continues to evolve, MRA may supplant arteriography as the first-line vascular study in this patient population.

Vascular Injuries

■ The mechanism of arterial injury varies with the type of dislocation.
  ■ Anterior dislocations typically produce a traction injury to the artery, resulting in an intimal tear.
  ■ Vascular injuries associated with posterior dislocations, however, are frequently complete arterial tears.
■ Regardless of the direction of the dislocation, vascular injury should always be suspected and evaluated.
  ■ Delay in diagnosis of major arterial injuries is a significant contributor to high amputation rates.
■ Detailed history and physical examination include the following:
  ■ A history of ischemia (pain, paresthesias, paralysis, pallor, and diminished limb temperature)
  ■ Assessment of the pulses by palpation, Doppler, and ankle-brachial indices when pulse status is questionable.
  ■ Evaluation of both distal perfusion and motor and neurologic function.
■ Regardless of the mechanism or position of the tibia, prompt reduction is needed.
  ■ If, after reduction, there is an asymmetrical vascular examination between the two lower extremities, urgent vascular studies should be obtained.

  ■ These variables must be reassessed on a frequent basis to evaluate for changes in the immediate period after closed reduction.
  ■ Any abnormalities or asymmetry should be investigated further.
■ The presence of pulses does not eliminate the possibility of vascular compromise.
■ Misdiagnosis of vascularity and subsequent delay in arterial repair based on palpable peripheral pulses and/or capillary refill is possible; thus, liberal or mandatory angiographic studies in cases of knee dislocations are often recommended.
  ■ Arguments for this approach have emphasized the risks of missed arterial injury, including muscle ischemia and limb amputation.
  ■ Others note that normal pulses, Doppler signals, and capillary refill after initial closed reduction do not rule out a vascular injury that progresses over time causing late vascular compromise.
■ Regarding management of patients with hard signs of limb ischemia, arteriography is not indicated in cases with an obviously ischemic limb, as there is a danger in delaying vascular repair. Arteriography may be useful if more than one level of injury exists.
  ■ This can often be accomplished with an intraoperative angiogram before vascular exploration.
  ■ Emergent vascular reconstruction with a reverse saphenous vein graft is the treatment of choice for an ischemic limb before a knee dislocation.
■ Patients for whom angiography is absolutely indicated are those whose pulses are abnormal or asymmetric but with no evidence of limb ischemia and those who have developed a change in their vascular status before serial examinations.

Nerve Injuries

■ A high incidence of nerve injury exists before knee dislocation. No consensus has been reached regarding management of these lesions.
■ Multiple anatomic factors contribute to the propensity of peroneal nerve injury during knee dislocation.
  ■ There is only 0.5 cm of excursion of the peroneal nerve at the fibular head during knee motion.
  ■ There is also a significantly smaller ratio of epineural tissue to axonal tissue in this nerve compared with other peripheral nerves, making it prone to stretch injuries.
■ During knee reconstruction, exploration of the peroneal nerve usually reveals that it is in continuity, although rupture may still exist.
  ■ A widespread zone of injury is typically encountered, which correlates with the poor results that have been documented after observation of complete nerve palsies.
■ Potential nerve injury evaluation includes the following:
  ■ Documentation of paresthesias, sensory changes, and motor function
  ■ Sequential neurologic evaluation over the first 48 hours and repeat evaluations 1 and 2 weeks after injury

- This is imperative because motor grades are often acutely reduced after dislocation secondary to pain alone.
    - In addition, delayed neurologic compromise may develop from swelling, hematoma, or direct compression from a splint or a cast.
- Needle electromyography (EMG) is performed to check the status of the motor axons in the peroneal nerve.
    - EMG changes that indicate axon disruption include fibrillation potentials, positive sharp waves, and absence of activity on voluntary effort or proximal nerve stimulation.
    - Typically, these changes may not appear for 2 to 3 weeks after injury, so EMG is of limited use before this time.
    - Absence of signs of denervation in a paralyzed muscle after 3 weeks indicates a neurapraxic lesion, and any identifiable voluntary motor unit axon potentials exclude nerve rupture.
    - Serial EMGs are also helpful in following recovery.
- Three options exist for operative intervention of peroneal nerve palsies: neurolysis alone, primary repair, or neuroma excision with nerve grafting.
- Observation is the treatment of choice for all incomplete peroneal nerve palsies because complete recovery is likely.
- If nerve rupture is identified at the time of ligamentous reconstruction, nerve reconstruction should be considered approximately 3 months after the original operation.
    - Acute repairs should be avoided, unless a primary repair can be performed under no tension.
- If, at exploration, the nerve appears to be normal, electrical studies should be obtained as a baseline 4 to 6 weeks after the injury.
    - If no contraction exists in the tibialis anterior at 3 months, electrophysiologic testing should be repeated and neurolysis or nerve reconstruction considered.
- The chance for success declines dramatically between 9 and 12 months after the original neurologic insult.

TREATMENT

Nonsurgical Treatment

Indications
- When the ACL and PCL are disrupted in the adult population, it is usually in the midsubstance of the ligament and, therefore, reconstruction is performed.
- When the posterior lateral corner has been injured, it can be repaired but often needs augmentation with autograft or allograft tissue.
- When the MCL is disrupted, the treatment is usually nonoperative, thus allowing it to heal in a brace before reconstruction of the other damaged ligaments.
- Multiple-ligament knee injuries in specific circumstances warrant nonoperative treatment:

- Critically ill patients unable to tolerate a surgical procedure
- Patients with grossly contaminated wounds or significant soft-tissue injuries around the prospective surgical site
- Elderly sedentary patient

Methods
- A long-leg or cylinder cast can be used.
- A long-leg knee brace locked in extension allows easy access and evaluation of the injured extremity.
    - This is especially helpful if there are significant wounds about the knee that a cast would conceal.
    - This is also helpful for a critically ill patient.
- If a cast or brace does not afford enough stability to maintain the knee in a reduced position, a knee-spanning external fixator may be necessary.
    - The external fixator also provides better access to soft tissue injuries if it can be positioned away from contaminated wounds.
- Regardless of the type of nonsurgical management, frequent radiographs should be obtained to verify continued reduction of the knee.

Surgical Treatment

- Surgical reconstruction is frequently advocated with the advent of improved surgical techniques, including better procurement, sterilization, and storage of allograft tissue, better graft fixation methods, arthroscopically assisted ligament reconstruction, and increased understanding of the ligamentous anatomy and biomechanics around the knee.
    - Improved ligamentous stability of the knee, as well as improved function postoperatively, have been achieved with these techniques.
- Few reports of combined ACL/PCL reconstruction are available in the literature, but surgical reconstruction appears to afford at least the same results (is not better) as direct repair of the ligaments.
    - It is imperative to address associated MCL or posterior lateral corner injury as well, or the results of ACL/PCL reconstruction alone will be less than optimal.
- Our preferred approach to combined ACL/PCL injuries is an arthroscopic ACL/PCL reconstruction using the transtibial technique, with collateral/capsular ligament surgery as indicated.
    - Not all cases are amenable to the arthroscopic approach; many patients with multiple ligament knee injuries suffer multiple trauma with multiple-system involvement; thus, the operating surgeon must assess each case individually.
- Surgical timing is dependent on:
    - Vascular status
    - Reduction stability
    - Skin condition
    - Systemic injuries
    - Open versus closed knee injury
    - Meniscus and articular surface injuries
    - Other orthopaedic injuries
    - Collateral/capsular ligaments involved

- Most ACL/PCL/MCL injuries can be treated with bracing of the MCL followed by arthroscopic combined ACL/PCL reconstruction in 4 to 6 weeks after healing of the MCL.
  - Certain cases may require repair or reconstruction of the medial structures and must be assessed on an individual basis.
- ACL/PCL/posterolateral repair reconstruction performed between 2 and 3 weeks postinjury allows healing of capsular tissues to permit an arthroscopic approach, and still permits primary repair of injured posterolateral structures.
- Open multiple ligament knee injuries/dislocations may require staged procedures.
  - The collateral/capsular structures are repaired after thorough irrigation and debridement.
  - The combined ACL/PCL reconstruction is performed at a later date, after wound healing has occurred.
  - Care must be taken in all cases of delayed reconstruction that the tibiofemoral joint is reduced.

Graft Selection
- The ideal graft material should be strong, easy to pass, readily available, provide secure fixation, and have low donor site morbidity.
- The available options in the United States are autograft and allograft sources.
- Our preferred graft for the PCL is the Achilles tendon allograft because of its large cross-sectional area and strength, absence of donor site morbidity, and easy passage with secure fixation.
- We prefer Achilles tendon allograft or bone–patellar tendon–bone allograft for the ACL reconstruction.
- The preferred graft material for the posterolateral corner is a split biceps tendon transfer, or free autograft (semitendinosus) or allograft (Achilles tendon) tissue when the biceps tendon is not available.
- Cases requiring MCL and posteromedial corner surgery may have primary repair, reconstruction, or a combination of both.
- Our preferred method for MCL and posteromedial reconstructions is a posteromedial capsular advancement with autograft or allograft supplementation as needed.

Surgical Approach
- Our preferred surgical approach is a single-stage arthroscopic combined ACL/PCL reconstruction using the transtibial technique with collateral/capsular ligament surgery as indicated.
- The posterolateral corner is repaired then augmented with a split biceps tendon transfer, biceps tendon transfer, semitendinosus free graft, or allograft tissue.
- Acute medial injuries not amenable to brace treatment undergo primary repair, and posteromedial capsular shift, or allograft reconstruction as indicated.
- The operating surgeon must be prepared to convert to a dry arthroscopic procedure, or open procedure if fluid extravasation becomes a problem.

Surgical Technique
- The patient is positioned supine on the operating room table.
  - The surgical leg hangs over the side of the operating table, and the well leg is supported by the fully extended operating table.
  - A lateral post is used for control of the surgical leg. We do not use a leg holder.
- The surgery is done under tourniquet control unless prior arterial or venous repair contraindicates the use of a tourniquet.
- Fluid inflow is by gravity. We do not use an arthroscopic fluid pump.
- Allograft tissue is prepared before bringing the patient into the operating room.
- Arthroscopic instruments are placed with the inflow in the superior lateral portal, arthroscope in the inferior lateral patellar portal, and instruments in the inferior medial patellar portal.
- An accessory extracapsular extra-articular posteromedial safety incision is used to protect the neurovascular structures and to confirm the accuracy of tibial tunnel placement (Fig. 27-6).
- The notchplasty is performed first and consists of ACL and PCL stump debridement, bone removal, and contouring of the medial wall of the lateral femoral condyle and the intercondylar roof. This allows visualization of the over the top position and prevents ACL graft impingement throughout the full range of motion.
- Specially curved PCL instruments are used to elevate the capsule from the posterior aspect of the tibia (Fig. 27-7).
- The PCL tibial and femoral tunnels are created with the help of a PCL/ACL drill guide (Fig. 27-8).
  - The transtibial PCL tunnel goes from the anteromedial aspect of the proximal tibial 1 cm below

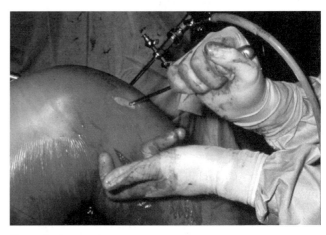

Figure 27-6 A 1- to 2-cm extracapsular posterior medial safety incision allows the surgeon's finger to protect the neurovascular structures, and confirm the position of instruments on the posterior aspect of the proximal tibia. (From Fanelli GC, Giannotti BF, Edson CJ. Current concepts review. The posterior cruciate ligament arthroscopic evaluation and treatment. Arthroscopy 1994;10: 673–688.)

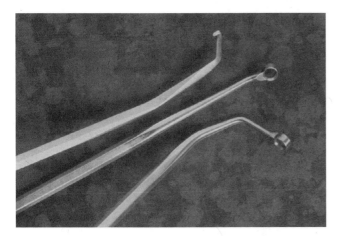

Figure 27-7 Specially curved PCL reconstruction instruments used to elevate the capsule from the posterior aspect of the tibial ridge during PCL reconstruction. Posterior capsular elevation is critical in transtibial PCL reconstruction because it facilitates accurate PCL tibial tunnel placement and subsequent graft passage. (Courtesy of Arthrotek, Inc., Warsaw, Indiana.)

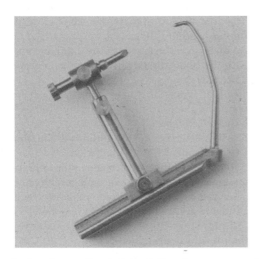

Figure 27-8 The Fanelli PCL/ACL drill guide system is used to precisely create both the PCL femoral and tibial tunnels, and the ACL single incision technique and double incision technique tunnels. The drill guide is positioned for the PCL tibial tunnel so that a guide wire enters the anteromedial aspect of the proximal tibia approximately 1 cm below the tibial tubercle, at a point midway between the posteromedial border of the tibia and the tibial crest anteriorly. The guidewire exits in the inferior lateral aspect of the PCL tibial anatomical insertion site. The guide is positioned for the PCL femoral tunnel, so the guidewire enters the medial aspect of the medial femoral condyle midway between the medial femoral condyle articular margin and the medial epicondyle, 2 cm proximal to the medial femoral condyle distal articular surface (joint line). The guidewire exits through the center of the stump of the anterolateral bundle of the PCL. The drill guide is positioned for the single incision endoscopic ACL technique, so that the guidewire enters the anteromedial surface of the proximal tibia approximately 1 cm proximal to the tibial tubercle at a point midway between the posteromedial border of the tibia and the tibial crest anteriorly. The guidewire exits through the center of the stump of the tibial ACL insertion. (Courtesy of Arthrotek, Inc., Warsaw, Indiana.)

the tibial tubercle to exit in the inferior lateral aspect of the PCL anatomic insertion site.

The PCL femoral tunnel originates externally between the medial femoral epicondyle and the medial femoral condylar articular surface to emerge through the center of the stump of the anterolateral bundle of the PCL.

- The PCL graft is positioned and anchored on the femoral or tibial side and left free on the opposite side.
- The ACL tunnels are created using the single incision technique.
  - The tibial tunnel begins externally at a point 1 cm proximal to the tibial tubercle on the anteromedial surface of the proximal tibia to emerge through the center of the stump if the ACL tibial footprint.
  - The femoral tunnel is positioned next to the over-the-top position on the medial wall of the lateral femoral condyle near the ACL anatomic insertion site.
  - The tunnel is created to leave a 1 to 2 mm posterior cortical wall so interference fixation can be used.
  - The ACL graft is positioned and anchored on the femoral side, with the tibial side left free (Fig. 27-9).

Split Biceps Tendon Transfer to the Lateral Femoral Epicondyle for Posterolateral Reconstruction (Fig. 27-10)

- For this procedure, the proximal tibiofibular joint, the posterolateral capsular attachments to the common bi-

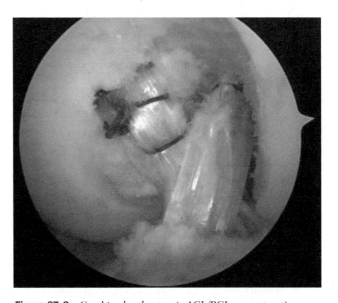

Figure 27-9 Combined arthroscopic ACL/PCL reconstruction using Achilles tendon allograft. The tunnels are precisely created to reproduce the anatomic insertion sites of the anterolateral bundle of the PCL and the anatomical insertion sites of the ACL. Correct and accurate tunnel placement is essential for successful combined ACL/PCL reconstructions. The Achilles tendon allograft is preferred because of its large cross-sectional area, strength, and absence of donor site morbidity.

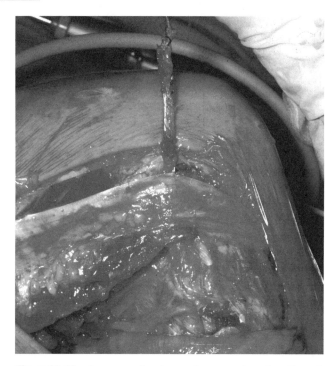

Figure 27-10 One surgical technique for posterolateral and lateral reconstruction is the split biceps tendon transfer, combined with posterolateral capsular shift and primary repair of injured structures as indicated. The split biceps tendon transfer uses anatomical insertion sites and preserves the dynamic function of the long head and common biceps femoris tendon.

ceps tendon, and the biceps femoris tendon insertion into the fibular head must be intact.

■ This technique creates a new popliteofibular ligament and LCL, tightens the posterolateral capsule and provides a post of strong autogenous tissue to reinforce the posterolateral corner.
  ■ A lateral hockey stick incision is made.
  ■ The peroneal nerve is dissected free and protected throughout the procedure.
  ■ The long head and common biceps femoris tendon are isolated, and the anterior two thirds is separated from the short head muscle.
  ■ The tendon is detached proximal and left attached distally to its anatomic insertion site on the fibular head. The strip of biceps tendon should be 12 to 14 cm long.
  ■ The iliotibial band is incised in line with its fibers, and the fibular collateral ligament and popliteus tendons are exposed.
  ■ A drill hole is made 1 cm anterior to the fibular collateral ligament femoral insertion.
  ■ A longitudinal incision is made in the lateral capsule just posterior to the fibular collateral ligament.
  ■ The split biceps tendon is passed medial to the iliotibial band and secured to the lateral femoral epicondylar region with a screw and spiked ligament washer at the previously described point.

  ■ The residual tail of the transferred split biceps tendon is passed medial to the iliotibial band and secured to the fibular head.
  ■ The posterolateral capsule that had been previously incised is then shifted and sewn into the strut of transferred biceps tendon to eliminate posterolateral capsular redundancy.

Posterolateral Reconstruction with Free Graft Figure-of-eight Technique

■ This technique uses semitendinosus autograft or allograft, Achilles tendon allograft, or other soft-tissue allograft material.
  ■ A curvilinear incision is made in the lateral aspect of the knee extending from the lateral femoral epicondyle to the interval between Gerdy's tubercle and the fibular head.
  ■ The fibular head is exposed and a tunnel is created in an anterior to posterior direction at the area of maximal fibular diameter.
    ■ The tunnel is created by passing a guide pin followed by a cannulated drill, usually 7 mm in diameter.
    ■ The peroneal nerve is protected during tunnel creation and throughout the procedure.
  ■ The free tendon graft is then passed through the fibular head drill hole.
  ■ An incision is then made in the iliotibial band in line with the fibers directly overlying the lateral femoral epicondyle.
  ■ The graft material is passed medial to the iliotibial band and the limbs of the graft are crossed to form a figure-of-eight.
  ■ A drill hole is made 1 cm anterior to the fibular collateral ligament femoral insertion.
  ■ A longitudinal incision is made in the lateral capsule just posterior to the fibular collateral ligament.
  ■ The graft material is passed medial to the iliotibial band and secured to the lateral femoral epicondylar region with a screw and spiked ligament washer at the previously described point.
  ■ The posterolateral capsule that had been previously incised is then shifted and sewn into the strut of figure-of-eight graft tissue material to eliminate posterolateral capsular redundancy.
  ■ The anterior and posterior limbs of the figure-of-eight graft material are sewn to each other to reinforce and tighten the construct. (Fig. 27-11).
  ■ The iliotibial band incision is closed. The procedures described are intended to eliminate posterolateral and varus rotational instabilities.

Posteromedial and Medial Reconstructions with a Medial Hockey Stick Incision (Fig. 27-12)

■ Care is taken to maintain adequate skin bridges between incisions.
  ■ The superficial MCL is exposed, and a longitudinal incision is made just posterior to the posterior border of the MCL.
    ■ Care is taken not to damage the medial meniscus during the capsular incision.

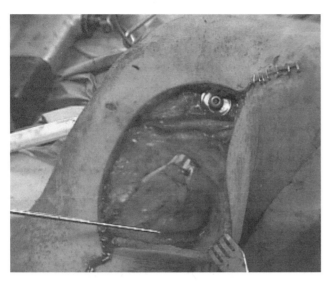

Figure 27-11 Another technique for posterolateral and lateral reconstruction is the allograft or autograft figure-of-eight reconstruction.

- The interval between the posteromedial capsule and medial meniscus is developed.
- The posteromedial capsule is shifted anterosuperiorly.
- The medial meniscus is repaired to the new capsular position, and the shifted capsule is sewn into the MCL.

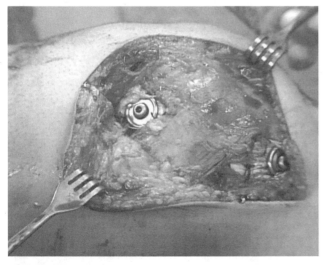

Figure 27-12 Severe medial side injuries are successfully treated with primary repair using suture anchor technique, combined with MCL reconstruction using allograft tissue combined with posteromedial capsular shift procedure. The broad anatomy of the Achilles tendon allograft can anatomically reconstruct the superficial MCL. The Achilles tendon allograft is secured to the anatomical insertion sites of the superficial MCL using screws and spiked ligament washers. The posteromedial capsule can then be secured to the allograft tissue to eliminate posteromedial capsular laxity. This technique will address all components of the medial side instability.

- When superficial MCL reconstruction is indicated, this is performed with allograft tissue or semitendinosus autograft.
- This graft material is attached at the anatomic insertion sites of the superficial MCL on the femur and tibia.
- The posteromedial capsular advancement is performed and sewn into the newly reconstructed MCL.

Graft Tensioning and Fixation
- The PCL is reconstructed first, followed by the ACL, followed by the posterolateral complex and/or posterior medial corner.

- The Arthrotek tensioning device is used for tensioning the ACL and PCL reconstructions (Fig. 27-13).
  - Tension is placed on the PCL graft distally, and the knee is cycled through a full range of motion 25 times to allow pretensioning and settling of the graft.
- The knee is placed in 70 to 90 degrees of flexion, a firm anterior drawer force is applied to the proximal tibia to restore the normal tibial step-off, and fixation is achieved on the tibial or femoral side of the PCL graft

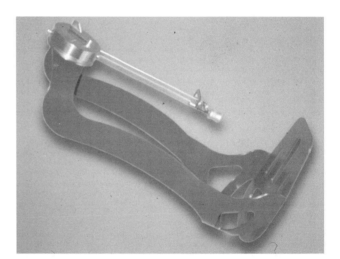

Figure 27-13 The mechanical graft knee ligament-tensioning device is used to precisely tension PCL and ACL grafts. During PCL reconstruction, the tensioning device is attached to the tibial end of the graft and the torque wrench ratchet set to 20 pounds. This restores the anatomical tibial step off. The knee is cycled through 25 full flexion-extension cycles, and with the knee at 0 degree of flexion, final PCL tibial fixation is achieved with a LactoSorb resorbable interference screw, as well as screw and spiked ligament washer for backup fixation. The tensioning device is applied to the ACL graft, set to 20 pounds, and the graft is tensioned with the knee in 70 degrees of flexion. Final ACL fixation is achieved with LactoSorb bioabsorbable interference screws and spiked ligament washer backup fixation. The mechanical tensioning device ensures consistent graft tensioning and eliminates graft advancement during interference screw insertion. It also restores the anatomical tibial step-off during PCL graft tensioning and applies a posterior drawer force during ACL graft tensioning. (Courtesy of Arthrotek, Inc., Warsaw, Indiana.)

with a screw and spiked ligament washer, and bioabsorbable interference screw.

■ The knee is then placed in 30 degrees of flexion, the tibial internally rotated, slight valgus force applied to the knee, and final tensioning and fixation of the posterolateral corner is achieved.

■ The knee is returned to 70 to 90 degrees of flexion, a posterior drawer force is applied to the proximal tibia with tension on the ACL graft, and final fixation is achieved of the ACL graft with a bioabsorbable interference screw, and spiked ligament washer backup fixation.

■ Reconstruction and tensioning of the MCL and posteromedial corner are performed after the ACP, PCL, and posterior lateral corner reconstructions, and are done in 30 degrees of knee flexion (Fig. 27-14).

Technical Hints

■ The posteromedial safety incision protects the neurovascular structures, confirms accurate tibial tunnel placement, and allows the surgical procedure to be done at an accelerated pace.

■ The single incision ACL reconstruction technique prevents lateral cortex crowding and eliminates multiple through and through drill holes in the distal femur reducing stress riser effect.

  ■ It is important to be aware of the two tibial tunnel directions and to have a 1-cm bone bridge between the PCL and ACL tibial tunnels (Fig. 27-15). This will reduce the possibility of fracture.

■ We have found it useful to use primary and backup fixation.

  ■ Primary fixation is with resorbable interference screws, and backup fixation is performed with a screw and spiked ligament washer.

  ■ Secure fixation is critical to the success of this surgical procedure.

■ Pitfalls are listed in Box 27-1.

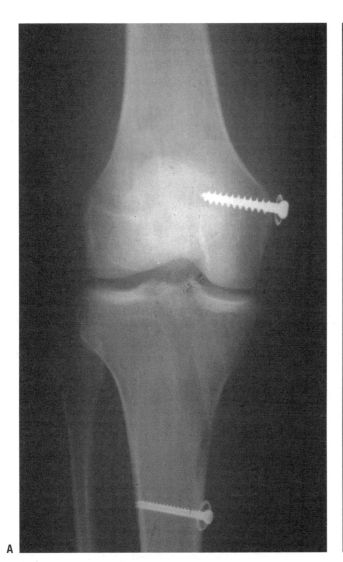
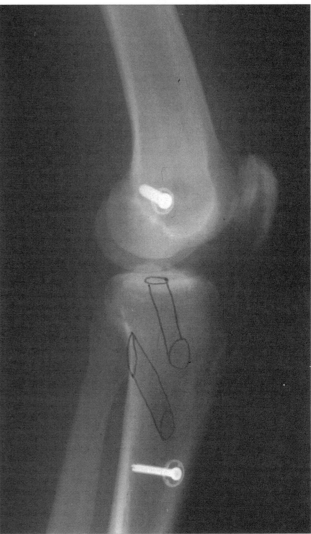

Figure 27-14   AP **(A)** and lateral **(B)** radiographs after combined ACL/PCL reconstruction. Note position of tibial tunnel on lateral x-ray. Tibial tunnel guidewire exits at the apex of the tibial ridge posteriorly, which places the graft at the anatomical tibial insertion site after the tibial tunnel is drilled.

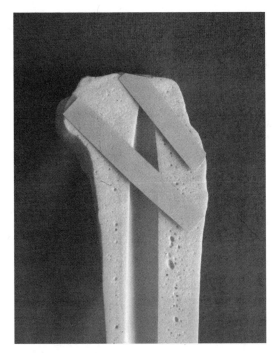

Figure 27-15 A model showing the tibial tunnel positions for combined ACL/PCL reconstructions. It is essential to have an adequate bone bridge between the two tunnels. (From Fanelli GC, Giannotti BF, Edson CJ. Current concepts review. The PCL arthroscopic evaluation and treatment. Arthroscopy 1994;10: 673–688.)

POSTOPERATIVE REHABILITATION

- The knee is kept in full extension, and a non-weight-bearing status is maintained for 6 weeks.
- Progressive range of motion occurs after postoperative week 6.
- The brace is unlocked at the end of 6 weeks and the crutches are discontinued after progression to full weight-bearing has been achieved.
- Progressive closed kinetic chain strength training and continued motion exercises are performed.

BOX 27-1 PITFALLS OF DIAGNOSING AND MANAGING MULTIPLE LIGAMENT INJURIES OF THE KNEE

- Failure to recognize and treat vascular injuries (both arterial and venous)
- Iatrogenic neurovascular injury at the time of reconstruction
- Iatrogenic tibial plateau fractures at the time of reconstruction
- Failure to recognize and treat all components of the instability
- Postoperative medial femoral condyle osteonecrosis
- Knee motion loss
- Postoperative anterior knee pain

- The brace is discontinued after the tenth week.
- Return to sports and heavy labor occurs after the ninth postoperative month, when sufficient strength and range of motion has returned.
- A loss of 10 to 15 degrees of terminal flexion can be expected in these complex knee ligament reconstructions.
  - This does not cause a functional problem for these patients and is not a cause for alarm.

RESULTS

- The 2- to 10-year results of 35 arthroscopically assisted combined ACL/PCL reconstructions suggest that combined ACL/PCL instabilities can be successfully treated with arthroscopic reconstruction and the appropriate collateral ligament surgery.
  - Significant improvement was noted from the preoperative condition at 2- to 10-year follow-up using objective parameters of knee ligament rating scales, arthrometer testing, stress radiography, and physical examination.
  - Postoperatively, these knees are not normal, but they are functionally stable.
- The 2- to 10-year results of chronic arthroscopically assisted combined PCL/posterolateral reconstructions indicate that chronic combined PCL/posterolateral instabilities could be successfully treated with arthroscopic PCL reconstruction using fresh frozen Achilles tendon allograft combined with posterolateral corner reconstruction using biceps tendon transfer combined with posterolateral capsular shift procedure.
  - Significant improvement is noted from the preoperative condition at 2- to 10-year follow-up using objective parameters of knee ligament rating scales, arthrometer testing, stress radiography, and physical examination.

SUGGESTED READING

Fanelli GC. The Multiple Ligament Injured Knee: A Practical Guide to Management. New York: Springer-Verlag, 2004.

Fanelli GC, Edson CJ. Arthroscopically assisted combined ACL/PCL reconstruction. 2–10 year follow-up. Arthroscopy 2002;18: 703–714.

Fanelli GC, Edson CJ. Arthroscopically assisted combined PCL-posterolateral reconstruction. 2–10 year follow-up. Arthroscopy 2004;20:339–345.

Fanelli GC, Edson CJ. PCL injuries in trauma patients. Part II. Arthroscopy 1995;11:526–529.

Fanelli GC, Feldmann DD. The use of allograft tissue in knee ligament reconstruction. In: Parisien JS, ed. Current Techniques in Arthroscopy, 3rd ed. Thieme, New York, 1998.

Fanelli GC, Gianotti BF, Edson CJ. Arthroscopically assisted combined anterior and posterior cruciate ligament reconstruction. Arthroscopy 1996;12:5–14.

Fanelli GC, Gianotti BF, Edson CJ. Arthroscopically assisted combined posterior cruciate ligament/posterior lateral complex reconstruction. Arthroscopy 1996;12:521–530.

Fanelli GC, Gianotti BF, Edson CJ. The posterior cruciate ligament arthroscopic evaluation and treatment. Arthroscopy 1994;10: 673–688.

Goitz RJ, Tomaino MM. Management of peroneal nerve injuries associated with knee dislocations. Am J Orthop 2003;32:14–16.

Irgang JJ, Harner CD. Loss of motion following knee ligament reconstruction. Sports Med 1995;19:150–159.

Jones RE, Smith EC, Bone GE. Vascular and orthopedic complications of knee dislocation. Surg Gynecol Obstet 1979;149:554–558.

Noyes FR, Barber-Westin SD. Reconstruction of the anterior and posterior cruciate ligaments after knee dislocation. Am J Sports Med 1997;25:769.

Potter HG, Weinstein M, Allen AA. Magnetic resonance imaging of the multiple-ligament injured knee. J Orthop Trauma 2002;16:330–339.

Seebacher JR, Inglis AE, Marshall DV, et al. The structure of the posterolateral aspect of the knee. J Bone Joint Surg Am 1982;64:536–541.

Shapiro MS, Freedman EL. Allograft reconstruction of the anterior and posterior cruciate ligaments after traumatic knee dislocation. Am J Sports Med 1995;23:580–587.

Shelbourne KD, Porter DA, Clingman JA, et al. Low-velocity knee dislocation. Orthop Rev 1991;20:995–1004.

Taft T, Almekinders L. The dislocated knee. In: Fu F, Harner C, Vince K, eds. Knee Surgery. Baltimore: Williams & Wilkins, 1994:837–858.

Warren LF, Marshall DVM. The supporting structures and layers on the medial side of the knee. J Bone Joint Surg Am 1979;61:56–62.

Wascher DC, Dvirnak PC, Decoster TA. Knee dislocation. Initial assessment and implications for treatment. J Orthop Trauma 1997;11:525–529.

PATELLOFEMORAL DISORDERS

BETH E. SHUBIN STEIN
CHRISTOPHER S. AHMAD

Patellofemoral disorders are extremely common, affecting up to 30% of young athletes in some reports. Although patellofemoral disorders are some of the most common problems seen in the sports medicine physician's office, they remain at times difficult and frustrating to manage for both the clinician and the patient. Recent advances in our understanding of patellofemoral biomechanics and improved imaging techniques have greatly enhanced our ability to diagnose even subtle injuries and to better characterize the extent of larger injuries. Treatments have also evolved and now include a variety of arthroscopic techniques for treating many of the pathologies encountered.

PATHOGENESIS

Etiology

Historically, many terms have been used to describe patella conditions, including chondromalacia patella, anterior knee pain, and "runner's knee," which have poorly described the pathology and thus are no longer in favor. Appreciating patellofemoral disorders requires knowledge of the relevant anatomy and biomechanics. The patella articulates with the trochlear groove of the distal femur. The cartilage thickness on the patella approaches 5 mm and is the thickest found anywhere in the body. Patellar biomechanics are governed by the articular geometry and dynamic and passive soft-tissue stabilizers (Fig. 28-1). The trochlea is elevated laterally, which helps resist lateral translation of the patella.

The dynamic forces that power knee extension act through the quadriceps and patellar tendons and create a resultant force vector that is directed laterally. The vastus medialis obliquus (VMO) is the primary medial dynamic stabilizer of the patella (Box 28-1). Passive stabilizing structures of the patella include the lateral retinaculum and the medial retinaculum. Of particular importance, the medial patellofemoral ligament (MPFL)—a discrete component of the medial retinaculum—provides up to 53% of the resistance to lateral patella translation and serves as the primary static restraint to lateral dislocation.

Forces approaching seven times body weight act across the patella during routine activities. With these huge forces acting across the patella, small aberrations in bone geometry, cartilage surfaces, dynamic or passive restraints, or lower-extremity alignment can alter the delicate balance of the patellofemoral joint (PFJ), thereby resulting in subtle or extensive pathology. Patellofemoral problems in athletes generally can be divided into those problems associated with instability and those due to overuse. Most clinicians believe that patellofemoral syndrome is, indeed, a multifactorial disorder.

Epidemiology

Although supportive data are lacking, it is believed that patellofemoral problems associated with overuse affect women more frequently than men. As is true with the overuse disorders, the epidemiological characteristics and natu-

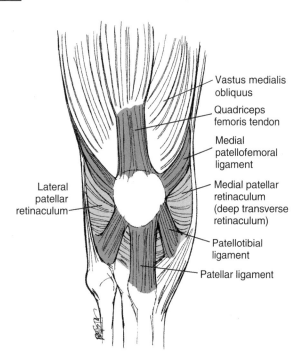

Figure 28-1 Many forces act on the patella to govern its motion. The vastus medialis obliquus is the main dynamic medial stabilizer of the patella. The medial patellofemoral ligament is the primary static medial restraint to lateral dislocation. (From Hendrickson T. Massage for Orthopaedic Conditions. Baltimore: Lippincott Williams & Wilkins, 2003.)

ral history of patients with patellar instability are also poorly described. Reports indicate that approximately 17% of all first-time dislocators will experience recurrent dislocations versus the more than 50% of prior dislocators who will go on to further episodes of dislocation or subluxation.

Pathophysiology

The classification of patellofemoral pathology is given in Box 28-2.

Overuse

Repeated knee flexion and extension typical of running or stair climbing can cause excessive pressure between the patella and the trochlea, leading to pain that may persist, even after stopping the aggravating activity. Frequently, the pain will lead to inhibition of the quadriceps, causing it to "shut down" and further contribute to the patient's symptoms.

BOX 28-1 PATELLA-STABILIZING STRUCTURES

- Trochlea groove geometry (static)
- Vastus medialis obliquus (dynamic)
- Medial patellofemoral ligament (static)
- Medial retinaculum (static)
- Patellomeniscal and patellotibial ligament complex (static)

BOX 28-2 CLASSIFICATION OF PATELLOFEMORAL PATHOLOGY

Trauma
Acute trauma
    Direct impact (contusion)
    Fracture
    Dislocation
    Tendon rupture
Repetitive trauma/overuse
    Enthesopathies
    Prepatellar bursitis
    Apophysitis
        Osgood-Schlatter
        Sindig-Larsen-Johnsen

Malalignment
Lateral patellar compression syndrome
Patellar instability
Osteochondritis desiccans

Biomechanics

As the patella tracks up and down in the femoral groove, it also tends to rotate and tilt such that, at different degrees of knee flexion, contact areas on the patella and the femur change in location and magnitude. Several anatomical and biomechanical factors can result in altered lower-extremity alignment and disturb the delicate balance of forces acting on the patella (Box 28-3).

The hindfoot normally pronates from heel strike until foot-flat, causing obligatory internal tibial rotation. Alterations in foot mechanics may affect tibial rotation, thereby affecting patellofemoral biomechanics. At the hip, abductor and external rotator weaknesses can lead to internal rotation of the hip and pelvic tilt, which results in lateral tracking of the patella. The VMO is the dynamic medial stabilizer of the patella and if atrophic or hypoplastic may lead to lateral tracking of the patella (Fig. 28-1). An excessively tight lateral retinaculum may cause the patella to tilt laterally, thereby placing excessive stresses on the lateral side of the PFJ (Fig. 28-2).

Acute Trauma

Trauma can range from a direct impact, such as a dashboard injury, to a noncontact twisting injury, such as is seen in

---

BOX 28-3 ANATOMICAL FACTORS CONTRIBUTING TO LOWER-EXTREMITY MALALIGNMENT

- Pes plano valgus
- Tibial torsion
- Genu valgum
- Hypoplastic lateral trochlea
- Excessive femoral anteversion
- Weak hip abductors/external rotators

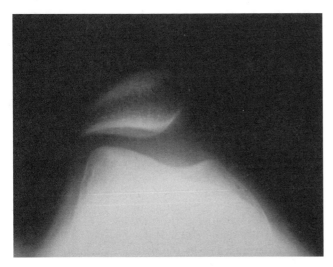

Figure 28-2 Merchant axial radiograph demonstrating lateral patellar tilt and subluxation.

cutting sports. Direct impact trauma often causes cartilage crush injuries, whereas the twisting mechanism is generally associated with a subluxation or dislocation that results in a shearing injury to the cartilage, typically on the medial patella and/or lateral trochlea. In addition to the cartilage injuries associated with instability, the medial soft-tissue stabilizing structures are also injured, placing the athlete at increased risk for future instability episodes.

DIAGNOSIS

History and Physical Examination

- Initial history should differentiate symptoms of pain from those of instability.
    - Repetitive overuse injury is suggested by insidious onset of pain.
    - Pain originating from the PFJ is suggested by anterior pain with prolonged knee flexion (the classic "movie theater" sign) or anterior pain with ascending or descending stairs.
    - A history of instability is usually associated with a traumatic weight-bearing or twisting event followed by the onset of acute pain.
    - Often, patients do not report a frank dislocation or subluxation event unless specifically questioned.
    - Direct patellar trauma such as dashboard injuries or contact with the ground should also be elicited from the history and may indicate an acute chondral injury.
- The history is used to concentrate the physical examination to specific areas of the lower extremity.
- Systematic evaluation of factors that influence lower-extremity alignment—including assessment of the position of the hips, knees, and feet—is critical (Box 28-3).
- Palpation for tenderness is performed systematically to identify injured structures.
    - Structures palpated include the lateral retinaculum, medial retinaculum, MPFL attachments to the me-

dial femoral epicondyle and patella, the medial and lateral patellar facets, and the inferior pole of the patella.
    - Direct compression of the patella into the trochlea at various degrees of knee flexion may elicit pain and localize articular cartilage injuries (Fig. 28-3).
- The features listed in Box 28-3, which may be contributing to lower-extremity malalignment, should be assessed.
- In particular, muscular imbalance at the hip can also affect alignment at the knee and should not be overlooked.
    - Patellofemoral forces may be influenced by lower-extremity flexibility.
    - Flexibility should be assessed for quadriceps, hamstrings, gastrocsoleus, iliotibial band (ITB), hip flexors, and hip external rotators.
    - Because of the prominent attachments of the ITB to the patella through the lateral retinaculum, careful evaluation and treatment of ITB tightness is essential.
    - Ober's test for ITB flexibility is performed with the patient lying on his/her side.
        - The down hip is flexed to stabilize the pelvis.
        - The upper leg is moved sequentially into maximal hip flexion, abduction, and extension.
        - The leg is then positioned into adduction by gravity, and the degree of adduction is noted, as well as pain localized to the lateral patella.
- Quadriceps flexibility is measured with the patient prone to stabilize the pelvis to prevent hip flexion.
    - Femoral anteversion may be measured in this position by keeping the knee flexed to 90 degrees and rotating the leg internally until the greater trochanter is maximally prominent laterally.
    - Hamstring flexibility is measured by the popliteal angle in the supine position with the hip at 90 degrees of flexion.
    - Quadriceps muscle weakness is measured by observ-

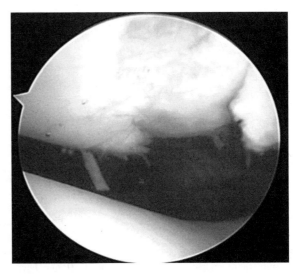

Figure 28-3 Articular cartilage defect on the medial facet of the patella sustained after a traumatic patellar dislocation.

ing gross atrophy and measuring thigh circumference.

■ VMO dyssynchrony may be observed when VMO contraction lags slightly behind the vastus lateralis with active quadriceps contraction.

■ Tightness or looseness of the passive medial and lateral stabilizers is assessed by measuring patellar mobility.

■ Patella translation is graded as the number of quadrants that the patella can be translated medially and laterally.

■ Passive patellar tilt is graded as less than neutral, neutral, or greater than neutral.

■ Passive patellar tilt less than neutral indicates a tight lateral retinaculum.

■ The Q-angle is measured from the anterior superior iliac spine to the midpatella, to the tibial tubercle, and reflects the lateral force on the patella.

■ A normal Q-angle is less than 15 degrees (Fig. 28-4).

■ In cases of gross lateral tracking of the patella, the Q-angle may be falsely reduced and thus misleading.

■ The tubercle-sulcus angle is measured with the patient seated and the knee flexed to 90 degrees.

■ The position of the tibial tubercle relative to the midpatella is observed, and lateralization of the tubercle past the midpatella indicates malalignment.

■ The J-sign refers to the inverted J-course of a patella

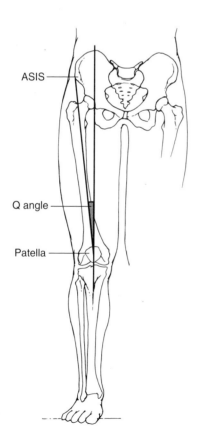

Figure 28-4   The Q-angle is measured from the anterior superior iliac spine to the midpatella, to the tibial tubercle. (From Oates CA. Kinesiology: The Mechanics and Pathomechanics of Human Movement. Baltimore: Lippincott Williams & Wilkins, 2004.)

that begins lateral to the trochlea and moves suddenly medially to enter the trochlea and is a sign of lateral patellar tracking during initiation of flexion.

■ Patellofemoral crepitus is elicited by palpation while placing the knee through a range of motion and is indicative of cartilage wear.

■ The presence and magnitude of knee effusion are assessed as well.

■ If the history is consistent with an acute traumatic event, indicating that the patient has sustained a recent subluxation or dislocation, the physical examination will likely reveal an effusion, possible ecchymosis over the injured medial stabilizers of the knee, tenderness over the MPFL and medial retinaculum, and severe patellar apprehension to lateral translation.

■ Patellar apprehension is the sensation of impending dislocation felt by the patient as a lateral force is applied to the patella with the leg in extension and can indicate underlying patellar instability.

■ Chondral injury is suggested by crepitus or gross palpation of a loose body.

■ The first-time dislocator may have some evidence of lower-extremity malalignment or, more often, a normal alignment.

■ Physical examination is summarized in Box 28-4.

Radiologic Examination

■ Radiologic workup for the athlete with patellofemoral pain should begin with a full set of plain radiographs, including a weight-bearing anteroposterior, lateral view (knee flexed to 30 degrees), and a merchant axial view at 30 or 45 degrees of knee flexion.

■ The lateral view is helpful in determining patellar height and rotation (Fig. 28-5).

■ The axial view offers information about patellofemoral alignment from tilt to subluxation, as well as

---

BOX 28-4 SUMMARY OF PHYSICAL EXAMINATION FOR PATELLOFEMORAL DISORDERS

Inspection
■ Q-angle
■ J-sign
■ Tubercle-sulcus angle
Palpation
■ Crepitus
■ Patellar facets
■ Tendons
■ Retinaculum
Provocative maneuvers
■ Lateral patellar apprehension
Patellar mobility (glide)
Flexibility
■ Hip flexors
■ Quadriceps
■ Hamstrings

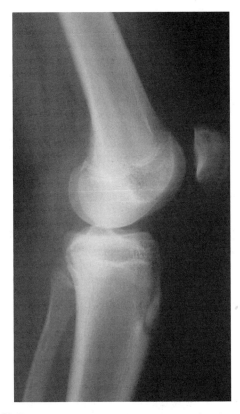

Figure 28-5 Lateral radiograph of an adolescent female with recurrent instability demonstrating open tibial tubercle apophysis and significant patella alta.

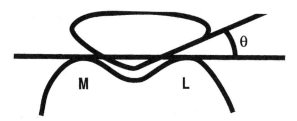

Figure 28-7 To evaluate patellar tilt, a line is drawn along the lateral facet of the patella and second line is drawn across the femoral condyles. In a normal knee, the angle of these lines (θ) should open laterally (L). If the lines are parallel or if they open medially (M), there is lateral patellar tilt.

visualizing the PFJ spaces and assessing cartilage wear (Fig. 28-6).

- In cases of patellofemoral pain due to overuse, plain radiographs are often all that is needed.
- Patients may have normal radiographs or may have subtle patellar tilt on the axial view.
- In cases of trauma and instability, radiographs may show loose bodies associated with osteochondral injuries (though these are rarely picked up on plain radiographs), subluxation of the patella on the axial view from the disruption of the medial stabilizers, or even avulsion fractures indicating ligament injury.
- Axial views are useful in evaluating subluxation, patellar deformity, avulsion fragments, joint space narrowing, subchondral sclerosis, osteophytes, and occasionally osteochondritis dissecans.

- Computed tomography (CT) is more sensitive than plain radiography in assessing patellar alignment.
    - The advantage of CT is that there is no image overlap

allowing more precise points of reference for measurements.

- To determine patellar tilt, a line is drawn on the axial cut (CT or plain radiograph) along the lateral facet of the patella, and a second line is drawn across the femoral condyles.
    - In a normal knee, the angle of these lines should open laterally.
    - If the lines are parallel or if they open medially, then there is lateral patellar tilt (Fig. 28-7).

- Magnetic resonance imaging (MRI) is a useful modality for visualizing the cartilage and soft-tissue structures.
    - In patients with continued complaints of patellofemoral pain without instability, MRI can demonstrate subtle cartilage thinning and asymmetric wear.
    - In cases of instability or trauma, MRI is useful in evaluating the integrity of the medial stabilizers, including the MPFL and VMO, as well as looking for any chondral injuries to the patella or the trochlea (Fig. 28-8).

- Diagnostic workup of patellofemoral disorders is summarized in Algorithm 28-1.

SPECIFIC DISORDERS

Lateral Patellar Compression Syndrome

- Nonoperative treatment consists of activity modification, nonsteroidal anti-inflammatory drugs (NSAIDs), physical therapy, taping, and bracing.
- Activity modification eliminates the repetitive insult. NSAIDS are used to reduce the pain, as well as the inflammation.

Figure 28-6 Bilateral merchant axial radiographs. The right knee displays patellar tilt with mild subluxation. The left knee has tilt with lateral patellar joint space narrowing and osteophytes resulting from cartilage loss.

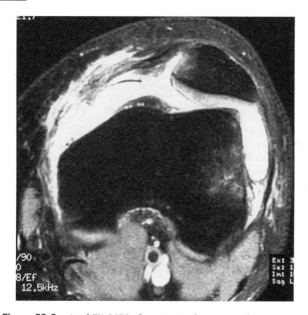

Figure 28-8   Axial T2 MRI of a patient who sustained a traumatic patellar dislocation. The medial patellofemoral ligament is torn off its origin at the medial epicondyle. In addition, there is bone edema in both the medial patellar facet and lateral trochlea resulting from the force of relocation. These are the most common locations of articular cartilage injuries after traumatic dislocations.

■ Bracing and taping are used to reduce the lateral stress on the patella by pulling the patella medially and may improve extensor function during weight-bearing activities.

■ Physical therapy is aimed at strengthening the quadriceps (specifically the VMO) and the hip abductors/external rotators, as well as stretching the tight lateral structures (the ITB and retinaculum) in an effort to restore balance to the delicate patellofemoral articulation.

■ If excessive foot pronation is noted, corrective orthotics may be used to restore a more normal plantigrade foot strike.

Traumatic Instability

■ Patients who present with traumatic instability can be divided into those with loose bodies and chondral injuries and those without.

■ For patients who sustain a chondral injury at the time of dislocation/relocation, there is little role for nonoperative treatment.

　■ The loose body needs to be recovered and if possible replaced and fixed if it is a substantial portion of the articular surface of the patella or trochlea.

　■ If it cannot be reduced and fixed, it needs to be removed and the cartilage defect treated with the options listed in Box 28-5.

■ In patients who sustain acute patella dislocations (APD) without the presence of loose bodies, the general consensus is a nonoperative approach as the first-line treatment (Box 28-6).

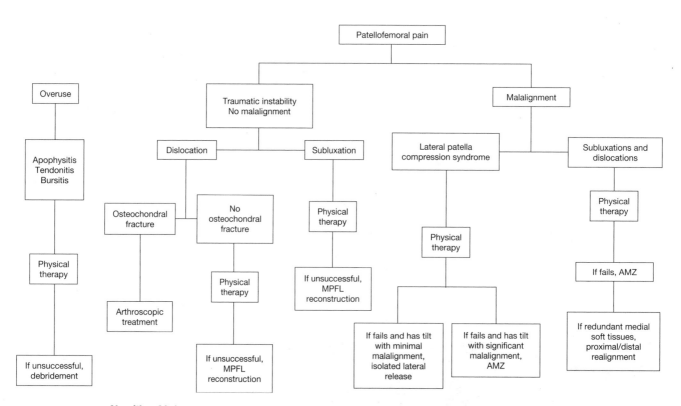

Algorithm 28-1   Diagnosis and management of patellar pain. MPFL, medial patellofemoral ligament; AMZ, anteromedialization.

BOX 28-5 SURGICAL TREATMENT OPTIONS FOR ARTICULAR CARTILAGE LESIONS

- Marrow stimulation techniques (microfracture vs. abrasion chondroplasty)
- Osteochondral autograft transplant
- Allograft osteochondral plugs
- Autologous chondrocyte implantation

- Initial management includes aspiration of the hemarthrosis if the knee exhibits a tense, painful effusion.
- A knee immobilizer is used to rest the knee and prevent further instability during recovery.
- Ice and NSAIDs are used to reduce swelling, and physical therapy is directed at obtaining normal range of motion, followed by strengthening the secondary stabilizers of the patella (VMO), as well as the rest of the surrounding muscle groups.
- These patients should be advised that they may return to sports when they have achieved a knee that is not swollen or painful and has full range of motion and full strength.
  - This may take up to 6 to 12 weeks.

Patellar Tilt

- Patellar tilt is characterized by anterior knee pain without instability.
- Examination reveals decreased patella translation and tilt.
- Imaging studies reveal patella tilt often combined with radiographic subluxation.
- Nonoperative treatment is usually successful and is designed at stretching the tight lateral structures, and strengthening the dynamic medial stabilizers.
  - Bracing, NSAIDs, and core strengthening enhance the treatment.
- Patients with pain despite nonoperative treatment are candidates for arthroscopic lateral release.
- Isolated lateral release is not appropriate for patients with a history of lateral patellar instability (subluxations or dislocations).

BOX 28-6 INITIAL MANAGEMENT OF ACUTE PATELLAR DISLOCATIONS

- Aspiration of the hemarthrosis
- Immobilization
- Ice
- Nonsteroidal anti-inflammatory drugs
- Supervised physical therapy

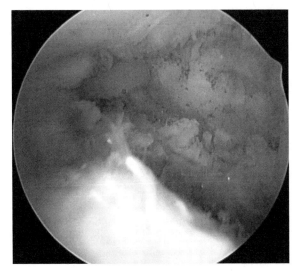

Figure 28-9 Arthroscopic picture of a lateral release. The camera is in the inferolateral portal looking superiorly, and the electrocautery device is placed through the superolateral portal to allow adequate visualization of the structures being released.

- Technically, the lateral release must include the entire retinaculum without extending too far proximally and weakening the vastus lateralis (Fig. 28-9).
- Lateral retinacular release was previously popular for treating all patellofemoral pain, but the indications have been narrowed.
  - Lateral release is now restricted to treating those patients with pain, a tight lateral retinaculum, and lateral tilt and who have not had any instability episodes (either subluxations or dislocations).
  - Surgery is indicated in this group only when nonoperative treatment has failed.
- Surgical technique involves diagnostic arthroscopy, chondroplasty as indicated, and release of the lateral retinaculum, taking care to avoid compromising the extensor mechanism.
  - Meticulous hemostasis should be obtained with the tourniquet released because hemarthrosis is the most common postoperative complication.
  - Inappropriate indications or release extending too far proximally involving the vastus lateralis obliquus can cause postoperative medial patellar subluxation.

Patellar Instability

- In first-time dislocators who sustain osteochondral injuries, all efforts are made to recover the fragment and fix it.
  - If the fragment is unable to be salvaged, then the surgeon needs to address the cartilage defect.
  - Several options exist for treating such articular lesions (Box 28-5).
- In patients without osteochondral fractures who have failed conservative treatment for instability, the surgical treatment is tailored to the underlying cause of the recurrent instability.

- Three categories of treatment are considered:
  - Proximal realignment for patients who are skeletally immature and have a dysplastic femoral trochlea and weak medial stabilizers, but who do not have overwhelming malalignment.
  - Distal realignment for patients with significant malalignment (i.e., Q-angle greater than 20 degrees) and or patellar chondral injuries that need to be unloaded.
  - Combined proximal and distal realignment when malalignment exists with deficient medial soft-tissue stabilizers.

Proximal Realignment

- In cases in which there is minimal bony malalignment, surgery is aimed at reconstructing the soft-tissue stabilizers (i.e., MPFL reconstructions or proximal realignment [medial imbrication]).
- MPFL reconstructions use allograft or autograft tissue fixed at the adductor tubercle and at the medial border of the patella at the native ligament anatomic insertions.
  - The graft is fixed on the femoral side and then tunneled under the soft tissue to the patella.
  - A medial force is applied to the patella to balance it within the trochlea because it is tensioned and fixed on the patellar side.
- Indications for performing a proximal realignment procedure include patellar instability with minimal bony malalignment and instability in the setting of a deficient medial retinaculum and VMO.
- Contraindications include medial chondral injuries to either the medial patella or trochlea that would receive greater load bearing with realignment.
- Medial imbrication can be performed open or arthroscopically.

- Open techniques involve creating a medial arthrotomy, followed by imbrication of the medial soft tissues.
  - Care should be taken to avoid creating medial subluxation with overaggressive medialization.
- Arthroscopic techniques for tightening redundant tissue with sutures have improved as instruments have evolved making arthroscopic medial imbrication a viable alternative for some patients (Fig. 28-10).

Distal Realignment

- Indications for distal realignment include chronic pain from lateral patellar subluxation and excessive lateral pressure syndrome with or without chondral wear.
- In addition, instability associated with malalignment or failed proximal realignment is an indication for a distal procedure.
- When there is tubercle malalignment with no symptomatic cartilage lesions, a straight medial tubercle transfer can be performed.
- Anteromedial tibial tubercle transfer (also called anteromedialization) restores patella tracking and unloads the lateral patella and trochlea (Fig. 28-11).
- Postoperatively, full weight-bearing should be avoided for approximately 6 weeks (until bony healing is noted on radiographs) in order to avoid fracture.
- Results after anteromedial tibial tubercle transfer are best with distal and lateral patellar cartilage lesions; results are not as good when the lesions are located on the proximal (direct impact and/or blunt injury) and medial facets.
- Arthroscopy before performing the osteotomy will help determine the degree of medialization and anteriorization needed to unload the patella.

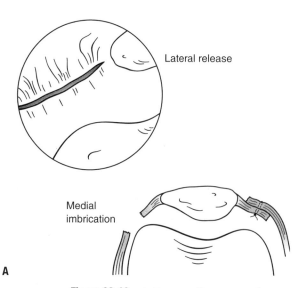

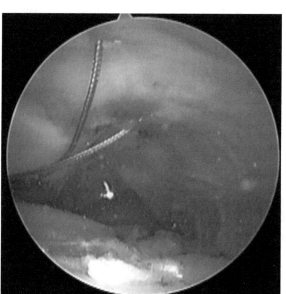

Figure 28-10 A: Diagram illustrating arthroscopic lateral release and medial imbrication. B: Arthroscopic view of medial suture placement for imbrication.

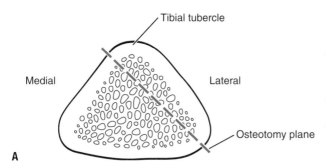

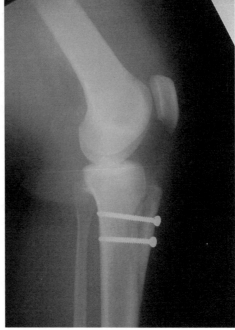

Figure 28-11   A: Axial diagram illustrating oblique osteotomy of a tibial tubercle transfer. **B:** Lateral radiograph of a patient who underwent a tibial tubercle anteromedialization. Fixation is achieved with two 4.5 cortical screws.

Acute Patellar Dislocation

- APD occurs most commonly in the second decade of life.
    - Factors predisposing patients to instability include patella alta, VMO dysplasia, generalized ligamentous laxity, increased Q-angle, tight ITB, genu valgum, and hypoplastic lateral trochlea.
    - The natural history of patellar dislocation treated with nonoperative measures results in recurrent instability in as many as 15% to 44% of patients.
- The pathology resulting from APD includes tearing of the medial retinaculum, VMO, and MPFL.
    - Osteochondral lesions are common and tend to occur on the medial patellar facet and lateral femoral trochlea.
- MRI is useful in the diagnosis of osteochondral and chondral injuries, as well as MPFL and VMO injuries.
- Management of APD is controversial, though most clinicians favor nonoperative treatment for the first-time dislocator.
- Improved understanding of the pathoanatomy of APD and studies showing high recurrence rates has stimulated recent interest in acute repair.
    - Most often, the MPFL is torn from its attachment on the distal femur. This can be repaired with suture anchors via a small incision (Fig. 28-12).
    - In addition, the VMO can be repaired anatomically (Fig. 28-13) and this may decrease the risk for redislocation, but follow-up studies and long-term outcome data are lacking for this method of treatment.

Other Patella-related Problems

Prepatellar Bursitis

- Prepatellar bursitis can be caused by acute trauma or repetitive trauma.

- Treatment includes ice, compression, short-term immobilization, activity modification, and NSAIDs.
- Bursal aspiration may be attempted, but care should be taken to prevent turning an aseptic bursitis into an infected bursitis.
- Surgery is rarely needed but may be indicated when extensive nonoperative treatment fails and can be performed open or by bursoscopy.

Patellar Tendinitis

- Patellar tendonitis (often referred to as "jumper's knee") results from a chronic overload in the patellar ligament near the insertion on the lower pole of the patella.
- This condition most commonly occurs in athletes involved in repetitive jumping activities such as basketball or volleyball.
- Plain radiographs may appear normal, but MRI and ultrasound reveal focal changes in the tendon signal and tendon hypertrophy.
- Palpation over the inferior pole of the patella is tender, reproducing the patient's symptoms.
- Examination of the lower extremity includes careful assessment of the flexibility of the lumbar spine, as well as the hamstring tendons, because stiffness may predispose the athlete toward infrapatellar tendonitis.
- Ultrasonography can diagnose the site of the infrapatellar tendonitis and quantify the size of the hypoechoic lesion.
- Initial treatment of infrapatellar tendonitis includes rest, activity modification, anti-inflammatory medications, and physical therapy.
- Early stages of patellar tendonitis generally respond to conservative treatment with resolution of the symptoms.
- When complaints of pain occur not only during sport-

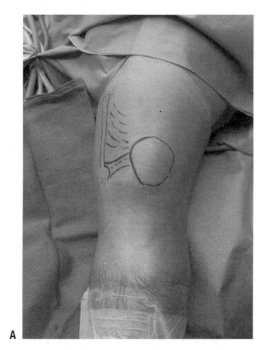
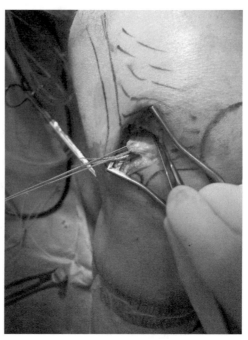

Figure 28-12   **A:** Medial patellofemoral ligament (MPFL), vastus medialis obliquus, and adductor magnus tendon outlined before acute repair. **B:** MPFL tear identified from femoral attachment and tagged for repair.

ing activities but also at rest, conservative treatment may fail to allow the athlete to return to his or her sport.

■ Surgical treatment is indicated in fewer than 5% of athletes who present with symptoms of infrapatellar tendonitis.

■ It consists of a direct approach to the inferior pole of the patella, with resection and debridement of the pathological area of tendon degeneration.

■ After a period of immobilization and restricted weight-bearing, rehabilitation is advanced gradually.

■ Full return to activities without restrictions is possible between 4 and 6 months postoperatively.

Patellar Osteochondritis Desiccans

■ Osteochondritis desiccans (OCD) is a disease in which a piece of cartilage and its underlying subchondral bone separate from the rest of the articular surface.

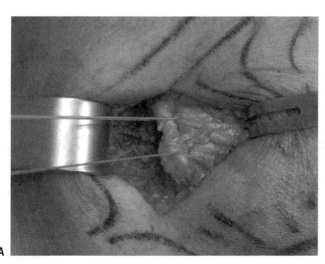
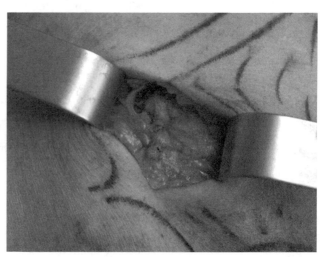

Figure 28-13   Vastus medialis obiquus tear identified and tagged **(A)** and anatomically repaired **(B)**.

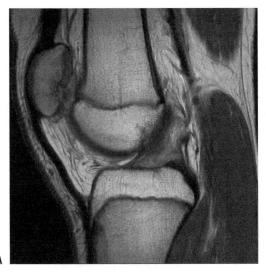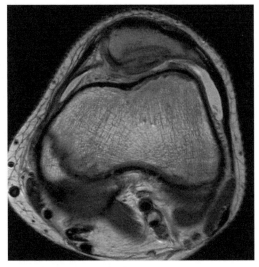

Figure 28-14   **A:** Sagittal T1 MRI of a patient with a patellar osteochondritis dessicans lesion. **B:** Axial T1 MRI of the same patient demonstrating cartilage surface irregularity overlying the osteochondritis dessicans lesion.

- The knee is the most common location for an OCD lesion, although the patella is not usually affected.
- Patients with patellar OCD usually present in their 20s and 30s, though the disorder may present later in life.
- The etiology of OCD is not fully understood.
  - Trauma and ischemia have both been implicated as possible causes for OCD, though neither has been directly proven to be responsible for the disease.
- Men are more frequently affected than women by OCD lesions.
- Often OCD is asymptomatic and is found incidentally on radiographs.
- Treatment is based on patient symptoms and stability of the OCD fragment.
- MRI is useful in determining the stability of the fragment as well as evaluating the integrity of the overlying cartilage (Fig. 28-14).
- If the fragment is well attached with an intact articular surface and the patient's complaints are limited to pain without mechanical symptoms, treatment usually consists of a trial of non- or partial weight-bearing to unload the lesion.
- If the lesion is loose or detached from its bony bed and the patient complains of mechanical locking or catching, then operative treatment is indicated.
- Surgery is aimed at retrieving the fragment if it is loose and trying to fix it in its bed to save the overlying cartilage.
- If the cartilage is soft or has degenerative changes, the fragment is removed and the cartilage defect treated (Box 28-5).
- Postoperative treatment is aimed at protecting the fragment or treated defect from load.
- The patella sees little load when the knee is extended, so the knee is braced in extension to prevent excessive pressure.
- Crutches are used to aid in non-weight-bearing for the

first 4 weeks, then progressing to full weight-bearing by 6 weeks.
- Physical therapy is started to prevent stiffness, with limits on flexion.
- During the first 4 weeks, the knee is ranged from 0 to 60 degrees, progressing to 90 degrees at 4 weeks and then to full motion after 6 weeks.
- Athletes can generally expect to return to their sport between 4 and 6 months postoperatively.

SUGGESTED READING

Ahmad CS, Shubin Stein BE, Matuz D, et al. Immediate surgical repair of the medial patellar stabilizers for acute patellar dislocation. A review of eight cases. Am J Sports Med 2000;28:804–810.

Atkin DM, Fithian DC, Marangi KS, et al. Characteristics of patients with primary acute lateral patellar dislocation and their recovery within the first 6 months of injury. Am J Sports Med 2000;28: 472–479.

Elias DA, White LM, Fithian DC. Acute lateral patellar dislocation at MR imaging: Injury patterns of medial patellar soft-tissue restraints and osteochondral injuries of the inferomedial patella. Radiology 2002;225:736–743.

Fithian DC, Paxton EW, Post WR, et al. Lateral retinacular release: a survey of the International Patellofemoral Study Group. Arthroscopy 2004;20:463–468.

Fithian DC, Paxton EW, Stone ML, et al. Epidemiology and natural history of acute patellar dislocation. Am J Sports Med 2004;32: 1114–1121.

Fulkerson JP, Becker GJ, Meaney JA, et al. Anteromedial tibial tubercle transfer without bone graft. Am J Sports Med 1990;18:490–496.

Maenpaa H, Huhtala H, Lehto MU. Recurrence after patellar dislocation. Redislocation in 37/75 patients followed for 6–24 years. Acta Orthop Scand 1997;68:424–426.

Merchant AC. Patellofemoral imaging. Clin Orthop 2001;389:15–21.

Murray TF, Dupont JY, Fulkerson JP. Axial and lateral radiographs in evaluating patellofemoral malalignment. Am J Sports Med 1999; 27:580–584.

Pidoriano AJ, Weinstein RN, Buuck DA, et al. Correlation of patellar articular lesions with results from anteromedial tibial tubercle transfer. Am J Sports Med 1997;25:533–537.

Sallay PI, Poggi J, Speer KP, et al. Acute dislocation of the patella. A correlative pathoanatomic study. Am J Sports Med 1996;24:52–60.

MENISCAL INJURIES

JOHN A. DOUGLAS
NICHOLAS A. SGAGLIONE

The medial and lateral menisci of the knee contribute to optimal knee function and joint stabilization through load sharing, stress distribution, anteroposterior stability, articular cartilage nutrition, joint congruence, prevention of synovial impingement, and proprioception. The menisci deepen the articular surfaces of the tibial plateau providing shock absorption and compensate for gross incongruity between the tibia and femoral articulating surfaces. The menisci also contribute to joint lubrication and help distribute synovial fluid throughout the joint, aiding in the homeostasis of articular cartilage. As the knee moves from flexion to extension, the menisci act as stabilizers and allow for a smooth coupled force transmission to occur, thus not functioning within a pure single-plane hinge, but rather a more complex mechanical joint capable of gliding/rotatory motion.

STRUCTURE AND FUNCTION

The meniscus is a crescent-shaped, specialized fibrocartilaginous structure. It is roughly triangular in cross section and covers one half to two thirds of the articular surface of the corresponding tibial plateau (Fig. 29-1). Menisci are composed of dense, tightly woven collagen fibers arranged in a pattern that allows for great elasticity and a remarkable ability to withstand compression forces. Its extracellular matrix (ECM) is composed of a complex three-dimensional interlacing network consisting of proteoglycans (which primarily function to give the meniscus its viscoelastic com-

pressive properties), water, and collagen fibers interspersed with fibrochondrocytes. The principal collagen type of the ECM is type I collagen, composing more than 90% of the fibers, with the remainder consisting of small amounts of types II, III, V, and VI. The majority of these fibers are oriented circumferentially, with radial and perforating fibers also present. The inner two thirds of the menisci are composed of a combination of radial and circumferential fibers, whereas the outer peripheral one third has a predominance of circumferential fibers (Fig. 29-2).

Weight-bearing produces forces across the knee that result in compression of the menisci, which thereby places the circumferential fibers under tension. Similar to metal hoops placed around a wooden barrel, the circumferential tension that is generated in response to compression counteracts the outward radial forces acting against the menisci. This generated peripheral meniscal tension ("hoop stress concept")—in conjunction with the strong bony attachments at the anterior and posterior horns—ensures efficient tibiofemoral load transmission and prevents meniscal extrusion (Fig. 29-3). Violation of the circumferential fiber structure either through pathologic tearing or surgical excision leads to significant disruption of the meniscal biomechanics with alteration in the normal distribution and dissipation of compressive loads and hoop stress conversion. In addition to the circumferential fiber band, the radial and random perforating fiber ultrastructure also contributes to optimal meniscal mechanics and function. The radial fibers act as intrasubstance tie rods and resist against longitudinal

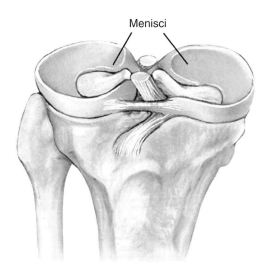

Figure 29-1 The meniscus is a crescent-shaped fibrocartilagenous structure that lies between the femur and tibia. Each knee has two menisci: one medial and one lateral. Together, they cushion the joint by distributing downward forces outward and away from the central anchor points of the menisci. (Courtesy of the Anatomical Chart Co.)

forces that tend to split the meniscal tissue, while random perforating fibers are important in the distribution of shear stress. Fibrochondrocytes are responsible for the synthesis and maintenance of the ECM and are essential in the process of meniscal healing.

The outer peripheral edges of the menisci are convex,

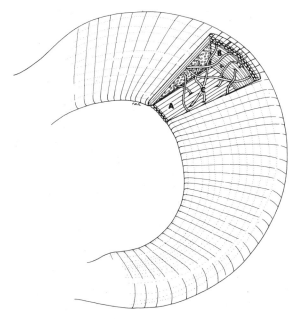

Figure 29-2 Orientation of meniscus collagen fiber. A: Radial fibers. B: Circumferential fibers. C: Perforating fibers. (From Shahriaree H. O'Connor's Textbook of Arthroscopic Surgery. Philadelphia: JB Lippincott, 1984.)

fixed, and attach to the inner capsule of the knee joint and to the corresponding tibia plateau via the coronary ligaments except at the popliteal hiatus laterally. The lateral meniscus at the popliteal hiatus is relatively avascular because of its lack of adjacent capsular attachments. The medial meniscus has a thickened capsular attachment that is most prominent at the body of the meniscus and is structurally consistent with the deep medial collateral ligament (MCL). The inner central edges of the menisci are concave and taper to a thin unattached edge. The inferior surface of each meniscus is flat, corresponding to the underlying tibia plateau, whereas the superior surface is concave and tapered, corresponding to the contour of the femoral condyle. The most peripheral aspect of the meniscus is the meniscosynovial junction, which extends from the anterior horn to the posterior horn. This is a transitional zone where there is a shift from predominantly type I circumferential collagen fibers to capsular fibers. The meniscus blood supply in this area is derived primarily from a circumferentially arranged perimeniscal capillary plexus that branches from the medial and lateral inferior and superior geniculate arteries. This capillary plexus penetrates approximately 10% to 30% of the medial and 10% to 25% of the lateral meniscus and is considered the "red-on-red zone" (red–red) and has the greatest healing potential (Fig. 29-4). The avascular inner two thirds of the meniscus, known as the "white-on white-zone," receives its nutrition from the synovial fluid through diffusion or mechanical pumping and has poor healing potential. Between these two "zones" is a variable vascular area known as the "red-on-white" zone (red–white) that has intermediate healing potential. This transitional zone can be located 3 to 5 mm from the meniscosynovial junction. The menisci contain both free nerve endings and corpuscular mechanoreceptors and may act as a source of proprioceptive feedback for the knee joint.

The medial meniscus is approximately 4 cm in size and is essentially C-shaped. It is larger in radius and diameter and narrower in body than the lateral meniscus, with the posterior horn bearing more of the weight of the meniscus than the anterior horn. The average width of this meniscus is 10 mm, with an average thickness of 3 to 5 mm, and it covers approximately 64% of the plateau. The lateral meniscus is more circular in shape, covering up to 84% of the articular surface of the tibial plateau. It is smaller in diameter, wider in body, and more mobile than the medial meniscus. The average width is 12 to 13 mm, with an average thickness of 5 mm that is overall more uniform laterally compared with the medial meniscus that has a more variable thickness throughout its length. The lateral meniscus is more mobile and can translate up to 9 to 11 mm, with an average excursion of 11.2 mm from 0 to 120 degrees of flexion. The medial meniscus, which is less mobile can translate up to 2 to 5 mm on the tibia, with an average of 5.1 mm of excursion from 0 to 120 degrees of flexion.

A unique feature of the lateral meniscus is the anterior and posterior meniscofemoral ligaments, which consist of the ligament of Humphrey anterior to and the ligament of Wrisberg posterior to the posterior cruciate ligament. These ligaments are inconsistent in their size and presence and have been reported to be absent in 30% of individuals. In

Joint load

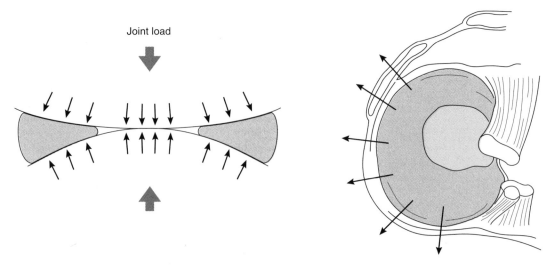

Figure 29-3 The role of hoop tension in menisci. Hoop tension generated by the menisci help keep it located between the tibia and femur cushioning the joint during load transmission. (After Grood ES. Meniscal function. Adv Orthop Surg 1984;7:193.)

the 70% of knees noted to have meniscofemoral ligaments, the Wrisberg ligament (posterior meniscofemoral ligament) is more commonly present than the anterior ligament of Humphrey (Fig. 29-5).

The shape of the medial and lateral menisci improves the congruency of the articulating surfaces and increases the surface area of joint contact, thus adding load transmission across the knee joint. With knee extension, the menisci are responsible for transmission of 50% to 70% of knee joint force; this increases to 85% with 90 degrees of knee flexion. The medial meniscus has been shown to act as an important secondary restraint to the anterior translation of the tibia,

specifically in the presence of anterior cruciate ligament (ACL) deficiency.

In isolated meniscal injuries, the lateral meniscus is injured less commonly than the medial meniscus (lateral meniscal tears are more commonly seen in association with acute ACL injuries). It is more mobile than the medial meniscus and can have fiber attachments to both cruciate ligaments. Both menisci follow the tibia during flexion and extension. The menisci move anterior with extension and posterior with flexion, with both the popliteus muscle laterally, by way of the arcuate ligament, and the semimembranosus muscle medially retracting the posterior horns of the menisci posteriorly during flexion. However, during rotation, the menisci follow the femur and move on the tibia. The lateral meniscus can, by way of the meniscofemoral ligament attachments, move with the lateral femoral condyle during flexion and extension, thus preventing the meniscus from being caught between the condyle of the femur and the plateau of the tibia. In contrast, the medial meniscus has no meniscofemoral ligaments, and with a more restrained tibial attachment, it tends to follow the tibia, and hence has a higher probability of sustaining shear stresses (and associated tearing) between the femoral condyle and the tibia plateau during rotation (Fig. 29-6).

PATHOPHYSIOLOGY

Acute tears of the menisci most commonly occur secondary to a rotational and compressive load placed on the knee as it moves from a flexed to an extended position. The combination of compression and rotation results in shear stresses that tear the meniscal tissue. The most common location of this lesion is the posterior horn of the medial meniscus, with a vertical longitudinal tear being the most common type of tear pattern.

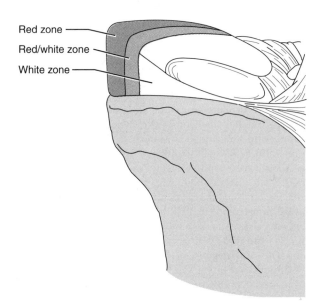

Red zone
Red/white zone
White zone

Figure 29-4 Zones of meniscal vascularity. (After Sgaglione NA. Meniscus repair: update on new techniques. Tech Knee Surg 2002; 1:113–127.)

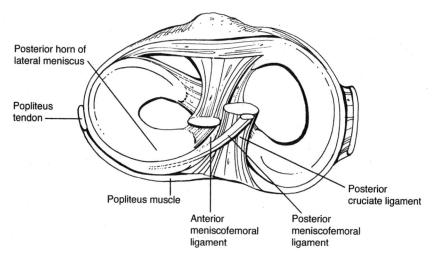

Figure 29-5 Superior view of the tibia condyles. Lateral meniscus is smaller in diameter, wider in body, thicker at the periphery, and more mobile. It is attached posteriorly to the medial femoral condyle by the anterior and posterior meniscofemoral ligaments and to the popliteus muscle.

EPIDEMIOLOGY

The mean annual incidence of meniscal tears is 60 to 70 per 100,000. The overall male to female ratio for meniscus tears ranges from 2.5:1 to 4:1, with a peak incidence occurring in males between 31 and 40 years of age. Meniscal tears constitute 50% of surgical injuries to the knee with medial tears being more common then lateral tears. The medial meniscus is more commonly injured in the stable knee or in the chronic ACL-deficient knee, whereas the lateral meniscus is more commonly injured in association with an acute ACL tear. Younger patients participating in

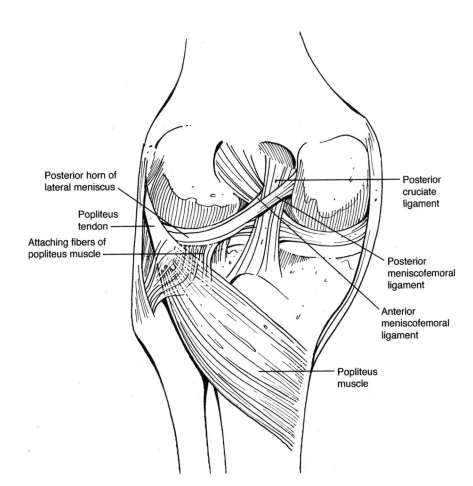

Figure 29-6 Posterior view of the knee. Lateral meniscus attaches posteriorly to the medial femoral condyle by the anterior and posterior meniscofemoral ligaments and to the popliteus muscle.

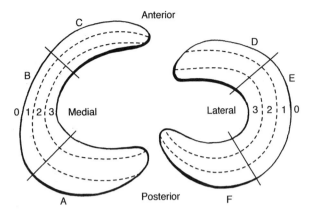

Figure 29-7 Zone classification of the meniscus. Posterior third zone of the medial menisci is lettered *A,* and moving in a clockwise direction in thirds, middle third zone is letter *B,* and the anterior third zone is letter *C,* etc. Here *0* is the meniscosynovial junction (the periphery), *1* is the outer third region of the menisci, *2* is the middle third region of the menisci, and *3* is the inner third region of the menisci.

sporting events are more prone to acute traumatic meniscal tears in comparison with older patients who tend to present with complex degenerative tears of insidious onset. Acute traumatic tears in the younger patient population are generally located at the periphery and are longitudinal in nature and often repairable. Tears that present in the absence of trauma and in older patients (usually greater than 40 years of age) tend to be degenerative tears, are often complex, and may have a horizontal cleavage component. They are generally not repairable.

CLASSIFICATION

Tears can be classified according to their location in relation to the vascular supply of the meniscus and whether that location is at the anterior, middle, or posterior third of the meniscus. A zone classification system has been devised by Cooper to provide consistent clinical documentation of meniscal tear patterns and to standardize descriptions of the locations of these tears. The menisci are divided into three radial zones anteriorly to posteriorly and four circumferential zones extending from the periphery to the inner aspect of the meniscus (Fig. 29-7). Tears are further classified according to their morphology and tear pattern relative to the tibial plateau (Fig. 29-8). Horizontal tears extend parallel to the transaxial plane of the tibia plateau, whereas vertical tears extend perpendicular to that plane. Vertical tears that propagate in a direct centrifugal direction from the inner to the outer aspect of the meniscus are called "radial (or transverse) tears," whereas those that propagate circumferentially in an anteroposterior direction are called "longitudinal tears." Oblique vertical (flap or parrot beak) tears by definition extend in a plane that is neither radial nor circumferential to the meniscus. A bucket-handle tear is essentially a vertical longitudinal tear that has gapped and can be further classified as displaced or nondisplaced. Complex (or degenerative) tears may include several geometric tear patterns and are for the most part associated with frayed, less viable meniscal tissue fragments.

Horizontal Tears

Horizontal meniscal tears, also known as horizontal cleavage tears, occur in all age groups but are seen more com-

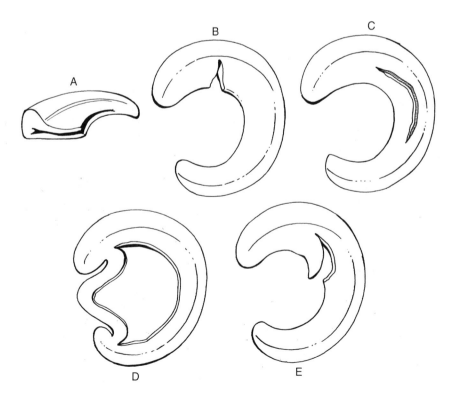

Figure 29-8 Meniscal tear patterns.
A: Horizontal tear. **B:** Radial tear.
C: Longitudinal tear. **D:** Bucket-handle tear.
E: Oblique tear.

monly in older patients, with a peak incidence of 31 to 50 years in men and 51 to 60 years of age in women. Horizontal tears occur most commonly in the posterior aspect of the medial meniscus. When this tear pattern is noted in the lateral meniscus, it may be associated with lateral meniscal cysts. The mechanism of injury is thought to be secondary to shear forces between the superior and inferior surfaces of the meniscus that tend to cause separation of the upper and lower segments of the tear. Initial tears may be confined to the substance of the meniscus without meniscal surface communication. With repeated traumatic episodes, an intrasubstance tear may extend to the articular surface communicating with the meniscal surface, or multiple tears may occur in the horizontal plane.

Repeated applied load to a meniscal tear can result in tear propagation, fragment displacement, and edge instability. These events can lead to mechanical symptoms including locking and catching with increased pain and effusion. Excision of the unstable portions of the meniscus is performed and does not usually require complete excision.

Longitudinal Tears

Vertical longitudinal tears are most commonly traumatic in origin and occur more often in younger individuals, with a peak incidence of 21 to 30 years of age in men and 11 to 20 years of age in women. They are noted more frequently medially in isolated cases and laterally in association with ACL tears. Longitudinal tears may be partial or complete and are often noted near the periphery, which heightens the indications for repair. Partial tears are generally confined to the posterior aspect of the meniscus, extending anteriorly with subsequent reinjury to the meniscus. Complete tears may produce locking of the knee joint if the inner portion of the meniscus tear site displaces into the intercondylar notch. This is more commonly noted with displaced bucket-handle–type tears.

Radial (Transverse) Tears

Radial tears are found in younger patients, with a peak incidence of 11 to 20 years of age in men and 51 to 70 years of age in women. They are usually traumatic, particularly when noted in the posterior horn of the lateral meniscus in younger patients. Function is compromised during load transmission in tears that extend to the periphery because of the disruption of the circumferential fibers and associated hoop stresses. Repairs of radial tears that extend to the periphery have the potential to heal because of the peripheral blood supply. Traditionally, repairs of radial tears were not recommended; however, more recent studies have indicated that, with more advanced repair techniques, clinical success may be achieved after full-thickness radial tear repairs (particularly of the posterior horn of the lateral meniscus).

Bucket-handle Tears

Bucket-handle tears are vertical longitudinal tears in which the central segment displaces medially. Bucket-handle tears theoretically maintain good healing potential after repair; however, chronic bucket-handle tears may be associated with tissue deformation, fraying, and complex radial components that make them less amenable to successful repair.

Oblique (Flap or Parrot Beak) Tears

Flap tears occur with a peak incidence of 31 to 40 years of age in men and 61 to 70 years of age in women. They are oblique tears that occur most commonly at the posterior horn of the medial meniscus and are anteriorly based. Initially, they may represent the anterior portion of a split buckle-handle tear or early complex tear in progression. As a result of the geometric complexity of these tears and the loss of associated tissue integrity, these tears are usually excised.

Complex (Degenerative) Tears

A complex tear is composed of two or more tear patterns and is the most common of all meniscal lesions, accounting for nearly 30% of all tears with a peak incidence of 41 to 50 years of age in men and 61 to 70 years of age in women. These tears may not be associated with any history of trauma and may have an insidious onset. Complex degenerative tears are frequently seen in association with other degenerative changes within the joint. In addition, complex degenerative tears usually have minimal to no healing potential and generally are not amenable to repair (Table 29-1 and Box 29-1).

DIAGNOSIS

History

- The history of previous knee symptoms or injury should be elicited along with any history of previous treatment or surgery.
- Questions regarding age, occupation, functional activity levels, patients' goals and expectations, and previous medical history should be defined.

TABLE 29-1 SUMMARY OF TEAR PATTERNS AND REPAIR POTENTIAL

Tear Pattern	Repair Potential
Horizontal	Not repairable Excise unstable superior or inferior segment
Longitudinal	Repairable
Radial (transverse)	Potentially repairable
Bucket handle	Repairable
Oblique (flap or parrot beak)	Not repairable Excise
Complex (degenerative)	Not repairable Excise if symptomatic

BOX 29-1 SUMMARY OF STABLE VERSUS UNSTABLE TEAR PATTERNS

Stable Tears
- Partial thickness tears that measure less than half the height of the meniscus
- Tears in the vascular periphery smaller than 7 to 10 mm in length, with excursion less than 3 to 5 mm during probing
- Radial tears measuring 5 mm or less
- Horizontal cleavage tears that do not appear to be causing symptoms

Unstable Tears
- Any tear unstable to probing that results in excursion of >3 to 5 mm or that can be displaced into the weight-bearing aspect of the joint, catching between the superior condyle and the tibial plateau

- A patient's history may not be associated with any one single traumatic event but rather repetitive overload, particularly in cases of degenerative meniscal tearing.
- Meniscal tears may occur secondary to contact or non-contact mechanisms.
- History often reveals a twisting injury that may or may not be associated with moderate swelling, loss of motion, and mechanical symptoms of catching or locking.
- Patients with meniscal tears often complain of pain localized to the joint line or referred to the popliteal region worse with knee flexion and weight-bearing.
- They may have mechanical symptoms—which are defined as popping, locking, buckling, or catching—if the meniscal tear is associated with any unstable fragment.

Physical Examination

- A thorough examination includes inspection, palpation and range-of-motion testing, followed by specific provocative maneuvers and meniscal-specific tests.
- The clinician should always examine the uninjured extremity for comparison, followed by the injured side.
- The knee joint should be inspected for effusion and atrophy of the quadriceps musculature.
  - The joint line and soft tissues should be inspected for soft-tissue swelling, which may be indicative of a parameniscal cyst.
  - Examination must include palpation of all bony prominences and manual examination of all ligamentous structures, including the ACL, the posterior cruciate ligament, the MCL, and the lateral collateral ligament.
  - A comprehensive examination of the patellofemoral joint should be conducted to rule out concomitant pathology or other sources of knee pain.
  - The joint line should be palpated for tenderness.
- The medial meniscus may be evaluated by internally rotating the tibia.
  - This maneuver allows the medial edge of the meniscus to become prominent and palpable on examina-

tion, and medial joint line tenderness suggests medial meniscal pathology.
- The lateral meniscus should be palpated with the knee in slight flexion or a figure-of-four position.
- Range-of-motion testing should document any loss of flexion or extension, because if a bucket-handle tear is present, the joint may be locked with full extension blocked.
- Provocative signs such as pain with squatting may also be indicative of a posterior horn meniscus tear.
- Numerous compression rotation tests have been described, but the McMurray and Apley's compression and distraction tests are the most commonly used in the diagnosis of meniscus tears.

McMurray Test
- The McMurray test is performed with the patient lying supine on the examination table with the lower extremity in a neutral position (Fig. 29-9).
  - The examiner places one hand on the knee with the thumb and thenar aspect of the palm on the lateral aspect of the joint and the fingers over the medial joint line.
  - The second hand is placed on the plantar part of the heel of the patient.
  - The examiner next flexes the knee up, followed by internal and external rotation of the leg.
  - A valgus stress is applied to the joint by pushing on the lateral aspect of the knee, followed by externally rotating the leg.
  - The knee is then slowly extended as the examiner palpates the medial joint line.
- Any painful, palpable, or audible click on extension is suggestive of a tear of the medial meniscus.
- If the tibia is rotated internally while applying a varus stress, the lateral meniscus can be examined similarly.

Apley's Compression and Distraction Test
- Apley's compression and distraction test is performed with the patient in the prone position and the examiner's knee placed over the posterior portion of the patient's thigh to stabilize it (Fig. 29-10).
  - The affected leg is flexed 90 degrees at the knee joint.
  - The examiner next grasps the heel and rotates the tibia internally and externally while applying a downward force on the foot.
  - Pain on either the medial or lateral side during compression and rotation is significant for a meniscal tear on the corresponding side.
- The distraction portion of this test is performed with the patient in the same position (Fig. 29-11).
  - Upward traction is applied to the leg by pulling up on the foot while the tibia is rotated internally and externally on the femur.
  - This maneuver reduces pressure on the meniscus and applies pressure to the collateral ligaments.
- If a specific collateral ligament injury is present, the patient may complain of pain on the corresponding ipsilateral side, whereas if the meniscus is the sole source

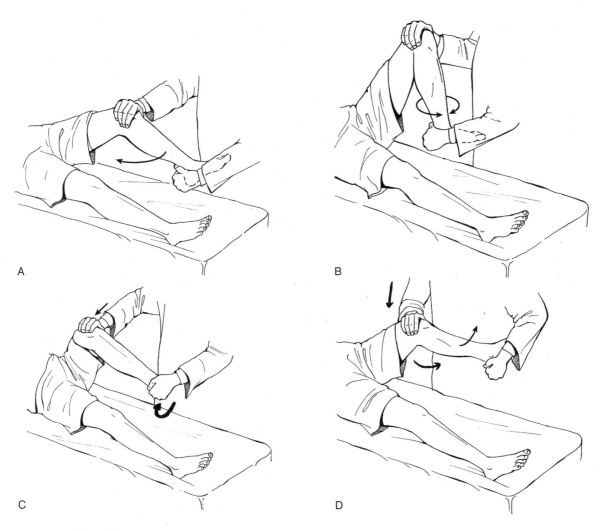

Figure 29-9 The McMurray test. **A:** With patient supine, flex the knee. **B:** Holding flexion, internally and externally rotate the tibia to loosen the knee joint. **C:** Holding flexion, apply a valgus stress to the knee and externally rotate the leg. **D:** Slowly extend the knee while palpating the medial joint line. A palpable, audible, or painful click during extension is suggestive of a torn medial meniscus.

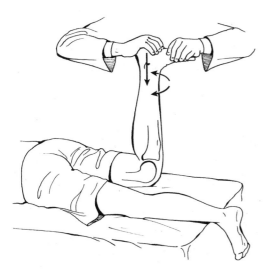

Figure 29-10 Apley's compression test for meniscal tears. With the patient prone and affected leg flexed 90 degrees, grasp and compress the heel while internally and externally rotating the tibia.

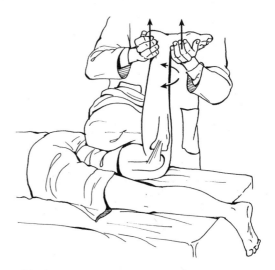

Figure 29-11 Apley's distraction test for ligamentous injury. With the patient in the same position, upward traction is applied to the leg while internally and externally rotating the tibia.

of pain, the distraction portion of the test will presumably be negative.

Radiologic Examination

- Imaging studies, such as radiographs and magnetic resonance imaging (MRI), should be used by the physician as adjuncts to a comprehensive history and physical examination.
- Diagnostic testing should first begin with radiographs of the knee.
- Plain radiographs are important in defining any bony pathology that may mimic a meniscus tear in symptoms, and in evaluation of the knee joint for any joint space narrowing.
- Four views are routinely obtained: a 30- or 45-degree posteroanterior flexion weight-bearing view, a true lateral weight-bearing view, a notch view, and a patella skyline view.
  - Articular cartilage wear is often more advanced in the posterior aspect of the femoral condyles; hence, the posteroanterior weight-bearing flexion view allows the physician a more precise method of assessing articular cartilage wear and determining joint space narrowing.
  - The notch view allows for more accurate assessment of osteochondritis dissecans (OCD) lesions.
  - The patella skyline view allows evaluation of the patellofemoral joint and any malalignment that may contribute to knee pain.
- MRI is not always indicated in isolated meniscus pathology if the diagnosis has been confirmed through history and physical.
- If there remains a question as to the diagnosis, MRI is the diagnostic procedure of choice to confirm meniscal pathology.
- MRI classifications of meniscal pathology have been defined.
  - A complete tear is commonly associated with a grade III high-signal intensity that communicates with the articular surface of the meniscus.
  - MRI findings in which a grade I or II signal is noted have high-signal intensity within the meniscus that does not communicate with or extend to the articular surface of the meniscus.

- Surgical intervention is usually reserved for symptomatic meniscal tears that are noted to be associated with complete tearing and grade III MRI signal intensity.
- MRI is also useful in cases where other ligamentous, articular cartilage, or bony disorders (such as osteonecrosis) are suspected.

TREATMENT

Approach to Meniscal Pathology

Principles of Repair

- If tissue viability and tear pattern lends itself to repair, then meniscal preservation should be considered.
- In younger patients who are undergoing concomitant ACL reconstruction, meniscal preservation through repair should be considered.

Principles of Resection

- In menisci not deemed repairable, partial meniscectomy should be conducted with the goal to remove all damaged and unstable meniscal fragments. Several important guidelines should be followed when carrying out a partial meniscectomy:
  - All efforts should be made to preserve as much normal meniscus tissue as possible.
  - Hypermobile meniscal pathologic fragments should be excised, leaving a smooth contour in the meniscus with no incongruous edges.
  - Residual tissue edges should be probed often to assess stability of the meniscus.
  - The meniscosynovial junction and adjacent articular cartilage surfaces should be protected at all times.
  - In summary, the goal of meniscal resection is to excise back to a normal stable rim, inspecting and identifying any unstable residual fragments (Fig. 29-12).
- Any remaining fragments that can be pulled into the joint and become secondarily entrapped between the weight-bearing aspect of the tibia and femur may cause persistent symptoms and precipitate localized articular damage as a result of increased focal compression forces across the articular surface.
- A higher incidence of associated chondromalacia has been reported in those patients with a history of unstable meniscal lesions of greater than 3 months duration.

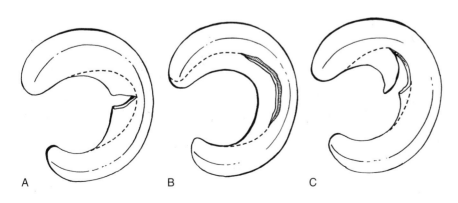

A   B   C

Fig 29-12 Balancing meniscal resection **(A)** with a radial tear, **(B)** with a longitudinal tear, and **(C)** with a flap tear. (After Newman AP, Daniels AU, Burks RT. Principles and decision making in meniscal surgery. Arthroscopy 1993;9:43.)

Resection versus Repair

- When considering repair versus resection, the ultimate clinical surgical decision is based on several factors, including activity level, overall health, patient compliance, and status of articular cartilage in the involved compartment.
- The benefits of any repair must always be weighed against the risks when counseling a patient regarding meniscal surgery.
- The potential long-term benefits of meniscus repair are clearly related to chondroprotection; however, the risks of repair include more extensive surgical intervention, including rehabilitation and recovery, stiffness and re-tears, or failures of the repair site to adequately heal.
- These risks may rise proportionately with age and thus should be taken into consideration during preoperative planning.
- Treatment must be individualized to the patient's significant goals and expectations.

Nonsurgical Treatment

- In the approach to meniscal tears, the clinician may use a working algorithm for the treatment of meniscal lesions (Algorithm 29-1).
- A stable peripheral longitudinal tear measuring less than 7 to 10 mm has the potential to heal by itself and may be left alone.
- Stable asymptomatic peripheral tears seen at the time of ACL reconstruction can continue to participate in load transmission and may be treated with abrasion and or trephination.
- After conservative management, the patient may be symptomatically improved over 6 weeks with the ability to return to normal activity after 3 months.
- If symptoms such as pain, tenderness, or effusion persist after this time, further treatment is indicated, and arthroscopy is advised.

Surgical Treatment

- The indications for more urgent arthroscopic intervention may include more significant mechanical symptoms and specifically locking, which can lead to articular cartilage damage from the increased focal pressure generated by the meniscal fragment, particularly during weight-bearing.
  - Patients who present with severe antalgia, marked pain, joint-line tenderness, and a large effusion may also be candidates for more immediate arthroscopic intervention.
  - Professional athletes, competitive recreational athletes, and laborers who rely on their lower extremities may not wish to delay surgical intervention; taking into account recovery times in these patients, arthroscopy may be indicated sooner rather than later to return these individuals back to work or sports quicker.
- During arthroscopy, the goal is to preserve as much normal meniscal tissue as possible while removing or repairing all tissue capable of contributing to subsequent symptoms.
- Difficult decisions must sometimes be made regarding menisci that have two or more segmental tears.
- One tear may be repairable and the other may not.
  - One clinical example involves a longitudinal tear near the periphery with an inner, central radial component. In this case, the radial component is excised with the longitudinal component repaired if it is in the vascular periphery and justified. Longitudinal tears located in the red–white zone, 3 to 5 mm from the meniscosynovial junction, may be repaired, depending on clinical indications (age of patient, articular cartilage status, etc.) and whether adequate healing stimulation is provided.
  - A second clinical example involves multiple longitudinal tears frequently seen in conjunction with ACL

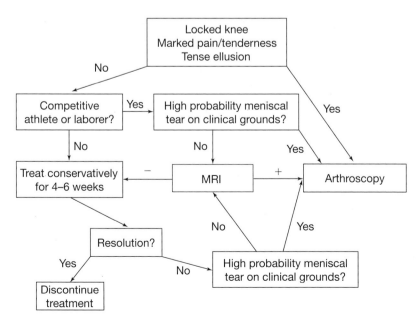

Algorithm 29-1 Decision to proceed to arthroscopy, MRI. (After Newman AP, Daniels AU, Burks RT. Principles and decision making in meniscal surgery. Arthroscopy 1993;9:44.)

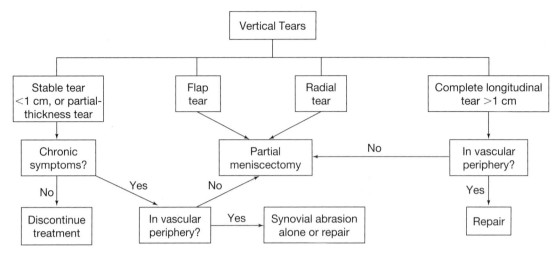

Algorithm 29-2 Management of vertical tears. (After Newman AP, Daniels AU, Burks RT. Principles and decision making in meniscal surgery. Arthroscopy 1993;9:44.)

injuries. In this case, those longitudinal tears in the white zone are resected, whereas tears in the other two zones may be repaired.

- The remaining repaired and contoured peripheral meniscus should be at least 3 to 4 mm in width to maintain load transmission capability and to justify the potential morbidity associated with repair.
- If the remaining meniscus measures 2 mm or less in width at its narrowest portion, repair yields little benefit in load transmission, and resection of the tear should be conducted instead (see Algorithms 29-2 and 29-3).
- In the older patient, it is important that the surgeon distinguish knee pain and symptoms secondary to osteo-

arthritis versus knee pain secondary to a truly symptomatic degenerative tear.
- Many degenerative tears are asymptomatic, and resection may not be indicated in all patients.
  - Because chondral pain may not be relieved by meniscectomy, symptoms may persist after the procedure.
- MRI studies should not be the primary focus of the physician's decision making because most studies are abnormal as a result of normal age-related changes.
- Decision making is usually based on the presence or absence of mechanical symptoms.
- If the patient has a history of an acute injury, followed by a brief period of pain and swelling, and if the radiographs show nominal degenerative articular changes with a neutral alignment of the knee axis, then partial meniscectomy may be an effective treatment (Algorithm 29-4).

Meniscal Resection Techniques

- Traditionally, instruments used for resection have included various angled hand-held punches, arthroscopic scissors, and mechanical shavers.
- Technological advances in the field of arthroscopy have allowed for the development of instruments that have improved the efficiency of arthroscopic procedures and access to the menisci, as well as allowing for smoother contouring of resected menisci.

Meniscal Rasping and Trephination Techniques

- Incomplete and stable tears can be stimulated to heal through rasping and trephination.
- The ideal tear selection involves a tear in the vascularized periphery in a patient with an acute ACL injury that is smaller than 7 to 10 mm in length and associated excursion <3 to 5 mm during probing.
- The abrasion technique involves a motorized shaver or meniscal rasp that is used to lightly abrade both the tibial and femoral sides of the tear site and adjacent

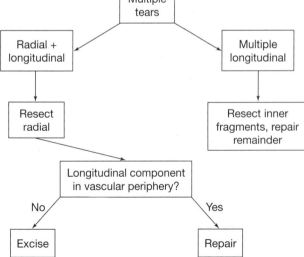

Algorithm 29-3 Management of multiple tears. (After Newman AP, Daniels AU, Burks RT. Principles and decision making in meniscal surgery. Arthroscopy 1993;9:44.)

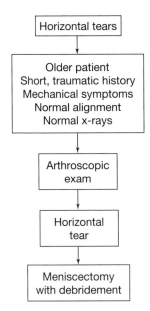

```
┌─────────────────┐
│ Horizontal tears │
└─────────────────┘
         ↓
┌─────────────────────┐
│   Older patient     │
│ Short, traumatic    │
│ history             │
│ Mechanical symptoms │
│ Normal alignment    │
│ Normal x-rays       │
└─────────────────────┘
         ↓
┌─────────────────┐
│  Arthroscopic   │
│     exam        │
└─────────────────┘
         ↓
┌─────────────────┐
│   Horizontal    │
│     tear        │
└─────────────────┘
         ↓
┌─────────────────┐
│ Meniscectomy    │
│ with debridement│
└─────────────────┘
```

Algorithm 29-4   Management of horizontal tears. (After Newman AP, Daniels AU, Burks RT. Principles and decision making in meniscal surgery. Arthroscopy 1993;9:44.)

meniscosynovial junction to stimulate vascularity for meniscal healing.

■ Trephination may be conducted to create small vascular access channels using an 18-gauge spinal needle.

■ The needle is placed through the skin or through arthroscopic portals and pierces the periphery of the meniscus traveling radially through the meniscus and tear site toward the inner rim.

   ■ Caution should be taken to avoid piercing the meniscal surface to limit further injury to the tissue.

■ Trephination promotes vascular access channels, enabling capillary ingrowth from the more vascularized peripheral tissues to the otherwise avascular inner third of the meniscus.

Meniscal Repair Techniques

■ When a meniscal tear is identified and surgical indications are met, then preservation of the meniscus through repair is preferred to help maintain articular cartilage integrity, particularly in younger, active individuals and in those undergoing associated ACL reconstruction.

■ Numerous arthroscopic-assisted meniscal repair methods exist to conduct the repair and include outside-in, inside-out, all-inside, and all-arthroscopic fixator implant and suture-based techniques.

■ There are various combinations of these methods known as hybridized techniques that may also be used.

■ The ultimate technique chosen generally depends on the tear type, size, site, displacement and, more importantly, surgeon preference.

Arthroscopic Outside-in Technique

■ The outside-in meniscal repair technique is generally recommended for tears of the anterior one-third and middle one-third regions of the meniscus, as well as for radial tears.

■ This technique reduces the risk of neurovascular injury by staying well anterior to the posterior horn, avoiding injury to the posterior neurovascular bundle.

■ The repair is performed under direct arthroscopic visualization.

■ It may be performed using several 18-gauge cannulated spinal needles placed 3 to 5 mm apart.

■ The needles are passed percutaneously from outside to inside the knee joint, passing centrally and radially through the peripheral meniscus and the tear site, and exiting the meniscus tear to achieve a vertical, oblique, or horizontal mattress suture configuration (tear pattern permitting).

■ An absorbable monofilament suture may be used with the individual suture strand tail remaining in the ipsilateral compartment of the knee.

■ A second needle with a wire retriever trocar can then be passed through the tear and visualized arthroscopically.

■ An arthroscopic grasping device can then be used to pull the free end of suture 1 through the looped intraarticular wire retriever, thereby passing a vertical or horizontal mattress suture.

■ After the sutures are tensioned up against the capsule, a 3- to 5-mm horizontal skin incision is made near the suture strand exit portals, and blunt dissection is carried down to the capsule using a hemostat.

■ With a nerve probe, the sutures are hooked and pulled out of this accessory incision site to properly tie and tension the sutures down against the adjacent capsule.

■ Knot tying should be advanced from a posterior to anterior direction if several sets of sutures are used in the repair.

■ The advantages of this technique include the use of a minimally invasive incision and safe and easy access to the anterior and middle third regions of the meniscus with the ability to place various suture patterns based on the tear pattern visualized.

■ This technique may also be used for displaced bucket-handle tears as a sole means of repair or used as an adjunct hybrid method for reducing and provisionally stabilizing displaced bucket-handle tears that are being repaired using other methods (inside-out or all-arthroscopic).

■ The disadvantages include the separate incision needed to capture and tie down the sutures against the capsule, and the technique's limited access to repair posterior horn tears, as well as the potential injury to the neurovascular structures here.

Arthroscopy-assisted Inside-out Technique

■ The inside-out meniscal repair technique involves arthroscopic-assisted passage of sutures on double-loaded "2-0" or "0" nonabsorbable suture on extra long flexible needles.

■ The technique requires specific cannulas for needle passage through the posterior, middle, and anterior third regions of the meniscus.

■ An accessory posterolateral or posteromedial incision is used to capture the repair needles and suture and for neurovascular structure protection, particularly if the posterior third of the meniscus is repaired.

- This technique can be conducted using single- or double-lumen, zone-specific cannulae that are placed through arthroscopic portals and up to the tear site.
- Double-armed sutures with long flexible needles are passed through the cannulae and across the tear site and out the accessory incisions of the knee.
- The risk of neurovascular injury is minimized through the use of contralateral arthroscopic portals and needle-directed vectors, as well as through proper placement of the accessory incisions and precise needle capture after passage through the capsule.
- Both posteromedial and posterolateral incisions are made beginning at the level of the joint line and extending one third above and two thirds below the joint for a total distance of 4 to 6 cm.
- After dissection is completed down to the corresponding capsule, a contoured "spoon" retractor or similar proprietary popliteal retractor is inserted anterior to and deep to the gastrocnemius to allow for visualization of the exiting needles.
- The posteromedial incision is made posterior to the MCL and above the level of the sartorius muscle.
- The dissection is continued anterior to the semimembranosus and deep to the medial head of the gastrocnemius muscle using blunt sweeping dissection.
- A popliteal retractor is then placed against the corresponding capsule.
- The posterolateral incision is made with the knee in 90 degrees of flexion, allowing the peroneal nerve to move posteriorly.
  - The incision is just posterior to the lateral collateral ligament, staying anterior to the fibular collateral ligament and biceps femoris tendon.
- The interval between the iliotibial band and biceps tendon is developed, and dissection is continued deep and anterior to the lateral head of the gastrocnemius, thus exposing the posterolateral capsule for placement of the popliteal retractor.
- After placement of the repair sutures through the cannulae, they are then tied to the corresponding capsule while arthroscopically viewing the tensioning and seating of the meniscus tear site.
- The medial meniscal repair sutures are tied with the knee in 20 to 30 degrees of flexion to avoid tethering the capsule and limiting extension, whereas the lateral sutures are tied with the knee in 90 degrees of flexion moving the peroneal nerve, popliteus, and lateral inferior geniculate artery posterior to the repair site.
- The advantages of using an arthroscopy-assisted inside-out technique include the ability to predictably place vertical mattress sutures across the tear site and the potential to effectively access the middle and posterior regions of the meniscus.
  - In meniscal allograft cases, this technique optimizes the anchoring of the transplanted tissue to the native meniscal rim and capsule.
- The disadvantages of using an inside-out technique include the difficulty associated with needle passage through the capsule and its proximity to the neurovascular bundle, as well as the potential morbidity associated with the accessory incisions and dissection down to the corresponding capsule.

All-arthroscopic Fixation Technique (First-generation Devices)

- Multiple meniscal repair fixator devices are currently available that allow for an all-arthroscopic approach to repairing meniscal tears.
- Most devices have a reverse-barbed fish-hook design that allows for compression of vertical longitudinal tears.
- These fixators are made of bioabsorbable copolymer materials composed of various amounts of poly-L-lactic acid, and poly-D-lactic acid.
- The fixation technique involves identification of the tear site and measurement of the tear distance from the periphery to allow for selection of an appropriate length fixator.
- Various specific delivery cannulae systems can be placed perpendicular to the meniscal surface, allowing for provisional reduction of the tear.
- The implant fixators are then usually inserted at 3- to 5-mm intervals apart across the tear site and perpendicular to the tear to maximally compress the tear site.
- Care must be taken to ensure that the particular fixator head is seated completely flush to the meniscus or countersunk to reduce the risk of loss of fixation and articular cartilage injury.
- The optimal tear pattern using this fixation method is a vertical longitudinal tear pattern in the red–white zone of the posterior horn of the meniscus.

All-arthroscopic Suture Fixation Technique (Second-generation Devices)

- This technique uses either two absorbable or nonabsorbable suture anchors, with attached nonabsorbable sutures noted between the anchors.
- Each anchor is passed, using a delivery system, through the meniscus on each side of the tear and secured to the peripheral rim.
- Sutures from adjacent anchors can be either arthroscopically tied together or, depending on the system, they may come pretied, allowing the surgeon to simply pull on the free end of the knot extracapsularly and "cinching" the meniscus tear site down.
- The advantage of these newer generation systems is that repair can be accomplished using sutures without the need for accessory posteromedial or posterolateral incisions.
- Disadvantages include the cost of the device and the learning curve associated with adopting its use.

Fibrin Clot Technique

- The insertion of an exogenous autologous fibrin clot is based on the concept that the concentrated platelet-rich material may provide a scaffold for repair and blood-associated chemotactic and mitogenic mediators, including platelet-derived growth factor that may promote tear site healing.
- The indications for use of a fibrin clot include meniscus repair conducted as an isolated repair or in revision repairs.
- The technique requires sterilely obtaining 30 to 50 mL of venous blood from the patient and then transferring

TABLE 29-2 REPAIR TECHNIQUES AND THEIR GENERAL INDICATIONS

Repair Technique	Generalized Indications
Outside-in technique	Anterior horn tears Middle-third tears Radial tears
Inside-out technique	Posterior horn tears Middle-third tears Bucket-handle tears Peripheral capsular tears Meniscal allografts
All arthroscopic nonsuture fixation technique (arrows or first-generation devices)	Posterior horn tears Vertical, longitudinal tears Tears with >2 to 3 mm rim width
All arthroscopic hybrid suture fixation technique (suture-based or second-generation devices)	Posterior horn tears Middle-third tears Bucket-handle tears Radial tears

it to a sterile glass container and stirring it with a sintered glass rod for 3 to 5 minutes.

■ After formation of a clot to the glass rod, the remaining blood is decanted off, and the clot is gently rinsed and blotted dry.
■ Meniscus repair sutures are left loosely approximated, and the arthroscopic fluid pressure is turned down while the clot is inserted under arthroscopic visualization using a grasper placed in the lumen of a 5-mm diameter cannula with its diaphragm removed.
■ The cannula is placed in the arthroscopic portal that provides the best access to the repair site.
■ The clot is then inserted at the repair site onto one of the loosely approximated repair sutures, adjacent to the tibial surface of the tear.
■ The repair sutures are then tied securing the clot.

Conclusions

■ Numerous meniscal repair techniques continue to evolve, and each technique may be associated with certain advantages and disadvantages.
■ Hybridized techniques involving the utilization of more than one technique in meniscal repair may also be used in select cases.
■ Ultimately, the surgeon's preference and comfort level with a particular technique should prevail when deciding which technique or techniques to use.
■ Table 29-2 provides a summary of these repair techniques and their general indications.

REHABILITATION

■ Rehabilitation protocols should take into consideration three main issues: knee motion, weight-bearing, and return to sports.

■ The authors' preferred postoperative regimen for isolated meniscal repairs is similar to the protocol used for patellar tendon autograft ACL reconstruction.
  ■ In the operating room, patients are placed in a long-leg hinged knee brace or knee immobilizer locked in extension and are partial weight-bearing as tolerated with crutches.
  ■ The crutches are discontinued once the patient has adequate leg and quadriceps control, when pain and effusion subside, and when gait mechanics and comfort permits (usually 3 to 4 weeks).
  ■ Range of motion from 0 to 90 degrees is encouraged on postoperative day 1, with progression of motion encouraged as tolerated within guidelines set.
  ■ Generally, flexion is limited to 90 degrees for the first 3 weeks after repair of nondisplaced meniscus tears and for 4 to 6 weeks after repair of displaced bucket-handle tears and meniscal transplants to protect these complex repairs/reconstructions.
■ A successful functional rehabilitation protocol also involves lower-extremity strengthening exercises that are started immediately to help restore adequate quadriceps firing.
■ Each patient functionally should be progressed, depending on comfort with range of motion, restoration of strength, and ability to perform functional and sport-specific drills.
■ For an isolated meniscal repair, return to pivoting sports is dictated by clinical examination and may range from 4 to 6 months when the patient no longer has point tenderness over the repair site and when the knee demonstrates no effusion, full extension, and painless terminal flexion.
■ Each factor in a case—including type of repair, surgical technique, and concomitant procedures—should be considered as far as individualizing the prescribed rehabilitation protocol.

MENISCUS REPLACEMENT

Despite improvements in our ability to repair meniscal lesions, meniscectomy still remains the most common orthopaedic knee procedure performed. Outcome studies have shown that meniscal resection can increase the incidence of degenerative osteoarthritis. Every effort should be made to repair meniscal tears and preserve meniscal tissue when injury occurs here. There will be cases, however, in which meniscectomy is indicated; in these cases, meniscal allograft transplantation may be indicated if the postmeniscectomy patient remains symptomatic after attempted conservative treatment.

Indications

■ A primary indication for meniscal allograft transplantation is the symptomatic patient who has undergone a previous meniscectomy with persistent pain in the involved compartment and who has failed nonoperative treatment.

BOX 29-2 INDICATIONS AND CONTRAINDICATIONS FOR MENISCAL ALLOGRAFT TRANSPLANTATION

Indications
- Skeletal maturity up to age 50 years
- No obesity
- Postmeniscectomy symptoms of pain, swelling, and catching in corresponding compartment
- Mechanical meniscal disorder; not from synovial, infectious, neoplastic, rheumatological, or other metabolic disease
- Intact immune system
- Stable ligaments as noted by physical examination and/or magnetic resonance
- Absence of an intact meniscal rim
- Normal tibiofemoral alignment on weight-bearing radiographs
- No significant osteoarthritis; less than grade III chondral wear as defined by the Outerbridge classification system
- Concomitant ligament reconstruction, articular surface resurfacing, or realignment surgery
- Patient compliance with rehabilitation and postoperative protocol

Contraindications
- Painless meniscal-deficient compartment
- Skeletal immaturity
- Obesity: body mass index >30
- Unstable knee as a result of ligament patholaxity
- Malalignment: varus in medial compartment and valgus in lateral compartment
- Osteoarthritis or other, degenerative, infectious, neoplastic, rheumatological, synovial, or collagen vascular-mediated joint diseases
- Grade III and IV chondral wear
- Immune deficiency
- Arthrofibrosis

- The patient must have normal knee alignment, a stable joint, and articular cartilage must be intact with less than grade 3 (Outerbridge) chondromalacia noted.
- The second most common indication is in the patient with an ACL-deficient knee undergoing reconstruction that has a concomitant meniscal deficiency that would preclude satisfactory stabilization (Box 29-2).
- There is no current role for meniscus transplantation in the "at-risk" asymptomatic patient who has undergone total or subtotal meniscectomy.
- Enthusiasm may exist to treat the young asymptomatic patient prophylactically in an attempt to prevent irreversible chondral changes that may develop over time.
  - However, sufficient long-term chondroprotection data to support this argument remain lacking.
- Risks include anesthesia related complications, possible allograft failure and rejection, tearing and shrinkage, converting from a pain-free condition to a painful status, and the risk of exposure to disease transmission from allograft tissue.

Contraindications

- Contraindications to meniscus allograft transplantation include those patients whose symptoms are not localized in the meniscal-deficient compartment or in patients who have associated grade III or greater chondral pathology in the ipsilateral compartment.

- Significant partial thickness chondral lesions involving fragmentation and fissuring greater than 0.5 inches in diameter (grade III) or lesions in which subchondral bone is exposed have had a negative effect on the transplant's survival.
- Other contraindications include the knee joint with malalignment that is uncorrected or uncorrectable, ligament instability that is not corrected or uncorrectable, and patients who are unwilling to participate in the postoperative rehabilitation protocol fully.
- Relative contraindications include excessive weight, age >50 years old, and a history of previous infections (Box 29-2).

FUTURE DIRECTIONS AND TECHNOLOGIES

In the past 20 years, technological advances have allowed for better understanding of meniscal structure, function, and pathophysiology. However, further research is needed to help improve our ability to uniformly achieve meniscal preservation and restoration to deliver articular cartilage chondroprotection more precisely. Improved methods of fixation and repair have already become mainstream and will continue to improve. New developments on the horizon involve the use of biologic and nonbiological adhesives that have demonstrated improved mechanical strength and sealant characteristics in animal models. Application and use of bioactive growth factors are areas of much excitement and promise. More and more work is being done in the area of tissue engineering and molecular genetics, and gene-modified research is expanding. Ultimately, these developments may extend and broaden the indications for repair to avascular tear sites and may increase the potential for meniscal preservation.

SUGGESTED READING

Andrish JT. Meniscal injuries in children and adolescents: diagnosis and management. J Am Acad Orthop Surg 1996;4:231–237.

Arnoczky SP, Warren RF. The microvasculature of the meniscus and its response to injury: an experimental study in the dog. Am J Sports Med 1983;11:131–141.

Barber FA, Harding NR. Meniscal repair rehabilitation. Instr Course Lect. 2000;49:207–210.

Cooper DE, Arnoczky SP, Warren RF. Arthroscopic meniscal repair. Clin Sports Med 1990;9:589–607.

Greis PE, Bardana DD, Holmstrom MC, et al. Meniscal injury. I. Basic science and evaluation. J Am Acad Orthop Surg 2002;10:168–176.

Levy M, Torzilli P, Warren R. The effect of medial meniscectomy on anterior-posterior motion of the knee. J Bone Joint Surg Am 1982; 64:883–888.

Newman AP, Daniels AU, Burks RT. Principles and decision making in meniscal surgery. Arthroscopy 1993;9:33–51.

Poehling GG, Ruch DS, Chabon SJ. The landscape of meniscal injuries. Clin Sports Med 1990;9:539–549.

Radin E, de Lamotte F, Maquet P. Role of the menisci in the distribution of stress in the knee. Clin Orthop 1984;185:290–294.

Renstrom P, Johnson RJ. Anatomy and biomechanics of the menisci. Clin Sports Med 1990;9:523–538.

Rodeo SA, Warren RF. Meniscal repair using the outside-to-inside technique. Clin Sports Med 1996;15:469–481.

Sgaglione NA. Meniscus repair: update on new techniques. Tech Knee Surg 2002;1:113–127.

Sgaglione NA. Meniscal transplant: bone block technique for medial meniscus. Op Tech Sports Med 2002;10:136–143.

Sgaglione NA, Steadman JR, Shaffer B, et al. Current concepts in meniscus surgery: resection to replacement. Arthroscopy 2003;19: 161–188.

ARTICULAR CARTILAGE INJURIES

TAMARA K. PYLAWKA
RICHARD W. KANG
BRIAN J. COLE

The articular cartilage of diarthrodial joints serves several important functions: joint lubrication, stress distribution to subchondral bone to minimize peak stress, and provision of a smooth low-friction surface. Repetitive and acute impact, as well as torsional joint loading can damage articular cartilage surfaces of the knee joint. Injury to articular cartilage can lead to pain, swelling, joint dysfunction, and possibly progressive joint degeneration. Nonsurgical treatment options include oral medications, simple bracing, and physical therapy. Surgical interventions range from simple arthroscopic debridement to complex tissue engineering, including autologous chondrocyte implantation. To determine the proper treatment option, each patient's age, intensity of symptoms, activity level, and lesion characteristics should be considered. The purpose of this chapter is to provide a comprehensive overview of the etiology, diagnosis, and management of articular cartilage lesions.

EPIDEMIOLOGY

Chondral lesions affect approximately 900,000 Americans each year, leading to more than 200,000 surgical procedures to treat high-grade lesions (grade III or IV), as described in the classification section of this chapter. Curl et al. completed a retrospective review of 31,516 arthroscopies and identified chondral lesions in 63% of cases, of which 41% were grade III and 19% were grade IV. Hjelle et al. prospectively evaluated 1,000 knee arthroscopies and identified chondral or osteochondral lesions in 61% of the patients, with 55% classified as grade III and 5% as grade IV. Chondral or osteochondral lesions vary in size and can occur in isolation or exist as multiple lesions in a single joint. Articular cartilage damage of the knee joint most commonly occurs in the weight-bearing zone of the medial femoral condyle (58% of all cartilage lesions in the knee). Other commonly affected zones include the weight-bearing zones of the lateral femoral condyle and patellofemoral joint.

ORGANIZATION AND COMPOSITION

Articular cartilage consists of a large extracellular matrix (ECM) with highly specialized cells (chondrocytes) sparsely distributed throughout the tissue, composing approximately 10% of the total wet weight of the tissue (Fig. 30-1). Chondrocytes are responsible for the homeostasis of articular cartilage, including synthesis, secretion, and maintenance of the ECM. This homeostasis is partially regulated by chondrocyte metabolic activity that responds to various agents, including (but not limited to) cytokines, growth fac-

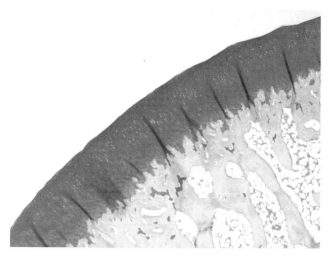

Figure 30-1   Photomicrograph demonstrating normal architecture of articular surface and the relationship to subchondral bone (safranin-O stain, ×4). (Courtesy of James Williams, PhD.)

tors, and hydrostatic and mechanical pressure changes. The principal components of the ECM include water (65% to 80% of total weight), proteoglycans (aggrecan, 4% to 7% of the total wet weight), and collagens (primarily type II, 10% to 20% of the total wet weight), with other proteins and glycoproteins in lesser amounts. Water content of articular cartilage is nonhomogeneously distributed, varying with the distance from the articular surface. Most water is contained in the molecular pore space of the ECM and concentrated at the surface and is partly responsible for joint lubrication. Water is able to move throughout the tissue by a pressure gradient or compression of the tissue. The majority of proteoglycans in cartilage are the large aggregating type (aggrecan) (Fig. 30-2). Proteoglycans are large, complex macromolecules and consist of a protein core with extensive polysaccharide (glycosaminoglycan) chains linked to this core. The role of proteoglycan is to bind water and enable cartilage to withstand large compressive loads. Collagens (mainly type II) are structural molecules distributed throughout cartilage, with fibril size and concentration vary-

ing throughout the tissue. Collagen provides cartilage the tensile strength needed to withstand shear forces. Articular cartilage is further subdivided into four distinct zones: superficial, transitional, deep, and calcified (Table 30-1, Fig. 30-3).

INJURY AND REPAIR

Acute articular cartilage injuries that lead to mechanical damage to cellular and matrix components can occur through blunt trauma, penetrating injury, friction abrasion, or abrupt changes of forces across the joint. Repair response depends on depth of penetration, volume of cartilage involved, and surface area involved. Articular cartilage lacks vascular, nervous, and lymphatic elements. It has a relatively low turnover rate, with only a limited ability to heal. Cartilage tends only to heal if the injury is minor; otherwise, for more extensive injury, restoration of the articular surface and functional capacity are dependent on surgical intervention. Injuries that do not penetrate the subchondral bone do not repair well, whereas injuries that extend into the depth of the subchondral bone initiate a vascular proliferative response through the release of mesenchymal cells of the bone marrow, leading to fibrocartilage repair tissue that consists primarily of type I collagen (Fig. 30-4). Although this method of repair may restore the articular surface, fibrocartilage is structurally and biomechanically inferior to native articular cartilage and thus is predisposed to future breakdown.

CLASSIFICATION

The mechanics and natural history of acute articular surface injuries are not well understood, but such injuries may result in isolated cartilage injuries known as a focal chondral defects, which are associated with varying grades of cartilage loss. Osteoarthritis is a progressive degenerative condition that shows a nonlinear increase in prevalence after the age of 50 years. Grossly, osteoarthritis appears as diffuse fraying, fibrillation and thinning of the articular cartilage. Chondromalacia describes the gross appearance of cartilage

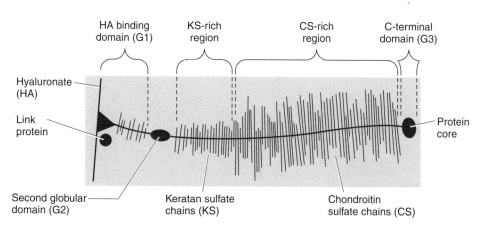

Figure 30-2   Schematic of PG aggregate molecule.

TABLE 30-1 ORGANIZATION OF ARTICULAR CARTILAGE

Zone	Chondrocyte	Collagen	Proteoglycan	Water	Properties
Superficial	Elongated in shape, horizontal to surface	Thin, parallel to surface, compact	Lowest concentration	Highest concentration	▪ Low fluid permeability ▪ Provides resistance to shear forces ▪ Secretes lubricating proteins ▪ Thinnest zone
Transitional	Oblique shape, randomly distributed, sparse	Larger diameter, less organized	↓ Highest	↓ Lowest	▪ Less stiff than superficial zone ▪ Distributes compressive loads to subchondral bone
Deep	Spherical shape, arranged in columns	Perpendicular to surface, extending into calcified zone			▪ Anchors cartilage to subchondral bone ▪ Partially calcified
Tidemark calcified	▪ Separates deep zone (cartilage) from calcified zone (subchondral bone) ▪ Small cells in cartilaginous matrix with apatitic salts ▪ Collagen fibers from deep zone penetrate calcified cartilage				

damage, including softening and fissuring to variable depths of cartilage involvement (Table 30-2). The extent of chondromalacia can be graded with arthroscopic evaluation using the Outerbridge classification scheme (Fig. 30-5). A more recent modification by the International Cartilage Repair Society classifies chondral injuries into five distinct grades (Table 30-3).

PATHOPHYSIOLOGY

Normal articular cartilage (2 to 4 mm thick) can withstand loads of up to five times body weight. Articular cartilage injuries can be separated into three types: partial thickness injuries, full thickness injuries, and osteochondral fractures.

Partial thickness articular cartilage injuries are defined by damage to the cells and matrix components limited to superficial articular involvement. This type of damage is most characterized by decreased proteoglycan (PG) concentration and increased hydration. These conditions are strongly correlated with a decrease in cartilage stiffness and an increase in hydraulic permeability leading to greater loads transmitted to the collagen–PG matrix, which increases ECM damage. Furthermore, breakdown of the ECM may lead to greater force transmitted to the underlying bone that eventually leads to bone remodeling. It has been postulated that chondrocytes can restore the matrix as long as enough viable cells exist to ensure that the rate of PG loss does not exceed the rate of synthesis and the collagen network remains intact.

Full thickness articular cartilage injuries are defined by

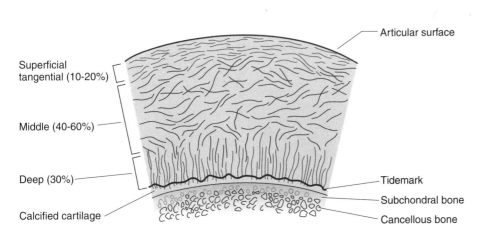

Figure 30-3 Schematic of zones of articular cartilage.

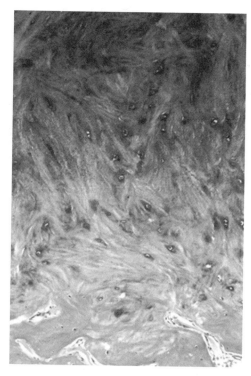

Figure 30-4 Photomicrograph of biopsy from fibrocartilage fill after marrow stimulation technique demonstrating a distinct lack of organizational structure and poor PG staining (hematoxylin and eosin, ×10).

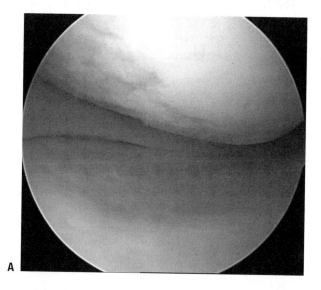

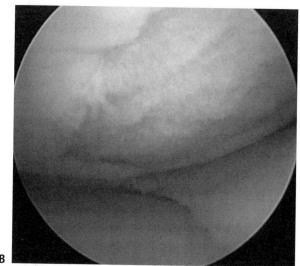

Figure 30-5 **A:** Arthroscopic photograph demonstrating an Outerbridge grade III lesion of the medial femoral condyle. **B:** Arthroscopic photograph demonstrating an Outerbridge grade IV lesion of the medial femoral condyle.

visible mechanical disruption limited to articular cartilage. These injuries are characterized as (but not limited to) chondral fissures, flaps, fractures, and chondrocyte damage. Lack of vascular integration, and therefore lack of migration, of mesenchymal stem cells to the damaged area limits the repair of this type of injury. Mild repair occurs as chondrocytes start proliferating and synthesizing additional ECM; however, this response is short lived, and defects remain only partially healed. Thus, normal articular cartilage that is adjacent to the damaged site may undergo additional loading forces predisposing it to degeneration over time.

Osteochondral injuries are defined by a visible mechanical disruption of articular cartilage and subchondral bone. Such injuries occur when there is an acute assault on the

cartilage, leading to a fracture that penetrates deep into the subchondral bone. Subsequent hemorrhage and fibrin clot formation elicit an inflammatory reaction. The clot extends into the cartilage defect and releases vasoactive mediators and growth factors, such as transforming growth factor-β and platelet-derived growth factor, both implemented in the repair of such osteochondral defects. The resulting chondral repair tissue is a mixture of normal hyaline cartilage and fibrocartilage and is less stiff and more permeable than normal articular cartilage. Such repair tissue rarely persists and may show evidence of deterioration with depletion of PGs, increased hydration, fragmentation and fibrillation, and loss of chondrocyte-like cells. Alternatively, osteochondritis dissecans is a condition that may be developmental

TABLE 30-2 OUTERBRIDGE CLASSIFICATION OF CHONDRAL INJURIES

Grade	Description
I	Softening and swelling of cartilage
II	Fissures and fragmentation in an area $^1/_2$ inch or less in diameter
III	Fissuring and fragmentation in an area with more than $^1/_2$-inch diameter involvement
IV	Erosion of cartilage down to subchondral bone

TABLE 30-3 MODIFIED INTERNATIONAL CARTILAGE REPAIR SOCIETY CLASSIFICATION SYSTEM FOR CHONDRAL INJURY

Grade	Description
0	Normal cartilage
I	Superficial fissuring, softening
II	Less than $1/2$ cartilage depth
III	Greater than $1/2$ cartilage depth up to and not including subchondral plate
IV	Penetration through subchondral plate, exposing subchondral bone

in nature and may exist as a chronic osteochondral defect with no demonstrable evidence of a healing response (Fig. 30-6).

DIAGNOSIS

History and Physical Examination

- In general, the history, physical examination, plain radiographs, and surgical history can provide enough information to make the appropriate diagnosis.
- Cartilage injuries can occur in isolation or in association with concomitant pathology, such as varus or valgus mal-

alignment, patellofemoral malalignment, ligamentous instability, and meniscal deficiency.
  - Acute full-thickness chondral or osteochondral injuries commonly present with a loose body and/or mechanical symptom.
  - When chronic, symptoms may include localized pain, swelling, and a spectrum of mechanical symptoms (locking, catching, crepitus).
- An extensive history should be completed, including the onset of symptoms (insidious or traumatic), the mechanism of injury, previous injuries, previous surgical intervention, and symptom-provoking activities.
- A comprehensive musculoskeletal examination should be performed to better assess for concurrent pathology that would alter the treatment plan.
  - Range-of-motion testing is usually normal in patients with isolated focal chondral defects; however, adaptive gait patterns—such as in-toeing, out-toeing, or a flexed-knee gait—may develop as the patient compensates to shift weight away from the affected area.

Radiologic Examination

- Plain radiographs remain the most effective tool for initial evaluation of the joint.
  - Typical plain films include 45-degree flexion weight-bearing posteroanterior, patellofemoral, and non-weight-bearing lateral projections.
  - These views allow assessment of joint space narrowing, subchondral sclerosis, osteophytes, and cysts.
- Other tools, such as magnetic resonance imaging, offer information concerning the articular surface, subchondral bone, knee ligaments, and menisci. However, magnetic resonance imaging generally tends to underestimate the degree of cartilage abnormalities seen at the time of arthroscopy.
- The role of the bone scan remains controversial because isolated articular surface defects that do not penetrate subchondral bone may not be identified.
- Despite advances in the aforementioned imaging techniques, arthroscopy still remains as the gold standard for diagnosis of articular cartilage injuries.

TREATMENT

Nonsurgical Treatment

- Nonsurgical management includes oral medications, physical modalities (physical therapy, weight loss), bracing (knee sleeve and unloader brace), and injections (corticosteroids and hyaluronic acid derivatives).
- Such management is often ineffective in highly active and symptomatic patients and may only prove beneficial in low-demand patients, patients wishing to avoid or delay surgery, or patients with advanced degenerative osteoarthritis (a contraindication for articular cartilage restoration procedures).
- Traditionally, treatment of articular cartilage lesions has included a combination of nonsteroidal anti-inflamma-

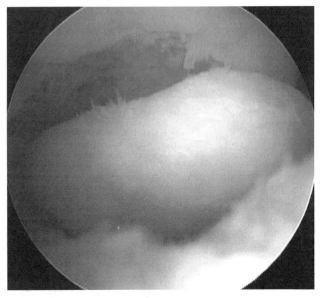

Figure 30-6 Arthroscopic photograph of a lesion of osteochondritis dissecans with a loose fragment remaining in situ.

tory drugs, activity modification, and oral chondroprotective agents such as glucosamine or chondroitin sulfate.

- Glucosamine stimulates chondrocyte and synoviocyte activities, whereas chondroitin inhibits degradative enzymes and prevents fibrin thrombus formation in periarticular tissue. These substances improve pain, joint line tenderness, range of motion, and walking speed. No clinical data, however, show that these oral agents affect the mechanical properties or biochemical consistency of articular cartilage.

- If nonsurgical management fails, a referral to an orthopaedic surgeon should be considered.
  - Indications that would suggest this type of referral are included in Box 30-1.

Surgical Treatment

- Treatment options to restore the articular cartilage surface involve consideration of many factors: defect size,

---

BOX 30-1 INDICATIONS FOR REFERRAL TO AN ORTHOPAEDIC SURGEON

- High-energy injury with direct trauma to the knee
- Acute motion loss
- Gross deformity of joint
- Acute neurovascular deficit
- Mechanical symptom (catching, locking, sensation of a loose body, crepitus)
- Failed nonsurgical management greater than 3 months in duration
- Repeated giving way or complaints of instability

---

depth, location, chronicity, response to previous treatment, concomitant pathology, patient age, physical demand level, and patient expectations.

- Articular cartilage lesions of similar size may have many surgical options with no general consensus among orthopaedic surgeons.

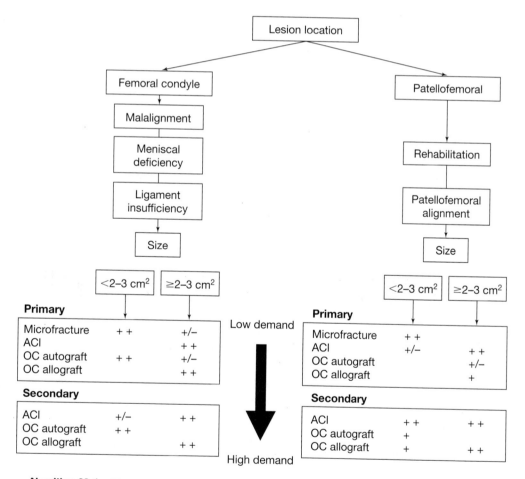

Algorithm 30-1   The treatment of femoral condyle lesions is predicated first on correction of malalignment, meniscal deficiency, and ligament insufficiency. Treatment of patellofemoral lesions is predicated on exhaustive rehabilitative efforts followed by evaluation for malalignment. Defect size, patient physical demand level, and whether the treatment is primary or secondary determine the subsequent treatment option. OC, osteochondral; ACI, autologous chondrocyte implantation.

- The treatment algorithm (Algorithm 30-1) should be regarded as an overview of surgical decision making and is dynamically evolving as longer-term data emerge about the indications and outcomes of cartilage repair procedures.
- Treatment of articular cartilage lesions and can be grouped into three categories: palliative, reparative, and restorative (Table 30-4).
- The goals of these procedures are to reduce symptoms, improve joint congruence by restoring the articular surface, and prevent further cartilage degeneration.
- Management of associated pathology such as malalignment, ligament insufficiency, or meniscal deficiency is mandatory for maximum relief of symptoms.

Palliative Treatment

- Palliative treatments include arthroscopic debridement and lavage, as well as thermal chondroplasty.
- Arthroscopic debridement and lavage is considered only as a palliative first-line treatment for articular damage and for treatment of the incidental or small cartilage defect (<2 cm^2).
    - Simple irrigation to remove debris may temporarily improve symptoms in up to 70% of cases, and when combined with chondroplasty, the success rate may initially increase.
    - These techniques are used to remove degenerative debris, inflammatory cytokines (i.e., interleukin-1α), and proteases, all of which contribute to cartilage breakdown.
    - Postoperative rehabilitation involves weight-bearing as tolerated and strengthening exercises.
    - Table 30-5 provides a summary of outcomes data for arthroscopic debridement and lavage.
    - Limitations of debridement include the inability to definitively manage the chondral defect and the general inability to contour, smooth, or stabilize the articular surface.
- Thermal chondroplasty (laser, radio frequency energy) of superficial chondral defects allows more precise contouring of the articular surface.
    - Depth of chondrocyte death has been shown to extend deeper than the chondrocyte loss expected with mechanical shaving alone.
    - These concerns leave this procedure to be considered as investigational by many orthopaedic surgeons.

Reparative Treatment

- Reparative treatments involve surgical penetration of subchondral bone to allow for migration of marrow elements (including mesenchymal stem cells), resulting in surgically induced fibrin clot and subsequent fibrocartilage formation in the area of chondral defect.
- Several types of treatments use this technique, including microfracture, subchondral drilling, and abrasion arthroplasty.
    - These procedures are recommended in active patients and moderate symptoms with smaller lesions (<2 cm^2) or in lower-demand patients with larger lesions (>2 cm^2).
- Microfracture is the preferred marrow stimulation technique because it creates less thermal energy, compared with drilling, and provides a controlled depth of penetration with holes made perpendicular to the subchondral plate.
    - Defect preparation is critical and is performed by violating the calcified layer at the base of the lesion with a curette or shaver and creating vertical "shoulders" of normal surrounding cartilage.
    - Perforations are made close together (usually 3 to 4 mm apart), with care taken not to fracture the subchondral bone plate (Fig. 30-7).

TABLE 30-4 SURGICAL MANAGEMENT OF CHONDRAL LESIONS

Procedure	Ideal Indications	Outcome
Arthroscopic debridement and lavage	Minimal symptoms, short-term relief	Palliative
Thermal chondroplasty (laser, radio frequency energy)	Investigational, partial thickness defects Used in combination with debridement	Palliative
Marrow-stimulating techniques	Smaller lesions, persistent pain	Reparative
Autologous chondrocyte implantation	Small and large lesions with or without subchondral bone loss	Reparative or restorative
Osteochondral autograft/mosaicplasty	Smaller lesions, persistent pain	Restorative
Osteochondral allograft	Larger lesions with subchondral bone loss	Restorative

TABLE 30-5 RESULTS OF ARTHROSCOPIC DEBRIDEMENT AND LAVAGE

Study	Follow-up	Number of Patients	Results
Sprague (1981)	14 mo	78	74% good 26% fair/poor
Baumgaertner et al. (1990)	33 mo	49	52% good 48% fair/poor
Timoney et al. (1990)	4 yr	109	63% good 37% fair/poor
Hubbard (1996)	4.5 yr	76 knees	Debridement Lysholm score: 28 Lavage Lysholm score: 4
McGinley et al. (1999)	10 yr	77: all candidates for total knee replacement	Postdebridement: 67% did not require total knee arthroplasty; 33% required total knee arthroplasty
Owens et al. (2002)	2 yr	20 bRFE 19 AD	Fulkerson score 12 mo: 80 AD, 87.9 bRFE 24 mo: 77.5 AD, 86.6 bRFE
Fond et al.(2002)	2 and 5 yr	36 patients	HSS score 2 yr: 88% good 5 yr: 69% good
Jackson et al. (2003)	4–6 yr	121 cases 71 advanced arthritic group Retrospective	87% of the advanced arthritic cases were improved

AD, arthroscopic debridement; bRFE, bipolar radio frequency energy; HSS, Hospital for Special Surgery.

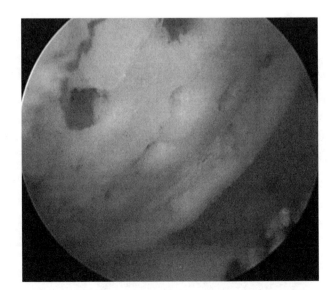

Figure 30-7 Arthroscopic photograph demonstrating microfracture technique performed for a grade IV lesion. The lesion was prepared by debriding the calcified cartilage. Next, microfracture awls were used to penetrate the subchondral bone.

- For femoral condyle or tibial lesions, postoperative rehabilitation consists of protected weight-bearing for 6 to 8 weeks and may include continuous passive motion.
- Table 30-6 summarizes the outcomes studies for microfracture.

Restorative Treatment

- Restorative techniques involve tissue engineering (autologous chondrocyte implantation [ACI]) and osteochondral grafting.
- ACI is a two-stage procedure involving a biopsy of normal articular cartilage (300 to 500 mg), usually obtained through an arthroscopic procedure, in which the cartilage is harvested from a minor load-bearing area (upper medial femoral condyle or intercondylar notch).
  - These chondrocytes are then cultured in vitro and implanted into the chondral defect beneath a periosteal patch during a second-stage procedure that requires an arthrotomy (Fig. 30-8).
  - This restorative procedure results in "hyaline-like" cartilage, which is believed to be biomechanically superior to fibrocartilage.
  - Postoperative rehabilitation entails continuous passive motion and protected weight bearing for up to 6 weeks.

TABLE 30-6 RESULTS OF MICROFRACTURE

Study	Follow-up	Number of Patients	Results
Blevins et al. (1998)	4 yr	140 recreational athletes	54 second-look arthroscopies yielded 35% with surface unchanged
Gill et al. (1998)	6 (2–12) yr	103 patients	86% return to sport 40 second-look arthroscopies yielded 50% normal
Steadman et al. (2003)	11.3 (7–17) yr	71 knees	80% improved Lysholm score 59 → 89 Tegner score 6 → 9
Miller et al. (2004)	2.6 (2–5) yr	81 patients	Lysholm score 53.8 → 83 Tegner score 2.9 → 4.5

- ACI is most often used as a secondary procedure for the treatment of medium-to-large focal chondral defects (>2 cm²).
- Table 30-7 summarizes the outcomes studies for ACI.

- Osteochondral grafts restore the articular surface by implanting a cylindrical plug of subchondral bone and articular cartilage.
    - The source of the tissue can be from the host (autograft) or from a cadaveric donor (allograft).
        - Several challenges face both autograft and allograft transplants: edge integration, restoring three-dimensional surface contour, and graft availability.
    - Osteochondral autografts are advantageous by virtue of using the patient's own tissue, which eliminates immunological concerns.
    - This technique is limited by the size of the graft (<2 cm²) and involves obtaining the donor osteochondral graft from a non-weight-bearing area of the joint and placing it into the prepared defect site (Fig. 30-9).
    - The major risk involved with this technique is plug failure and donor site morbidity, which increases as the size of the harvested plug increases.
    - Postoperative rehabilitation includes early range of motion and non-weight-bearing for 2 weeks with an increase to full weight-bearing from 2 to 6 weeks.
    - Indications for use of this technique include pri-

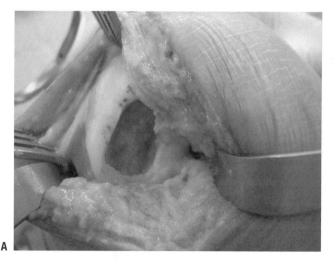
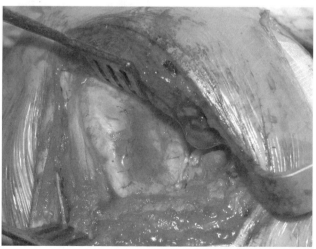

A   B

Figure 30-8 Intraoperative photographs demonstrating autologous chondrocyte implantation. Large lateral femoral condyle focal cartilage defect prepared (**A**) before suturing of the periosteal patch and sealing with fibrin glue (**B**).

TABLE 30-7 RESULTS OF AUTOLOGOUS CHONDROCYTE IMPLANTATION (ACI)

Study	Follow-up	Number of Patients	Results
Brittberg et al. (1994)	39 mo	23	6 excellent 8 good
Minas (2001)	1–2 yr	66	60% patient satisfaction
Peterson et al. (2002)	2–7 yr	61	89% good/excellent
Ochi et al. (2002)	3 yr	28 knees	93% good/excellent outcomes
Henderson et al. (2003)	3 and 12 mo	37	IKDC: 88% improvement at 12 mo MR score at 12 mo: 82% nearly normal cartilage Second-look biopsies: 70% hyaline-like material
Bentley et al. (2003)	19 mo	100	Modified Cincinnati and Stanmore: 88% good/excellent for ACI 69% good/excellent for mosaicplasty Arthroscopy (1 yr): 82% good/excellent repair for ACI 34% good/excellent for mosaicplasty
Yates (2003)	12 mo	24	78% good/excellent

IKDC, International Knee Documentation Committee; MR, magnetic resonance.

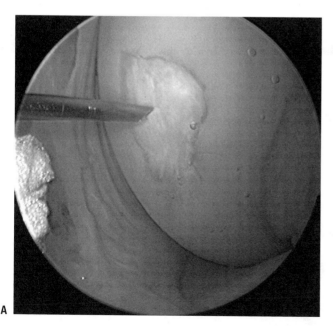
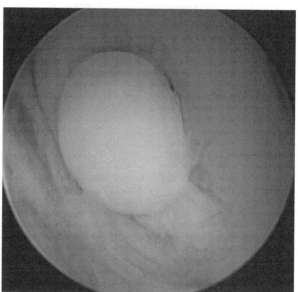

Figure 30-9 Arthroscopic photograph of a lesion treated previously with microfracture **(A)** being revised with a 10-mm diameter osteochondral autograft plug **(B)**.

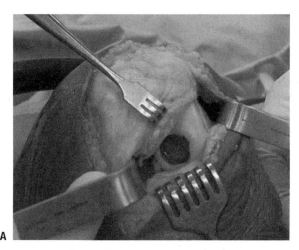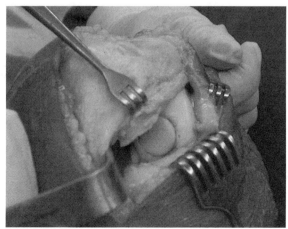

A   B

Figure 30-10   Intraoperative photograph of a defect **(A)** prepared to receive a fresh osteochondral allograft transplant measuring 20 mm in diameter **(B)**.

mary treatment of smaller lesions considered symptomatic and for similarly sized lesions for which a microfracture or possibly prior ACI procedure has failed.

- Osteochondral allografts are used to treat larger defects (>2 cm²) that are difficult to treat with other methods.
  - Allografts involve the transplantation of mature, normal hyaline cartilage with intact native architecture and viable chondrocytes.
  - Because the graft includes subchondral bone, any disorder with associated bone loss (avascular necrosis, osteochondral fracture, and osteo-

chondritis dissecans) may also be restored (Fig. 30-10).

- Major concerns such as tissue matching and immunologic suppression are unnecessary because the allograft tissue is avascular and alymphatic.
- Graft preservation techniques include fresh, frozen, and prolonged cold preserved.
- Fresh allografts must be used within 3 to 5 days of procurement. Thus, logistic concerns become an issue.
- Frozen grafts can be stored and shipped on demand, potentially alleviating scheduling issues.

TABLE 30-8   RESULTS OF OSTEOCHONDRAL AUTOGRAFTS

Study	Number of Patients	Location	Mean Follow-up	Results
Hangody et al. (1998)	57	F, P	2 yr	91% good/excellent
Kish et al. (1999)	52	F: competitive athletes	>1 yr	100% good/excellent 63% returned to full sports 31% returned to sports at lower level 90% <30-year-old returned to full sports 23% ≥30-year-old returned to full sports
Bradley et al. (1999)	145	NA	1.5 yr	43% good/excellent 43% fair 12% poor
Hangody and Fules (2001)	461 93 24	F P, Tr T	>1 yr >1 yr >1 yr	92% good/excellent 81% good/excellent 80% good/excellent
Jakob et al. (2002)	52	Knee	2 yr	86% good/excellent
Hangody and Fules (2001)	831	F, T, P, Tr	10 yr	F = 92% good/excellent T = 87% good/excellent P, Tr = 79% good/excellent

F, femur; P, patella; Tr, trochlea; T, tibia.

TABLE 30-9 RESULTS OF OSTEOCHONDRAL ALLOGRAFTS

Study	Number of Patients	Mean Age (yr)	Location	Mean Follow-up	Results
Meyers (1984)	21	16–50	H	63 mo	80% success
Meyers et al. (1989)	39	38	F,T,P	3.6 yr	78% success 22% failure
Garret (1994)	17	20	F	3.5 yr	94% success
Gross (1997)	123	35	F,T,P	7.5 yr	85% success
Chu et al. (1999)	55	35	F,T,P	75 mo	76% good/excellent 16% failure
Bugbee (2000)	122	34	F	5 yr	91% success rate at 5 yr 75% success rate at 10 yr 5% failure
Aubin et al. (2001)	60	27	F	10 yr	84% good/excellent 20% failure
Shasha et al. (2003)	65	NA	T	12 yr	Kaplan-Meier Survival Rate: 5 years–95% 10 years–80% 15 years–65% 20 years–46%

H, hip (femoral head); F, femur; Tr, trochlea; P, patella; T, tibia.

However, frozen osteochondral tissue lacks cellular viability.

- The prolonged cold preservation method increases the "shelf-life" of the graft to at least 28 days and alleviates the scheduling difficulties while maintaining cell viability (78% at 28 days preservation); however, chondrocyte suppression remains an issue.
- Incorporation and healing of allografts depend on creeping substitution of host bone to allograft bone.
- Postoperative rehabilitation consists of immediate continuous passive motion and protected weight-bearing for 6 to 8 weeks.
- This procedure is most often used as a secondary treatment option in patients who have failed previous attempts at cartilage repair.
- Tables 30-8 and 30-9 summarize the outcomes studies for osteochondral autograft and allograft transplants.

SUGGESTED READING

Brittberg M. Evaluation of cartilage injuries and cartilage repair. Osteologie 2000;9:17–25.

Brittberg M, Lindahl A, Nilsson A, et al. Treatment of deep cartilage defects in the knee with autologous chondrocyte transplantation. N Engl J Med 1994;331:889–895.

Buckwalter JA. Articular cartilage injuries. Clin Orthop 2002;402:21–37.

Buckwalter JA, Hunzinker EB, Rosenberg LC, et al. Articular cartilage: composition, structure, response to injury, and methods of facilitation repair. In: Ewing JW (ed), Articular Cartilage and Knee Joint Function: Basic Science and Arthroscopy. New York: Raven Press, 1990:19–56.

Bugbee WD. Fresh osteochondral allografting. Op Tech Sports Med 2000;8:158–162.

Caplan A, Elyaderani M, Mochizuki Y, et al. Overview of cartilage repair and regeneration: principles of cartilage repair and regeneration. Clin Orthop 1997;342:254–269.

Chu CR, Convery FR, Akeson WH, et al. Articular cartilage transplantation. Clinical results in the knee. Clin Orthop 1999;360:159–168.

Curl W, Krome J, Gordon E, et al. Cartilage injuries: a review of 31,516 knee arthroscopies. Arthroscopy 1997;13:456–460.

Edwards RB, Lu Y, Markel MD. The basic science of thermally assisted chondroplasty. Clin Sports Med 2002;21:619–647.

Hjelle K, Solheim E, Strand T, et al. Articular cartilage defects in 1,000 knee arthroscopies. Arthroscopy 2002;18:730–734.

Kish G, Modis L, Hangody L. Osteochondral mosaicplasty for the treatment of focal chondral and osteochondral lesions of the knee and talus in the athlete. Rationale, indications, techniques and results. Clin Sports Med 1999;18:45–66.

Mandelbaum BR, Romanelli DA, Knapp TP. Articular cartilage repair: assessment and classification. Op Tech Sports Med 8:90–97.

Miller BS, Steadman JR, Briggs KK, et al. Patient satisfaction and outcome after microfracture of the degenerative knee. J Knee Surg 2004;17:13–17.

Peterson L, Brittberg M, Kiviranta I, et al. Autologous chondrocyte transplantation: biomechanics and long-term durability. Am J Sports Med 2002;30:2–12.

Poole A. What type of cartilage repair are we attempting to attain? J Bone Joint Surg Am 2003;85:40–44.

Sprague NF. Arthroscopic debridement for degenerative knee joint disease. Clin Orthop 1981;160:118–123.

Steadman JR, Rodkey WG, Rodrigo JJ. Microfracture: surgical technique and rehabilitation to treat chondral defects. Clin Orthop 2001;391:S362–S369.

31

OVERUSE INJURIES OF THE LEG

KEVIN A. NADEL
ANTHONY A. SCHEPSIS

Overuse injuries of the lower extremity are commonly seen in the sports medicine clinic. Fortunately, only a handful of injured athletes present with a problem that requires surgical intervention to return to the field of play. In this chapter, we will focus on the more commonly seen overuse injuries that affect the athlete: stress fractures, medial tibial syndrome, exertional compartment syndrome, and popliteal artery entrapment syndrome.

STRESS FRACTURES OF THE TIBIA AND FIBULA

Also known as "insufficiency fractures," "march fractures," and "fatigue fractures," stress fractures are common overuse injuries found in the lower extremity. Stress fractures were first described in 1855 in soldiers following long marches. These fractures can be caused by any activity that requires repetitive stress from running, jumping, or prolonged walking, and as such, they are commonly found in athletes and military recruits. The highest incidence of stress fractures is found in the lower extremity, with the tibia representing the most commonly involved bone.

Pathogenesis

Etiology and Epidemiology

The cause of stress fractures is multifactorial. Factors that increase the occurrence of stress fractures in athletes are the type of athletic activity, patient's general health and overall fitness level, biomechanical anatomic differences, hormonal or nutritional imbalances, sleep deprivation, collagen or metabolic bone disorders, advancing age, gender, and footwear.

The biomechanical factors that may predispose athletes to stress fractures are leg-length discrepancy, high longitudinal arch of the foot, excessive subtalar pronation, a narrow tibia, greater passive external rotation at the hip, and smaller bone cross-sectional geometry. Pronated feet are most commonly found in athletes with tibial and fibular stress fractures. This is related to the increased tibial torsion during the support phase of running that has been shown to occur with excessive pronation. Cavus feet are rarely associated with these fractures.

Leg-length discrepancy has been shown to increase the incidence of stress fractures. In one study of athletes with recurrent stress fractures, a leg-length discrepancy was found in 83% of patients in the study group.

The "female athlete triad" of eating disorder, amenorrhea, and osteoporosis has been clearly established. Female athletes are more likely to have menstrual irregularities than are women in the general population. The decreased bone mineral density from the hypoestrogenic state likely leads to an increased incidence of stress fractures.

Male endurance athletes may also be prone to stress fractures, since they have been shown to have abnormally low sex hormone levels. Increased osteoclast production and bone resorption result from a loss of testosterone inhibition of the osteoclast-stimulating cytokine interleukin-6.

The incidence of stress fractures in the general population is reported to be less than 1%, but the incidence in athletes is much higher. Reports of stress fractures in the literature have widely varied statistics based on the differences in the populations described. One consistent finding is that the tibia is the most common site of stress fractures, representing up to 75% in some series Among these, the most common are fractures in the posteromedial cortex in the proximal third of the tibia on the compression side; fractures in the middle third affecting the anterior cortex on the tension side are only occasionally seen.

The fibula is less commonly affected, accounting for 5% to 13% of cases in athletes. Fractures in the fibula are much more common in the distal third than in the proximal third. Stress fractures of the medial malleolus have only been reported in 23 cases.

It is generally believed that women are at increased risk of developing stress fractures. One study of track and field athletes showed men and women to be at equal risk of developing stress fractures, which was supported by a study of military recruits that showed an incidence of stress fractures in men of 6.1% and 5.3%. However, in a study of female naval recruits, there was an incidence of 8.4% in women, but only 2.3% in men.

Athletes involved in certain sports are at increased risk of stress fractures. Running is by far the most common sport resulting in stress fractures, which account for 4.7% to 15.6% of all injuries to runners. Basketball, volleyball, and gymnastics are also associated with a high incidence of stress fractures. It was also demonstrated that military recruits who transition from a primarily non-weight-bearing sport, such as swimming, are more likely to develop stress fractures during training than recruits who played primarily weight-bearing sports like basketball. In one large review, 16.6% of all stress fractures were bilateral. Another important risk factor is history of a previous stress fracture.

Pathophysiology

Repetitive, submaximal loads on bone lead to an imbalance between bone resorption and remodeling. The normal response of bone to mechanical loads is to increase the rate of remodeling, but there is a lag before normal remodeling occurs, allowing bone to become weakened if the inciting activity is continued at a strenuous level. Microdamage that accumulates in this weakened region can propagate and coalesce into a stress fracture if repetitive loading continues.

The location and magnitude of this microdamage, leading to the common posteromedial tibial stress fractures, is explained by two theories. The first suggests that the shock absorption of the lower extremity is reduced by muscle weakness from fatigue, leading to increased strain on the bone. The second theory proposes that stress fractures result from highly concentrated muscle action upon specific points in bone, which comes with particular repetitive tasks, producing enough force to create a stress fracture.

Stress fractures in the anterior cortex of the tibia are found on the tension side of the bone, where the posterior muscles apply constant tension to the hypovascular anterior cortex. Since the fibula has a limited role in weight-bearing, stress fractures in this location are also most likely the result of muscle traction and torsional forces.

Micromotion of the fibula from rhythmic contraction of the long toe flexors in activities such as distance running may cause distal fibula stress fractures.

It has been proposed that proximal fibular fractures are the result of loading the lower extremity with the knee flexed and the ankle dorsiflexed, as would occur with jumping from a squatting position. Action of the biceps femoris may also play a role.

Medial malleolar stress fractures are most likely caused by repetitive impingement of the talus on the medial malleolus during ankle dorsiflexion and tibial rotation.

Diagnosis (Algorithm 31-1)

Physical Examination and History
- Athletes with stress fractures typically present with insidious onset of pain.
  - The athlete first experiences a dull ache that is aggravated by activity.
  - Initially, rest relieves the pain, but sometimes athletes experience rest pain or night pain, especially after strenuous activity.
  - Eventually, the pain will progress, become more focal, and may lead to cessation of exercise.
- Pain with tibial stress fractures is most commonly experienced in the proximal metaphysis, although central-third diaphyseal pain can alert the examiner to the more troublesome stress fracture in the anterior cortex of the tibia.
- It is important to evaluate the athlete's general health and to be cognizant of any nutritional or hormonal imbalances.
  - Weight changes and menstrual irregularities should be noted.
  - It is also valuable to analyze the athlete's training regimen, especially for type and condition of footwear, changes in training surface, or any recent changes in intensity, duration, or frequency.
- A complete examination should include evaluation for any biomechanical abnormalities, such as limb length discrepancy, excessive subtalar pronation, high arches, and muscle imbalances.
- Athletes will occasionally note localized swelling or erythema, and the examiner may find palpable thickening of the periosteum or a discrete fibrous mass.
- The single-leg hop test is useful in reproducing the pain experienced by athletes during exertion and may also be helpful in predicting when an athlete is ready to return to unrestricted pain-free activity.
- A high clinical suspicion of stress fracture in anyone engaged in a sport involving repetitive running or jumping is important since physical examination findings can be variable and any delay in diagnosis can lead to increased morbidity.

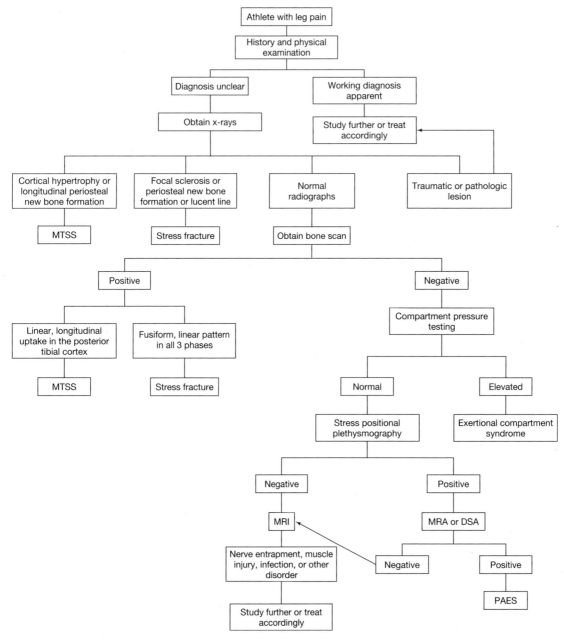

Algorithm 31-1   Diagnosis of overuse injuries of the lower extremity. (After Pell RF, Khanuja HS, Cooley GR. Leg pain in the running athlete. J Am Acad Othop Surg 2004;12:396–404.)

Radiologic Examination

Radiographs

■ Although initial radiographs are often normal when an athlete initially presents with a stress fracture, their role as an initial diagnostic aid is appropriate.

■ Radiographs may be positive within a few weeks, although some never show any radiographic changes even when followed for a long period of time.

■ Periosteal new bone formation (Fig. 31-1), focal sclerosis, a crack in the cortex, or even a complete fracture may be evident on later films.

■ Chronic stress fractures may show intramedullary sclerosis or cystic changes on radiography.

■ With anterior tibial cortex fractures, a wedge or V-shaped defect may be seen in the middle third of the anterior cortex.

  ■ The characteristic "dreaded black line" (Fig. 31-2) may be seen once the cortex hypertrophies and the cortex widens, which some feel represents a pseudarthrosis.

■ Stress fractures of the medial malleolus, when seen on radiographs, typically are present as a vertical fracture line from the junction of the tibial plafond and medial

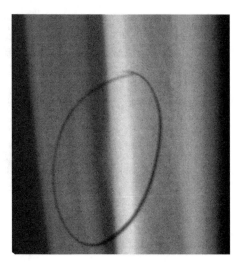

Figure 31-1 Periosteal new bone formation in a healing tibial stress fracture.

malleolus, although it may run obliquely from this area to the distal tibial metaphysis.

Bone Scanning
- Bone scintigraphy is especially useful in the diagnosis of stress fractures.
- Despite having slightly lower specificity than radiographs, bone scans are nearly 100% sensitive in diagnosing stress fractures and may be positive as early as 48 to 72 hours after onset of symptoms (Fig. 31-3).

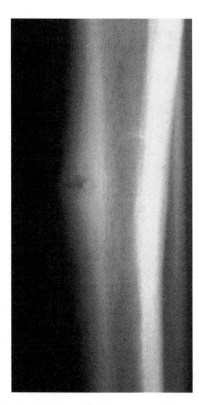

Figure 31-2 "Dreaded black line" representing stress fracture in anterior cortex of the tibial diaphysis.

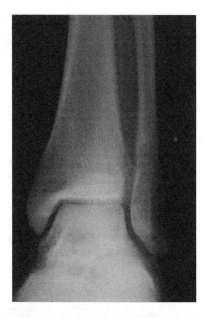

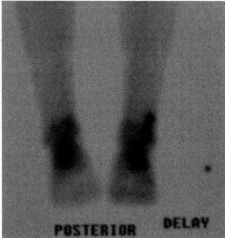

Figure 31-3 X-ray and bone scan of stress fracture of the distal fibula.

- Triple-phase bone scans—with angiogram (phase I), blood pool (phase II), and delayed static images (phase III)—monitor accumulation of radionucleotide markers at the site of increased metabolic activity, as is seen in stress fractures secondary to mechanical disturbances.
- Acute stress fractures are positive in all three phases, although soft-tissue injuries, such as medial tibial stress syndrome, typically show increased uptake only in the first two phases.
- Stress fractures also show smaller fusiform lesions as compared with medial tibial stress syndrome (MTSS).
- Bone scan can also be useful in diagnosing nonunion of a stress fracture, appearing as an area of low activity.
- The accuracy and sensitivity of bone scans can be enhanced with high-resolution views of suspected areas and comparison scans of the uninvolved, contralateral limb.
- Stress fracture findings on scintigraphy follow a characteristic pattern, as is shown in Table 31-1.

TABLE 31-1 NATURAL HISTORY OF STRESS FRACTURE IMAGING

Stage	Time Frame	Appearance
Acute	2–4 wk	All three phases show diffuse increased activity; no discrete fracture line seen on radiograph
Subacute	4–12 wk	Angiogram phase slowly decreases to normal; blood pool still positive and distinct fracture line noted on delayed radiographs
Healing	12 wk to 2 yr	Angiogram phase and blood pool normal; delayed slowly becomes negative (by year 1, 60% to 80%; by year 2, 90% normal)

(Adapted from Martire JR. The role of nuclear medicine bone scans in evaluating pain in athletic injuries. Clin Sports Med 1982;6:713–737.)

Other Studies

- Computed tomography (CT), ultrasound, and thermography have all been used in diagnosis with variable results, although it is believed that CT scans are even less sensitive than radiographs in diagnosing stress fractures.
- Magnetic resonance imaging (MRI) studies may have a role in the diagnostic workup of patients with suspected stress fractures and may aid in distinguishing stress fractures in a bone scan positive region from a suspected bone tumor or infectious process.
- MRI has the advantage of being noninvasive and aids in early diagnosis, since changes can be seen during the early stages of stress fractures.
- Common findings on MRI include endosteal and periosteal new bone formation, soft-tissue edema, and increased bone marrow density; T_2-weighted and STIR images may be particularly useful in the acute setting.
- Fat-suppressed MRI images have also been shown to aid in distinguishing stress fractures from MTSS. MRI may also be useful in the diagnosis of longitudinally oriented stress fractures.

Treatment

Nonsurgical Treatment

- The first step in treating stress fractures is to identify and correct any factors that are placing the athlete at risk.
- Training errors, improper technique, poor conditioning, and inadequate footwear should all be identified.
- Athletes should train in shoes that are appropriate for their foot type. Athletes with low arches should select shoes that provide stability and motion control, whereas those with high arches should select cushioned shoes.

TABLE 31-2 NONOPERATIVE MANAGEMENT OF STRESS FRACTURES

Phase	Management
I	• Modified rest, allowing weight-bearing with daily activities • Pain control with nonsteroidal anti-inflammatory drugs, ice, and local modalities • Stretching and strengthening exercises • Cross-training with cycling, swimming, or pool running
II	• Continuation of phase I objectives • Gradual reintroduction of activity on an alternate-day basis • Pain used as a guide to assess progress and increase workload • Modification of risk factors

- Pain control with nonsteroidal anti-inflammatory medications, along with rotating ice and heat, may be beneficial, although this has not been shown to improve recovery time (Table 31-2).
- Calcium supplementation may be of benefit to women.
- It is essential that the athlete avoid the offending or painful activity. A structured plan of treatment with two phases will reliably result in a successful outcome in athletes with stress fractures.
- Patient compliance and motivation are essential to successful treatment.
- The duration of treatment depends on clinical resolution of pain and radiographic evidence of fracture healing.
- Athletes progress to phase II once they have been free of pain for at least 10 to 14 days.
- When considering patient factors, biomechanical shoe orthoses have been suggested to aid in treatment of stress fractures.
  - Although custom biomechanical shoe orthoses worn within military boots have been reported to reduce the incidence of stress fractures by 50% in infantry recruits, such orthoses, both soft and semirigid, showed no benefit in athletes wearing running shoes.
- Another consideration that has shown promise in improving recovery time is an Aircast pneumatic leg brace, which may return athletes to unrestricted activity in less than half the time required if no brace is used. Traditional casting may also be used to relieve stress with weight-bearing on the affected lower extremity.
  - The benefit of using an Aircast pneumatic leg brace has been shown in two studies.
    - In one study, athletes using a brace resumed unrestricted activity at 5.3 weeks from the onset of treatment, which was significantly faster than with traditional treatment, which required 12 weeks before return to full activity.

- In the other study, athletes using these braces were able to start light activity in 7 days, compared with 21 days for athletes treated without a brace. There was no significant difference between the two groups with respect to resolution of swelling, tenderness at the fracture site to palpation, percussion, or vibration. Using the single-leg hop test, athletes in the brace group became pain-free at a median 14 days, compared with 45 days for the athletes treated without a brace. The athletes were able to return to full activity in their sport and did not feel that the brace impeded their performance.
  - Aircast bracing with full weight-bearing is also advocated in the treatment of medial malleolus stress fractures. Athletes are expected to progress to full participation in 6 to 8 weeks.
- The use of a pulsed electromagnetic field has shown some promise in the treatment of delayed union and nonunion of tibial fractures and may be of benefit in tension-sided fractures in the tibia.
- In athletes with fractures of the anterior tibial cortex, it is especially important that athletes do not return to activity until evidence exists of cortical bridging on radiography.
  - These fractures have gone on to completion from minimal contact long after they were felt to be healed.

Surgical Treatment

- Although most stress fractures reliably heal with nonoperative management, certain fractures are prone to delayed union, nonunion, and fracture completion. In these cases, surgical treatment may be warranted.
- Stress fractures in the anterior cortex of the tibial shaft often prove to be challenging to treat.
  - This region of the tibia is vulnerable to nonunion due to poor vascularity and increased tension because of morphologic bowing of the tibia and strong pull of the posterior musculature.
  - Surgical intervention is indicated if nonoperative management for 4 to 6 months fails to heal the fracture.
  - A bone scan with minimal activity in the area of the stress fracture or findings of nonunion and chronic changes on the radiograph, such as intramedullary sclerosis or cystic changes, also suggest that operative management will be necessary.
  - Once the "dreaded black line" is present, likelihood of nonunion and the need for surgical intervention are greatly increased.
  - Earlier surgical treatment may also be appropriate in elite athletes with this high-risk fracture, especially if little or no evidence of healing is seen after 3 months of nonoperative management.
- Surgical options for stress fractures of the anterior diaphyseal cortex of the tibia are drilling at the fracture site, bone grafting, and the now-favored treatment for this fracture type, intramedullary fixation (Fig. 31-4).
- Stress fractures of the medial malleolus are also prone to nonunion due to high shear forces at the fracture site and may require operative management.

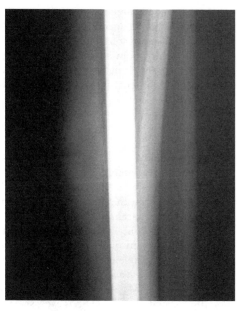

Figure 31-4 Intramedullary fixation of a stress fracture of the anterior cortex of the tibial diaphysis. (Courtesy of Robert Arciero, MD, Farmington, CT.)

- Internal fixation with two cancellous screws is advocated when a radiograph shows a complete fracture line.
- Bone grafting may be indicated if there is evidence of fracture displacement or nonunion.
- An athlete who suffers this injury in the middle of a season should also be treated with open reduction internal fixation.
- Range-of-motion exercises can begin shortly after surgery, with running started at 6 weeks and return to full activity allowed at 8 weeks postoperatively.

Results

The great majority of stress fractures of the tibia and fibula heal reliably with nonoperative treatment. Stress fractures of the tibia and fibula typically heal in 6 to 20 weeks if complete cortical disruption has not occurred.

Of special consideration is the high rate of delayed union seen with stress fractures in the anterior cortex of the tibial shaft. With sufficient patience, these fractures may be able to heal without requiring operative intervention. However, most tibial stress fractures in this area have a challenging natural history. When athletes do undergo intramedullary fixation for these fractures, a successful outcome can be expected.

MEDIAL TIBIAL STRESS SYNDROME

MTSS is the most common overuse injury causing leg pain found in athletes. Also referred to as shin splints, this has been defined by the American Medical Association as "pain and discomfort in the leg from repetitive running on hard surface or forcible, excessive use of foot flexors; diagnosis should be limited to musculotendinous inflammations, excluding fracture or ischemic disorder." Pain is characteristically located in the distal posteromedial aspect of the tibia, starting as a dull, aching pain after exercise and gradually becoming worse as the inciting activity is continued. Rest is the mainstay of treatment, but surgery is occasionally needed in recalcitrant cases.

Pathogenesis

Etiology and Epidemiology

Repetitive impact activity combined with hyperpronation of the foot has been implicated as the cause of MTSS. MTSS can be related to any activity that involves running, jumping, or sustained walking or marching. Improper training techniques, insufficient warm-up, exercise on hard or uneven surfaces, abrupt increase in duration or intensity of exercise, change in footwear, skeletal malalignment, and muscle imbalance or inflexibility have all been described as inciting factors in the genesis of MTSS. The skeletal abnormality most commonly associated with MTSS is excessive foot pronation. Forefoot and hindfoot varus alignment occur more frequently among patients with MTSS, predisposing them to dynamic hyperpronation of the subtalar joint. MTSS is commonly bilateral.

MTSS is very common among runners, accounting for 13% to 17.3% of all running injuries. In one study of high school runners, the overall incidence of MTSS was found to be 12%. In this group, females were at a much higher risk than males. Female predominance was also shown in a study of military recruits, where females were twice more likely to develop MTSS than males. The overall incidence in this study was much higher at 35%.

Pathophysiology

Leading theories on the pathophysiology of MTSS relate the pain to traction periostitis or a bone stress reaction. Unaccustomed eccentric contraction of the plantar flexors and foot invertors in a hyperpronated foot leads to excessive strain in the region of the medial tibia. The muscle originally believed to most commonly produce this increased load was the posterior tibialis. However, the function and anatomy of the soleus, flexor digitorum longus, and medial crural fascia more accurately account for the location of pain in this condition.

MTSS has traditionally been considered a traction periostitis, resulting from muscle or fascial traction on the periosteum. Records of surgical histology are sparse in the literature. According to one report, chronic inflammatory infiltration along with thickening and tension of the crural fascial were found at the time of surgery.

Although vasculitis and increased medial periosteal formation have been suggested as causative agents for MTSS, recent evidence suggests that it is more likely the result of a bone stress reaction. MTSS may not be as benign or self-limiting as the inflammatory mechanism of traction periostitis suggests. The idea that repetitive microtrauma leads to a bone stress injury has led some to hypothesize that MTSS and stress fractures are related along a continuum of bone microdamage and reparative processes, where MTSS is a milder form in this spectrum.

Diagnosis (Algorithm 31-1)

Physical Examination and History

■ Diagnosis of MTSS is largely based on clinical history and location of the pain.
  ▪ Pain with MTSS is most commonly described as a dull ache along the posteromedial border of the middle to distal tibia.
  ▪ It is first experienced during or immediately after a workout and gradually becomes worse over a period of days of weeks.
  ▪ Initially, rest usually relieves the pain.
  ▪ As the inciting activity is continued, pain becomes more severe, appears earlier during exercise, and can occur at rest.
  ▪ Because the pain is progressive, it will eventually impair athletic performance and may limit daily activities.
■ The physical examination finding most consistent with MTSS is pain with palpation of the posteromedial border of the tibia.
  ▪ This area of tenderness can span as much as a third of the tibia in a region centered at the junction of the middle and distal thirds of the leg.
  ▪ The diffuse nature of the tenderness helps distinguish this condition from stress fractures.
  ▪ There is usually no associated swelling.
  ▪ Peripheral pulses and neurologic examination are normal.
  ▪ Range of motion of the foot and ankle does not produce pain.
  ▪ Muscle strength is preserved, although resisted ankle plantar flexion and toe raises may elicit pain.

Radiologic Examination

■ Radiographs of the lower extremity are usually normal, although cortical hypertrophy or longitudinal periosteal new bone formation with scalloping along the posteromedial border of the tibia is found in some patients.
■ The delayed images of three-phase bone scintigraphy demonstrate a linear, longitudinal uptake in the posterior tibial cortex (Fig. 31-5).
  ▪ This test can produce false-negative results in patients with MTSS, but it can exclude stress fractures, and the diagnosis of MTSS can still be made on the basis of a consistent history and physical examination.
■ MRI has also been shown to be a useful tool in the diagnosis of MTSS, especially in acute cases.
  ▪ In a prospective study of diagnostic imaging for acute MTSS (less than 3 months of symptoms), a three-phase bone scan had a sensitivity of 84% and a specificity of 33%, whereas MRI had a sensitivity of 79% and a specificity of 33%. When the results of these tests were correlated, the diagnostic sensitivity was 95% and specificity was 67%. Incidentally, the MRI findings in this study supported the mechanism of a bone stress reaction, showing periosteal fluid and endosteal changes in both the posteromedial and anteromedial tibia.

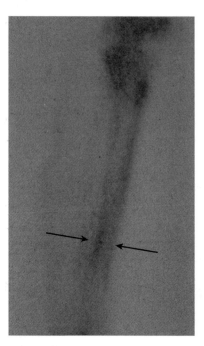

Figure 31-5 Bone scan showing linear uptake on the delayed images in the posterior tibial cortex in a patient with medial tibial stress syndrome.

Treatment

Nonoperative Treatment

- Surgery is almost never indicated in patients with MTSS.
- Treatment should be centered around relative rest, avoiding the inciting activity.
- Involvement in activities that do not cause pain, such as swimming or cycling, may be an option for patients who wish to remain active.
- A short period of rest may be all that is required to allow the patient to gradually return to activities over a 3- to 6-week period.
- Alteration in training schedule or intensity, change in footwear or training surface, heel cord stretching, and treatment with anti-inflammatory medication should also be tried in the course of treatment.
- Patients with excessive pronation of the foot should be fitted with orthotics.
- Physical therapy with modalities such as ultrasound and iontophoresis may be beneficial in more chronic cases.

Surgical Treatment

- Surgery should be reserved for recalcitrant cases.
  - Some advocate at least 12 months of conservative treatment, whereas others recommend that the athlete have at least two episodes of symptom recurrence after prolonged periods of rest.
- Regardless of the approach, patients with MTSS reliably heal with nonoperative measures, and surgery should be used only as a last resort in the treatment of this condition.
- If surgery is to be undertaken, fasciotomy of the posterior compartment, possibly combined with cauterization of the tibial edge, is advocated.

Postoperative Management

- Weight-bearing as tolerated with the assistance of crutches is allowed postoperatively.
- The patient is encouraged to start range-of-motion exercises for the ankle and knee right away.
- A compressive dressing is left in place for 3 days, and crutches are used for 3 to 5 days.
- Stretching and strengthening exercises are performed for the first 6 weeks, at which point a gradual return to jogging is allowed.
- Full return to activities is allowed between 2 to 3 months postoperatively, although it may take up to 12 months.

Results

Relative rest with a gradual return to exercise and sports routinely yields positive results in patients with MTSS. In those patients who do go on to require surgery, success is varied among the reports in the literature. In the first report of fasciotomy and periosteal release, good results with ability to begin effective training 1 month after surgery were found in all 11 patients.

Other reports have been less favorable. A report of nine patients with MTSS treated with posterior compartment fasciotomy showed only five who were pain-free, although two of the others reported some pain relief with the procedure. In a study that included periosteal cauterization with fasciotomy, 78% were completely better and 14% had significant improvement. In another report of fasciotomy without detachment of the soleus bridge, a majority of patients had improvement from their preoperative condition, but only 29% had satisfactory results. With release of the soleus bridge and periosteal cauterization combined with fasciotomy, patients with MTSS had significant reduction of pain, with only one patient reporting an increase in pain. Sixty-nine percent of these patients had good or excellent results, but only 41% were able to return to their presymptom level of activity. Potential complications of surgical management include infection, hematoma, neurovascular injury, and recurrence.

EXERTIONAL COMPARTMENT SYNDROME

Exertional compartment syndrome (ECS) most commonly afflicts young athletes involved in running sports. Lower leg pain from transient increases in intercompartmental pressure is usually relieved shortly after cessation of the exercise. Most commonly, the anterior and deep posterior compartments are involved. If the athlete wishes to continue the offending activity, surgical intervention is often necessary.

Pathogenesis

Etiology and Epidemiology

The etiology for ECS is unknown and likely multifactorial. The syndrome often affects bilateral lower extremities, and incidence is equal in males and females. Although the anterior and deep posterior compartments are affected more commonly, it is not unusual to have involvement of the lateral and superficial posterior compartments, usually in concert with involvement of the adjacent compartment. Running athletes commonly experience exercise-induced pain, but in athletes suspected of having ECS, only 14% to 27% were found to have increased intercompartmental pressures during and after exercise. Incidence reported in the literature appears to be quite variable due to differences in the study populations with respect to age, sex, and type of activity, as well as in the practice habits of the authors involved. It is clear, however, that this is predominately a problem of young, active people.

Pathophysiology

Although the etiology can be multifactorial, it is generally agreed that transient ischemia at the capillary level is the responsible culprit for symptoms. Compartment syndromes, in general, occur when increased tissue pressure within the compartment compromises the circulation and function of the contents of the compartment. During exercise, muscles only get blood flow during the relaxation phase of exercise. With muscle contraction, the pressures are much higher than the capillary perfusion pressures, leading to decreased blood perfusion of muscle tissue. Although this theory has been called into question by several studies, it has been shown that patients with ECS have significantly greater maximum relative deoxygenation during exercise. It was also demonstrated that there is a longer recovery time to return to the pre-exercise level of oxygenation in patients with ECS.

Diagnosis (Algorithm 31-1)

Physical Examination and History

- Exertional leg pain may be secondary to many causes; therefore, as in most orthopaedic conditions, a careful history, physical examination, imaging studies, and compartment pressure studies are paramount in making the diagnosis.
  - The patient usually begins to experience a dull ache, crampiness, fullness, or a pressure sensation in the affected compartment that occurs after he has been exercising for a period of time.
    - Although this period of time is variable from patient to patient, it usually has a predictable onset for that particular patient.
  - Pain is usually localized to the entire affected compartment and usually increases to the point where activity has to be stopped.
  - The pain is characteristically felt in the soft tissues rather than in the bone.
  - If pain is more bony in origin and persists despite cessation of exercise, stress fractures or periositis (medial tibial syndrome) should be considered.
- In many cases, as symptoms become more chronic, the onset of symptoms can come on quicker and meet maximum tolerability in a shorter time period.
- Sensory or motor disturbances sometimes occur, more commonly when the anterior compartment is affected.

- Transient "floppiness" of the ankle or a feeling of instability in the ankle and sensory disturbances in the distribution of the superficial peroneal nerve can occur when the anterior compartment is affected.
  - This usually occurs more commonly when the athlete tries to push through the pain.
- Typically, cessation of exercise will relieve pain, with more severe pain diminishing over 10 to 15 minutes, but a dull, low level of symptoms can continue for a significant period of time.
  - Classically, the discomfort will virtually disappear until exercise once again commences.
- Examination at rest is usually not helpful.
  - Most of the patients are young, healthy athletes who are symptomatic when they come into the office, making history of paramount importance in the suspicion of the diagnosis.
  - In some cases, the athletes may be overconditioned with hypertrophy of the muscles and a compartment that cannot tolerate the 20% increase in volume that is typically seen with exercise.
- It is important to look for fascial hernias, more typically seen in patients with anterior and/or lateral compartment syndrome (15% to 60% of patients).
  - Hernias usually can be best demonstrated with the patients standing on their heel with active dorsiflexion of the foot.
  - Fascial hernias most likely represent an enlargement of the foramen through which the superficial peroneal nerve exits through the lateral intermuscular septum to become superficial.
  - These hernias, therefore, are typically seen at the junction of the middle and distal thirds of the leg.
- It is important to examine the whole extremity, including alignment, range of motion, and stability of the knee and ankle, as well as postural foot abnormalities.
  - Manual testing usually reveals no weakness.
  - Careful palpation of the bone is paramount to rule out a stress fracture.
  - A careful examination of the distal pulses is important, although most of these athletes are young and do not have vascular claudication. However, dynamic popliteal artery entrapment can be confused with ECS.
- It is worthwhile to examine the patient after reproduction of symptoms.
  - This can be done either at the time of compartment pressure testing or by having the patient leave the office and run up and down stairs until the symptoms are reproduced.
  - This will often help to substantiate the patient's history and will help the physician localize the symptoms, particularly if sensory disturbances and motor weakness transiently occur.
- In general, pain with anterior ECS tends to be well localized to the anterior compartment.
  - In a patient with posterior ECS, however, the pain may be poorly localized. It thus becomes even more important to rule out bony or vascular etiologies in these cases.

In patients with profound peroneal nerve symptoms with marked weakness of dorsiflexion after exercise, peroneal nerve entrapment at the fibular head should also be expected.

- A Tinel's sign can usually be elicited in this location in these cases, and nerve conduction velocities of the peroneal nerve across the fibular head at rest and after exercise can confirm the diagnosis.

Diagnostic Tests

- Bony abnormalities should be ruled out routinely with anteroposterior and lateral radiographs of the leg.
  - Chronic stress fractures can often be seen in these radiographs, but not always.
- A technetium bone scan can be useful, particularly in patients with any bony tenderness or posterior symptoms.
- The key test in the diagnostic workup is the recording of intracompartmental pressures.
  - The most clinically useful measurements are to test the pressure before exercise, immediately after exercise, and then 5 minutes after exercise.
  - The most practical method is repeated needle insertion via a commercially available slit catheter (Fig. 31-6).
    - It is crucial that the catheter be inserted in muscle and not in fascia or tendon. The leg must also be tested in a consistent position. Since foot position can affect the pressure measurement, testing should be performed with the patient supine and the ankle in neutral position. The skin and subcutaneous tissue should be anesthetized

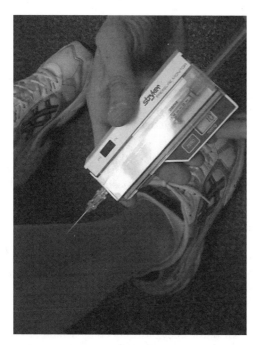

Figure 31-6 This commercially available testing device is easy to calibrate and use. (Courtesy of Stryker Corporation, Kalamazoo, MI).

first with a longer-acting anesthetic that will last the duration of the pressure testing.

- For the anterior compartment, the catheter should be placed within the muscle belly of the tibialis anterior. A useful landmark is the junction of the proximal and middle third of the leg, approximately 2 cm lateral to the tibial crest.
- For the lateral compartment, which is tested less commonly, the catheter is inserted at the same level, just over the fibular shaft in the muscle belly of the peroneals.
- For the superficial posterior compartment, placement of the catheter within the fleshy part of the medial head of the gastrocnemius at the junction of the proximal and middle third of the leg is easiest.
- Pressure testing for the deep posterior compartment is the most difficult. The most volume of muscle is in the proximal portion of the deep posterior compartment; however, placement of the catheter blindly in this location can be hazardous because of adjacent blood vessels. The catheter should be carefully inserted into the flexor digitorum longus muscle just posterior to the tibial shaft at the junction of the middle and distal thirds of the leg, at the location where the soleus bridge ends. The catheter is angled proximally. Having the patient contract and relax the muscle will ensure to the examiner that the catheter is in the proper location.
- To test the subcompartments of the lower leg, particularly the tibialis posterior compartment, CT imaging or ultrasound guidance is necessary.
- After resting pressures are obtained, the patient is instructed to run on the treadmill at an increasing cadence and incline until symptoms are maximally reproduced.
  - It is crucial that symptoms are maximally reproduced and the patient can no longer run before postexercise pressure measurements are recorded.
  - A set of measurements is taken immediately after cessation of exercise, followed by 5 minutes later by another set.
  - The pressure criteria set forth by Pedowitz et al. (1990) are the most useful. The presence of one or more of the parameters in Table 31-3 is diagnostic for ECS.

Treatment

Surgical Treatment

Indications and Contraindications

- Once a patient is diagnosed with ECS based on history, physical examination, and compartment pressure testing, there really are only two choices: modify activities to alleviate symptoms or surgical fasciotomy.
- The more competitive and avid the athlete, the more likely the individual is to undergo surgery.

TABLE 31-3 EXERTIONAL COMPARTMENT SYNDROME PRESSURE CRITERIA

Time	Pressure (mm Hg)
Rest	≥15
1 min postexercise	≥30
5 min postexercise	≥20

The presence of one or more of the parameters is diagnostic.
(Adapted from Pedowitz RA, Hargens AR, Mubarak SJ, Gershuni DH. Modified criteria for the objective diagnosis of chronic compartment syndrome of the leg. Am J Sports Med 1990;18:35–40.)

■ Although different surgical choices have been advocated, it is generally agreed that fasciotomy of the affected compartment is the treatment of choice.
■ Contraindications to surgical management:
  ▪ Any vascular insufficiency of the lower extremity
  ▪ Extensive varicosities over the affected compartment
  ▪ Poor skin circulation
  ▪ A patient unwilling to accept the risks of any potential surgical complications or the potential for an unsuccessful outcome

Technique
Release of the Anterior and Lateral Compartments
■ One skin incision is used to release both the anterior and lateral compartments of the leg.
■ The major structure at risk is the superficial peroneal nerve, which generally exits through the lateral intermuscular septum approximately 10 cm proximal to the lateral malleolus and becomes superficial at the junction of the middle and distal thirds of the leg, although there is significant anatomic variation.
■ The patient is placed in the supine position on the operating table, and a tourniquet is applied to the proximal thigh.
■ The leg is divided into thirds and marked at the junction of the middle and distal thirds of the lower leg.
■ A 4- to 5-cm incision is made, with this mark (about 10 cm proximal to the lateral malleolus) being the center point.
■ The incision is made halfway between the tibial crest and anterior border of the fibula.
  ▪ This is usually 3 cm lateral to the tibial crest and roughly centered over the lateral intermuscular septum, where the superficial peroneal nerve will be exiting.
■ In cases where a fascial hernia is present, the incision should always be centered over this.
■ Looking closely for the superficial peroneal nerve, a transverse fascial incision is made from the tibial crest, across the septum, to the peroneal muscles.
  ▪ The superficial peroneal nerve should always be identified and explored proximally and distally into its branches.

■ Performing a partial fasciectomy by removing a 1-cm strip of fascia may prevent regrowth of fascia and return of symptoms.
■ Soft tissue is dissected free both superficial and deep to the fascia before fasciotomy.
■ Fasciotomy of the anterior compartment is then performed approximately 1 cm lateral to the tibial with long fasciotomy scissors, allowing access to the most proximal portion of the compartment.
  ▪ The tips of the scissors are pointed anterior to avoid the superficial peroneal nerve.
■ In very large patients, it may be advisable to make a small 2-cm counterincision proximally in order to adequately complete the fasciotomy.
■ Fasciotomy of the lateral compartment is performed in a similar fashion at the most posterior extent of the transverse fascial incision.
  ▪ This should be done as lateral as possible, with the tips of the scissors pointed posterior to avoid any branches of the superficial peroneal nerve.
■ Lateral fascial release should be 1 to 2 cm anterior to the fibula.
■ The tourniquet is deflated and hemostasis achieved using electrocautery.
  ▪ Marked bleeding can lead to extensive fibrosis and failure of the procedure.
■ The use of suture material should be minimized.
  ▪ Subcutaneous tissue is closed with an interrupted 2-0 absorbable suture and the skin with a subcuticular nonabsorbable suture that can be removed 2 weeks postoperatively.
■ A large, compressive dressing is applied with large ABD pads over the whole extent of the compartments that have been released, with ace bandages from toes to knee.

Release of the Superficial and Deep Posterior Compartments
■ A 6-cm incision is made 2 cm posterior to the posteromedial border of the tibia, centered at the junction of the middle and distal thirds of the lower leg.
■ Care must be taken to identify the saphenous nerve and vein.
■ A transverse incision is made going from the posteromedial border of the tibia, crossing the septum separating the deep and superficial posterior compartments.
■ The superficial fascia is first split at the posterior part of the wound, releasing the superficial compartment proximally and distally, with the tips of the scissors pointed posteriorly.
■ Both heads of the gastrocnemius have separate compartments, so if there is a compartment syndrome definitely involving the heads of the gastrocnemius, a separate small incision may be necessary to release the fascia over the lateral head.
■ Release of the deep posterior compartment, particularly proximally, is the most difficult and hazardous of any of the fascial releases. The most common sequela is deep venous bleeding.

- The deep fascia is identified in the distal third of the leg, where the deep posterior compartment becomes superficial distal to the end of the soleus bridge.
- When dividing the fascia proximally, it is crucial to have long retractors lifting up the soleus bridge and to free up all the soft tissue off of the fascia.
- The fascia covering the flexor digitorum longus is incised through its length going proximally, being cognizant of the location of the saphenous nerve.
- Deeper dissection to expose and release the subcompartment over the posterior tibial muscle is more hazardous and controversial.
- With posterior releases, it is particularly important to achieve hemostasis before wound closure.

Alternative Techniques
- As described by Leversedge et al. (2002), arthroscopically assisted fasciotomy is used not only to minimize the size of the incision, but also to minimize the amount of postoperative scar formation, potentially decreasing the chance of recurrence.
  - Early reports have been promising, but more experience is necessary before this technique can be recommended.
- In revision cases, fasciotomy and partial fasciectomy is combined with removal of all fibroproliferative scar, exploration, decompression of the superficial peroneal nerve, and bathing the deep tissues in a dilute steroid solution before closure with minimal nonabsorbable suture.

Postoperative Management
- In unilateral cases, patients should remain non-weight-bearing for approximately 1 week to control swelling.
- In bilateral cases, weight-bearing is allowed as tolerated with the use of two crutches for the first week, gradually discontinuing the use of crutches during the second week.
  - A compressive dressing is maintained for the first 3 to 4 days.
- Immediate range-of-motion exercises for the knee and ankle are prescribed. After the sutures are removed at the 10- to 14-day mark, stretching exercises and isometric strengthening exercises are started.
- Stationary bicycling is allowed at 2 weeks postoperatively.
- In general, patients with isolated anterior compartment fasciotomies have the quickest rehabilitation, and usually these patients can resume running within 6 to 8 weeks after surgery.
- Patients who have deep posterior compartment or four-compartment release usually require at least 12 weeks of rehabilitation before running is permitted.

Results

In general, the results of fasciotomy for anterior ECS enjoy the highest success rate. Because it is virtually impossible to release completely all of the subcompartments of the deep posterior compartment without a massive dissection, and because this problem is sometimes multifactorial in nature, probably tends to lower success rates in these groups. One study showed a 90% to 95% success rate in patients with anterior compartment fasciotomy and 70% to 80% success rate with deep posterior compartment fasciotomy.

The main pitfalls occur around neurovascular injury. At risk anteriorly is the superficial peroneal nerve. Posteriorly, there is a rich vascular network. Bleeding issues, both venous and arterial, are much more common. The major vessels are at risk in the deep posterior compartment. Patients with marked bleeding and postoperative swelling are predisposed to extensive fibrosis and failure of the procedure. Recurrences are most often related to the thick fibroproliferative scar that forms around the incision and can generate local high pressures and entrap the superficial peroneal nerve. Recurrences and failures are more common in women.

With recurrent cases, results are best in those patients with evidence of superficial peroneal nerve entrapment. In one series of revision surgeries, only 50% of patients who did not have nerve entrapment had a successful outcome. It is important to distinguish failures (patients that never got better after the index procedure) from recurrences (patients who had an initial successful result with gradual deterioration secondary to the formation of fibroproliferative scar and/or nerve entrapment).

POPLITEAL ARTERY ENTRAPMENT SYNDROME

Entrapment of the popliteal artery can occur as a result of either congenital musculotendinous variations in the development of the medial head of the gastrocnemius and popliteus muscles or in dynamic situations with no evidence of anatomic abnormalities. These latter "functional" forms are most closely related to hypertrophy of the medial head of the gastrocnemius associated with repetitive overuse in athletes. This condition may lead to lower-leg claudication and, in rare circumstances, can lead to limb-threatening ischemia. Nonoperative measures do not reliably provide relief, and a variety of operative interventions have been suggested.

Pathogenesis

Etiology and Epidemiology
Popliteal artery entrapment syndrome (PAES) was first described in 1879 by a medical student who described an anatomical variant of the course of the popliteal artery in a leg amputated for gangrene. The significance of the alteration in the normal anatomy of the popliteal fossa relating to pathologic impingement of the popliteal artery was not fully recognized until almost a century later, when this syndrome was described by Love and Whelan.

The cause of PAES relates either to variation in the course of the popliteal artery or to hypertrophy of the calf musculature. Both mechanisms lead to entrapment of the popliteal artery, resulting in the characteristic syndrome. Intermittent occlusion of the popliteal artery occurs with

TABLE 31-4 CLASSIFICATION OF PAES

Type	Description
I	Marked medial deviation of the popliteal artery around a normal medial head of the gastrocnemius muscle
II	Medial head of gastrocnemius has more lateral and inferior attachments in the intercondylar region or lateral aspect of the medial femoral condyle, displacing the medial popliteal artery
III	Aberrant accessory slip from the medial head of the gastrocnemius or fibrous band entraps the normally positioned popliteal artery
IV	Popliteal artery lies in its deep, primitive position, entrapped by a fibrous band or the popliteus muscle
V	In addition to findings of any of the first four types, the popliteal vein is also entrapped
VI	"Functional" entrapment by the hypertrophied medial head of the gastrocnemius; no anatomic abnormality

(Adapted from Levien LJ, Veller MG. Popliteal artery entrapment syndrome: more common than previously recognized. J Vasc Surg 1999;30:587–598. Atilla S, Ilgit ET, Akpek S, et al. MR imaging and MR angiography in popliteal artery entrapment syndrome. Eur Radiol 1998l;8:1025–1029.)

each plantar flexion motion and may lead to degeneration of the artery with resultant intimal damage.

A classification scheme to describe the various causes of PAES is given in Table 31-4. Type I entrapment is the most common form, occurring in 57% of cases in one study. The entrapment mechanism has been documented to involve the popliteal vein in up to a third of PAES cases.

Type VI, or functional, entrapment is most likely in the athletic population a result of hypertrophy of the medial head of the gastrocnemius secondary to repetitive and forceful ankle plantar flexion against resistance, as occurs in running and jumping activities. The gastrocnemius is one of the chief plantar flexors of the ankle, providing propulsion during walking, running, and jumping. Athletes at particular risk of overtraining and overdeveloping the muscles in the calf are involved in basketball, soccer, volleyball, and cross-country running. A similar pattern of repetitive contraction of the calf muscles is also seen in drivers of heavy vehicles, and PAES should be considered in any patient in such a job when presenting with lower leg claudication. Functional entrapment has also been related to hypertrophy of the soleus, plantaris, and semimembranosus.

The incidence of PAES is unknown and believed to occur in 0.17% to 3.5% of the population. PAES occurs more commonly in men and is generally seen in patients 20 to 40 years old. It is bilateral in up to 76% of cases; thus, it is recommended that the contralateral limb be screened even when asymptomatic.

Pathophysiology

Anatomic forms of PAES are related to the developmental anatomy of the popliteal fossa. As the limb bud develops, the medial head of the gastrocnemius muscle migrates medially across the popliteal fossa and attaches to the posterior surface of the medial femoral condyle. This migration occurs at the same stage in development as the rearrangement of the arterial structures in the lower leg. If the order of migration and formation do not occur in the normal stepwise fashion, an abnormal anatomic relationship results.

The repetitive trauma to the vessel that results from lower leg overuse, in both the anatomical and functional forms, leads to the characteristic symptoms of PAES and can eventually result in intimal injury with subsequent thrombosis, aneurysm formation, and acute limb-threatening ischemia. This highlights the importance of a high clinical suspicion when a young patient presents with lower leg claudication.

Diagnosis (Algorithm 31-1)

Physical Examination and History

- PAES can be associated with a wide range of symptoms.
- Characteristic complaints are aching pain after strenuous activity that resolves after a few minutes of rest, rapid limb fatigue, cramping in the calf, paresthesias, swelling, blanching, or coldness in the foot.
  - In one series, claudication was the only symptom in 65%; paresthesias were found in 14%, and rest pain or trophic changes were found in 11%.
- Onset is often insidious but can occur suddenly during intense exercise.
- Repetitive jumping or uphill running most predictably aggravates symptoms.
- Athletes with ECS often present with similar complaints, but their symptoms typically are present for a longer period of time after exercise than in those patients with PAES.
- Physical signs are often absent at rest.
- The most characteristic finding in patients with PAES is diminished ankle pulses upon maneuvers that cause contraction of the gastrocnemius: plantar flexion of the foot against resistance, passive dorsiflexion, and knee hyperextension.
  - This finding should be interpreted with caution because it is often found in asymptomatic individuals.
- Patients may show evidence of an overdeveloped gastrocnemius muscle.
- Alteration of the ankle-brachial index of more than 0.2 is suggestive of popliteal artery entrapment.

Radiologic Examination

- Duplex ultrasonography was originally the diagnostic test of choice for PAES.
- Reduced blood flow in the foot upon provocative maneuvers is suggestive of popliteal artery entrapment, but there is an unacceptably high rate of false-positive results with this test, and it is unable to distinguish the underlying cause of the disorder.
- Contrast arteriography has also been used in the diagnostic workup, but more precise findings are capable

with digital-subtraction arteriography and magnetic resonance angiography.

- With these tests, medial deviation of the popliteal artery, segmental occlusion, and poststenotic dilatation may be seen.
- Intrinsic arterial lesions associated with degeneration in later forms of the disease can be identified by either technique, but magnetic resonance angiography has the advantage of being noninvasive and can reveal the anatomic abnormality, leading to entrapment.

Treatment

Surgical Treatment

- Nonoperative measures have not been found to be of benefit in patients with symptomatic entrapment.
- Avoidance of aggravating activities may provide some relief; however, patients are at risk of progression to acute popliteal artery occlusion, especially when PAES is secondary to an anatomic abnormality.
- Although the indications for surgery in individuals with minor or absent symptoms are unclear, surgery is recommended in any symptomatic patient who demonstrates an anatomical or functional entrapment of the popliteal artery.
- If no evidence of damage to the popliteal artery is present, simple release of the popliteal artery by myectomy of the medial head of the gastrocnemius and any abnormal slips of muscle or fascia are sufficient.
  - Because of its importance as a knee flexor and role in limiting knee hyperextension, reattachment of the medial head to the medial femoral condyle after release is recommended.
  - This has been shown to reduce rehabilitation time and improve performance postoperatively.
  - Simple release of the medial head may also allow it to reattach in a nonanatomic position and continue to exert pressure on the popliteal vessels.
- In cases in which arterial damage is evident, expedient treatment with interposition vein grafting has shown the best results, as compared with local therapies such as endarterectomy, angioplasty, and vein patching.
- Although anatomy is not as well visualized, using a medial approach in young athletes with functional entrapment allows a sufficient release of the offending musculotendinous tissue and allows an early return to sports.

- When bypass grafting is necessary or in revision cases, a posterior S-shaped approach affords the best view of the structures of the popliteal fossa.

Postoperative Management

- In cases in which arterial repair is not indicated, a splint maintaining the knee in 30 degrees of flexion is applied, and quadriceps exercises are encouraged immediately.
- Ambulation with crutch assistance is started at 1 week.
  - Crutches are used until normal weight-bearing and gait is achieved.
- At 2 weeks, the splint may be removed, and the patient is allowed to ride a stationary bike and perform kickboard exercises in the pool.
- Light jogging can begin at 3 to 4 weeks postoperatively, and full recovery is expected in 2 to 3 months.

Results

Since PAES is not a common disorder, few clinical series are present in the literature.

In one review, 9 of 12 patients treated surgically had complete relief of claudication and paresthetic symptoms, whereas the other three were significantly improved by surgery. In another series, athletes who were compelled to stop their sporting activities as a result of PAES were able to resume sports after postoperative recovery. In patients with intrinsic arterial damage, long-term patency after aneurysm repair and saphenous vein grafting was excellent.

SUGGESTED READING

Detmer DE. Chronic shin splints: classification and management of medial tibial stress syndrome. Sports Med 1986;3:436–446.

Detmer DE, Sharpe K, Sufit RL, et al. Chronic compartment syndrome: diagnosis, management, and outcomes. Am J Sports Med 1985;13:162–170.

Korpelainen R, Orava S, Karpakka J, et al. Risk factors for recurrent stress fractures in athletes. Am J Sports Med 2001;29:304–310.

Leversedge FJ, Casey PJ, Seiler JG, et al. Endoscopically assisted fasciotomy: description of technique and in vitro assessment of lower-leg compartment decompression. Am J Sports Med 2002;30:272–278.

Matheson GO, Clement DB, McKenzie DC, et al. Stress fractures in athletes: a study of 320 cases. Am J Sports Med 1987;15:46–58.

Pedowitz RA, Hargens AR, Mubarak SJ, et al. Modified criteria for the objective diagnosis of chronic compartment syndrome of the leg. Am J Sports Med 1990;18:35–40.

Rorabeck CH, Fowler PJ, Nott L. The results of fasciotomy in management of chronic exertional compartment syndrome. Am J Sports Med 1988;16:224–227.

Rupani HD, Holder LE, Espinola DA, et al. Three-phase radionuclide bone imaging in sports medicine. Radiology 1985;156:187–196.

Turnipseed WD. Popliteal entrapment syndrome. J Vasc Surg 2002;35:910–915.

ANKLE INJURIES

BRIAN D. BUSCONI
NICOLA A. DEANGELIS
HEATHER KILLIE
TIMOTHY J. MARQUEEN

ANATOMY

Ankle stability is provided by three primary entities: bony, ligamentous, and muscular (dynamic). Although they all work together, they are discussed separately to gain full appreciation of their contributions. In general, the ankle is a complex hinge joint consisting of three bones (the tibia, fibula, and talus) and three ligamentous complexes (medial, lateral, and syndesmotic).

Bony Anatomy

Bony stability occurs through the tibiotalar articulation. This articulation consists of the tibia, fibula, and talus. The tibia and fibula provide the mortise surrounding the talus.

Tibia

The tibia flares distally to form the majority of the superior articular surface of the ankle. The lower end of the tibia has five surfaces. The most important of these are the inferior (tibial plafond) and the medial malleolus, which is located anteromedially. The plafond is a mostly concave surface when viewed laterally to allow for articulation with the talar dome. There is a central prominence that results in a significant reduction in contact area between the tibia and talus with as little as 1 mm of subluxation. It is wider laterally than it is medially, and the posterior surface is lower than the anterior surface. The medial malleolus is an apophysis formed by two colliculi: the anterior and posterior. The superficial deltoid ligament attaches to the smaller, anterior

colliculus and the deep deltoid attaches to the posterior colliculus and intercollicular groove.

The anterior and posterior aspects of the distal tibia serve as attachment points for the syndesmotic ligament complex. The posterior aspect of the distal tibia is often referred to as the posterior malleolus when describing trimalleolar ankle fractures and is important with regard to posterior stability. Posterolaterally, the tibia forms a groove called the incisura to accommodate the fibula.

Fibula

The fibula flares distally to form the lateral malleolus. The tip of the lateral malleolus is located more posteriorly and distal than that of the medial malleolus. The lateral malleolus contains the lateral articular surface of the ankle. The lateral malleolus and distal fibular shaft serve as attachment sites for many of the ligamentous supports of the ankle. Along the shaft of the medial fibula, the interosseous membrane, anterior-inferior tibiofibular ligament (AITFL) and posterior-inferior tibiofibular ligament (PITFL) all insert and form the complex known as the syndesmotic ligament complex. The lateral malleolus slopes outward distally and extends approximately 1 cm more distal than the medial malleolus. As the ankle is brought into dorsiflexion, the fibula externally rotates and migrates proximally to accommodate the talus in the intercrural space.

Talus

The talus is composed of three parts: the body, neck, and head. The talus is intercalated between the tibia and fibula to form the tibiotalar joint. It has several unique properties. Sixty percent to 70% of the talus is covered by cartilage. At any one time, it is only two thirds covered by the tibial plafond, the rest is left uncovered. It is anchored within the foot and ankle by strong ligamentous attachments both subtalar and intermalleolar. With the exception of the extensor digitorum brevis, there are no muscular attachments to the talus. Because there are very few soft-tissue attachments and its blood supply is tenuous, the talus is quite susceptible to devascularization, nonunion of fractures, and avascular necrosis. The talus is wider anteriorly than posteriorly. This unique shape confers stability to the ankle joint in dorsiflexion.

Ligamentous Anatomy

Ligamentous support of the ankle is provided primarily by the medial deltoid ligament, the lateral ankle ligaments, and secondarily by the syndesmotic ligament complex (Fig. 32-1).

Lateral Ankle Ligament Complex

This complex consists of three primary ligaments, the anterior talofibular ligament (ATFL), the calcaneofibular ligament (CFL), and the posterior talofibular ligament (PTFL). Each of these ligaments are under varied tension throughout ankle range of motion, making the lateral tibiotalar articulation flexible in comparison with the rigid medial aspect.

The ATFL is composed of two bands, which are confluent with the anterior joint capsule. It originates on the anterior lateral malleolus and inserts onto the anterior articular facet of the talus at the junction of the talar neck and head. Normally, the ligament is 2 mm thick, 6 to 8 mm wide, and 15 to 20 mm long. Its function is to provide stability to the ankle when it is plantarflexed and inverted. In a neutral ankle position, the ATFL also serves to limit internal rotation and anterior translation of the talus. The ATFL is the weakest of the three ligaments and is the most commonly injured ligament in a lateral ankle sprain.

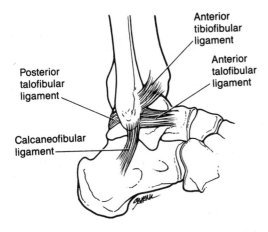

Figure 32-1   Lateral collateral ligaments of the ankle and the anterior syndesmotic ligament. (From Bucholz RW, Heckman JD. Rockwood & Green's Fractures in Adults, 5th ed. Philadelphia: Lippincott Williams & Wilkins, 2001.)

The CFL originates just distal and posterior to the ATFL on the lateral malleolus. It courses posteriorly to insert on the posterior-superior peroneal tubercle of the calcaneus. Because it also crosses the subtalar joint, the CFL plays a role in stabilizing this joint as well. Like the ATFL, the CFL is contiguous with the ankle capsule, but the CFL often can be seen as a distinct band. It is usually 3 to 5 mm thick, 4 to 8 mm wide, and 2 to 3 cm long. Generally, it forms an angle of 105 degrees with the ATFL. Due to its position in the ankle, the CFL is taut in neutral and becomes tighter as the ankle is dorsiflexed. This makes the CFL more susceptible to injury with dorsiflexion and inversion of the ankle.

The PTFL essentially is a thickening of the posterior ankle capsule, which has its origin on the posterior-medial surface of the lateral malleolus. It courses horizontally and broadly inserts onto the posterior talus. The PTFL is the stoutest portion of the lateral ligament complex. Thus, injury to the PTFL is very rare. Its primary role is to limit the end point of dorsiflexion. However, when the ATFL has been disrupted, the PTFL may serve a more important function in limiting internal rotation of the talus.

Medial Deltoid Ligament

There are two portions of the deltoid ligament: the thin superficial layer and the thick deep layer. The superficial layer originates on the anterior colliculus and has multiple insertion sites, including the sustentaculum tali and the spring ligament. The deep layer is a synovium-covered, intra-articular structure. It originates on the posterior colliculus and intercollicular groove and inserts on the nonarticular area of the talus medially. Like the lateral ligaments, the deep deltoid is confluent with the ankle capsule. The deep deltoid ligament is the primary medial stabilizer of the ankle. However, both superficial and deep deltoid ligaments act to limit eversion of the ankle. If the lateral ligaments are disrupted, the deep layer in particular will act as a secondary stabilizer to anterior and lateral migration of the talus. In general, injury to the deltoid requires significant force.

Syndesmotic Ligament Complex

The interosseous ligament, the AITFL, the PITFL, and the transverse tibiofibular ligament form the syndesmotic ligament complex.

Of these structures, the most commonly injured ligament is the AITFL. It courses from the anterolateral tubercle of the tibia to the distal fibular shaft at a 45-degree angle. The PITFL is composed of superficial and deep layers that course obliquely from the posterolateral tubercle of the tibia to the posterior aspect of the fibula. Its primary function is to deepen the ankle joint. The interosseous ligament is the primary connection between the tibia and fibula. It is a thickening of the interosseus membrane and usually runs transversely approximately 1 to 2 cm above the tibial plafond. Superiorly, it becomes confluent with the interosseous membrane. The syndesmotic complex, along with the deep deltoid ligament, is largely responsible for the structural integrity of the ankle. The syndesmotic complex acts to maintain the tibiofibular relationship throughout the arc of ankle motion. It does not confer a great deal of stability to the ankle when it is uninjured. However, when the lateral ligaments are torn, the syndesmotic ligaments do help to prevent excessive external rotation of the fibula when the ankle is dorsiflexed.

Muscular Anatomy

Peroneus Longus and Brevis

The peroneus brevis and longus muscles are the primary dynamic stabilizers of the ankle. Their role is to provide eversion strength to the ankle to prevent inversion injury. They are also directly involved in the proprioception reflex essential to ankle stability. The origin of the tendons is on the lateral fibula. From here, they course posterior to the fibula and wrap around the lateral malleolus in the fibular (or peroneal) groove. Here, the tendons are held in place by the superior peroneal retinaculum, which helps to prevent subluxation of the tendons, especially in plantarflexion. After coursing through the groove, the peroneus brevis inserts onto the base of the fifth metatarsal. In contrast, the peroneus longus travels plantar toward the medial foot to insert onto the base of the first metatarsal and medial cuneiform. The deep peroneal nerve innervates these muscles. Their role in pathology and etiology of chronic ankle instability will be discussed in a later section.

Posteriorly, the Achilles tendon crosses the ankle joint to insert on the calcaneal tuberosity. The sural nerve runs lateral to this tendon, and the plantaris tendon runs along its medial aspect. Posteromedially, the tibialis posterior, flexor digitorum longus, posterior tibial artery and vein, tibial nerve, and the flexor hallucis longus pass behind the medial malleolus as they course to the foot. The saphenous vein and nerve lie anterior to the medial malleolus. The anterior tibial tendon, anterior tibial artery, deep peroneal nerve, extensor hallucis longus, extensor digitorum longus, and superficial peroneal nerve pass across the anterior aspect of the ankle.

Tibiotalar Articulation

This articulation is exceptional in many ways. First of all, the bimalleolar construct is rigid medially but mobile laterally. As the ankle is placed in dorsiflexion, the distal fibula externally rotates and migrates superiorly to allow the wider anterior portion of the talus to also externally rotate and "lock" into position. Therefore, when the ankle is dorsiflexed, it is more stable than in plantarflexion; hence, the increased incidence of ligamentous injuries to the ankle in a position of plantar flexion. When the ankle is dorsiflexed, there are increased contact stresses placed both on the medial and lateral tibial plafonds. When a vertical force is applied to the ankle in this position, a fracture of the plafond or talus is more likely than a ligamentous injury. Furthermore, contact stresses of the ankle are dramatically altered by as little as 1 mm of lateral talar shift.

BIOMECHANICS

In most ankles, motion consists of simple rotation around an axis formed by the medial and lateral malleoli. This axis is somewhat oblique and, as a result, talar motion is analogous to a portion of a cone. The mortise and talus are nar-

rower posteriorly, allowing congruence throughout a range of motion. Average ankle extremes of motion are 30 degrees of dorsiflexion and 45 degrees of plantarflexion. Ten degrees of dorsiflexion are all that is required for activities of daily living, but full dorsiflexion is needed for many sporting activities. The obliquity of the ankle's axis of rotation results in a greater radius of curvature on the lateral side during ankle range of motion and causes internal rotation of the foot with plantar flexion and external rotation with dorsiflexion.

CHRONIC ANKLE PAIN

There are myriad causes for chronic ankle pain, creating a challenge to the orthopaedic surgeon. A thorough history and physical are essential in differentiating the etiology of ankle pain.

To properly assess all patients with ankle pain, certain clues from the history must be gleaned. These include preceding traumatic events (past or present), location of pain, pain exacerbators, comorbid systemic diseases (i.e., gout, rheumatoid arthritis, osteoarthritis, or diabetes,) timing of pain (morning vs. nighttime), and previous surgery.

A thorough examination of the foot and ankle is essential to diagnosis of chronic ankle pain. Typically, the examination should start with gross inspection for edema, alignment, and ecchymosis. Foot position with weight-bearing and gait should also be analyzed. This will help to delineate underlying pathology. Neurovascular examination can help to discern if the underlying pain is secondary to claudication, vascular insufficiency, or undiagnosed peripheral neuropathy. Last, both active and passive range of motion, as well as ligamentous and strength testing, should be performed.

INSTABILITY

As noted previously, ankle sprains are among the most common sports injury. It has been estimated that 27,000 ankle sprains occur in the United States each day. Of these, approximately 20% to 40% will have persistent pain or a sense of instability. Patients participating in certain "cutting" sports (i.e., soccer and basketball) are at an even higher risk of recurrent injury or persistent instability.

The cause of ankle instability is multifactorial. Contributing factors include peroneal weakness/atrophy, ligamentous laxity, loss of proprioception, adhesion formation/stiffness, and inflammation.

Instability can be classified as mechanical or functional instability or both. Eventually, all patients with symptomatic instability will likely have both mechanical and functional instabilities. Functional instability is defined as a subjective feeling of giving way with frequent ankle sprains and a feeling of inability to control ankle motion. However, physical examination may reveal no objective increase in range of motion. This is in contrast to mechanical instability, which by definition means ankle range of motion is beyond the normal physiologic range. Excessive range of motion has been described by the following criteria: (1) anterior translation with anterior drawer testing of greater than 1 cm or 3 mm more than the unaffected side, and (2) greater than 5 to 10 degrees of lateral talar tilt or a 3-degree difference from the unaffected side. Although these figures serve as a general reference, measurements are quite subjective. Therefore, they should not be used as an absolute guide for treatment. Rather, treatment is based on clinical assessment and, to a lesser extent, imaging studies.

Diagnosis

History and Physical Examination

- Patients with chronic ankle instability often report a history of multiple sprains, vague lateral ankle pain (with or without medial pain), a sense of giving way with activity (especially on uneven surfaces), and intermittent swelling.
- They usually have asymptomatic intervals where they are able to participate in normal activities.
- Physical examination may be nonspecific and may not demonstrate gross instability of the ankle.
- Range-of-motion and provocative testing, such as anterior drawer testing and strength testing, should be performed.
- The anterior drawer test assesses ATFL competence.
    - It is performed with the ankle in slight plantar flexion with the patient in a sitting position to relax the calf muscles.
    - While stabilizing the leg with one hand, an anterolateral force is applied to the heel with the other.
- Talar tilt, another provocative test, primarily tests ATFL and CFL competence (Fig. 32-2).
    - It is performed with the ankle in plantar flexion, and an inversion force is applied to the middle and hind foot.
    - In thin patients and those with dramatic tilt, a sulcus may be palpated on the anterolateral aspect of the ankle.
    - This test is especially difficult to interpret, however.

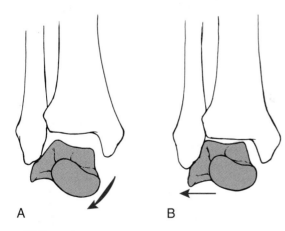

Figure 32-2 Stability of the ankle joint is assessed by examining talar tilt **(A)**, which is the medial or lateral rotation of the talus about an AP axis, and talar shift **(B)**, which is the translation of the talus in a medial or lateral direction. (From Oatis CA. Kinesiology: The Mechanics and Pathomechanics of Human Movement. Baltimore: Lippincott Williams & Wilkins, 2004.)

Radiologic Examination

- Radiographic evaluation begins with standard anteroposterior (AP), mortise, and lateral views to rule out fracture, posttraumatic changes, and osteochondral lesions.
- Weight-bearing views/stress views may aid in the diagnosis of instability as well.
- To assess instability more accurately, the contralateral ankle should also be x-rayed for comparison.
- Anterior translation produced by an anterior drawer may be seen on a lateral x-ray, and talar tilt may be seen on a mortise view.
- Stress x-rays are often difficult to obtain due to pain and guarding, as well as inadequate x-ray technique. Therefore, they are of limited value in the treatment algorithm.
- Magnetic resonance imaging (MRI) studies may also be used in the evaluation of instability, since ligamentous structures are well seen on MRI.
    - The primary use of MRI is to rule out other potential causes of pain and instability, such as occult fracture, osteochondral lesions, masses, or tendon injuries.

Treatment

Nonsurgical Treatment

- Treatment of all ankle instability should begin conservatively with the use of physical therapy and semirigid ankle orthoses.
    - Although some studies have shown a benefit to bracing athletes, their true benefit is still debated.
    - In general, studies have shown that the use of semirigid ankle braces, or taping to a lesser extent, will help to prevent primary and recurrent ankle sprains.
- Physical therapy is essential in treating ankle sprain both in acute and chronic settings.
- The goals of therapy are to improve dynamic stabilization to the ankle by strengthening the peroneal muscles, to restore proprioception (neuromuscular control), and to improve range of motion to the ankle.
- Proprioception training is done on balance boards or ankle disc exercisers.
    - Although balance board training has not been shown to prevent initial ankle sprains, one recent prospective study in volleyball players showed a possible benefit to balance board therapy in preventing reinjury of the ankle.
    - The theory behind proprioceptive training is that there is a prolonged reaction time in the peroneal muscles after injury (i.e., decreased proprioception and weakness). If the muscles are "retrained" and strengthened, then patients may not feel a sense of giving way. In other words, proprioception training restores functional stability.
    - To be successful, functional training should be combined with strengthening and agility training.

Surgical Treatment

- If a 10-week course of physical therapy fails to alleviate symptoms, or restore mechanical and functional stability, surgery should be considered.

- Surgical options are numerous and are often classified based on anatomic or nonanatomic reconstruction.
  - Anatomic reconstruction includes Brostrom repair, the Gould modification, and local tissue augmentation techniques.
  - Nonanatomic reconstruction includes the use of peroneus brevis or other autogenous tendon grafts for the Watson Jones, Chrisman-Snook, and Evans procedures.
- Whereas most patients (80% to 90%) will do well with direct anatomic repair, there are some predictors of poor outcome.
  - These include patients with hindfoot varus malalignment, excessive ligamentous laxity elsewhere, associated ankle arthritis, and high-performance athletes or obese patients.
  - This particular group should be considered for a nonanatomic reconstruction.
  - These procedures also have very good results but they may limit dorsiflexion and inversion since the normal biomechanics are not necessarily restored.

Postoperative Management
- Regardless of the technique used, patients should be splinted for 1 week postoperatively and thereafter placed in a short leg–walking cast or boot.
- After a total of 2 to 3 weeks of immobilization, progressive plantar flexion is allowed.
- Range of motion with supervised physical therapy is increased over a 6-week course, followed by progressive proprioceptive training and strengthening.
- Full activity may be resumed after 3 to 6 months.

ANKLE IMPINGEMENT

Anterolateral Impingement

Ankle impingement is the result of posttraumatic synovitis with associated synovial thickening.

Wolin et al. were the first to describe the development of a "meniscoid" mass between the fibula and the talus. It was felt that this mass was hyalinized connective tissue from the talofibular joint capsule or ATFL. In addition, the ATFL may become interposed between the lateral malleolus and the lateral aspect of the talus. This was described as the "lateral gutter syndrome." Later workers questioned the hyalinization theory. Current thinking has led to the concept of chronic synovitis and scar tissue leading to impingement. An inversion sprain results in torn ligaments that do not heal completely. Repetitive motion leads to inflammation of the ligament ends, causing synovitis and scar tissue development. These conditions ultimately cause joint impingement and manifests clinically as chronic ankle pain. The three major sites are the superior border of the ATFL, the distal portion of the ATFL, and the lateral talar dome.

Diagnosis
History and Physical Examination
- Patients usually have a history of chronic ankle sprains.
- They will complain of pain along the anterolateral aspect of the ankle, especially with ankle dorsiflexion.
- Pain is usually absent at rest and present with most activities particularly sports.
- There may also be symptoms of instability.
- Pain may also be present along the medial and posterior areas of the ankle.
- On physical examination, tenderness is elicited at the anterolateral corner of the talar dome and the lateral gutter.
  - Care should be taken to differentiate this from sinus tarsi pain.
- Relief of pain with an injection of local anesthetic at the point of tenderness supports the diagnosis of ankle impingement.

Radiologic Examination
- Plain radiographs show mild spurs, calcification, and joint space narrowing in 50%.
- Stress radiographs are usually normal.
- MRI may be helpful as a diagnostic aid demonstrating thickening of the anterior joint capsule.

Treatment
- Conservative treatment may be considered initially, including nonsteroidal anti-inflammatory drugs (NSAIDs), rest, steroid injections, physical therapy, and braces/orthotics.
- An indication for operative intervention is persistent pain for 3 to 6 months, which is unresponsive to conservative treatment.
- Before surgery, it is important to rule out other causes of chronic lateral ankle pain.
- Ankle arthroscopy can be diagnostic as well as therapeutic.
  - Through standard arthroscopic portals and resection of synovitis, scar, fibrosis, and loose bodies can be performed.
  - Meniscoid tissue may also be debrided but care should taken not to excise normal ligamentous tissue.
- Postoperatively, the patient is kept non-weight-bearing in a posterior splint for 5 to 7 days.
  - Weight-bearing may begin in a removable brace following this.
  - Physical therapy is started 2 to 3 weeks after surgery.
    - Therapy started too early runs the risk of recurrence of the patient's symptoms.
  - The patient may return to full activity in 1 to 2 months.

Results

Liu et al. (1994) treated 55 patients for anterolateral ankle impingement. Good to excellent results were noted in 87%, with 98% patient satisfaction. Eighty-four percent returned to their previous sports. Meislin et al. (1993) reported on a series of 29 patients treated arthroscopically for synovial impingement of the ankle. Follow-up was 25 months. Twenty-six of the 29 patients had good-to-excellent results. Similar results were also reported by Martin et al. (1989).

Posterior Impingement

Posterior impingement is less common than anterior impingement. The mechanism of injury is plantar flexion. An external rotation injury may also cause this problem.

Diagnosis

- Symptoms include pain and tenderness along the posterior and posterolateral aspects of the ankle and hindfoot.
- Pain may also localize to the region anterior to the retrocalcaneal bursa.
- The pain is made worse by going down stairs and by going into a plantar flexed position.
- Occasionally, mechanical symptoms such as locking may be present.
- Physical examination confirms pain at the posterolateral aspect of the ankle, as well as anterior to the retrocalcaneal bursa.
- Pain is exacerbated more by plantar flexion rather than dorsiflexion.
- Radiographs may demonstrate ossicle or evidence of avulsion injuries.
- MRI can aid in diagnosis.

Treatment

- Initial conservative treatment is similar to that of anterior impingement.
- Surgery is indicated is the patient is still symptomatic after 3 to 6 months of conservative management.
- Arthroscopic debridement of synovitis and scarring along the posterior ligaments may be conducted through the standard anterior portals.
- On occasion, the posterolateral portal may be needed.
- Postoperative care is similar to that of anterior impingement.

Results

Reports of clinical results are limited, with only isolated cases being described. Lohrer and Arentz (2004) described a case of posterolateral impingement in a top-level field hockey player. After arthroscopic resection and rehabilitation, the player returned to full activity within 2 months.

Syndesmotic Impingement

Soft-tissue impingement after injury to the syndesmosis is uncommon but may be underdiagnosed. External rotation of the foot and ankle is the chief mechanism of injury. Hyperdorsiflexion may also cause this injury.

Diagnosis

- Patients may note pain along the AITFL or anterior syndesmotic ligament.
- Symptoms may sometimes be present along the PITFL.
- In addition, activities that create an external rotational stress on the ankle, such as cutting or pivoting, may induce pain.
- On physical examination, tenderness will be localized over the AITFL with less pain noted over the ATFL or the anterolateral gutter.
- The squeeze and external rotation tests may also be positive.
- Plain radiographs, including stress views, may show evidence of previous injury but are usually nondiagnostic.
- MRI can help define the extent of the syndesmotic injury.

Treatment

- Conservative management is similar to other types of ankle impingement.
- Surgery is indicated if pain persists even after 3 to 6 months of nonsurgical treatment.
- Treatment includes debridement of inflamed synovial tissue and scar along the AITFL, the tibiofibular joint, the interosseus membrane, the PITFL, and the lateral gutter.
- Care should also taken to evaluate the synovial recess behind the AITFL.
- Management after surgery is similar to other types of impingement.
- Published results are limited but appear to be similar to outcomes for anterolateral impingement.

Bony Impingement

Bony impingement of the ankle involves osteophytes along the anterior aspect of the tibia and talus that become entrapped during ankle dorsiflexion. This condition is sometimes called "footballer's ankle" or "soccer player's ankle." The mechanism of injury is thought to be due to changes resulting from traction on the joint capsule as the foot is repeatedly forced into extreme plantar flexion. Repetitive capsular strain leads to calcific deposits developing along capsular lines. Osteophytes may also form as a result of degenerative joint disease or previous trauma. Repetitive dorsiflexion causes subchondral injury and resultant new bone formation. These lesions most commonly form at the anterior lip of the tibia and the anterior neck of the talus.

Soccer players and dancers are the most common athletes to develop this condition. However, osteophytes may develop after athletic trauma to the ankle in any sport. Bony impingement typically develops over a prolonged period of 10 years or more and has a high incidence in dancers and football players.

A classification system for bony impingement is shown in Table 32-1.

Diagnosis

History and Physical Examination

- Patients usually note pain, especially after activity, as the first symptom.
  - It usually starts initially as a vague discomfort, often brought on by ankle dorsiflexion.

TABLE 32-1 CLASSIFICATION OF BONY IMPINGEMENT

Grade	Description
1	Synovial impingement
2	Osteochondral reaction exostosis
3	Severe exostosis with or without fragmentation
4	Pantalocrural osteoarthritic destruction

(Adapted from Scranton PE, McDermott JE. Anterior tibial spurs: a comparison of open versus arthroscopic debridement. Foot Ankle 1992;13:125–129.)

- As the condition progresses, the pain tends to become sharper and more localized over the anterior aspect of the ankle.
    - Tenderness over the anterior ankle and joint swelling also develops.
- Other complaints include catching, locking, and decreased range of motion, which may be demonstrable on examination.
- Physical examination confirms pain and tenderness along the anterior ankle especially over the central aspect of the tibia.
- Tenderness can sometimes be noted medially, laterally, or posteriorly.

Radiologic Examination

- Plain radiographs demonstrate the osteophytes quite easily, especially on the lateral view (Fig. 32-3).
- Weight-bearing stress views in maximal dorsiflexion may also show the impingement.
- Bone scans can help differentiate symptomatic impingement from a fracture or nonunion.
- Computed tomography (CT) scanning, especially with sagittal reconstructions, is the most useful imaging modality for demonstrating the size, extent, and location of the lesions.
    - CT analysis has shown that the spurs often do not overlap.
    - The talar spur tends to be medial, and the tibial spur is usually lateral to the joint midline.
    - The tibial spur also tends to be wider than the talar spur.
    - The talar spur may extend medially off the edge of the talar neck.

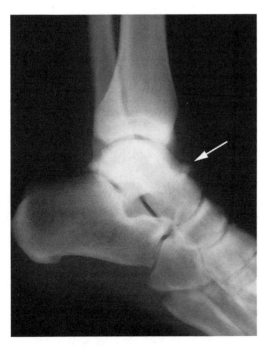

Figure 32-3 Impingement exostoses of the tibial plafond and talus. (From Koval KJ, Zuckerman JD. Atlas of Orthopaedic Surgery: A Multimedia Reference. Philadelphia: Lippincott Williams & Wilkins, 2004.)

- Tibial spurs secondary to impingement are usually localized anteriorly, whereas spurs due to degenerative joint disease tend to be more widespread.
- MRI and arthrograms are not considered as helpful.

Treatment

- Conservative treatment consists of heel lifts, rest, activity modification, and physical therapy.
- Indications for surgery include persistent pain, loss of motion, and mechanical symptoms.
- Arthroscopic removal of impinging osteophytes may be accomplished using both anterior and posterior portals.
    - A variety of instruments may be used including burrs, rongeurs, osteotomes, elevators, and graspers.
    - Partial synovectomy may be needed is a significant amount of synovitis is encountered.
    - An intraoperative lateral ankle radiograph may help assess the adequacy of osteophyte resection.
- Postoperatively, the patient is placed in a posterior splint for 5 to 7 days.
- Range of motion is encouraged after splint removal.
- Physical therapy may be started 1 to 2 weeks postoperatively.
- Most patients are able to return to regular activity in 2 to 3 months.

Results.   Ogilvie-Harris et al. (1993) treated a series of 17 patients with good results. There were significant improvements in pain, swelling, stiffness, limping, and activity level. Dorsiflexion improved more than plantar flexion. Scranton and McDermott (1992) also describe good results with surgical treatment. Ogilvie-Harris et al. (1995) also treated 27 patients, most of whom had ankle osteoarthritis also with good results. Seventeen patients showed significant improvements in pain, swelling, stiffness, and activity level.

Os Trigonum Syndrome

Os trigonum syndrome can be a cause of posterior ankle pain. The os trigonum is a secondary ossification center of the talus. It lies lateral to the groove for the flexor hallucis longus (FHL) tendon (Fig. 32-4). A cartilage connection may or may not attach the os trigonum to the talus. The os trigonum has been reported to be present in 1.7% to 7% of normal, asymptomatic feet.

Os trigonum syndrome is usually seen in ballerinas and athletic individuals. The mechanism of injury is forced plantar flexion with resultant impingement of the os trigonum against the posterior aspect of the tibial plafond. FHL tendinitis may also coexist.

Diagnosis

History and Physical Examination

- The diagnosis of os trigonum syndrome is based on history, physical examination, and image findings.
- Patients usually present with a gradual onset of pain, especially in the anterior aspect of the retrocalcaneal space.
- Pain is recreated by forced plantar flexion of the ankle.
- On physical examination, pain may be elicited by direct pressure over the posterior lip of the talus.

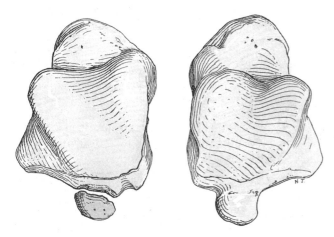

Figure 32-4 The lateral (posterior) tubercle of the talus has a separate center of ossification, which appears from ages 7 to 13 years. When this fails to fuse with the body of the talus, as in the left bone of this pair, it is called os trigonum. (From Grant's Atlas of Anatomy. Baltimore: Lippincott Williams & Wilkins, 2002.)

Radiologic Examination

- The os trigonum may be visible on plain radiographs.
- Stress views with the ankle in plantar flexion can demonstrate the posterior impingement.
- Three-phase bone scanning may show increased tracer activity in the case of a symptomatic nonunion.
  - However, not all os trigonum with positive bone scans are symptomatic.
- CT scanning can provide more detailed visualization, especially of a fibrous union or nonunion.
- MRI imaging may demonstrate edema within the os trigonum fragment, as well as fluid around it.

Treatment

- Nonoperative treatment consists of NSAIDs, activity modification, and sometimes immobilization.
- Surgical treatment may be indicated if nonsurgical management fails.
- Excision can be performed arthroscopically.
  - The os trigonum is visualized through the anterolateral portal, and instrumentation is usually performed through the posterolateral portal.
  - Excision is performed using arthroscopic banana knives, curettes, and graspers.
  - Care should be taken to avoid injury to the FHL tendon and the posteromedial neurovascular structures.
- Surgical treatment is usually successful.

PERONEAL TENDON INJURIES

The peroneal tendons pass posterior to the fibula and are restrained by the superior peroneal retinaculum. The pero-

neus longus and brevis muscles originate in the lateral compartment from the intermuscular septum and the lower two thirds of the fibula. The peroneus brevis tendon lies closest to the bone in the peroneal groove of the posterior fibula. The peroneus brevis inserts on the styloid process of the fifth metatarsal. It is the strongest abductor and evertor of the foot and is a secondary flexor of the ankle. The peroneus longus tendon passes posterior to the fibula deep to the peroneus brevis. It then passes below the trochlear process of the calcaneus and then turns beneath the cuboid in the cubital sulcus. The peroneus longus then inserts into the base of the first metatarsal and the cuneiforms. It acts as a depressor of the first metatarsal head. In addition, it acts as a pronator and abductor of the foot and plantarflexor of the ankle.

TENDINITIS

Acute tendinitis is commonly due to overuse. Tendinitis of the peroneus brevis presents with swelling and tenderness along the course of the sheath. Inflammation of the peroneus longus tendon presents with pain over the lateral calcaneus, especially when rising onto the ball of the foot when running, cutting, or turning. Tenderness may be elicited over the tendon as it passes from the trochlea lateralis under the cuboid.

Chronic tendinitis develops over a course of weeks to months and may be associated with tears of the tendon. MRI may be helpful in confirming the diagnosis.

Treatment

- Treatment consists of rest, ice treatment, and NSAIDs. Severe cases may require a period of immobilization in a cast or boot.
- Orthotics such as a lateral heel wedge can help symptoms by limiting tendon excursion.
- Physical therapy emphasizing peroneal strengthening and flexibility is usually helpful.
- Taping, bracing, and proper warmup is also recommended.
- Surgical intervention is indicated for refractory cases.
- Procedures include tenosynovectomy, repair of longitudinal tendon tears, and treatment of related conditions such as instability and arthritis.

TEARS

Peroneal tendon tears may be acute or chronic in nature, with the latter being more common.

ACUTE TEARS

The peroneus brevis tendon is prone to tearing as a result of its position between the peroneus longus and fibula, which represents an area of relative hypovascularity. The tear is usually 2 to 5 cm in length along the deep side of the tendon. It usually begins at or just distal to the lateral malleolus and may extend proximally. Tears tend to be longitudinal and are referred to as "split tears."

The etiology includes overuse and direct trauma. These causes may be compounded by the presence of other conditions, such as degenerative joint disease, ankle instability, and fractures of the fibula or calcaneus.

Diagnosis

History and Physical Examination
- Patients will report an insidious onset of lateral ankle pain.
- Physical findings include tenderness along the course of the tendon, pain that appears out of proportion for the degree of ankle instability if present, and sometimes a varus deformity.

Radiologic Examination
- Plain radiographs are used to evaluate bony alignment and to rule out osseus pathology.
- MRI is useful in diagnosis of the tendon tear.
  - Findings include disruption of the tendon and fluid within the tendon sheath.

Treatment
- Treatment depends on the severity of the symptoms.
  - Mild cases may respond to NSAIDs, stretching, physical therapy, ankle bracing, and shoe modification, such as a lateral heel wedge or outflare.
  - More severe symptoms, as well as those cases unresponsive to conservative treatment, may require surgery.
- Surgical treatment options include tenosynovectomy, debridement, repair of longitudinal tears, and tubularization of the remaining tendon segment.
- Correction of associated conditions is also undertaken.
- Acute ruptures that are complete need surgical repair.
- Tendon grafting may be needed.
- Postoperatively, tear repairs not requiring tendon graft are immobilized for 2 weeks, followed by a walker boot allowing increased range of motion.
- An Aircast is used at 6 weeks postoperatively. A fitted ankle brace is then used during athletic activity.

Chronic Tears

Chronic tears of the peroneus longus tendon tend to be longitudinal in configuration.

Diagnosis
- Symptoms such as pain and tenderness are present over the course of the tendon and the os perineum.
- Imaging evaluation is similar to that of acute tears.

Treatment
- Incomplete tears may be treated nonoperatively, including immobilization for 2 weeks, NSAIDs, physical therapy, Aircast, and lace-up brace.
  - A more rigid orthosis may be helpful because it helps limit pronation.
- Complete tears and those refractory to conservative care usually require surgery.
- Surgical treatment includes tenosynovectomy, debridement of all degenerative tissue, tendon repair, and correction of other associated conditions.

- In chronic cases, the tendon may be retracted and will require mobilization and advancement.
- Tendon graft may be necessary to bridge or augment the defect.
- If the tendon cannot be advanced or reconstructed satisfactorily, then resection of the torn or scarred tendon segments or fractured os peroneum is indicated.
- After resection, tenodesis of the proximal and distal ends to the lateral calcaneus or to the peroneus brevis tendon may be necessary.

Rupture

Acute ruptures of the peroneus longus tendon usually occur as a result of avulsion fractures through the os peroneum.

Diagnosis
- Symptoms may precede the actual injury by several weeks.
- Physical examination may demonstrate loss of active foot eversion and a varus alignment.
- Plain radiographs may show proximal migration of the bony os, which is attached to the proximal tendon stump.
- MRI may show the intratendinous disruption, as well as other associated conditions, such as an associated peroneus brevis tear.

Treatment
- Patients with minimal symptoms or functional deficit may be treated conservatively.
- More severe cases require direct repair with possible graft augmentation.
- Postoperatively, patients are kept non-weight-bearing in a short leg cast for 3 weeks.
- This is followed by a walker for increased range of motion.
- Strengthening and physical therapy are commenced at 6 weeks after surgery.

Subluxation/Dislocation

Peroneal tendon subluxation/dislocation involves anterior displacement of the tendons with respect to the fibula. In the case of subluxation, the tendons never pass completely in front of the fibula. It is a rare injury and can be an occult event; thus it is often overlooked. The cause is generally traumatic, with disruption of the superior peroneal retinaculum. The mechanism of injury is a sudden, forceful contraction of the peroneal muscles with associated rapid plantar flexion and inversion of the foot and ankle. Ninety-seven percent of cases occur during athletic activity. Seventy-one percent are associated with snow skiing, and 7% occur with football. Other sports in which dislocation may occur include soccer, ice skating, and basketball. Anatomic variation, especially a shallow peroneal groove, may contribute to this condition. In an anatomic study, the configuration of the groove was described as convex (7%), flat (11%), and concave (82%). Factors that increase the lateral pull on the tendons also increase the risk of tendon dislocation and include pes planus, hindfoot valgus, lax superficial peroneal retinaculum, and recurrent ankle sprains.

TABLE 32-2 CLASSIFICATION OF ACUTE PERONEAL TENDON DISLOCATIONS

Grade	Description
I	Retinaculum stripped away from the lateral fibula
II	Cartilaginous ridge avulsion of the lateral fibula
III	Bony avulsion of the posterolateral fibula

(Adapted from Eckert WR, Davis EA Jr. Acute rupture of the peroneal retinaculum. J Bone Joint Surg Am 1976;58:670–672.)

A classification system for acute peroneal tendon dislocations is given in Table 32-2.

Diagnosis

History and Physical Examination
- Patients may complain of pain in the retromalleolar area of the ankle, a snapping sensation, or a feeling of instability.
- Physical examination may reveal pain and swelling along the posterior aspect of the distal fibula.
- There may also be pain with resisted foot/ankle dorsiflexion and eversion.
- The dislocated tendons may be palpable, although this may be difficult in the presence of acute swelling.
- Active eversion may demonstrate actual tendon subluxation or dislocation.
- Differential diagnosis includes an ankle sprain, but the pain and swelling is typically along the anterior aspect of the fibula.

Radiologic Examination
- Plain radiographs are taken to rule out other injuries and pathology.
- The presence of a "rim fracture," which is a fleck of bone off the lateral malleolus, is diagnostic of disruption of the superior peroneal retinaculum, thus raising the concern for possible tendon dislocation.
- MRI examination can be helpful but is not considered a routine part of the evaluation.

Treatment

Nonsurgical Treatment
- Patients with asymptomatic subluxation do not require treatment.
- Conservative management would consist of a non-weight-bearing cast with the ankle in slight plantar flexion and eversion for 6 to 8 weeks.
- This is followed by aggressive physical therapy.

Surgical Treatment
- Surgical treatment is indicated for those in which the subluxation/dislocation is symptomatic or adversely affects performance, as well as for those who have failed conservative measures.
- General surgical treatment includes tenosynovectomy and debridement, repair of tendon tears, and reduction of the tendons to their anatomic positions.
- Bony procedures attempt to restore the retrofibular sulcus either by deepening the groove and by performing a bone block procedure.
- Soft tissue procedures are directed at repairing and/or reconstructing the superior peroneal retinaculum.
- The superior peroneal retinaculum may be reattached to the malleolar ridge, plicated if attenuated, or reinforced with a sling made from a strip of Achilles tendon.
- Other tissues that may be used to reinforce the retinaculum include periosteum, the peroneus brevis, the peroneus quartus, or the plantaris.
- The tendons may also be rerouted under the calcaneofibular ligament.
- Postoperatively, the foot/ankle is immobilized for 2 to 3 weeks with increased range of motion allowed in a boot.
- The patient is then started on a physical therapy program emphasizing strength and flexibility, followed by a gradual return to regular activities.

ACHILLES TENDON INJURIES

Injury to the Achilles tendon is the most common form of tendinosis in athletes. Overall incidence ranges from 6.5% to 18%. It represents 20% of all foot tendinoses and 11% of all running injuries.

The Achilles tendon is the thickest and strongest tendon in the body. It is formed by the confluence of the soleus and gastrocnemius muscles, approximately 15 cm proximal to the heel. The tendon inserts on the calcaneus distal to the posterior superior calcaneal tuberosity on the inferior portion.

The Achilles tendon is not surrounded by a synovial sheath but rather by a paratenon. The blood supply to the tendon is from muscular branches that run longitudinally along its length. Vessels from the surrounding paratenon, bone, and periosteum also supply the tendon. A relatively hypovascular zone is present 2 to 6 cm proximal to the tendon insertion.

TENDINITIS

Three categories of tendinitis are described. Peritendinitis is inflammation of the paratenon with fibrin adhesions between the paratendon and the tendon. There is no associated tendinosis. Peritendinitis with tendinosis consists of inflammation of both structures. The tendon is thicker and softer than normal. Tendinosis is degeneration of the tendon characterized by mucinoid degeneration, central necrosis, and lipomatous infiltration.

The pathophysiology is one of accumulated repetitive microtrauma. This results in paratenon inflammation that can also involve the tendon. Prolonged inflammation can result in fibrosis and scarring of the paratenon. This results in hypovascularity of the tendon due to restricted blood flow. This causes degenerative changes in the tendon. Histologically, the tendon shows a noninflammatory picture characterized by collagen fiber disorientation, scattered vascular ingrowth, and areas of necrosis and calcification.

The etiology of Achilles tendinosis is multifactorial. Training errors, especially in runners, can account for up to 75% of cases. The common denominator is muscle fatigue and glycogen depletion, resulting in excess stretching and microtears in the tendon. Common training errors include an increase in training mileage, resumption of training after an extended period of inactivity, a sudden increase in the intensity of training, repetitive heel running, repetitive hill running, running on uneven or slippery terrain, and use of athletic shoes with inadequate heel wedges. Anatomic factors resulting in extremity malalignment also may contribute to the problem. This includes excessive foot pronation, hindfoot varus, forefoot varus/cavus feet, talipes equines, and tibia vara. Tight heel cords and tight hamstrings may also play a role.

Diagnosis

History and Physical Examination

- Clinically, patients present with pain localized to the Achilles tendon region several centimeters proximal to the insertion.
- The pain is brought on by activity and relieved by rest.
- Diffuse, fusiform swelling, and thickening are noted on palpation.
- There may also be palpable crepitus.
- Chronic tendinitis may also have pain at rest as well.
- Tendinosis can be asymptomatic and is characterized by palpable thickening or nodularity in the tendon 4 to 6 cm proximal to the tendon insertion.
- Associated pain is usually secondary to peritendinitis.
- Acute tendinitis is defined as symptoms for less than 2 weeks.
- Subacute tendinitis has symptoms for 3 to 6 weeks and chronic tendinitis for more than 6 weeks.
- Differential considerations include retrocalcaneal bursitis and superficial tendo-Achilles bursitis ("pump bump").

Radiologic Examination

- Radiographs of the ankle may show calcification within the tendon or in the soft tissue around the tendon.
- MRI demonstrates increased signal intensity within the tendon.

Treatment

Nonsurgical Treatment

- Conservative treatment includes rest.
- With severe symptoms, treatment in a non-weight-bearing cast for 1 to 2 weeks may be indicated.
- Activity modification includes decreasing a runner's weekly mileage, as well as avoidance of hills, banked roads, and uneven surfaces.
- Flexible shoes with a molded Achilles pad, as well a 1/4 to 3/8 inch heel lift, may help.
- Night splints can also be used.
- Regular NSAID use is recommended.

- Physical therapy treatment includes ice massage, contrast baths, ultrasound, and a heel cord stretching program.
- Orthotics are used to correct any alignment problems.
- Nonsurgical therapy may be augmented by brisement, which is mechanical lysis of adhesions.
  - This procedure involves rapid injection of a local anesthetic (5 to 15 mL) into the subperitenon space.
- This is followed by aggressive range-of-motion exercises.
- Brisement has been proposed for the treatment of acute peritendinitis.
- Steroid injections should be avoided.

Surgical Treatment

- Indications for surgical treatment include failure of 6 months of conservative treatment and the presence of significant mucoid degenerative nodules.
- Open treatment of peritendinitis involves tenolysis through a medial incision.
  - Debridement and excision of degenerative paratenon tissue are performed.
  - This is performed along the medial, lateral, and posterior aspects of the paratenon.
  - The anterior aspect along with the associated fatty tissue are preserved, as this is a source of blood supply for the tendon.
- Treatment of tendinosis consists of making a longitudinal incision in the paratenon and examining the tendon.
  - If grossly normal, several longitudinal incisions are made in the tendon.
  - If the tendon is abnormal, the degenerative areas are excised and the defects closed.
  - Large defects may require extensive debridement.
  - These areas may be reinforced with a plantaris tendon, flexor digitorum communis tendon, or a turn-down flap.
  - Any tears are repaired primarily.
- Postoperatively, patients with debridement of small defects may be immobilized for 2 weeks.
- Patients with larger defects should be immobilized for 4 to 6 weeks.

Results

Results after operative treatment are generally good. Schepsis and Leach (1987) reported on the results of 45 patients with a good-to-excellent outcome in 89%. Release of the sheath was performed in 15 cases, excision of calcified areas in 4 patients, and debridement of partial tears and tendon repair in 9 cases.

RUPTURE

Partial Rupture

Partial ruptures of the Achilles tendon typically occurs in well-trained athletes and are usually secondary to trauma. They usually occur on the lateral side. Partial ruptures may be longitudinal, transverse, or combination. They are sometimes misdiagnosed as chronic Achilles tendinosis. MRI evaluation may help in confirming the diagnosis.

Treatment

- Small partial ruptures may be treated nonsurgically using heel lifts, ice, and rest.
- Surgical treatment is indicated if conservative treatment fails.
- Treatment options include primary repair and excision with reconstruction.
- Immediate repair is recommended for large partial tears.

Complete Rupture

Complete Achilles tendon ruptures usually occur in middle-aged, overweight males who are in poor athletic condition. They are commonly involved in intermittent recreational sports requiring sudden acceleration or jumping, such as basketball, tennis, snow skiing, and badminton. Sixty-two percent of ruptures occurred in professional or white collar workers with sedentary jobs. Males are more commonly involved than females, with a ratio of 2 to 12:1. Other risk factors include local and systemic steroid use, tendon hypovascularity, and chronic long-standing tendinosis.

The mechanism of injury is landing with the foot in a dorsiflexed position, resulting in a sudden sprain. Other mechanisms include pushing off with the knee extended or direct trauma to the tendon when the muscle is strongly contracted.

Diagnosis

- Patients classically describe hearing or feeling a "pop" in the Achilles region with minimal discomfort.
- Weakness with push-off is also noted. Pain and swelling may be noted later.
- Occasionally, the patient may be asymptomatic
- On physical examination, a defect in the tendon may be palpable, which may be more apparent with gentle dorsiflexion of the foot (Fig. 32-5).
- The Thompson test is performed with the patient prone and the knee flexed.

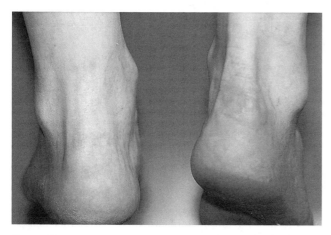

Figure 32-5 The patient's ruptured left Achilles tendon appears thickened and less distinct than the normal right side, and the patient is unable to plantarflex the left foot. (From Fleisher GR, Ludwig S, Baskin MN. Atlas of Pediatric Emergency Medicine. Philadelphia: Lippincott Williams & Wilkins, 2004.)

- A positive test is noted when squeezing the calf will not result in passive plantar flexion of the foot in the face of a complete tendon rupture.
- However, the plantaris may give a false-negative.
  - The patient will demonstrate an inability to do a single heel raise and absence of or weakness with resisted foot plantar flexion.
  - The patient may still be able to demonstrate some degree of active foot plantar flexion when not weight-bearing due to the posterior tibialis, the toe flexors, and the peroneal muscles.
- Other diagnostic tests include O'Brien's needle test and the Copeland test.

Treatment

- Treatment remains controversial.
- The advantage of nonsurgical treatment is avoidance of the complications associated with surgery.
  - The rerupture rate is higher at 10% to 30%.
  - In addition, there are problems with decreased strength, as well as ankle stiffness.
- Proponents of surgical repair point to a lower rerupture rate of 2% to 3%, as well as increased strength and tension.
  - The complication rate can be up to 8%.
  - Potential complications include wound infection, tissue necrosis, sural nerve injury, suture granulomas, stiffness, and pulmonary embolus.

Nonsurgical Treatment

- Nonsurgical treatment is currently reserved for patients who are elderly, extremely sedentary, or have comorbid medical conditions that represent a high risk for anesthesia and surgery.
- Patients who do not want surgery may also be treated conservatively.
- Treatment consists of casting initially with a long leg cast with the knee flexed and the ankle in equinus for 2 to 3 weeks.
- This is followed by treatment in a short leg cast for at least 8 weeks.
- The patient is kept non-weight-bearing for the first 6 weeks.

Surgical Treatment

- Primary repair is suitable in the acute setting with good return of strength, endurance, and power.
- Techniques include simple end-to-end repair, three-bundle suture, and suture weave.
- Percutaneous suture repair is a technique of primary repair while attempting to avoid the potential problems of open surgery.
- Repair with augmentation techniques include suture plus plantaris weave, suture plus gastroc fascia turndown flap, or the use of one or two rotated gastroc flaps.
- Reconstruction may use endogenous or exogenous material.
  - Endogenous tissue includes gastroc fascia/tendon, flexor digitorum longus, or the peroneus brevis.

- Exogenous materials used include carbon fiber, Martex mesh, and PLA.

INSERTIONAL TENDINITIS

Insertional Achilles tendinitis is an inflammatory condition of the pre-Achilles bursa resulting in posterior heel pain. It may be associated with a Haglund deformity, which is a prominence of the superior calcaneal tuberosity. Other names for this condition include pump bump, winter heel, knobby heels, calcaneus altus, high-brow heels, and cucumber heels.

The etiology is the use of a shoe with a rigid heel counter. The upper edge of the heel counter-contacts the heel, resulting in chronic pressure on the posterior heel. There is increased stress on the Achilles tendon and the associated bursa. The result is painful swelling overlying the insertion of the tendon, as well as thickened skin and callous formation. Pathologically, there is inflammation of the retrocalcaneal bursa with or without bony erosion. There may be calcific tendinitis as well. The Haglund deformity can also impinge on the insertion of the Achilles tendon and the retrocalcaneal bursa, thus contributing to the inflammatory process.

Diagnosis

- Radiographs may be normal or may demonstrate the prominent posterior superior calcaneal tuberosity.
- Methods to evaluate the size of the Haglund deformity include the parallel pitch lines and measuring of the posterior calcaneal angle.

Treatment

Nonsurgical Treatment

- Nonoperative treatment is recommended initially.
- This consists of shoe modifications, including a heel lift (internal or external), heel cup, a felt pad to decrease the pressure of the heel counter, and removal or softening of the heel counter.
- Activity modification, such as decreasing the amount of weekly mileage for runners, is helpful.
- NSAIDs and local steroid injections can aid in reducing the tissue inflammation.

Surgical Treatment

- Surgical management is indicated if conservative treatment is unsuccessful.
- Through a medial incision, the retrocalcaneal bursa and posterior superior calcaneal tuberosity are excised.
- Calcific deposits and areas of degeneration in the Achilles tendon are excised.
- Studies have shown that 50% of the tendon may be resected without risk of rupture of the remaining tendon.
  - If more than 50% is resected, tendon transfer, such as the FHL, is suggested to reinforce it.
- The Achilles tendon insertion may be elevated and reattached as necessary.
- Destabilization of the tendon should be avoided in high-performance athletes, however.

- Splint or cast immobilization is done for 3 weeks postoperatively.
- This is followed by use of a range-of-motion walker and physical therapy.

Results

Sammarco (1994) reported on the results of conservative and surgical treatment. The nonsurgical group had 13 patients with 17 heels. All patients had resolution of their symptoms with minimal or no residual problems. Five had excellent results, and 12 had good results. The surgical group consisted of 26 patients with 34 heels. All had failed conservative treatment. Good-to-excellent results were noted in 32 cases. Although most were nonathletes, all patients returned to work or former activities.

OSTEOCHONDRAL LESIONS

OSTEOCHONDRAL LESIONS OF THE TALUS

An osteochondral lesion of the talus (OLT) is the pathologic loss of the chondral or osteochondral surface of the talar dome. Historically, it has been referred to by a variety of terms, many of which evolved in an attempt to define the etiology of the lesion. Previous terminology included transchondral fracture, osteochondritis desiccans, osteochondral fracture, talar dome fracture, and flake fracture. Currently, the most accepted term is "osteochondral lesion of the talus."

Overall, OLT is a relatively uncommon condition. It constitutes approximately 4% of all osteochondral lesions and 0.9% of all talus fractures. The average age is 20 to 30 years old. The majority of patients are male. Medial dome lesions are more common than lateral ones. OLT occurs bilaterally in 10% of cases.

Etiology

The etiology is controversial. The primary competing theories are trauma and spontaneous osteonecrosis. These lesions have been proposed to be the result of a pathologic fracture occurring in bone that was necrotic secondary to ischemia. The fact that trauma is not documented in every case lends credence to this theory. In addition, multiple affected members have been noted in the same family. Bilaterality as described suggests a systemic mechanism. Finally, OLT has similar risk factors as other forms of osteonecrosis, such as alcohol abuse, steroids, emboli, and other hereditary and endocrine factors.

Trauma, however, remains the most common cause of OLT. Both gross macrotrauma and repetitive microtrauma can play a role. OLT lesions have been reported in 6.5% of patients who have suffered an ankle sprain. Furthermore, some form of chondral injury may occur in as many as 50% of patients. Despite this high incidence, misdiagnosis or delayed diagnosis has been reported to be as high as 81%. Medial dome lesions are more common than lateral lesions. Sixty-four percent of medial lesions and nearly 100% of lateral ones are the result of trauma. Medial lesions are thought to be due to repetitive overuse, whereas lateral lesions are caused by acute trauma.

The mechanism of injury is different for medial lesions compared with lateral lesions. Medial lesions are produced by an inversion force applied to a plantar flexed foot with the tibia externally rotated. The posteromedial edge of the talar dome contacts the posteromedial tip of the tibia, resulting in a shearing injury. Lesions tend to be in the middle or posterior third of the medial dome (Fig. 32-6). They tend to be relatively deep, cup-shaped, and nondisplaced.

Lateral lesions are the result of an inversion force to a dorsiflexed foot with the tibia in internal rotation. The anterolateral talar margin impacts the articular surface of the medial aspect of the fibula, creating shear and compressive forces. These injuries tend to be in the middle or anterior third of the lateral talar dome (Fig. 32-7). Lateral lesions are usually shallow, wafer-shaped, and are often displaced.

Classification

Pritsch et al. (1986) originally developed a staging system based on the condition of the articular cartilage as viewed arthroscopically. Correlation was made with CT and MRI

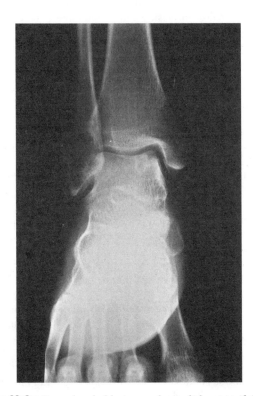

Figure 32-6   Osteochondral lesion on the medial aspect of the talus. (From Koval KJ, Zuckerman, JD. Atlas of Orthopaedic Surgery: A Multimedia Reference. Philadelphia: Lippincott Williams & Wilkins, 2004.)

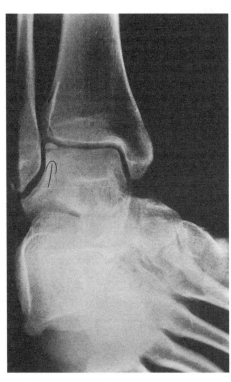

Figure 32-7   Osteochondral lesion on the lateral aspect of the talus. (From Koval KJ, Zuckerman JD. Atlas of Orthopaedic Surgery: A Multimedia Reference. Philadelphia: Lippincott Williams & Wilkins, 2004.)

findings. Arthroscopic classification does not always correlate with radiographic and CT scan findings.

Before advanced imaging modalities, staging of OLT was done using plain radiographs. Pettine and Morrey (1987) described a four-stage system (Table 32-3). Berndt and Harty (1959) described a similar classification system that is also still used. It was also based on plain radiographs. They subclassified transchondral fractures by mechanism: those caused by avulsion and those caused by compression. They believed that OLT was primarily caused by trauma.

TABLE 32-3 PETTINE AND MORREY'S STAGING OF OSTEOCHONDRAL LESIONS OF THE TALUS

Stage	Description
I	Compression injury causing microscopic damage to the subchondral bone; radiographs are normal
II	Partially detached osteochondral fragment that is visible on radiographs
III	Osteochondral fragment completely detached but in anatomical position
IV	Detached fragment is also displaced and present somewhere else in the joint

(Adapted from Pettine KA, Morrey BF. Osteochondral fractures of the talus: a long-term follow-up. J Bone Joint Surg Br 1987;69:89–92.)

Anderson et al. (1989) proposed a classification based on MRI. In their study, they found MRI to be comparable with CT. MRI was better at imaging subtle trabecular lesions, and CT was superior at defining bony fragment position.

In 1993, Ferkel and Scaglione developed a CT scan staging system. It corresponded to the 1959 classification system of Berndt and Harty and incorporated information about the degree of osteonecrosis, subchondral cyst formation, and the degree of fragment displacement not appreciated on plain radiographs. Under this system, the common lesion was a stage III lesion.

Diagnosis

History and Physical Examination

- Patients with an osteochondral injury often give a history of an ankle sprain that sometimes includes a "popping feeling."
- If a severe ligament injury has occurred, the pain associated with this may mask the pain from the osteochondral lesion.
- Patients usually present with chronic ankle pain after an ankle sprain.
- Symptoms can be vague, mild, and intermittent and include stiffness, recurrent swelling, clicking, catching, and locking.
- Occasionally, patients will report symptoms of instability, such as giving way and persistent ankle inversion.
- Some patients may be totally symptomatic.
- Physical findings can be nonspecific.
- Tenderness is located along the medial or lateral aspect of the ankle but can be more generalized.
- Theoretically, the location of the lesion will determine the location of the pain and tenderness.
- Patients may also have pain with range of motion.
- A posteromedial OLT lesion may cause pain anteriorly with plantar flexion and pain posteriorly with dorsiflexion.
- Lateral lesions can elicit posterior pain with direct pressure or with forced plantar flexion.
- Other findings include decreased range of motion, swelling, and mechanical catching and locking.
- Weakness and instability may also be demonstrated.
- If there is persistent pain, swelling, and mechanical symptoms, further evaluation is warranted.

Radiologic Examination

- Routine plain radiographs—including AP, lateral, and mortise views—may be normal.
- Maximal plantar and dorsiflexion mortise views may show the talar dome lesion.
  - Anterolateral lesions are best seen on the dorsiflexion view, and posteromedial lesions can be seen on the plantar flexed view (see Figs. 32-6 and 32-7).
- If plain films do not show the osteochondral lesion, a bone scan is a useful and inexpensive diagnostic aid. It is very sensitive but lacks specificity.
- MRI is also helpful when radiographs are normal and may help to identify injuries to the subchondral bone and cartilage.

- CT scanning is more useful for preoperative evaluation and is considered the test of choice for a known OLT.

Treatment

Nonsurgical Treatment

- The goal of treatment is an asymptomatic ankle.
- Nonoperative treatment is recommended to CT stage I and II lesions.
  - This applies to medial and lateral lesions.
- Nonoperative management is also recommended as initial treatment of medial stage III lesions.
- Treatment involves restricted weight-bearing and a cast or brace for 6 to 12 weeks.
- Complete non-weight-bearing is not considered necessary.
- The duration of treatment depends on multiple factors, including the size of the defect, the chronicity of the lesion, and the age of the patient.

Surgical Treatment

- Surgery is not recommended for an asymptomatic OLT.
- Surgery is indicated for stage III lesions on the medial side, which do not respond to nonoperative care.
- In addition, operative intervention is recommended for lateral stage III lesions, as well as medial and lateral stage IV injuries.
  - An exception to this recommendation is the young patient with open growth plates.
- Surgical treatment can be performed through open ankle arthrotomy using a medial malleolar osteotomy as necessary and ankle arthroscopy.
- Open treatment has problems is more soft-tissue damage, malleolar malunion, or nonunion and joint stiffness.
- Arthroscopic treatment allows improved access, better visualization of the joint surface, and less tissue trauma than open procedures.
- The keys to successful arthroscopic treatment are the use of anterior and posterior portals, small joint instrumentation, and adequate distraction of the ankle joint.
- Arthroscopic treatment starts with identification, inspection, and staging of the lesions.
- Definitive surgical treatment involves removal of loose bodies, unroofing and removal of separated loose osteochondral fragments, and stimulating development of new cartilage.
  - If the OLT is not loose, it is drilled.
  - Removal of soft, yet intact, cartilage is not recommended.
  - Loose lesions are excised, debrided, and drilled. This can be accomplished by a variety of curettes, graspers, shavers, burrs, and arthroscopic scalpels.
  - The lesion bed can be drilled using a small drill or Kirschner wire. Drilling is performed to a depth of about 10 mm at 3- to 5-mm spacing intervals. This is accomplished through a transtalar or transmalleolar approach.
    - A small joint ankle guide can be used with the transmalleolar approach.

- Intraoperative fluoroscopy may be a helpful aid, especially with the transtalar approach.
  - Drilling is recommended for lesions greater than 1 cm.
    - Abrasion arthroplasty may be adequate for lesions less than 1 cm.
  - Large, acute osteochondral fragments that can be anatomically reduced can be fixed with small screws, absorbable pins, Kirschner wires, or absorbable darts or arrows.
  - Medial malleolar osteotomy may be required for additional exposure.
- Microfracture is a relatively new technique for treating OLT.
  - Good clinical success has been reported using this technique to treat cartilage lesions in the knee.
  - Early results of this technique in the talus have been promising with regard to improving function and restoring cartilage.
  - If the talar articular surface is intact, bone graft may be placed via a transtalar approach. Bone graft is also used to pack cystic bony lesions.
- Osteochondral autologous transfer system (OATS) and mosaicplasty involve the transfer of osteochondral plugs to cover an osteochondral defect.
  - This technique involves using a large single plug (OATS) or multiple smaller plugs (mosaicplasty) to fill the lesion.
  - The donor site is the femoral trochlea or condyle in the knee.
  - A large, single plug allows for greater coverage with less fibrocartilage ingrowth but has the risk of greater donor site morbidity.
  - A large plug also has the capability of having a better press fit and thus may be more stable.
  - Conversely, mosaicplasty may have lower donor site morbidity but less defect coverage, with as much as 20% to 40% of the defect being filled with fibrocartilage.

Postoperative Management

- Postoperatively, a bulky compression dressing with a posterior splint is used with the foot in neutral position.
- The patient is kept non-weight-bearing for 2 weeks if the OLT is less than 1.5 cm in diameter and 6 to 8 weeks if the OLT is greater than 1.5 cm in diameter.
- Some will allow OATS/mosaicplasty patients to begin weight-bearing 3 to 4 weeks postsurgery.
- Therapy (including range of motion and strengthening) may begin after the soft tissues heal, which is about 1 week.
- Follow-up CT scan to assess the degree of healing can be done at 6 months.
- OATS/mosaicplasty may be evaluated by MRI or second-look arthroscopy.

Results

Arthroscopic treatment has less morbidity and patients tend to rehabilitate quicker. Short-term results of arthroscopic treatment show 75% to 90% good-to-excellent results. Fer-

kel and Scaglione (1993) reported 84% good-to-excellent results in a series of 59 patients treated arthroscopically. Average follow-up was 40 months. Open surgery showed 63% to 88% good-to-excellent results. In general, the prognosis and degree of success depend on the time interval between the time of injury and the time of treatment. Time delays of greater than 1 year tended to have a poorer outcome.

Hangody et al. (2001) reported 94% good-to-excellent results using mosaicplasty to treat osteochondral lesions greater than 10 mm in diameter. Thirty-six patients were included in this study. Follow-up ranged from 2 to 7 years. In a more recent study, Hangody and Fules (2003) reported on the results of autologous osteochondral mosaicplasty in 831 patients. They reported good-to-excellent results in 94%.

OSTEOCHONDRAL LESIONS OF THE TIBIA

- These are very rare.
- The etiology is unknown.
- Trauma is believed to the most common causal factor.
- Symptoms tend to be chronic and nonspecific.
- Plain radiographs are usually nondiagnostic.
- CT scanning can demonstrate the size and location of the lesion.
- MRI helps to assess the condition of the underlying bone, including the presence of edema and cystic fluid.
- MRI can sometimes determine if the articular cartilage surface is intact.
- Treatment is similar to that of OLT.
- Surgery is performed arthroscopically and includes drilling or microfracture of the lesion and bone grafting of bone cysts.

FRACTURES

Ankle fractures are among the most common injuries treated by orthopaedic surgeons, with an overall incidence in the United States of 250,000 per year. The goals in the treatment of ankle fractures, as with most other periarticular fractures, is joint stability, articular congruity, and near anatomic alignment. Poor reduction with resulting malunion is the most common reason for poor outcome in ankle fractures.

CLASSIFICATION

Indirect ankle fractures are usually classified in one of two ways. The Lauge-Hansen classification, first described in 1954, is based on the position of the foot at the time of injury and the subsequent deforming force. The Danis-Weber, or AO, classification, first described in 1966, is based on the level of the fibula fracture in relation to the tibial plafond. Ninety-five percent of ankle fractures fit into the Lauge-Hansen classification. The most common mechanism, accounting for 40% to 75 % of all ankle fractures, is supination-external rotation. This is a circular injury starting in the region of the anterior syndesmosis and progressing sequentially around to the medial side of the ankle. Pronation-external rotation injuries start medially and progress sequentially around the front of the ankle. Most pronation-external rotation injuries have a fibular fracture proximal to the syndesmosis and often result in syndesmotic instability. Translation ankle fractures are classified as either supination-adduction or pronation-abduction.

In the Danis-Weber classification system (Fig. 32-8), type A is a fibular fracture below the plafond, type B is a fibular fracture at the level of the plafond, and type C is a fibular fracture above the plafond. A supination-adduction injury corresponds to Weber A, pronation-abduction and supination-external rotation correspond to Weber B, and pronation-external rotation corresponds to Weber C.

Restoration of medial stability is a key factor in ankle fracture management. Isolated fibular fractures that do not disrupt the relationship between the tibia and the talus almost universally do well with operative or nonoperative management, as long as there is not significant malalignment or shortening. Up to 50% of ankle fractures result in articular surface injuries, typically of the talar dome. The extent of these injuries plays a role in outcomes as well.

DIAGNOSIS

History and Physical Examination

- A thorough history and physical examination are important in evaluating the patient with an ankle fracture.
- Mechanism of injury and medical comorbidities in particular are useful in guiding initial management and may influence final outcome and point to potential complications.
- Skin and soft tissue should be carefully evaluated for ecchymosis and swelling.
- Peripheral pulses and a distal neurovascular exam should be documented.
- Areas other than the ankle should be examined as well to rule out associated injuries.

Radiologic Examination

- Radiographic evaluation of the ankle consists of three views: anteroposterior, 15-degree internal oblique or mortise, and lateral.
- Full-length tibia and fibula radiographs and occasionally views of the foot may be necessary to completely evaluate bony injury.
- Several radiographic criteria have been established in attempt to identify unstable fracture patterns.
  - On a mortise radiograph, one important measurement is the medial clear space (Fig. 32-9).
  - Measured as the distance between the anterosuperior corner of the talus and the medial corner of the plafond, this value is used to predict injury to the deep deltoid ligament.
  - The medial clear space is between 1.7 and 3.7 mm in most people.

- Syndesmotic integrity can be assessed on both AP and mortise radiographs.
  - On an AP x-ray, the fibula should overlap the tibia by at least 1 cm, and the clear space between the two should be 5 mm or less.
  - On a mortise radiograph, the tibia and fibula should overlap by at least 1 mm.
- Fibular shortening can be assessed on either an AP or mortise radiograph by measuring the angle of a line perpendicular to the plafond and another line running from the tip of the two malleoli.
  - This angle should measure 83 degrees.
- Stress radiographs are often helpful in evaluating ankle stability with certain types of fractures.
  - In the presence of an isolated fibular fracture with a normal medial clear space, an external rotation stress mortise radiograph can be used to evaluate deep deltoid ligament competence.
  - Some experts advocate lateral stress radiographs in situations where syndesmotic instability is suspected but not evident on static x-rays.
- CT scanning is useful in high-energy ankle injuries and in evaluating malunions.
- MRI is best for evaluating soft-tissue and articular surface injuries.

TREATMENT

- In the clinical setting, determination of ankle stability is critical when planning fracture management.
- Typically, stable fractures can be treated nonoperatively with good results, whereas outcomes in the management of unstable ankles are often better with surgery.
- In general, isolated fractures of the lateral malleolus without evidence of medial injury or lateral talar shift will do well with nonoperative treatment.
  - Acceptable amounts of displacement and shortening are typically defined as 5 mm and less than 3 degrees difference in talocrural angle when compared with the uninjured ankle.
  - These fractures almost universally do well with casting and early weight-bearing.
- Isolated medial malleolar fractures must be carefully evaluated to avoid missing a proximal fibular fracture with an unstable syndesmosis.
  - A truly isolated nondisplaced medial malleolar fracture and usually can be treated nonoperatively, but displaced fractures typically require open reduction to avoid interposition of periosteum or deltoid ligament in the fracture.
  - Medial malleolar fractures have up to a 15% nonunion rate in the orthopaedic literature; this may in part be due to closed reduction of displaced fractures with unrecognized soft-tissue interposition.
- Bimalleolar, trimalleolar, and distal fibula fractures with disruption of the deep deltoid ligament often require operative management to restore stability.
  - In the presence of a distal fibular fracture with a normal medial clear space, an attempt should be

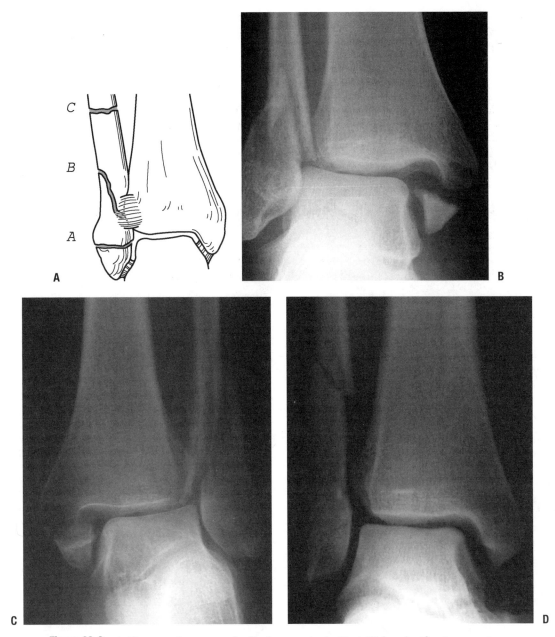

Figure 32-8   **A:** There are three types of ankle fractures in the Danis-Weber classification: type A, type B, and type C. **B:** An AP radiograph of a type A distal fibula fracture in which the fracture line is completely below the level of the syndesmosis. **C:** Radiograph of a type B ankle fracture in which the fibula fracture begins anteriorly at the level of the distal tibiofibular syndesmosis. **D:** A mortise radiograph of a type C injury with disruption of the syndesmosis up to the level of the fibula fracture, which is completely above the distal syndesmotic ligament complex. There is a medial deltoid ligament injury. (From Bucholz RW, Heckman JD. Rockwood & Green's Fractures in Adults, 5th ed. Philadelphia: Lippincott Williams & Wilkins, 2001.)

made to determine the integrity of deep deltoid ligament.

■ Recent evidence suggests that clinical signs of injury—such as swelling, ecchymosis, and tenderness—are not reliable, and stress radiographs or close follow-up to detect late subluxation may be necessary.

■ The goal of operative treatment of these fractures is anatomic reduction.

■ When the posterior malleolus is involved as well, greater than 25% involvement of the joint surface or more than 2 mm or articular step-off is a traditionally accepted cutoff for operative management.

■ When fixation of a distal fibula fracture results in

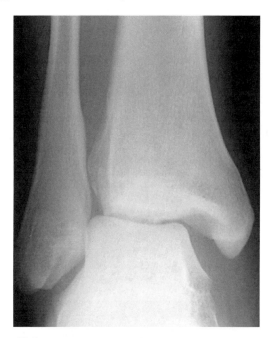

Figure 32-9 An external rotation stress view shows significant widening of the medial clear space, lateral shift of the talus, and distal tibiofibular diastasis indicating an unstable injury. (From Bucholz RW, Heckman JD. Rockwood & Green's Fractures in Adults, 5th ed. Philadelphia: Lippincott Williams & Wilkins, 2001.)

normalization of the medial clear space, there is no advantage to repairing the deltoid ligament.

- Fixation of syndesmotic injuries that accompany ankle fractures are somewhat controversial.
    - As a general rule, most fibular fractures above the tibial plafond will have a component of syndesmotic injury as well.
    - After fixation of medial and lateral fractures, the syndesmosis should be evaluated with intraoperative stress radiographs or C-arm images and fixed as necessary.
    - The usual goals of anatomic reduction of the fibula and restoration of the medial clear space still apply,

although fibular fractures more than 5 to 7 cm above the tibial plafond often do not need direct fixation.

SUGGESTED READING

Anderson JF, Crichton KJ, Gattan-Smith T, et al. Osteochondral fractures of the dome of the talus. J Bone Joint Surg Am 1989;71: 1143–1152.

Berndt AL, Harty M. Transchondral fractures (osteochondritis dessicans) of the talus. J Bone Joint Surg Am 1959;41:988–1020.

Eckert WR, Davis EA Jr. Acute rupture of the peroneal retinaculum. J Bone Joint Surg Am 1976;58:670–672.

Ferkel RD, Fasulo GJ. Arthroscopic treatment of ankle injuries. Orthop Clin 1994;25:17–32.

Ferkel RD, Scaglione NA. Arthroscopic treatment of osteochondral lesions of the talus: long term results. Orthop Trans 1993–1994; 17:1011.

Hangody I, Fules P. Autologous osteochondral mosaicplasty for the treatment of full-thickness defect of weight-bearing joints: ten years of experimental and clinical experience. J Bone Joint Surg Am 2003; 85(suppl 2):25–32.

Hangody L, Kish G, Modis L, et al. Mosaicplasty for the treatment of osteochondritis desiccans of the talus: two to seven year results in 36 patients. Foot Ankle Int 2001;22;552–558.

Liu SH, Raskin A, Osti L, et al. Arthroscopic treatment of anterolateral ankle impingement. Arthroscopy 1994;10:215–218.

Lohrer H, Arentz S. Posterior approach for arthroscopic treatment of posterolateral impingement syndrome of the ankle in a top-level field hockey player. Arthroscopy 2004;20:e15–e21.

Martin DF, Baker CL, Curl WW, et al. Operative ankle arthroscopy. Long term followup. Am J Sports Med 1989;17:16–23.

Meislin RJ, Rose DJ, Parisien JS, et al. Arthroscopic treatment of synovial impingement of the ankle. Am J Sports Med 1993;21:186–189.

Ogilvie-Harris DJ, Mahamed N, Demaziere A. Anterior impingement of the ankle treated by arthroscopic removal of bony spurs. J Bone Joint Surg Br 1993;75:437–440.

Ogilvie-Harris DJ, Sekyi-Out A. Arthroscopic debridement for the osteoarthritic ankle. Arthroscopy 1995;11:433–436.

Pettine KA, Morrey BF. Osteochondral fractures of the talus: a long-term follow-up. J Bone Joint Surg Br 1987;69:89–92.

Pritsch M, Horoshovski H, Farine I. Arthroscopic treatment of osteochondral lesion of the talus. J Bone Joint Surg Am 1986;68:862.

Sammarco GJ. Peroneal tendon injuries. Orthop Clin North Am 1994; 25:135–145.

Schepsis AA, Leach RE. Surgical management of Achilles tendinitis. Am J Sports Med 1987;15:308–315.

Scranton PE, McDermott JE. Anterior tibial spurs: a comparison of open versus arthroscopic debridement. Foot Ankle 1992;13: 125–129.

REHABILITATION IN SPORTS MEDICINE

MICHAEL M. REINOLD
ADAM C. OLSEN
KEVIN E. WILK

Rehabilitation is a multifaceted and ever-evolving process based on the basic science and general principles of tissue healing. The rehabilitation specialist must integrate the clinical diagnosis from the medical team with a full functional examination of the musculoskeletal system. The goal of rehabilitation is to enhance the recovery of injured tissues while avoiding stresses that may prove deleterious to the healing process. This is accomplished through a thorough understanding of the normal function, pathomechanics, and healing process of the specific tissue involved. The rehabilitation specialist must use current research and scientific evidence to establish guidelines to facilitate this process. In this chapter, we will overview the most current evidence-based principles of rehabilitation, with emphasis on clinical implication for sports medicine patients. The primary goal of this chapter is to discuss current concepts in rehabilitation.

PRINCIPLES

Successful rehabilitation begins with communication with the sports medicine team and the establishment of an accurate and differential diagnoses. The key to successful rehabilitation is communication; to facilitate this interaction, the physician and rehabilitation specialist must communi-

cate, providing information regarding the type of injury or surgical procedure performed, method of surgical fixation, the results of any diagnostic tests, the integrity and quality of the patient's tissue, and the expectations of the physician for that specific patient. This information is invaluable to the rehabilitation specialist in designing and implementing a rehabilitation program.

The rehabilitation specialist must also perform a thorough and systematic physical examination to determine specific functional impairments, such as loss of motion or decreased strength of involved joints or muscles. Furthermore, the rehabilitation specialist must identify all involved structures that may be contributing to the patient's loss of motion, such as a tight joint capsule or muscular tightness. To obtain a successful outcome, the rehabilitation specialist must identify and treat the causes of the dysfunction. Then a thorough rehabilitation program may be outlined to address the individual diagnosis and functional needs of the athlete. It is imperative that the rehabilitation program be individualized based on each patient's unique response to injury.

For a patient to progress from one rehabilitation phase to the next, he or she must fulfill specific criteria. This progression allows the program to be individualized on the basis of the patient's unique healing rate and constraints. Programs are oftentimes broken up into phases, such as acute postoperative or advanced strengthening phases, designed to emphasize goals that are specific to the proper timeframe of tissue healing at that particular point in rehabilitation. Each phase has its unique goals that must be met to progress to the next phase, such as restoring full range of motion (ROM) or normalizing arthrokinematics. Each patient may reach these milestones at different times, which promotes a criteria-based progression versus time-based progression. The progression also helps to assist in locating areas in which the patient may be improving slowly and may need additional attention.

A fundamental concept we use in developing a rehabilitation program at our center is to establish a differential diagnosis from the involved structures and causes contributing to the lesion. An example could be subacromial impingement. The cause of subacromial impingement is multifaceted. Some possible causes are capsular tightness, capsular hypermobility, scapula position, rotator cuff imbalances, etc. To treat this specific diagnosis successfully, the rehabilitation specialist must treat the causes of the problem, thus normalizing joint function.

CREATE A HEALING ENVIRONMENT

The basis for all rehabilitation programs is to facilitate healing. It is imperative that the clinician must promote healing but be careful not to overstress the healing tissue. This first principle involves not just the facilitation of healing but also avoidance of excessive stresses that may be disadvantageous for tissue healing throughout the rehabilitation process. This may be illustrated in the rehabilitation of articular cartilage lesions. Controlled motion and gradual weight-bearing progression are necessary to stimulate the healing process but must be progressed cautiously to avoid applying disadvantageous forces that will overload the tissue and inhibit healing. Thus, the program must be progressive and sequential, with each phase building from the prior. Attempting to have a patient progress too quickly may result in inflammation, soreness, and potentially tissue failure, whereas the controlled application of specific stresses can benefit healing tissues. Another example of this is the rehabilitation of the anterior cruciate ligament (ACL) reconstruction patient. The graft must undergo revascularization, as well as tissue remodeling before strenuous activities are allowed.

DECREASE PAIN AND EFFUSION

The first specific goal in most rehabilitation plans is to decrease the patient's pain and effusion resulting from the injury or pathology. Swelling at the injury site can stimulate sensory nerves, leading to a further increase in the athlete's perception of pain. Pain and inflammation also work as muscle inhibitors, causing disuse atrophy the longer the effusion is present.

Numerous authors have studied the effect of joint effusion on muscle inhibition. DeAndrade et al. (1965) reported that joint distention resulted in quadriceps muscle inhibition. A progressive decrease in quadriceps activity was noted as the knee exhibited increased distention. Spencer et al. (1984) found a similar decrease in quadriceps activation

with joint effusion. The authors reported the threshold for inhibition of the vastus medialis to be approximately 20 to 30 mL of joint effusion and 50 to 60 mL for the rectus femoris and vastus lateralis. Similar results have been reported within the literature.

In an unpublished study, the peak torque and electromyographic activity of the quadriceps musculature were measured while the knee joint was progressively effused. With the addition of 30 to 40 mL to the knee joint, quadriceps peak torque dramatically decreased by approximately 50% and continued to decrease with added effusion. Also, whereas the rectus femoris and vastus lateralis noted mild decreases in the muscle activity with the addition of joint effusion, the vastus medialis muscle activity decreased dramatically in proportion to the amount of joint effusion added. Vastus medialis oblique activity began to decrease with the addition of 20 mL, whereas the rectus femoris and vastus lateralis required approximately 60 mL before a reduction in muscle activity was noted.

Thus, the reduction in knee joint swelling is crucial to restore normal voluntary quadriceps activity. Treatment options for swelling reduction include elevation, cryotherapy, high-voltage electrical stimulation, and joint compression through the use of a knee sleeve or compression wrap (Fig. 33-1). In patients who have undergone certain procedures for the knee, such as a lateral retinacular release, a foam wedge, shaped to form around the lateral patella, can be used in conjunction with a wrap to provide increased compression around the lateral genicular artery. Patients presenting with chronic joint effusion may also benefit from a knee sleeve or compression wrap to apply constant pressure while performing everyday activities in an attempt to minimize joint effusion. Conversely, patients with acute inflammation can benefit from ice and elevation.

Pain may also play a role in the inhibition of muscle activity observed with joint effusion. In an examination of the electromyographic activity of the quadriceps in the acutely swollen and painful knee, an afferent block by local anesthesia was produced intraoperatively during medial

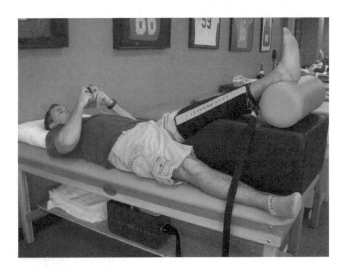

Figure 33-1 The application of cryotherapy and compression through a Game Ready commercial ice machine (Game Ready, Inc., Berkeley, CA) with high-voltage electrical stimulation (300 PV; Empi, Inc., St. Paul, MN) and elevation to minimize effusion.

meniscectomy. Patients in the control group reported significant pain postoperatively and pronounced inhibition of the quadriceps (30% to 76%). In contrast, patients with local anesthesia reported minimal pain and only mild quadriceps inhibition (5% to 31%). Thus, it appears that muscle inhibition may be attributed to a combination of joint pain and effusion.

Pain can be reduced passively through the use of cryotherapy and analgesic medication. Immediately after injury or surgery, the use of a commercial cold wrap can be extremely beneficial. Passive ROM may also provide neuromodulation of pain during acute or exacerbated conditions. Numerous studies have documented that passive range of motion exercises reduces the need for pain medication. Favorable results have been reported when continuous passive motion or manual passive ROM exercises are emphasized following repair of small, medium, or large tears of the rotator cuff. Therapeutic modalities such as ultrasound and electrical stimulation may also be used to control pain via the gate control theory.

The speed of progression in rehabilitation, particularly weight-bearing status and range of motion, may also affect pain and swelling. Therefore, any increase in pain of effusion in the involved joint is monitored as the patient progresses through rehabilitation and begins new exercises. This is monitored to assure that the pace of rehabilitation is appropriate and the tissue is not being overstressed. Persistent pain, inflammation, and swelling may have results in long-term complications involving range of motion, voluntary quadriceps control, and a delaying of the rehabilitation process; thus, it is imperative that these symptoms be minimized.

CONSIDER BIOLOGY

When progressing a patient through rehabilitation, thought must be given to the healing tissue itself. If a patient is progressing ahead of schedule and has no complaints, can that patient continue at an accelerated rate without compromising the long-term health of his or her tissues? Is an athlete returning to sport at 4 months mean a better outcome than 6 months? Several characteristics must be considered when deciding the appropriate speed of rehabilitation. The patient's age, genetics, nutrition, concomitant injuries, and unique healing characteristics can all affect the rehabilitation timeline. Injuries to the meniscus or collateral ligaments may require a slower rehabilitation process after ACL reconstruction. Not all concomitant injuries are visible. Several studies have reported that more than 80% of patients who sustain an acute ACL injury exhibit a bone bruise on magnetic resonance imaging. Patients with a bone bruise who underwent ACL reconstruction in one study required a longer period to reduce effusion and pain and to return muscle function. Additional effects may not be seen for years after the initial injury, such as articular cartilage lesions and the development of early knee osteoarthritis. Some authors believe that bone bruises resolve in several months, whereas others believe the homeostasis of the bone may be altered for much longer. The decisions made during rehabilitation may have significant effects on the metabolic

activity of the injury site and in the return to normal joint homeostasis. Risks of an accelerated rehabilitation must be evaluated for each patient, with careful consideration of the possible consequences. The rehabilitation specialist must be very careful when treating bone bruises. We recommend treating them with partial weight-bearing, ice, compression, and control aggressive loading for several months.

PREVENT THE DELETERIOUS EFFECTS OF IMMOBILIZATION

In the acute stages of healing, it is often necessary to restrict motion of the injured tissues to promote healing. Although restricted, strength and muscular girth are quickly lost, and joint contracture and loss of range of motion may occur. Furthermore, the combination of unloading and immobilization results in significant proteoglycan loss and weakening of the articular cartilage. The deleterious effects of immobilization must therefore be minimized, and immobilization should be avoided in almost all cases.

Immediate, controlled motion (Fig. 33-2) is critical to a successful outcome. Rehabilitation after ACL injury changed dramatically when it was found that patients who were taken through an accelerated program experienced a better outcome, including a decreased incidence of arthrofibrosis and quicker return to activity. Immobilization is avoided in rehabilitation, with a greater emphasis on controlled ROM in a protected range.

It is our belief that the controlled application of ROM during the early phases of ROM is beneficial to avoid long-

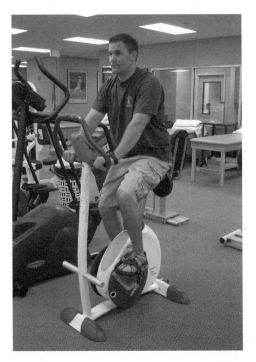

Figure 33-2 ROM performed on a Uni-Cam bicycle (Uni-Cam, Inc., Ramsey, NJ). The axis of the pedals may be adjusted to allow for a different ROM for each extremity during the exercise. This can be used to protect specific areas within the joint ROM.

term loss of motion and to stimulate the synthesis, organization, and alignment of collagen tissue. Other benefits of early passive ROM include the reduction of pain and swelling, facilitation of a more normal gait pattern, and stimulation of collagen and cartilage repair. With ACL subjects, during passive ROM, there is no strain on the ACL with 0 to 125 degrees of motion.

Passive motion is most often performed by a skilled clinician but can also be performed by a continuous passive motion (CPM) or by an isokinetic device set in the passive ROM setting. The use of a CPM after surgery has several benefits, including the avoidance of arthrofibrosis. In a study by Rodrigo et al. (1994), patients undergoing a microfracture procedure of the knee who used a CPM for the first 8 weeks demonstrated 85% good-to-excellent results versus a group of patients without CPM who only had 55% good-to-excellent results. In the case of rotator cuff–repaired patients, restoring passive ROM is critical to the successful outcome of these patients.

RETARD MUSCULAR ATROPHY

Rehabilitation should also emphasize the retardation of muscular atrophy and the facilitation of volitional muscle activity after an injury or surgical procedure. As previously described, a small increase in pain and/or joint effusion can decrease the voluntary control of surrounding musculature. This can significantly affect the patient's ability to control their limb and ambulate with a normal gait pattern.

Exercises designed to enhance muscular volition begin with basic isometric contractions of the involved muscles. This isometric contraction allows firing of the muscle fibers without joint motion. This is a safe, effective method of exercise during the early phases of rehabilitation. Isometric contractions are performed for each muscle at multiple static angles throughout the available ROM. Isometric contraction has also been shown to be one of the most efficient forms of exercise, increasing muscular tension and improving strength.

Muscle re-education with electrical muscle stimulation (EMS) may assist in restoring the patient's voluntary control of inhibited musculature. EMS is often applied concomitantly during isometric and isotonic exercises to increase the recruitment of muscle fibers during the contraction.

Snyder-Mackler et al. (1995) studied the effects of electrical stimulation on quadriceps muscle strength after ACL reconstruction. After a comparable 4-week training period, patients exercising with the adjunct of a high-intensity electrical stimulation unit exhibited quadriceps strength greater than 70% of the uninvolved lower extremity. Patients not using electrical stimulation presented with quadriceps strength of only 57% of the opposite knee at the same time period after surgery. The addition of neuromuscular electrical stimulation to postoperative exercises resulted in stronger quadriceps and more normal gait patterns than patients exercising without electrical stimulation. Several authors have also reported similar gains when integrating EMS into postoperative rehabilitation programs.

Another study evaluated the use of EMS of the external rotators in the first 2 weeks after mini open and arthroscopic rotator cuff repair surgery. The authors measured the amount of voluntary force generation by the patient during an isometric external rotation contraction with and without the application of EMS. Results revealed that patients were able to generate approximately 60% great force production while using the EMS. This was a significant increase in force with the use of EMS superimposed over the muscular contraction.

Biofeedback may also be used to enhance the voluntary control of the injured musculature. Biofeedback is used to allow the patient to monitor the amount of force production throughout the exercise. One study compared the use of electrical stimulation with biofeedback in the recovery of quadriceps strength after ACL reconstruction. Rehabilitation began immediately postsurgery and continued for the first 6 weeks postoperatively. Both groups produced a significant increase in quadriceps peak torque. The group of patients using biofeedback showed slightly greater peak torque output of the quadriceps than did the group using electrical stimulation.

Clinically, we use electrical stimulation immediately after injury or surgery while performing isometric and isotonic upper and lower-extremity exercises (Fig. 33-3A,B). Electrical stimulation is used before biofeedback when the patient presents acutely with the inability to activate the musculature. Once independent muscle activation is present, biofeedback may be used to facilitate further neuromuscular activation. However, EMS may still be used to recruit more motor units, thus resulting in greater strength gains. Therefore, we use EMS for several weeks (from 4 to 8 weeks) after ACL surgery or after selected shoulder surgeries. Conversely, biofeedback is used for patellofemoral patients when they are unable to actively recruit their vastus medialis (Fig. 33-3C). The patient must concentrate on neuromuscular control to independently activate the muscle during rehabilitation.

RESTORE MUSCULAR STRENGTH AND ENDURANCE

After volitional control of muscle activity is achieved, emphasis is placed on gradually restoring muscular strength. A baseline level of muscular strength is needed before the athlete can progress to the later stages of rehabilitation that include advanced neuromuscular control drills. Strengthening can be performed through a variety of different methods of isotonic exercise. Weight is gradually applied and increased as the athlete progressively improves in strength to ensure that the exercise is constantly challenging. Isotonic exercises are generally performed as either isolated joint movements (such as knee extension) or as multijoint movements (such as a squat). Furthermore, exercises may be performed in either an open kinetic chain (OKC) or closed kinetic chain (CKC) environment. OKC exercise can be defined as a movement where the distal extremity is not fixed, such as knee extension. Conversely, CKC exercise can be defined as a movement in which the distal extremity is fixed, such as the leg press. Each of these modes of exercise has a place in rehabilitation, although all have a different effect on not only muscular activity but also biomecha-

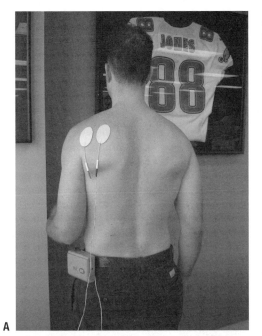

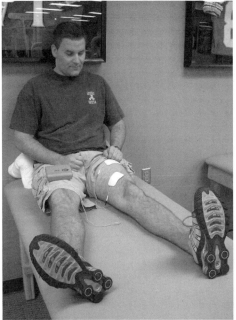

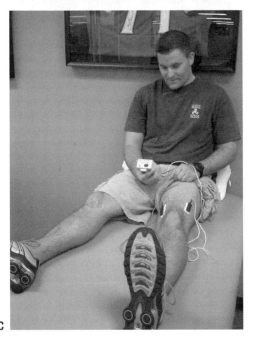

Figure 33-3   A: Neuromuscular electrical stimulation (300 PV; Empi, Inc., St. Paul, MN) of the infraspinatus during external rotation isometric exercise. **B:** Neuromuscular electrical stimulation (300 PV) of the quadriceps during isometric quadriceps setting exercise. **C:** Biofeedback (Pathway MR-20, Prometheus Group, Dover, NH) on the vastus medialis oblique and ventrolateral site during isometric quadriceps setting exercise to allow the patient to monitor the amount of muscle activity.

nics of the joint. Wilk et al. (1996) and Escamilla et al. (1998) studied the EMG activity and biomechanical stresses during OKC and CKC exercises for the lower extremities during various conditions. The authors noted that how the exercise is performed can significantly affect the exercise effect. For example, during the vertical squat, by increasing the subject's hip flexion, the EMG activity of the hamstrings is increased and the quads are slightly decreased. By performing a wall squat, the EMG activity of the quadriceps is extremely high and hamstrings are lower, significantly different than the vertical squat.

Witvrouw et al. (2000) prospectively studied the efficacy of OKC and CKC exercises during nonoperative patellofemoral rehabilitation. Sixty patients participated in a 5-week exercise program consisting of either OKC or CKC exercises. Subjective pain scores, functional ability, quadriceps and hamstring peak torque, and hamstring, quadriceps, and gastrocnemius flexibility were all recorded before and after rehabilitation, as well as 3 months proceeding. Both treatment groups reported a significant decrease in pain, an increase in muscle strength, and an increase in functional performance at 3 months after intervention.

Muscular endurance is also an important factor to emphasize in rehabilitation programs. Many of the activities in which athletes participate involve repetitive and microtraumatic events. Training the musculature to endure these events is necessary to prevent injuries. Fatigue has been shown to result in decreased proprioception and altered biomechanics of the joints, which may result in further pathology. Significant changes in throwing mechanics, joint stresses, and velocity occur during overhead pitching once the thrower has fatigued.

NORMALIZE SOFT-TISSUE MOBILITY AND FLEXIBILITY

Oftentimes, in rehabilitation, soft-tissue balance is emphasized. This applies to both the soft tissue around joints, such as the retinacular tissue surrounding the patella, but also the muscular flexibility around each joint. Any deviations in the balance of soft tissue forces will promote altered arthrokinematics and excessive forces to the joints. This can be easily illustrated in the patellofemoral patient who presents with excessive lateral pressure syndrome and clinical signs of patellar tilting and lateral displacement due to tightness of the lateral retinacular tissue.

Another example of balancing the soft tissue about a joint is at the glenohumeral joint. Wilk and Andrews (1994) have referred to this concept as "asymmetrical capsular tightness." This means that if one side of the joint capsule is tight, then the arthrokinematics of the joint will be significantly affected. Thus, if the inferior capsule is tight, then the humeral head will translate superior during active arm motions. This concept has been documented with tightness of the posterior glenohumeral joint.

Muscular flexibility is also vital to normal joint function by allowing the musculature to absorb force and align the joint in a neutral position. For example, soft-tissue tightness of the quadriceps musculature is a common occurrence in patients with patellar tendonitis and patellofemoral pain.

Witvrouw et al. (2000) prospectively studied the risk factors for the development of anterior knee pain in the athletic population over a 2-year period. A significant difference was noted in the flexibility of the quadriceps and gastrocnemius muscles between the group of subjects that developed patellofemoral pain and the control group, suggesting that athletes exhibiting tightness of specific muscles may be at risk for the development of patellofemoral disorders.

In the upper extremity, it is often common to see patients who present with tightness in the anterior structures, such as the pectoralis musculature, and consequently exhibiting a protracted, forward head posture. This can lead to several shoulder pathologies, such as impingement due to the protracted and anterior tilted scapular position. Furthermore, the authors believe a loss of internal rotation in most throwers is due to posterior rotator cuff tightness and osseous adaptation and not from tightness of the posterior glenohumeral joint.

RESTORE NEUROMUSCULAR CONTROL

Early proprioception and kinesthesia exercises are important for patients returning to sporting activities. Basic exercises designed to enhance the athlete's ability to detect the joint position and movement in space are performed to establish a baseline of motor learning for further neuromuscular control exercises that will be integrated during the later phases of rehabilitation. Dynamic stability refers to the ability to stabilize a joint during functional activities to avoid injuries. This involves neuromuscular control and the efferent (motor) output to afferent (sensory) stimulation from the mechanoreceptors.

The emphasis of rehabilitation programs has shifted over the past several years to focus on restoring proprioception, dynamic stability, and neuromuscular control in patients. The neuromuscular control system may have a critical effect on the prevention of serious knee injuries. Numerous authors have shown a decrease in proprioceptive and kinesthetic abilities after injury. Beard et al. (1994) examined the effects of applying a 100 N anterior shear force on ACL-deficient knees and noted a deficit in reflexive activation of the hamstring musculature. Furthermore, Wojtys and Huston (1994) examined the neuromuscular deficits in 40 normal subjects and 100 ACL-deficient subjects. In response to an anteriorly directed tibial force, the ACL-deficient group showed deficits in muscle timing and recruitment order. Proprioception deficits after shoulder dislocation have also been noted.

We routinely begin basic proprioceptive training during the early phases of rehabilitation, such as the second postoperative week after ACL reconstruction, pending adequate normalization of pain, swelling, and quadriceps control. Proprioceptive training initially begins with basic exercises, such as joint repositioning and CKC weight-shifting. Furthermore, gait and weight-bearing drills are altered for several months following ACL injury.

Joint repositioning drills begin with the athlete's eyes closed; the rehabilitation specialist passively moves the extremity in various planes of motion, pauses, and then returns the extremity to the starting position. The patient is then instructed to actively reposition the extremity to the previous location. The rehabilitation specialist may perform these joint repositioning activities in variable degrees throughout the available range of motion and notes the accuracy of the patient. Altering the patient's external stimulus such of vision and hearing may also provide increased challenge to the patient's proprioceptive system.

Weight shifts may be performed in the medial-lateral direction and in diagonal patterns. Mini squats are also performed early postoperatively. A force platform may be incorporated with weight shifts and mini squats to measure the amount of weight distribution between the involved and uninvolved extremity (Fig. 33-4). An elastic bandage worn postoperatively has a positive impact on proprioception and joint position sense, and thus our patients are encouraged to wear an elastic support wrap underneath their brace as well.

As the patient advances, mini squats are progressed onto an unstable surface, such as foam or a tilt board. The patient is instructed to squat down to approximately 25 to 30 degrees and hold the position for 2 to 3 seconds while stabilizing the tilt board. The greatest amount of hamstring and quadriceps cocontraction occurs at approximately 30 degrees of knee flexion during the squat. Squats may be performed with the tilt board positioned in the medial-lateral and anterior-posterior directions. Muscular contraction can decrease the anterior and posterior laxity in the knee joint by 275% to 450%. Also, there is an increased risk of ligamentous injury in knees with quadriceps to hamstring muscle

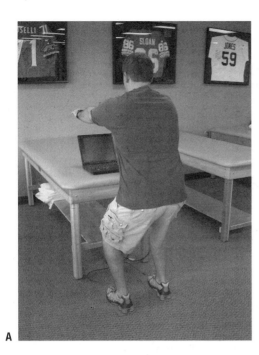
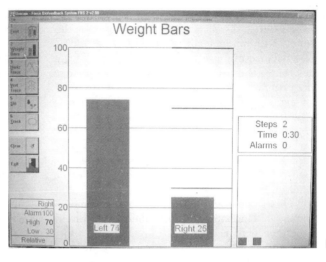

Figure 33-4 Mini squats on a force platform **(A)** that can provide objective feedback of the amount of weight distributed between lower extremities **(B)** (Balance Trainer, Uni-Cam, Inc., Ramsey, NJ).

strength imbalances. Thus, we believe by improving neuromuscular coactivation, stability is enhanced.

As proprioception is advanced, drills to encourage preparatory agonist-antagonist coactivation during functional activities are incorporated. These dynamic stabilization drills for the lower extremity begin with single leg stance on flat ground and unstable surfaces, cone stepping, and lateral lunge drills. The patient may perform forward, backward, and lateral cone step-over drills to facilitate gait training, enhance dynamic stability, and to train the hip to help control forces at the knee joint. The patient is instructed to raise the knee up to the level of the hip and step over a

series of cones, landing with a slightly flexed knee. These cone drills may also be performed at various speeds to train the lower extremity to dynamically stabilize with different amounts of momentum.

Lateral lunges are also performed with the patient instructed to lunge to the side, landing on a slightly flexed knee and holding that position for 1 to 2 sec before returning to the start position. We use a functional progression for the lateral lunges: straight-plane lateral lunges are performed first, progressing to multiple-plane/diagonal lunges, lateral lunges with rotation, and finally lateral lunges onto foam (Fig. 33-5). As the patient progresses, concentration

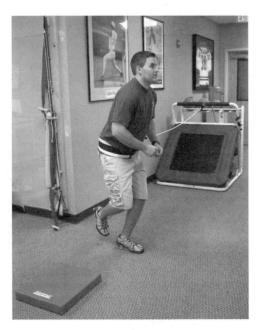
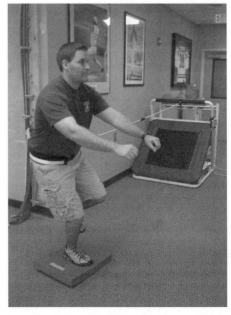

Figure 33-5 Lateral lunges using a sport cord onto an unstable surface.

may be distracted by including a ball toss with any of these exercises to challenge the preparatory stabilization of the lower extremity with minimal conscious awareness.

Single-leg balance exercises are progressed by altering the patient's center of gravity and incorporating movement of the upper extremity and the uninvolved lower extremity. The patient stands on a piece of foam with the knee slightly flexed and performs random flexion, extension, abduction, adduction, and diagonal movement patterns of the upper extremity while holding weighted balls and maintaining control of the knee joint (Fig. 33-6). The uninvolved lower extremity may also be moved in the anterior-posterior or medial-lateral directions while maintaining control of the joint. Finally, both upper and lower-extremity movements may be combined. The patient again stabilizes the flexed knee on a piece of foam as the upper extremity moves forward with simultaneous extension of the lower extremity. This movement is followed by the upper extremity extending while the lower extremity moves forward. These single-leg balance drills are used with extremity movement to provide mild variations of the patient's center of gravity, thus altering the amount of dynamic stabilization needed and recruiting various muscle groups to provide the majority of neuromuscular control. Medicine balls of progressive weight may be incorporated to provide further challenge to the neuromuscular control system.

Perturbation training may also be incorporated. Fitzgerald et al. (2000) examined the efficacy of perturbation training in the rehabilitation program of ACL-deficient knees. The authors reported that perturbation training resulted in more satisfactory outcomes and lessened the frequency of subsequent giving-way episodes in ACL-deficient knees. We incorporate perturbations while the patient performs double- or single-leg balance on a tilt board. While flexing the knee to approximately 30 degrees, the patient stabilizes the tilt board with an isometric hold at 30 degrees of flexion and throws and catches a lightweight medicine ball. The patient is instructed to stabilize the tilt board in reaction to the sudden outside force produced by the weighted ball. The rehabilitation specialist may also provide manual perturbations by striking the tilt board with his or her foot to create a sudden disturbance in the static support of the lower extremity, requiring the patient to stabilize the tilt board with dynamic muscular contractions (Fig. 33-7). Perturbations may also be performed during this drill by tapping the patient at their hips to provide proximal and distal perturbation forces.

Exercises such as balance beam walking, lunges onto an unstable surface, and step-up exercises while standing on an unstable surface are also used to strengthen the knee musculature while requiring the muscles located proximally and distally within the kinetic chain to stabilize and allow coordinated functional movement patterns.

Plyometric jumping drills may also be performed to facilitate dynamic stabilization and neuromuscular control of the knee joint. Plyometric exercises use the muscle's stretch-shortening properties to produce maximal concentric contraction after a rapid eccentric loading of the muscle tissues. Plyometric training is used to train the extremities to produce and dissipate forces to avoid injury (Fig. 33-8).

Hewett et al. (1999) examined the effects of a 6-week plyometric training program on the landing mechanics and strength of female athletes. The authors reported a 22% decrease in peak ground reaction forces and a 50% decrease in the abduction/adduction moments at the knee during landing. Also, a significant increase in hamstring isokinetic

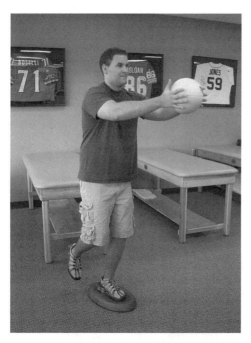

Figure 33-6   Single-leg balance on an unstable surface while incorporating alternating upper extremities movement with a weighted ball to alter the patient's center of gravity.

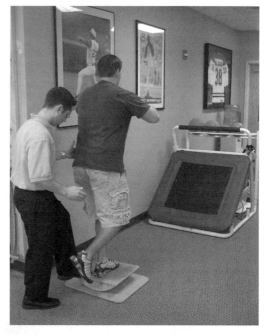

Figure 33-7   Single-leg balance on a tilt board while the patient tosses a ball against a rebound device. The rehabilitation specialist may create a perturbation by striking the board.

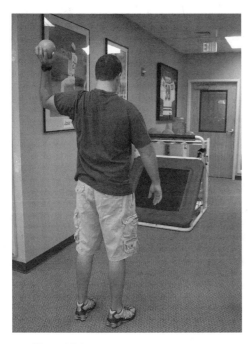

Figure 33-8   Upper extremity plyometrics.

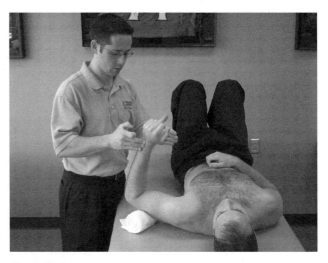

Figure 33-9   Rhythmic stabilization to promote co-contraction of the rotator cuff.

strength, hamstring to quadriceps ratio, and vertical jump height were reported.

Using the same plyometric program, Hewett et al. (1996) prospectively analyzed the effect of neuromuscular training on serious knee injuries in female athletes. The authors reported a statistically significant decrease in the amount of knee injuries in the trained group versus the control group.

The final aspect of rehabilitation regarding neuromuscular control involves enhancing muscular endurance. Proprioceptive and neuromuscular control has been shown to diminish once muscular fatigue occurs. Exercises such as cycling, stair climbing, and using an elliptical machine may be used for long durations to increase endurance as well as high-repetition, low-weight resistance strengthening. Additionally, we frequently recommend performing neuromuscular control drills toward the end of a treatment session, after cardiovascular training. This type of training is performed to challenge the neuromuscular control of the knee joint when the dynamic stabilizers have been adequately fatigued.

The enhancement of neuromuscular control is equally important in the upper extremity, and many of the previously described techniques can also be applied to the upper extremity. The excessive mobility and compromised static stability observed within the glenohumeral joint often result in numerous injuries to the capsulolabral and musculotendinous structures of the shoulder. Efficient dynamic stabilization and neuromuscular control of the glenohumeral joint are necessary for athletes to avoid injuries during competition.

Dynamic stabilization exercises for the upper extremity also begin with baseline proprioception and kinesthesia drills to maximize the athlete's awareness of joint position and movement in space. In addition to joint repositioning and CKC drills, rhythmic stabilizations are incorporated to facilitate cocontraction of the rotator cuff and dynamic stability of the glenohumeral joint. These exercises involve alternating isometric contractions designed to promote cocontraction and basic reactive neuromuscular control (Fig. 33-9). These dynamic stabilization techniques may be applied as the athlete progresses to provide advance challenge to the neuromuscular control system. As the athlete progresses, it is necessary to train the upper extremity to provide adequate dynamic stabilization in response to sudden forces, particularly at the end of ROM (Fig. 33-10). We refer to this as reactive neuromuscular control.

EMPHASIZE THE ENTIRE KINETIC CHAIN

Rehabilitation must be focused on not only regaining strength and neuromuscular control of the affected joint, but also including attention to the surrounding areas. For example, neuromuscular control of the shoulder involves stability of not only the glenohumeral joint, but also the scapulothoracic joint. The scapula serves to provide a stable base of support for muscular attachment and dynamically positions the glenohumeral joint during upper extremity movement. Scapular strength and stability are essential to proper function of the glenohumeral joint. Therefore, isotonic strengthening and dynamic stabilization of the scapula musculature should also be included into rehabilitation programs for the athlete's shoulder to ensure proximal stability. Furthermore, the core of the body should be emphasized to enhance scapular control.

Additionally, altered forces at the knee joint may be the result of several biomechanical faults both distal and proximal in the kinetic chain. These include rearfoot and tibial rotation distally and femoral rotation, hip control, and core stability proximally. We believe the way to control varus and valgus at the tibiofemoral joint is proximally (through pelvic and hip control), distally with foot mechanics (i.e., controlling hyperpronation, etc.), or both. Thus, we emphasize hip

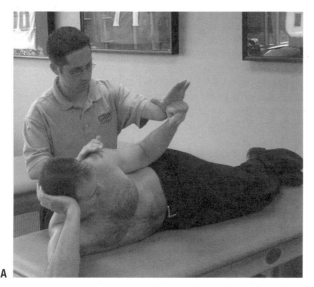 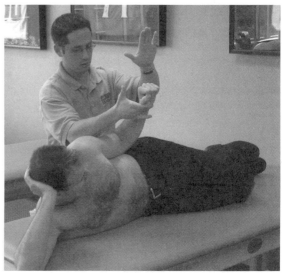

Figure 33-10   Manual resistance during side-lying external resistance. **A:** The rehabilitation specialist resisted both external rotation and retraction of the scapula. **B:** Rhythmic stabilizations may also be performed at end range.

rotation strengthening exercises and foot biomechanical correction.

Core stabilization drills are used to further enhance proximal stability with distal mobility of the extremities. Core stabilization is used based on the kinetic chain concept, in which imbalance within any point of the kinetic chain might result in pathology throughout. Movement patterns, such as throwing, require a precise interaction of the body's entire kinetic chain to perform efficiently. An imbalance of strength, flexibility, endurance, or stability may result in

fatigue, abnormal arthrokinematics, and subsequent compensation. Core stabilization is progressed using a multiphase approach, progressing from baseline core and trunk strengthening to intermediate core strengthening (Fig. 33-11) with distal mobility to advanced stabilization in sport-specific movement patterns (Fig. 33-12).

Also, during rehabilitation, it is important not to neglect

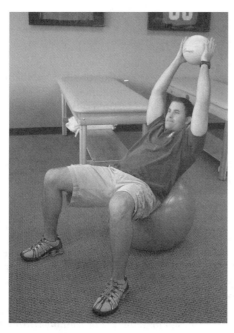

Figure 33-11   Abdominal exercises on a Swiss ball while holding a weighted ball.

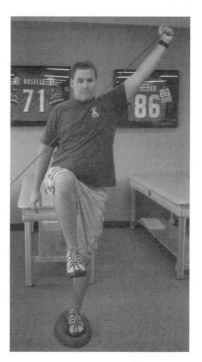

Figure 33-12   Proprioceptive neuromuscular facilitation exercise while standing on a piece of foam. This exercise incorporates strengthening, neuromuscular control, and core stabilization while simulating the stance position of baseball pitching.

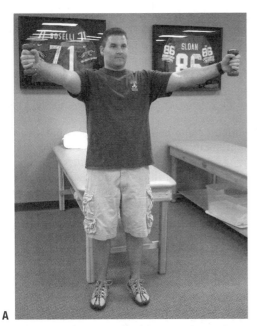
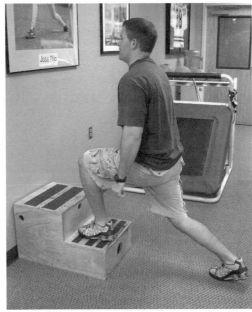

Figure 33-13   Examples of exercises performed bilaterally, the standing "full can" exercise **(A)** and forward lunging onto a box **(B)**.

the uninjured extremity. Studies have pointed to a crossover effect when the contralateral extremity is exercised, which may result in improvements in proprioception and strength. Preliminary studies at our center have shown a decrease in proprioception of the uninvolved extremity after ACL injury. This has also been reported with unilateral ankle sprains. It appears that the neuromuscular control system may have a certain amount of central mediating function that may be receptive to bilateral training techniques. Thus, when rehabilitating a patient with a joint injury, the rehabilitation specialist must consider the patient performing either bilateral exercises or unilateral reciprocal exercises (Fig. 33-13).

ENSURE GRADUAL RECONDITIONING THROUGH APPLIED LOADS AND STRESSES

Rehabilitation must be performed in a gradual manner. Tissues are best reconditioned through progressive loading and stressing. The rehabilitation process involves a progressive application of therapeutic exercises designed to gradually increase function in the athlete. As previously discussed, an overaggressive approach early within the rehabilitation program may result in increased pain, inflammation, and effusion. This simple concept may also be applied to the progression of strengthening exercises, proprioception training, neuromuscular control drills, functional drills, and sport-specific training. For example, exercises such as weight shifts and lunges are progressed from straight plane anterior-posterior or medial-lateral directions to involve multiplane and rotational movements. Two-legged exercises—such as leg press, knee extension, balance activities,

and plyometric jumps—are progressed to single-leg exercises. Thus, the progression through the postoperative rehabilitation program involves a gradual progression of applied and functional stresses. This progression is used to provide a healthy stimulus for healing tissues while ensuring that forces are gradually applied without causing damage. This ensures that the patient has ample time to develop the neuromuscular control and dynamic stabilization needed to perform these drills.

PROMOTE A GRADUAL RETURN TO FUNCTIONAL ACTIVITIES

After the successful completion of a rehabilitation program, the athlete must begin a gradual return to sporting activities. Interval sport programs (ISP) are designed to gradually return motion, function, and confidence to the athlete after injury or surgery by slowly progressing through graduated sport-specific activities. The goal of this phase is to gradually and progressively increase the functional demands on the athlete to return the patient to full, unrestricted sport or daily activities. The criteria established before a patient's return to sport activities are full-functional ROM, adequate static stability, satisfactory muscular strength and endurance (Fig. 33-14), adequate dynamic stability, and a satisfactory clinical examination. Once these criteria are successfully met, the patient may initiate a gradual return to sport activity in a controlled manner. Healing constraints based on surgical technique and fixation, as well as the patient's tissue status, should be considered before a functional program can be initiated.

The ISP is set up to minimize the chance of reinjury and emphasize precompetition warmup and stretching. Because

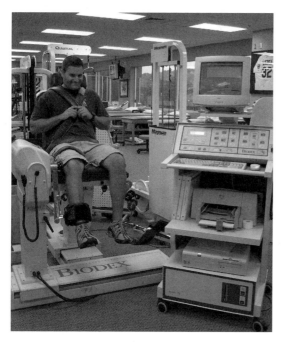

Figure 33-14 Strength testing on a Biodex isokinetic device (Biodex Corp., Shirley, NY).

there is an individual variability in all athletes, there is no set timetable for completion of the program. Variability will exist based on the skill level, goals, and injury of each athlete. ISPs may be developed based on the specific sport and stresses observed during these athletic activities. For example, overhead athletes perform an interval-throwing program that begins with a limited amount of throws using a flat-ground, long-toss program. As the distance of throws is progressed from 45, 60, 90, and 120 feet, the athlete may progress to begin throwing from a mound. Again, a gradual approach is applied by progressing amount and intensity of throws.

Other goals of this phase are to maintain the patient's muscular strength, dynamic stability, and functional motion established in the previous phase. A stretching and strengthening program should be performed on an ongoing basis to maintain and continue to improve on these goals. The rate of progression with functional activities is dictated by the patient's unique tolerance to the activities. Exercise must be performed at a tolerable level without overstressing the healing tissues; this is referred to as the patient's envelope of function.

The athlete's return to sport-specific drills progresses through a series of transitional drills designed to progressively challenge the neuromuscular control system. Pool running is performed before flat-ground running, backward and lateral running are performed before forward running, plyometrics are performed before running and cutting drills, and finally culminating in sport-specific agility drills. The integration of functional activities is necessary to train the injured patient to perform specific movement patterns necessary for everyday activities. The intention of sport-specific training is to simulate the functional activities associated with sports while incorporating peripheral afferent stimula-

tion with reflexive and preprogrammed muscle control and coactivation. Many of the drills—such as cone drills, lunges with sport cord, plyometrics drills, and the running and agility progression—may be modified based on the specific functional movement patterns associated with the patient's unique sport. Some of the sport-specific running and agility drills incorporated include side-shuffle, cariocas, sudden starts and stops, 45-degree cutting, 90-degree cutting, and various combinations of the previous drills. The specific movement patterns learned throughout the rehabilitation program are integrated to provide challenge in a controlled setting. These drills are performed to train the neuromuscular control system to perform during competition in a reflexive pattern to prevent injuries.

CONCLUSION

The rehabilitation process is based on our knowledge of the basic science of injury and tissue healing, as well as an understanding of the general principles discussed in this chapter. Team communication and the gradual application of these principles in a well-designed rehabilitation program based on the individual needs of each patient are essential to ensure successful results. The goal of this chapter was to discuss current concepts in the rehabilitation process.

The ultimate goal of the rehabilitation process is not getting the patient or athlete back to work or sport as fast as possible, but rather return the patient to function when it is safe and appropriate. For example, returning someone to running or jumping while the patient exhibits a femoral bone bruise will lead to long-term articular cartilage problems. The ultimate goal of rehabilitation is a healthy, asymptomatic patient 5 to 10 years after surgery, not just at 6 months.

SUGGESTED READING

Beard DJ, Kyberd PJ, Dodd CA, et al. Proprioception in the knee. J Bone Joint Surg Br 1994;76:992–993.

Beard DJ, Kyberd PJ, O'Connor JJ, et al. Reflex hamstring contraction latency in anterior cruciate ligament deficiency. J Orthop Res 1994; 12:219–228.

Buckwalter JA, Stanish WD, Rosier RN, et al. The increasing need for nonoperative treatment of patients with osteoarthritis. Clin Orthop Relat Res 2001;385:36–45.

Buckwalter JA. Articular cartilage: injuries and potential for healing. J Orthop Sports Phys Ther 1998;28:192–202.

Colwell CW, Morris BA. The influence of continuous passive motion on the results of total knee arthroplasty. Clin Orthop 1992;276: 225–228.

DeAndrade JR, Grant C, Dixon A. Joint distension and reflex muscle inhibition in the knee. J Bone Joint Surg Am 1965;47:313–320.

Dye SF, Wojtys EM, Fu FH, et al. Factors contributing to function of the knee joint after injury or reconstruction of the anterior cruciate ligament. Instr Course Lect 1999;48:185–198.

Escamilla RF, Fleisig GS, Zheng N, et al. Biomechanics of the knee during closed kinetic chain and open kinetic chain exercises. Med Sci Sports Exerc 1998;30:556–569.

Fitzgerald GK, Axe MJ, Snyder-Mackler L. The efficacy of perturbation training in nonoperative anterior cruciate ligament rehabilitation programs for physical active individuals. Phys Ther 2000;80: 128–140.

Hewett TE, Lindenfeld TN, Riccobene JV, et al. The effect of neuromuscular training on the incidence of knee injury in female athletes. A prospective study. Am J Sports Med 1999;27:699–706.

Hewett TE, Lindenfeld TN, Riccobene JV, et al. The effect of neuromuscular training on the incidence of knee injury in female athletes: a prospective study. Am J Sports Med 1999;27:699–706.

Hewett TE, Stroupe AL, Nance TA, et al. Plyometric training in female athletes. Decreased impact forces and increased hamstring torques. Am J Sports Med 1996;24:765–775.

Johnson DL, Urban WP, Caborn DNM, et al. Articular cartilage changes seen with magnetic resonance imaging-detected bone bruises associated with acute anterior cruciate ligament rupture. Am J Sports Med 1998;26:409–414.

Reinold MM, Wilk KE, Reed J, et al. Interval sport programs: Guidelines for baseball, tennis, and golf. J Orthop Sports Phys Ther 2002; 32:293–298.

Rodrigo JJ, Steadman JR, Sillman JF, et al. Improvement of full-thickness chondral defect healing in the human knee after debridement and microfracture using continuous passive motion. Am J Knee Surg 1994;7:109–116.

Skinner HB, Wyatt MP, Hodgdon JA, et al. Effect of fatigue on joint position sense of the knee. J Orthop Res 1986;4:112–118.

Snyder-Mackler L, Delitto A, Bailey SL, et al. Strength of the quadriceps femoris muscle and functional recovery after reconstruction of the anterior cruciate ligament: a prospective, randomized clinical trial of electrical stimulation. J Bone Joint Surg Am 1995;77: 1166–1173.

Spencer JD, Hayes KC, Alexander IJ. Knee joint effusion and quadriceps reflex inhibition in man. Arch Phys Med Rehabil 1984;65: 171–177.

Wilk KE. Are there speed limits in rehabilitation? J Orthop Sports Phys Ther 2005;35:50–51.

Wilk KE, Andrews JR. Rehabilitation following arthroscopic subacromial decompression. Orthopedics 1993;16:349–358.

Wilk KE, Escamilla RF, Fleisig GS, et al. A comparison of tibiofemoral joint forces and electromyographic activity during open and closed kinetic chain exercises. Am J Sports Med 1996;24:518–527.

Witvrouw EE, Lysens R, Bellemans J, et al. Intrinsic risk factors for the development of anterior knee pain in an athletic population. Am J Sports Med 2000;28:480–489.

Witvrouw E, Lysens R, Bellemans J, et al. Open versus closed kinetic chain exercises for patellofemoral pain. Am J Sports Med 2000;28: 687–694.

Wojtys EM, Huston LJ. Neuromuscular performance in normal and anterior cruciate ligament-deficient lower extremities. Am J Sports Med 1994;22:89–104.

STRENGTH AND CONDITIONING

STEPHEN E. LEMOS

Strength and conditioning are the essence of sport. It has been shown that training techniques have direct benefits and consequences for the athlete and their chosen sport. The understanding and science of strength and conditioning have defined the practices of professional and amateur athletes. Physicians should know how their patients, teams they cover, and communities are training to get an edge on the competition. They should learn the practices of team trainers and coaches. Physicians should continue to keep abreast of training lore, new trends in strength and conditioning, and new data on nutrition and supplements.

Strength and conditioning may be undertaken to improve or maintain performance and to prevent injury or recover from injury. Each goal requires specific exercise, rest, nutrition, and mindset to carry it out effectively. Healthy individuals may have sport-specific goals to improve or maintain performance that require specific direction to achieve them. Individuals participating in a sport with sport-specific injuries (i.e., soccer, sprained ankle) may benefit by a specific set of exercises to help prevent injury. Injured athletes, trying to return to sport after injury, will have specific needs and expectations that must be met with education and understanding.

Strength and conditioning comprise a complex interaction involving the gastrointestinal, respiratory, cardiovascular, and musculoskeletal systems. The gastrointestinal system supplies the fuel and building blocks to run and build the cardiovascular and musculoskeletal systems. The respiratory system benefits both resistance and endurance training. It supplies the blood with oxygen and takes out carbon dioxide. It also functions as an endocrine organ. The cardiovascular system supplies the musculoskeletal system with fuel to run it and the components to maintain, repair, and build it. The cardiovascular system itself responds and adjusts to activity and is as important to success at sport as the musculoskeletal system. The musculoskeletal system drives the individuals in sport. It is the interaction of these systems, with appropriate training of each, that will lead to maximizing the athlete for their chosen sport.

NUTRITION

Food and oxygen are the fuels that allow us to walk, run, jump, lift, throw, and think. Nutrition is important for all of us, but it is even more important to competitive athletes. Often, these individuals are most neglectful of what they consume or are poorly informed on what they should consume. Though increased attention has been focused on ergogenics aids, most of these supplements have no scientific basis for their use. In 2001, 30% of respondents (the National Collegiate Athletic Association [NCAA] Division IA varsity athletes) to a survey knew the correct percentage of carbohydrates (51% to 60%), 3% identified the correct percentage of protein (12% to 15%), and 11% recalled the correct percentage of fat (26% to 30%) based on a percentage of the kilocalories consumed per day. Seventy-nine percent of men and 65% of women indicated that they had used nutritional supplements during their college athletic career. Creatine was the most common supplement used, with men more likely to use it than women. Only 35% to

40% of the athletes correctly identified that vitamins were important for the regulation of metabolism, whereas there was a common misconception, especially among men, that they aided in weight gain.

The basic needs of the body for energy and for maintaining or building tissue are water, oxygen, carbohydrate, fat, protein, vitamins, and minerals. Athlete caloric intake can vary widely and is dependent on the daily energy expenditures and the body mass they must maintain. Male athletes have reported consuming between 10 and 25 MJ/day (2,500 to 6,000 cal/day). Female athletes, due to their decreased body mass, are expected to have a lower energy requirement. However, the calories they consume are reported to be 4 to 8 MJ/day (1,000 to 2,000 cal/day). Protein needs have been set at 1.2 to 1.6 g/kg/day (12% to 15% of total caloric intake) for both endurance- and resistance-trained athletes. Recent literature has found that protein supplementation in the elderly, combined with resistance training, can lead to increased strength and muscle mass when compared with controls. This has not been shown to be the case in their younger counterparts. Carbohydrate intake should represent between 50% and 60% of total caloric intake. For athletes needing to "carbohydrate load" before an event, an intake of 7 to 10 g of carbohydrate/kg/24 hours (50% to 80% of total energy intake) is recommended. Others feel that the same routine performed over a 72-hour period before the event is most beneficial. Last, fat should represent 26% to 30% of daily caloric requirement.

Nutritional Supplements

Creatine

Creatine is an over-the-counter (OTC) supplement that is taken as a 20 g/day load for 4 days and then a 2 g/day maintenance dose. It does appear to increase work capability over brief repetitive maximal exertions. Individual response does vary. It does not help endurance or maximal exertion for more than 60 seconds. Creatine appears relatively safe in a small number of studies. There is currently no good information on long-term use. There is some concern on how creatine may affect the heart and brain. There is no information on the use of creatine in adolescents. Early weight gain appears to be from water retention. There are anecdotal reports of cramping and hydration issues. There are sporadic reports of renal problems with creatine use.

Ephedra

Ephedra, originally taken off the shelves by the U.S. Food and Drug Administration (FDA), was allowed back in stores in 2005 as an OTC supplement. The fate of ephedra as an OTC supplement is unknown. It does not improve endurance or weight loss when used alone. Ephedra seems to improve endurance when combined with caffeine. This dietary supplement seems to improve weight loss when combined with caffeine in obese persons on dietary restrictions. No studies have shown weight loss in lean athletes, even when combined with caffeine.

Ephedra has many side effects, and controversy concerning its use has been expressed in the scientific community and the popular press. Ephedra is linked to serious adverse cardiovascular and central nervous system events such as hypertension, stroke, and sudden cardiac death. Effects experienced with ephedra intake are potentiated by the addition of caffeine; however, the FDA considers the combination of ephedra with caffeine unsafe. The International Olympic Committee and the NCAA ban systematic use of ephedra and ephedra with caffeine. The herbal forms of ephedra, in combination with caffeine found in OTC supplements, are not recommended.

Anabolic/Androgenic Steroids

Anabolic steroids have been shown to increase strength and muscle mass at high doses. They do not increase endurance performance. They exert their effects by acting like testosterone to build muscle, decrease the breakdown of muscle, and increase motivation due to the promotion of increased aggression. At supraphysiologic doses, the anticatabolic effect (prevention of muscle breakdown) may be more important than the anabolic effect. Oral preparations include methandrostenolone, stanozolol, oxandrolone, methyltestosterone, fluoxymesterone, and oxymetholone. Parental anabolic steroid preparations include nandrolene decanoate, nadrolone phenpropionate, testosterone enanthate, testosterone propionate, and testosterone cypionate.

There are many untoward side effects of anabolic steroid use. They lead to testicular atrophy and irreversible gynecomastia in males and irreversible virilization in females. Changes in lipid profiles for the worse and an elevation in blood pressure occur. Hepatic enzymes may elevate and jaundice, and hepatic malignancy may occur. The musculoskeletal system becomes susceptible to injury because the tendons have decreased tensile strength, which may lead to tendon rupture. The physis may fuse as well. Psychiatric concerns also exist, and addiction and dependence may occur with regular use of anabolic steroids.

Anabolic steroids are illegal, and illicit use is punishable as a felony. They are a schedule III controlled substance and are banned by all major sports and governing organizations. Anabolic steroids are condemned by both the American Academy of Pediatrics and the American College of Sports Medicine.

Androstenedione/Dehydroepiandrosterone

Androstenedione, or andro, has not been shown to increase testosterone production or strength with doses up to 100 mg. Andro taken at higher doses might increase testosterone, but this will cause an increase in estrogens at the same time. Dehydroepiandrosterone (DHEA) does not enhance performance and does not increase muscle strength.

Adverse changes occur in lipid profile. Increased estrogens exert their effects. At higher doses, the effects of increased androgens may be apparent. Andro may promote the growth of hormone-sensitive malignancies.

STRENGTH TRAINING

Up to 45% of the body is composed of skeletal muscle, which is characterized by fiber types. These fibers are classified as type I (slow twitch) or type II (fast twitch). Energy is provided for muscle contraction by aerobic and anaerobic respiration. Each energy-producing mechanism varies in its relative importance by fiber type and the demand of the task at hand. The muscle metabolizes glucose to produce lactic acid and energy in an anaerobic system, a very rapid source of energy. Glycogen is the primary fuel of aerobic respiration; where there is the presence of oxygen, energy is provided. Anaerobic respiration is primarily used in high-intensity, short-duration activities (i.e., sprinting). Aerobic respiration is primarily used for endurance activity (i.e., marathon running).

Skeletal muscles have general similarities and specific anatomic and physiologic variations that allow them to perform a specific task. Skeletal muscle has active and passive characteristics that aid in the development of tension. The BLIX curve (Fig. 34-1) demonstrates the total tension developed in a muscle is the sum of the voluntary active tension and passive tension. Muscle fibers have specific arrangements to improve the efficiency of force generated. Fiber pattern may be unipennate (all in same direction), bipennate (two directions), or multipennate (more than two different directions). Strength training depends solely on skeletal muscle adaptability. That is, if a muscle is stressed optimally during systematic training, it adapts and improves its function. Conversely, if a muscle is loaded suboptimally, its function deteriorates. A prime example of this is disuse atrophy that occurs with immobilization. Ideally, physical training will stress the body systematically to improve strength. Thus, three possible scenarios may occur with strength training. First, optimal stress occurs when the athlete exercises with appropriate loads and the muscle then adapts and increases in size and strength. Second, suboptimal stress occurs when no gains or decreases in muscle mass and strength are experienced. Third, overtraining and injury result from overloading muscles or having insufficient time between training sessions.

Strength training is used in virtually all athletic sports. Controversy surrounds what constitutes optimal strength training. It is important to identify dangerous practices in health clubs and in training rooms.

Physiology

The transport of oxygen by the respiratory and circulatory systems to the muscle mitochondria is essential for muscular function. Pulmonary ventilation is responsible for bringing oxygen to the bloodstream. Increased oxygen requirements during exercise are met by an increase in breathing rate and heart rate, which does not limit physical performance in healthy individuals. Oxygen must diffuse across the alveoli to reach the bloodstream. Conditioning can increase the number of alveoli available by improving lung aeration and the total surface area available for oxygen diffusion, thereby improving oxygen delivery to the bloodstream. The distribution of oxygen through the bloodstream to the skeletal muscle depends on cardiac output.

Skeletal muscle has a different physiological, histological, and biochemical make up based on fiber type. Fiber type within muscle is usually mixed; however, one type of fiber may predominate. Type I (slow twitch) fibers have relatively slow contraction times. This fiber type, based on its role, has large stores of triglycerides and is densely packed with mitochondria and myoglobin. Type I fibers have a low concentration of glycogen and associated glycolytic enzymes, as well as a low concentration of ATPase with a high pH (9.4) and use aerobic respiration (oxidative phosphorylation) for energy production. Type I fibers contain slow-type myosin chains, and the sarcomeres contain a wide Z-band. Type II fibers (fast twitch) have relatively faster contraction times and are needed for high-demand, short-duration activities and use anaerobic respiration to obtain energy. This shorter contraction time is obtained with fast-type myosin chains. Type II fibers have a lower density of mitochondria and hemoglobin. Type II fast-twitch fibers have been subdivided into four subtypes: IIA, IIB, IIC, and IIM. These divisions are based on the mitochondria and myoglobin content of the muscle fibers. Type IIA have a relatively higher myoglobin content than other type II subtypes and are recruited for moderate duration use.

EFFECTS OF PHYSICAL TRAINING ON MUSCLE

Endurance Training

In endurance exercise, myofibrils can respond to increased contractile activity by increasing their rates of synthesis of mitochondria and mitochondrial enzymes necessary of the aerobic pathway. A concomitant increase in muscle capillaries with increases in muscle myoglobin elevates concentrations of oxygen to aerobic respiration. Type IIB fibers demonstrated the smallest increase in the number of mitochondria when exposed to endurance training.

Endurance training also increases the muscle capacity to metabolize glycogen and fat. Fat may be used only through aerobic metabolism. Glycolysis is inhibited by fatty acid oxidation. This saves glycogen stores by having a greater portion of energy derived from fatty acid oxidation. Athletes derive a greater percentage of their energy from fatty acid than untrained individuals.

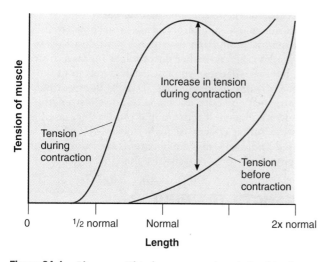

Figure 34-1 Blix curve. This demonstrates the relationship of muscle tension developed to precontraction muscle length and precontraction muscle tension.

Muscular Contraction and Exercise

There are three types of muscular contractions: isometric, isotonic, and isokinetic. Isometric exercise involves the application of a force without movement. Isotonic exercise involves force with movement. Isokinetic exercise involves the exertion of force at a constant speed.

Isometric Exercise

An isometric contraction occurs when a specific muscle contracts without movement of its associated joint. Isometric exercise increases strength at a specific joint angle at which the training is being affected. Subsequent research has shown that isometric exercise has limited applications in the training program of athletes. In the mid-1900s, isometric exercise was a popular form of strength training. If included with other techniques and training programs, isometric exercise may still have a role in training, especially rehabilitation (Fig. 34-2). Benefits of isometrics seem to occur during the early stages of training or rehabilitation. Optimal affect occurs with maximal contraction, and the duration contraction should be long enough to recruit as many fibers in the muscle group as possible. The greatest gains in strength occur when isometrics are practiced several times a day. As with other strength training techniques, excessive training will eventually lead to deterioration in performance (overtraining).

Isotonic Exercise

An isotonic muscle contraction occurs when the resistance or load remains constant throughout the contraction. Isotonic exercise is the most familiar strength training technique used. Isotonic loading methods include constant variable, eccentric, plyometric, and speed resistance.

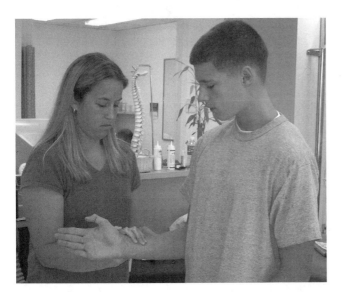

Figure 34-2 Isometric exercises. One advantage of isometric exercise is that it can be performed without assistance or with the assistance of the physical therapist as shown. When performed with the physical therapist, isometric exercises can help to delineate the patient's deficits. When used in athletics, isometrics can improve strength at a specific joint angle.

In constant resistance exercise, the load remains constant, but the difficulty in overcoming the resistance varies with the angle of the joint. For example, in a free-weight biceps curl, the weight is easier to lift as elbow flexion increases. Free weights (barbells and dumbbells) are the most common example. Isotonic training techniques continue to be the most popular with athletes, but many athletes supplement their training with other techniques.

There are many weight machines that attempt to load a muscle group uniformly throughout a range of motion. Variable-resistance exercise machines change the fulcrum as the joint moves so that the muscle receives a more similar load. This technique has not shown an improvement in strength training, compared with more traditional isotonic loading techniques.

An eccentric contraction occurs when a muscle lengthens while being loaded. Eccentric loading is then tension exerted during the lengthening of a muscle. During a dumbbell biceps curl, the muscles that created elbow flexion are eccentrically loaded as the bar is lowered. This technique often receives much attention and can be an effective training tool but has not been shown to be more effective than other techniques. Eccentric training can result in injury if not practiced carefully, and athletes should be judicious in its application.

Plyometric loading is implosion training, in which the muscles are loaded suddenly and forced to stretch before they can contract and illicit movement. Throwing a weighted ball at a trampoline or to an individual and then returning the ball to the thrower, allowing the throwing arm to go back in a reversal of the throwing motion and throwing back to the trampoline or individual is an example of plyometrics. Plyometrics, like eccentric loading, have been shown to increase muscle soreness and have an increased risk of injury. Plyometric exercises are a popular rehabilitation adjunct and are often used by jumping and throwing athletes (Fig. 34-3).

Proprioceptive neuromuscular facilitation or proprioceptive exercises are manual resistance exercise that uses a combination of isotonic and isometric loading. An example would be standing on a balance board in a one-leg stance on a foam rubber block and twisting on the other leg. Using a large balance ball has become popular with physical therapist and athletic trainers alike (Fig. 34-4). This technique is widely used by physical therapists and athletic trainers in the treatment and prevention of athletic injuries.

Isokinetic Exercise

An isokinetic muscle contraction occurs when a muscle shortens at the same speed. Thus, an isokinetic exercise controls the rate of muscle shortening. This involves a machine (isokinetic dynamometer) that exerts a force that equals that exerted by the individual. Isokinetic loading is popular, and at slow speeds, it has shown to be effective in increasing muscular strength at slow (less than or equal to 60 degrees/second) training speeds. An example of an isokinetic device is shown in Figure 34-5.

Muscular Adaptation

Muscle strength is directly related the to cross-sectional area of the muscle. Muscle strength, however, increases by

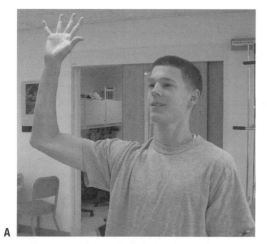

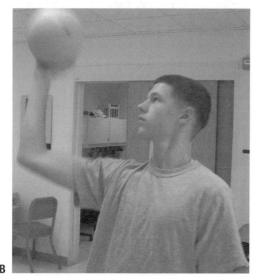

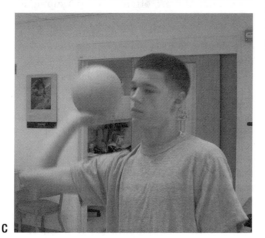

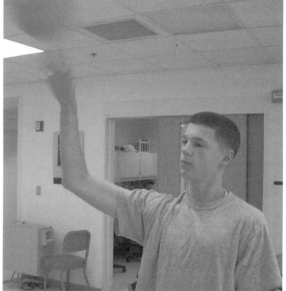

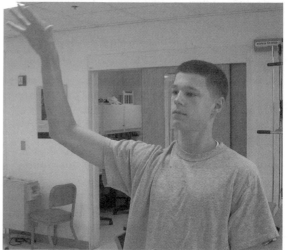

Figure 34-3 Plyometrics. This is a demonstration of implosion training of rotator cuff and periscapular muscles in overhead throwing athletes. There is a learning effect; therefore, it is imperative that the patient/athlete start with a very light weight when embarking on this training technique. A: First, the patient/athlete prepares to receive the weighted ball (in this case of upper extremity plyometrics). The subject receives the ball **(B)** and then goes through the desired motion, thereby eccentrically loading the rotator cuff and periscapular muscles **(C)**. **D,E:** The throw is completed on release of the ball and follow-through. The subject then prepares to receive the ball again.

increasing size and by increasing neuromuscular recruitment and increasing firing rates of their motor units. Age and gender are important determinants in the mechanisms involved in strength gains. After the age of 40, strength gains decrease dramatically in men and women, although gains are still achieved. Elderly men and women of all ages seem to increase strength mainly by neural adaptation (with

some hypertrophy), whereas young men rely more on increases in muscular size.

Training is important to develop threshold tension to increase strength. Distance runners tend to develop sarcoplasmic protein (oxidative enzymes, mitochondria mass, etc.), whereas weight lifters tend to develop contractile protein. Training programs should be designed with this in

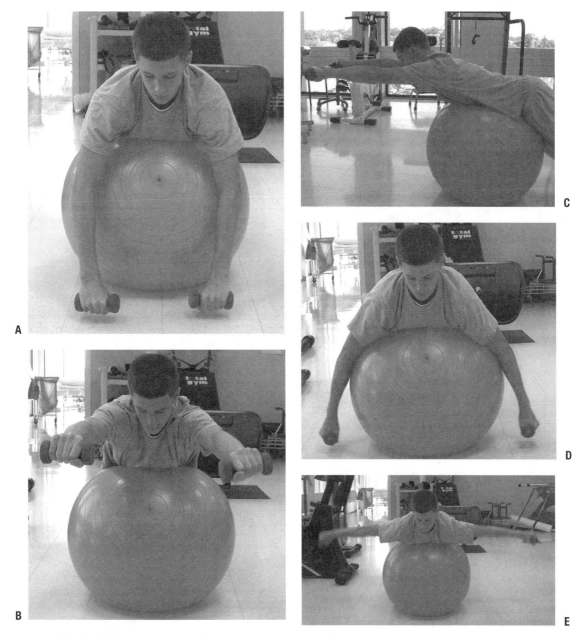

Figure 34-4   Proprioception with strength training. Periscapular and rotator cuff exercises can be combined with proprioceptive/balance work with the exercise ball. A–C: "Superman" exercises. D,E: Reverse flies.

mind so that the appropriate fiber types are stimulated and respond to enhance the performance of the athlete.

Muscles increase in cross-sectional area and strength after contractions near maximal tension. The intensity and duration of muscle tension influence the transport of amino acids into the cell, and this in turn influences the rate of protein synthesis. The ideal number of repetitions for strength training is between 4 and 12, and these should be performed in three or more sets. If fewer or greater numbers of repetitions are performed, strength gains are less. Sport-specific exercises are important to keep in mind when designing strength programs, because increased strength may be only one part of the desired improvement.

Muscles tend to adapt specifically to the nature of the exercise that is used to stress them. The strength and conditioning program should load the muscle in a similar manner in which they are to perform. Specific motor units are recruited within a muscle depending on the requirements of the contraction. The different fiber types have characteristic contractile properties. The slow-twitch fibers (red or type I fibers) are relatively fatigue resistant but have a lower tension capacity than the fast-twitch fibers (white or type II fibers). Fast-twitch fibers contract more rapidly and forcefully but are also less fatigue resistant. A motor unit contraction depends on the threshold of its alpha motor neuron. Low-threshold, slow-twitch fibers are recruited for

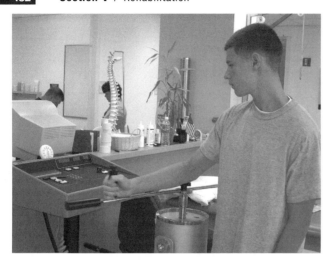

Figure 34-5 Isokinetic exercises. This is an example of an upper extremity device developed to apply a load at a specific uniform speed. It can be set to various angles and heights to accommodate patients and athletes and the specific muscle group tested.

low-intensity activity, which represent most human activity (i.e., walking, postural muscles). High-intensity/high-speed activities recruit fast twitch motor units, and this adaptation occurs as predominantly fast twitch muscles are recruited with high-velocity activities. Conversely, high-repetition/low-intensity stress recruits red oxidative slow-twitch fibers.

Training programs use this adaptation, and an athlete's muscle fiber type development appears to determine success in some sports. The amount of oxygen consumed per kilogram or Vo_2max, is increased in distance runners who have a high proportion of slow twitch muscles. Sprinters have a higher percentage of fast twitch muscle fibers.

The role of fiber type in sport is not clear. A diversity of muscle fiber type was found in the gastrocnemius of shot putters. Still, athletes who participate in explosive sports exhibit a higher fast-to-slow-twitch fiber area ratio than in a sedentary subject and endurance athletes despite this variability. In athletes who participate in high-intensity sports and have varied fiber type, they may excel due to individual differences in training intensity, and technique may counter their decreased relative percentage of fast-twitch fibers.

Cross-training is popular in the general recreational population; however, it appears that simultaneous participation in training programs designed to stimulate both strength and endurance will interfere with the ability to gain strength. Up to a 20% difference in strength has been observed in cross-trained subjects (strength and endurance) when compared with strength-trained subjects. The reverse has not been observed because strength training does not seem to have the same affect on endurance athletes.

A cross-sectional area of a muscle is directly related to its ability to develop tension. Whether increased muscle size occurs from hypertrophy (increased size of cells) or hyperplasia (increased number of cells), or both hypertrophy and hyperplasia, is not known. Muscle adaptation leading to increased cross-sectional area of the muscle is thought to occur primarily by increase in fiber size (hyper-

trophy). The contribution to increased cross-sectional area by increasing fiber number (hyperplasia) is only thought to occur in the neonatal period. Some investigators feel, however, that hyperplasia may be important later in life to increased muscle mass. "Fiber splitting" or hyperplasia has been proposed as a possible method to increase muscle mass. It is thought to primarily involve type IIB fibers. In this theory, the muscle fiber or cell splits longitudinally to increase fiber number.

Hypertrophy is still thought to be a major mechanism involved in enlarging muscle fiber size in response to the proper stimulus. Increased number and size of myofibrils increase muscle fiber size. Amino acid transport into cells is increased and enhances the amino acid incorporation into contractile proteins.

Biomechanical changes are observed during an increase in the cross sectional area of muscle during strength training. After high-intensity, slow-speed training using isokinetic loading, increases in muscle glycogen, creatine phosphate, ATP, ADP, creatine, phosphorylase, phosphofructokinase, and Krebs cycle enzyme activity occur. Training at faster speeds does not induce these changes. Resistance exercise must be progressively increased for constant gains and strength to occur. A protocol must be closely followed or overtraining will result. Strength-building exercises, which constantly increase resistance, can be counterproductive and can lead to overtraining.

Muscle Soreness

Muscle soreness that appears 24 to 48 hours after strenuous exercise is termed *delayed muscle soreness* and is an overuse injury that is commonly experienced. Eccentric muscle contractions are associated with delayed muscle soreness. Delayed muscle soreness should be distinguished from discomfort during exercise that is often associated with muscle fatigue and from painful involuntary cramps caused by strong contractions of susceptible muscles, such as the gastrocnemius. Delayed muscle soreness is characterized by a variable sense of discomfort in the muscles beginning several hours after exercise and reaching a maximum of 1 to 3 days. Patients usually demonstrate reduced activity and often display firm, swollen muscles. Peak swelling typically occurs 1 day or more after the exercises.

Swelling suggests increased intramuscular pressures are present and may be responsible in whole or in part for the pain experienced. Strength loss in the affected muscles is also common. In some cases, there can be up to a 50% loss in isometric strength immediately postexercise. This loss in strength usually lasts only a short time, however; measurable deficits can persist for up to 10 days. Torn tissue, muscle spasm, and connective tissue damage may cause muscle soreness after strength training.

A comparison of surface electromyograms to test the muscle spasms, myoglobin in the urine to test muscle damage theory, and measurement of the ratio of hydroxyproline to creatinine to assess disruption of the connective tissue elements supported the connective tissue theory of muscle soreness. Eccentrically loaded downhill runners demonstrated significant aberrations in serum enzymes that indicate muscle damage (creatine phosphokinase and lactate dehydrogenase) and disruption in cellular histology 1.5 to 2 days postexercise.

One accepted theory argues that mechanical factors are responsible for initial events leading to injury. High-intensity stresses within the muscle result in structural injury, such as sarcolemma damage that is accompanied by the influx of calcium. This damage to the sarcolemma is accompanied by diffusion of intracellular components into the interstitial and plasma. The phagocytic phase predominates as monocytes are converted to macrophages leading to an accumulation of histamine and kinins, as well as elevated pressure from tissue edema. This elevated pressure leads to an activation of receptors resulting in the painful sensation of delayed muscle soreness.

The structural abnormalities that accompany delayed muscle soreness include Z-ban streaming, A-band disruption, and myofibril misalignment. Soreness does not appear immediately after exercise despite muscle biopsies showing structural damage within an hour after exercise. These structural abnormalities are most severe 2 to 3 days after exercise and seem to occur primarily in the fast-twitch glycolytic (type IIB) fibers. Magnetic resonance imaging has demonstrated increased T_2 relaxation times lasting 2 to 3 months after the bout of exercise. Early changes in T_2 relaxation probably reflect changes in cell water resulting from edema and swelling. Muscle soreness has been shown to be directly associated with swollen muscle fibers in elevated muscle resting pressures 2 days after a single bout of eccentric exercise.

Serology studies have shown that exhausting exercise may be associated with an increased level of intramuscular enzymes in the serum. The increased levels of common indicators of muscle damage—such as creatine kinase, myoglobin, and lactate dehydrogenase—may correlate with the presence of muscle soreness. In addition, there are indications that connective tissue breakdown is also part of the syndrome of delayed muscle soreness. Increased levels of urinary hydroxyproline excretion, which are indicative of collagen or connective tissue breakdown, have been associated with delayed muscle soreness. Recent studies have shown that the structural damage that occurs with eccentric exercise is repairable. It appears that changes take place, which allows the involved muscles to become more resistant to damage from a subsequent bout of exercise. Delayed muscle soreness results from muscle injury and the breakdown of connective tissue. This mechanical event then leads to a release of multiple intracellular and extracellular factors. These injuries may result in an influx of fluid in the affected area, causing pressure, and local inflammatory response, causing pain.

Rest

Appropriate rest with exercise must occur at several levels. This rest must occur during the individual workout, between workouts, and before competition to ensure successful training. Rest is important for muscle recovery to maximize the tension and recruitment developed during the workout and to maximize between-workout gains. Despite the recognized importance of rest, the best interval has not been determined. In general, athlete strength training occurs with at least 1 to 2 days of rest between workouts on specific muscle groups. Detraining or loss of strength may result from as little as 3 days of inactivity. Other ways to rest muscle groups have been developed; however, no specific technique has proved superior.

Disuse Atrophy

A decline in muscle size and strength will accompany disuse, immobilization, and starvation. Disuse atrophy is another type of adaptation. Atrophy results in a decrease in both contractile and sarcoplasmic proteins. Disuse includes a cessation of exercise or change in exercise protocol and microgravity (space flight). Injury may result in atrophy without specific immobilization.

The rate of muscle atrophy is based on fiber type and does not occur at the same rate for each fiber type. Joint immobilization results in a faster rate of atrophy for slow-twitch fibers than fast-twitch muscle fibers. During rehabilitation, endurance—as well as strength—should be stressed because of the relative greater loss of slow-twitch muscle capacity. The position of the immobilized joint affects muscle length. When a muscle is fixed in a lengthened position, sarcomeres are added. If the muscle is immobilized in a shortened position, they are lost. A decrease in glycogen, adenosine triphosphate, creatine phosphate, and creatine also accompany muscle immobilization. Deconditioning of a strength athlete results in atrophy of fast- and slow-twitch fibers. An increase in mitochondrial volume and in maximal oxygen consumption in an elite power lifter during a 7-month detraining period has been observed. How endurance capacity of muscle improves during cessation of strength training, even in the absence of any endurance training, is not known.

TRAINING BASICS

There are three phases to a strength or conditioning session: warmup, workout, and cool down. Each plays a specific role in maximizing the workout.

Warmup increases the temperature of muscle to elevate the metabolic rate (Q^{10} effect) and increases the speed of muscle contraction. Preliminary exercise increases cardiac output and dilates muscle capillaries. Warmup stretching also aids in helping prepare muscle for activity. Proprioceptive and motor nerves are activated during warm up and this contribution may be important in preventing injury during exercise. Ten minutes of exercise is required to reach a steady-state muscle temperature. A time interval should exist between warmup and workout. Workouts are described, but they should begin gradually to work up to maximal output. This can be carried out even with strength work by performing high-repetition, lighter weight workout for the first set before doing heavier weight with fewer repetitions.

The cool-down period is often overlooked. This can involve a low-demand activity and stretching. A cool-down period may affectively minimize soreness and stiffness during the days after hard training or competition.

Endurance Training

Many types of training regimens exist to develop oxidative capacity and can be divided into two basic types: over distance training and high-intensity interval training. Both types of training appear to be important, and athletes can work through a range of combinations and variations of these two training types.

Overload occurs with physiological adaptations to increase endurance in response to appropriate stimuli. Manipulating two basic factors can vary endurance ability and overload: training intensity and training volume. Training volume is made up of training frequency and training duration.

The amount of adaptation and increased capacity is related to overload; the greater the overload, the greater the resulting adaptation and increase in functional capacity. A progressive increase in endurance training allows the time required for the physiological response. A gradual and discontinuous increase in training appears to increase athletic endurance performance best. This would include intense training sessions, followed by lighter training sessions and rest. Adequate rest each day of training is important, and hard training days should be interspersed with easy training days. Adaptation changes take place during rest; therefore, it is a very important part of training.

Endurance training increases Vo_2max and increases tissue aerobic capacity. Endurance athletes demonstrate very high values of Vo_2max. Despite this, increasing aerobic or mitochondrial capacity is more important than increasing Vo_2max in endurance athletes. In fact, Vo_2max actually correlates poorly with endurance performance. Many endurance athletes can use 90% of Vo_2 max for entire events, such as marathons and triathlons. This ability arises from internal mechanisms in muscles.

Over distance/endurance training consisting of sustaining a "sub-race pace" for an extended time and distance leads to increased mitochondrial concentration. Muscle mitochondria concentration correlates better with endurance ability than Vo_2max. Distance training develops the ability to use fats as fuels and the ability to protect mitochondria against damage during prolonged workouts.

It is as important to work on "race pace" as it is to develop aerobic capacity. Speed work fulfills that requirement and allows the athlete to recover. Speed work and interval training allow athletes to achieve a higher Vo_2max and race pace. It is training involving both quantity (overtraining/distance training) and quality (interval training/speed work), which allow endurance athletes to reach their goals.

Speed Work

Speed work or interval training is the best way to increase speed and maximize Vo_2max. Interval training has the benefit of training at close to competitive pace to improve technique, mitochondrial density, and Vo_2max.

Aerobic training along with high-intensity interval training uses the glycolytic system in muscle and will result in increased lactate acid formation. Lactic acid buildup stresses the athlete and helps acclimate the individual and improves mechanisms for its removal. Lactic acid removal occurs in the heart, red skeletal muscle, liver, and kidneys. The Cori cycle is the conversion of lactic acid to glucose (gluconeogenesis) and occurs primarily in the liver. Lactic acid removal is directly dependent on concentration, and interval training increases blood lactic acid levels, thereby stimulating the capacity to remove blood lactate levels.

As the competitive seasons approach, increasing interval/speed work and decreasing distance work will help to achieve peak performance.

Sprinting (intense, maximal activity lasting less than 30 seconds) requires an extreme degree of metabolic power. Energy for this power comes from a readily available and nonoxidative energy source present in muscle. The ability to recover rapidly is essential. Recovery is an aerobic process that can be improved through overdistance and interval training. Overdistance conditioning of sprinters may also reduce the incidence of injury.

Tapering before major competition is accomplished by decreasing training time, distance, and intensity. Tapering allows the athlete to recover and allow muscles to yield the full affect of adaptive responses. In addition, tapering before competition is sport-specific and can occur on several levels. Glycogen superconcentration in muscles is a 2- to 3-day process to regain maximum glycogen stores. In 5 to 7 days, nitrogen balance should return to zero from positive levels. The half-life of muscle respiratory proteins (mitochondria) indicates the adaptation period has a half-life of 2 weeks. Therefore, a layoff of more than 1 to 2 weeks should result in physiologic decay of fitness.

SUGGESTED READING

Abraham WM. Factors in delayed muscle soreness. Med Sci Sports 1977;9:11–20.

Arendt EA, ed. Orthopaedic Knowledge Update: Sports Medicine 2. Rosemont, IL: American Academy of Orthopaedic Surgeons, 1999: 37–42.

Brooks GA, Fahey TD, Baldwin KM, et al. Exercise Physiology: Human Bioenergetics and Its Applications, 3rd ed. New York: McGraw-Hill, 2000.

Burns RD, Schiller MR, Merrick MA, et al. Intercollegiate student athlete use of nutritional supplements and the role of athletic trainers and dietitians in nutrition counseling. J Am Diet Assoc 2004; 104:246–249.

Chandler TJ. Physiology of aerobic fitness/endurance. Instr Course Lect 1994;43:11–15.

Congeni J, Miller S. Supplements and drugs used to enhance athletic performance. Pediatr Clin North Am 2002;49:435–461.

Durell DL, Pujol TJ, Barnes JT. A survey of the scientific data and training methods utilized by collegiate strength and conditioning coaches. J Strength Cond Res 2003;17:368–373.

Faigenbaum AD. Strength training for children and adolescents. Clin Sports Med 2000;19:593–619.

George FJ. The athletic trainer's perspective. Clin Sports Med 1997; 16:361–374.

Goldberg AL. Mechanisms of growth and atrophy in skeletal muscle. In: Cassens RD, ed. Muscle Biology. New York: Marcel Dekker, 1972.

Hickson RC. Interference of strength development by simultaneously training for strength and endurance. Eur J Appl Physiol 1980;45: 255–263.

Koutedakis Y. Seasonal variation in fitness parameters in competitive athletes. Sports Med 1995;19:373–392.

Massey CD, Maneval MW, Phillips J, et al. An analysis of teaching and coaching behaviors of elite strength and conditioning coaches. J Strength Cond Res 2002;16:456–460.

Mazur LJ, Yetman RJ, Risser WL. Weight-training injuries. Common injuries and preventative methods. Sports Med 1993;16:57–63.

Rhea MR. Synthesizing strength and conditioning research: the meta-analysis. J Strength Cond Res 2004;18:921–923.

Shephard RJ. Exercise and training in women. Part I. Influence of gender on exercise and training responses. Can J Appl Physiol 2000; 25:19–34.

Sherry E, Wilson SF, eds. Oxford Handbook of Sports Medicine. Oxford, UK: Oxford Medical Publications, 1998.

INDEX

Page numbers followed by *a* indicate an algorithm, those followed by *b* indicate a box, those followed by *f* indicate a figure, and those followed by *t* indicate a table.

A

α-Blockers, for hypertension, 140
AAP (American Academy of Pediatrics), 28, 56
AATB (American Association of Tissue Banks), 116
A-band, 1–2
ABCs examination. *See* Airway, breathing, and circulation (ABCs) examination
Abdomen, in physical examination, 24
Abduction of shoulder, 178*f*, 179
Abduction traction technique, in posterior sternoclavicular joint dislocation, 265
β-*hemolytic Streptococcus*, group A, 159
Abscess, 159–160
Absolute contraindications, in metallic radial head fractures, 292*b*
Acceleration phase, 183, 183*f*, 201*t*, 209
Accessory anterior portal, in ankle arthroscopy, 130
Accessory navicular, 28
Accessory posterior portal, in ankle arthroscopy, 130
Acclimatization, 22
Acetaminophen
  for infectious mononucleosis, 165
  for viral upper respiratory infections, 163
Acetazolamide (Diamox), 38
Acetylcholine receptors, 4
Achilles tendon
  injuries, 14, 453–456
    insertional tendinitis in, 455–456
    tendinitis in, 453–454
  reconstruction of, 123–124, 123*f*
Achilles tendonitis, 76
ACI. *See* Autologous chondrocyte implantation (ACI)
AC joint. *See* Acromioclavicular (AC) joint
ACL. *See* Anterior cruciate ligament (ACL)
Acne, 160
Acne mechanica, 160
Acne vulgaris, grading and treatment of, 160*t*, 161*t*

Acquired immune deficiency syndrome (AIDS), steroids for, 36
Acquired instability of the shoulder, 214
Acquired stenosis, 102
Acromial arch, 245
Acromioclavicular (AC) joint
  anatomy of, 171–172, 171*f*, 254–255, 255*f*
  biomechanics of, 254–255, 255*f*
  complications in, 262
  coracoid process fractures in, 262
  diagnosis of, 257–258
  epidemiology of, 255–256
  etiology of, 256
  motion in, 171
  osteoarthritis in, 262
  pathophysiology and classification of, 256–257, 256*f*, 257*t*
  physeal injuries in, 262
  physical examination of
    compression test in, 192
    crossover impingement test in, 191, 191*f*
    distraction test in, 191–192, 191*f*
    piano key sign in, 192
  primary ligament restraints of, 255*b*
  research results about, 261–262
  soft-tissue allografts in, 117–118, 118*f*
  stability in, 171–172
  treatment of, 258–261
Acromion, ossification centers of, 246–247, 247*f*
Acromionectomy (radical), in subacromial impingement, 248
Acromioplasty, in subacromial impingement, 248
ACSM (American College of Sports Medicine), 46, 55
Actin, 44
Actions
  of amphetamines, 48
  of androstenedione, 36
  of β2-agonists, 38
  of branched-chain amino acids, 44
  of caffeine, 41–42
  of carbohydrate-protein combination, 46

of carbohydrates, 46
of chondroitin sulfate, 43
of creatine, 40
of dehydroepiandrosterone, 36
of ephedra, 42
of fats, 47
of glucosamine, 43
of glutamine, 45
of human growth hormone, 37
of steroids, 34
of testosterone, 33
of water and fluid replacement, 47
Active compression test, 26
Active mechanisms, in glenohumeral joint, 215
Activity modification
  in bony impingement, 450
  in os trigonum syndrome, 451
Acute avulsions of medial epicondyle, 298
Acute compartment syndrome, 9–10
Acute disc herniation, 102
Acute distal biceps ruptures, 119
Acute illness, clearance and, 28
Acute olecranon bursitis
  diagnosis of, 296
  treatment of, 297
Acute otitis media (AOM), 147
Acute patellar dislocation, 397*b*, 399, 400*f*
Acute peroneal tendon dislocation, 452–453, 453*t*
Acute tears, in peroneal tendon injuries, 451–452
Acute trauma
  metallic radial head fractures and, 292*b*
  patellofemoral disorders and, 392–393
Acyclovir
  for herpes simplex, 153
  for infectious mononucleosis, 165
Adduction traction technique, in posterior sternoclavicular joint dislocation, 265–266
Adenosine diphosphate (ADP), 6
Adenosine, 41
Adenosine triphosphate (ATP), 3, 6, 89
Adolescent athletes
  ankle injuries in, 76–79

Adolescent athletes (*contd.*)
  background about, 61
  elbow injuries in, 66
  foot injuries in, 79
  hip injuries in, 67–68
  knee injuries in, 68–76
  shoulder injuries in, 61–64
  spine injuries in, 66–67
  wrist injuries in, 64–66
ADP (Adenosine diphosphate), 6
Adrenocorticotropic hormone, 33
Adson's maneuver, 195–196, 195*f*
Adult lateral elbow, 308–313
Advanced Trauma Life Support
      guidelines, 273, 274
Adverse effects
  of amphetamines, 48
  of androstenedione, 36
  of β2-agonists, 38
  of β-hydroxy-β- methylbutyrate, 39
  of branched-chain amino acids, 45
  of caffeine, 42
  of carbohydrate-protein combination,
      46
  of carbohydrates, 46
  of chondroitin sulfate, 43
  of dehydroepiandrosterone, 36
  of ephedra, 43
  of fats, 47
  of glucosamine, 43
  of glutamine, 45
  of human growth hormone, 38
  of protein, 44
  of sports supplements, 40–41
  of steroid use, 34–35, 35*b*
  of testosterone, 33–34
  of 3,4,5-trihydroxystilbene, 37
  of water and fluid replacement, 47
Aerobic nonimpact exercise, in pelvis
      stress fracture, 327
Age/aging. *See also* Aging athletes
  anterior shoulder instability and,
      218, 219
  biomechanical effects on, 14
  ligaments and, 17
  stress fractures and, 106
Aggression, steroids and, 34
Aging athletes
  about, 81
  articular cartilage injuries and,
      83–84
  epidemiology of, 81–83
  expected physiologic results of,
      82–83
  joints and, 83
  muscle strains and, 84–85
  rehabilitation and, 85
  surgery and, 86
Aircast, in chronic peroneal tendon
      injuries, 452
Aircast pneumatic leg brace, in leg
      overuse injuries, 434–435
Air movement, 24
Airway, breathing, and circulation
      (ABCs) examination, 92
AITFL (Anterior-inferior tibiofibular
      ligament), 444

ALB (Anterolateral bundle), 362–363,
      363*f*
Alcohol, 23, 35, 49
Alendronate, 56
All-arthroscopic fixation technique
      (first-generation devices), in
      meniscal injuries, 414
All arthroscopic hybrid suture fixation
      technique, in meniscal
      injuries, 415*t*
All arthroscopic nonsuture fixation
      technique, in meniscal
      injuries, 415*t*
All-arthroscopic suture fixation
      technique (second-generation
      devices) in meniscal injuries,
      414
Allergies, 21
Allograft
  drawback of, 340*t*
  graft sources and, 345*t*
  tissues, 340
Allograft osteochondral plugs, in
      articular cartilage lesions,
      395*b*
Allylamines, for tinea, 157
ALPSA (Anterior labrum periosteal
      sleeve avulsion), 216, 216*f*
Amantadine, for influenza, 166
Ambulatory (office) examination, in
      spinal injuries, 97
Amenorrhea
  clearance and, 28–29
  eating disorders and, 53–56
  premature osteoporosis and, 53–56
  primary, 24, 55
  steroids and, 35
American Academy of Neurology, 91*t*
American Academy of Pediatrics
      (AAP), 28, 55
American Association of Tissue Banks
      (AATB), 116
American College of Obstetrics and
      Gynecology, 60
  guidelines for exercise during
      pregnancy and postpartum,
      59*b*
American College of Sports Medicine
      (ACSM), 44, 53
American Medical Association (AMA),
      guidelines for grading MCL or
      LCL complex injuries, 349*t*
American Orthopedic Society for
      Sports Medicine, 51, 88
American Shoulder and Elbow
      Surgeons, 177
Americans with Disabilities Act of
      1990, 30
Amino acids, 44–45
Aminoglutethimide (Cytadren), 37
Amoxicillin, for otitis media, 148
Amphetamines, 47–48
Anabolic/androgenic steroids, 476
Anabolic steroids, 7, 22–23, 32–33, 35
Anaerobic glycolysis, 6
Analgesics
  for barotrauma, 148

  for idiopathic brachial neuritis, 275
  for otitis externa, 147
  for otitis media, 148
Anaphylaxis, 21
Anatomic risk factors, anterior cruciate
      ligament injury and, 335–336
Anatomy
  of acromioclavicular (AC) joint,
      171–172, 171*f*, 254–255,
      255*f*
  of anterior cruciate ligament (ACL),
      333, 334*f*
  of axillary nerve, 277–278, 278*f*
  of brachial plexus, 272
  of glenohumeral and scapulothoracic
      motion, 172–175
  of hip, 320–323, 322*f*
  of ligaments, 16–17
  of long thoracic nerve, 281, 281*f*
  of medial collateral ligament complex
      of the knee, 349
  of medial epicondylitis, 313
  of multiple ligament-injured knee,
      376–378, 377*f*
  of musculocutaneous nerve, 147*f*,
      280
  of olecranon fractures, 285–286
  of pelvis, 320, 321*f*
  of posterior cruciate ligament,
      362–363, 363*f*
  of posterolateral corner, 354
  of rotator cuff, 244–245
  of rotator interval, 245
  of shoulder instability areas, 237*t*
  of spinal accessory nerve, 282, 283*f*
  of sternoclavicular (SC) joint,
      169–170, 170*f*, 262–263
  of suprascapular nerve, 275–276,
      275*f*
  of thigh, 320–323
  of upper extremity nerve, 268, 269*f*,
      270*f*
Anchor-first technique, in anterior
      shoulder instability, 224–226,
      225*f*
Androstenedione, 36, 476
Anemia, 143–144
Anesthetic infiltration, in nerve
      entrapment syndrome, 330
Anesthetic (local), in bursitis, 330
Angiofibroblastic hyperplasia, 14
Angiotensin-converting enzyme
      inhibitors, for hypertension,
      140
Anisocoria, 22, 24
Ankle. *See also* Ankle injuries; Bony
      anatomy of ankle; Chronic
      ankle pain
  arthroscopy of, 129–130
  gymnast, 78
  of immature and adolescent athletes,
      76–79
  physical examination of, 26
Ankle injuries
  Achilles tendon and
    insertional tendinitis in, 455–456

rupture in, 454–455
tendinitis in, 453–555
biomechanics of, 446
bony anatomy of ankle, 444
chronic pain and
ankle impingement in, 448–451
instability in, 446–448
fractures and
classification of, 459–460
diagnosis of, 460
treatment of, 460–462
ligamentous anatomy and
lateral ankle ligament complex in, 445
medial deltoid ligament in, 445
syndesmotic ligament complex in, 445–446
muscular anatomy and
peroneus longus and brevis in, 446
tibiotalar articulation in, 446
osteochondral lesions of the talus and
classification of, 457, 457t
diagnosis of, 457–459
etiology of, 456–457
osteochondral lesions of the tibia and, 459
peroneal tendon and
acute tears in, 451–453
chronic tears in, 452
subluxation/dislocation in, 452–453
tears in, 451
tendinitis in, 451
Anorexia nervosa, 23, 54b
Anterior acromioplasty, in subacromial impingement, 248
Anterior cruciate ligament (ACL), 14, 53, 115
acidity level of, 338t
anatomy of, 333, 334f
biomechanics of, 333–335, 334f, 335f
classification of, 336
diagnosis of, 337
epidemiology of, 335
etiology of, 335
injuries in female athletes, 57–60
interoperative complications in, 345
in knees, 348
laxity of, 336t
pathophysiology of, 335–336
postoperative complication in, 345–346
rehabilitation after surgery in, 346–347
results of surgery studies, 346t
soft-tissue allografts in, 120, 121f
tears, 69
treatment of, 337–345
Anterior drawer test, 193, 193f, 337t, 350
Anterior-inferior tibiofibular ligament (AITFL), 444
Anterior labrum periosteal sleeve avulsion (ALPSA), 216, 216f

Anterior ligament of Humphrey, 404, 405f
Anterior portals
in ankle arthroscopy, 129–130
in shoulder arthroscopy, 128
Anterior shoulder instability
categories of, 214–215
description of, 214
diagnosis of, 218–221, 221a
etiology and epidemiology of, 218
management of, 221a
mechanisms of, 215–218
pathogenesis of, 215–218
pathophysiology of, 215–218
postoperative management in, 227–230
sulcus sign in repair of, 235f
treatment of, 221–230
Anterior single-incision approach, in biceps tendon rupture and, 307
Anterior slide-test, for superior labral lesions, 204t
Anterior sternoclavicular (SC) joint dislocation, 264–265
Anterior-superior portal, in shoulder arthroscopy, 128
Anterior talofibular ligament (ATFL), 445
Anterior tibia stress fracture, 58f
Anterolateral bundle (ALB), 362–363, 363f
Anterolateral impingement, 448
Anterolateral portals, in knee arthroscopy, 125–126, 126f
Anteromedial portals, in knee arthroscopy, 125–126, 126f
Antibiotics
for cellulitis, 159
for chronic bursitis, 297
for folliculitis, 156
for impetigo, 155
for otitis extena, 147
for otitis media, 148
for travelers diarrhea, 143
Antidrug Abuse Act, 1988, 35
Antiestrogens, 37
Antihistamines
for barotrauma, 148
for exercise-induced anaphylaxis, 137
Anti-inflammatory drugs
for athletic pubalgia, 331
for osteoarthritis of the elbow, 303
for valgus extension overload, 305
Antilordotic (Boston) brace, for spondylolysis, 99
Antistaphylococcal penicillin, for impetigo, 155
Anxiety, 42, 43
AO classification of ankle fractures, 459
AOM (Acute otitis media), 147
Apley's compression and distraction test, 408, 409f, 410
Apophyseal injuries, 326, 326b
Apprehension test
for patellar instability, 74f

for shoulder instability, 26, 188f, 192, 192f, 204, 219
Aromatization, 34–35
Arrhythmogenic right ventricular dysplasia (ARVD), 141
Arteriogram, in upper extremity nerve injury, 271–272
Arthroplasty, 86
Arthroscopic acromioplasty, in subacromial impingement, 248
Arthroscopic debridement
in Bennett lesions, 211
in chondral lesions surgery, 424t, 425t
Arthroscopic lateral release, in adult lateral elbow, 309
Arthroscopic outside-in technique, in meniscal injuries, 413
Arthroscopic surgery
of the ankle, 129–132, 448
diagnostic
in posterior cruciate ligament injury, 368
in shoulder injury, 16;6
of the elbow, 131–133, 303, 305b
complications in, 131–133
portals in, 131–132, 131f
of the knee, 125–127
in multiple ligament-injured knee, 383–384
in osteochondral lesions of talus, 458
overview of, 125
of the shoulder, 128–129
techniques of
in adult lateral elbow, 309–310
in anterior shoulder instability, 221–222
Bankart repair, 224–227, 225f, 226f, 227f, 229t
assisted inside-out technique in meniscal injuries, 413–414
in full-thickness rotator cuff tears, 252
in internal impingement, 249
in multidirectional shoulder instability, 239
in osteochondritis dissecans, 76
in partial-thickness rotator cuff tears, 250
in posterior instability, 237–238, 238f
in subacromial decompression, 208
Arthroscopy Association of North America, 127
Arthrotek tensioning device, 387, 387f
Articular cartilage injuries
in aging athletes, 83–84
classification of, 419–420, 419f, 421f
diagnosis of, 422
epidemiology of, 418
organization and composition of, 418–419, 419f, 420f, 420t
pathophysiology of, 420–422

Articular cartilage injuries (*contd.*)
  repair of, 419, 421*f*
  treatment of, 422–429
Articular cartilage lesions, surgical
  treatment for, 397*b*
ARVD. *See* Arrhythmogenic right
  ventricular dysplasia (ARVD)
Asparagines, 45
Aspartate, 45
Associated knee tests, 337*t*
Associated posterior cruciate ligament
  injury, treatment of,
  373–374, 373*f*, 374*f*
Asthma
  clearance and, 29
  marijuana and, 49
Astringents, 13;9*t*
Antiestrogens, 37
ATFL (Anterior talofibular ligament),
  445
Athletes. *See also* Adolescent athletes;
  Female athletes; Immature
  athletes; Male athletes
  feet of, 157–158, 158*f*
  pediatric sport injuries of, 62*b*
Athletic considerations
  in acne, 160
  in community-acquired MRSA, 160
  in folliculitis, 157
  in herpes simplex, 154
  in impetigo, 155–156
  in infectious mononucleosis, 165
  in influenza, 166–167
  in streptococcal pharyngitis, 163
  in tinea, 157–159
  in viral upper respiratory infections,
  163–164
  in warts, 161
Athletic Drug Reference Book, 49
Athletic pubalgia, 331–332
ATP. *See* Adenosine triphosphate
  (ATP)
Atraumatic instability of the shoulder,
  215
Atrial fibrillation, hypertrophic
  cardiomyopathy (HCM) and,
  138
Atrophy, in muscle injury, 8–10
Augmentation technique, in rupture of
  Achilles tendon, 455
Auricular hematoma, 148–149, 149*f*
Auscultation, 24
Autograft, 345*t*
Autograft CA ligament, 261
Autologous chondrocyte implantation
  (ACI)
  in articular cartilage lesions, 395*b*
  in chondral lesions surgery, 424*t*,
  425
  surgery and, 427*t*
Avascular necrosis (AVN), 79
AVN. *See* Avascular necrosis (AVN)
Avulsion fracture, 218, 287, 287*f*, 326,
  326*b*
Axillary nerve injury
  anatomy of, 277–278, 278*f*

diagnosis of, 278–279
etiology of, 277–278
Axonotmesis, 269
Azithromycin
  for folliculitis, 159*t*
  for impetigo, 155, 159*t*
  for otitis media, 148
  for streptococcal pharyngitis, 163,
  164*t*
  for travelers diarrhea, 143

B
Babinski response, 97
Balloon venoplasty, in effort
  thrombosis, 211
Bandlike fracture line, in stress
  fracture, 109
Bankart lesion, 215–216, 215*f*
Bankart repair, in anterior shoulder
  instability surgery
  anchor-first technique in, 224–226,
  225*f*
  results of, 229*t*
  suture-first technique in, 226–227,
  226*f*
Banned or restricted drugs, 37–39
Barotrauma, 149
β²-adrenergic agonists, for exercise-
  induced bronchospasm (EIB),
  136
β²-Agonists, 40, 137
β-blockers
  as banned or restricted drug, 39
  for hypertension, 140
  for hypertrophic cardiomyopathy
  (HCM), 138
  for long QT syndrome, 139
β-hydroxy-β- methylbutyrate (HMB),
  40*t*, 41–47
BCAA. *See* Branched-chain amino
  acids (BCAA)
Beach chair position, in anterior
  shoulder instability, 222, 222*f*
Belly press test, 175*f*, 189–190, 190*f*,
  203*t*, 251
Bennett lesion, 211
"Bennies," 47–48
Benzoyl peroxide, 160*t*
Bernageau view, 232
Berthold, A., 33
Best motor response (M), in Glasgow
  coma scale, 92*t*
Biceps, long head of, 181, 181*f*
Biceps femoris, 354–355
Biceps load test, for glenoid labrum,
  195
Biceps Speed's test, 176*f*, 203*t*
Biceps tendon (BT), 172*f*. *See also*
  Biceps tendon (BT) rupture
  Speed's test for, 190, 190*f*
  Yergason's test for, 190, 190*f*
Biceps tendon (BT) rupture
  diagnosis of, 306–307
  pathophysiology of, 306
  treatment of, 307
Biochemistry of ligaments, 16–17
Biology, in sports medicine, 465

Biomechanical risk factors, anterior
  cruciate ligament injuries and,
  336
Biomechanical testing, for posterior
  cruciate ligament injury, 366
Biomechanics
  of acromioclavicular (AC) joint,
  254–255
  of ankle injuries, 446
  of anterior cruciate ligament (ACL),
  333–335, 334*f*, 335*f*
  of elbow injury, 285
  of ligaments, 17
  of multiple ligament-injured knee,
  376–378
  of patellofemoral disorders, 392,
  392*b*, 392*f*
  of the rotator cuff, 245–246
  of shoulder injuries, 200–201
  of skeletal muscles, 4–6
  of sternoclavicular (SC) joint,
  262–263
  of tendons, 13
  of throwing, 183–184, 183*f*
Biplanar osteotomy, in posterior
  cruciate ligament injury, 366
Bismuth subsalicylate, 143
Bisphosphonates, 56
Black individuals, stress fractures in,
  106
Blisters, 161
BLIX curve, 4–5, 6*f*, 477, 477*f*
Blood doping, 144
  erythropoietin and, 39
Blood pressure, 24, 26. *See also*
  Hypertension
BMD. *See* Bone mineral density
  (BMD)
Body fat analysis, 24
Body weight (BW), 182
Bone loss, anterior shoulder instability
  and, 218
Bone mineral density (BMD)
  osteoporosis and, 55
  reproductive function and, 56
  stress fractures and, 106, 107
Bone-patellar-bone Harvest, in anterior
  cruciate ligament injury, 341
Bone-patellar tendon-bone (BTB)
  grafts, 339, 340*t*
Bone remodeling, in stress fractures,
  105
Bone scanning
  in osteitis pubis, 327
  in stress fractures, 433, 433*f*, 434*t*
Bone scintigraphy, 433
Bone-to-bone fixation, in anterior
  cruciate ligament injury,
  340–341
Bony anatomy of ankle
  fibula in, 444
  talus in, 444–445
  tibia in, 444
Bony avulsions knee injury, 379
Bony impingement, 449–450, 449*t*
Bony injuries

avulsion fractures and apophyseal injuries in, 326
fracture and dislocation in, 325
osteitis pubis in, 327
slipped capital femoral epiphysis in, 386
stress fractures in, 326–327
Braces/bracing
for acute peroneal tendon injuries, 452
for anterior cruciate ligament injuries, 335, 338
for anterolateral impingement, 448
for articular cartilage injuries, 422, 86
for juvenile disc herniation, 67
lace-up, for chronic peroneal tendon injuries, 452
for lateral patellar compression syndrome, 395, 396
for medial collateral ligament complex injuries, 351
for osteochondral lesions of talus, 458
for patellar tilt, 397
for spondylolysis, 67
for tendinitis, 451
Brachial plexopathy, 266
Brachial plexus injuries, 268, 270f
anatomy of, 270f, 272
diagnosis of, 273–274
etiology of, 273, 273f
stretch test for, 195
treatment of, 274
Branched-chain amino acids (BCAA), 40t, 44–45
Breast
cancer, 37
steroids and, 35
Brisement, in tendinitis, 454
Bronchitis, marijuana and, 49
Brown adipose cells, 38
Brown-Sequard, C., 33
BT. See Biceps tendon (BT)
BTB grafts (Bone-patellar tendon-bone grafts), 339, 340t
Bucket-handle meniscal tears, 407, 407t
Bulbocavernosus reflex, in spinal injuries, 97
Bulimia nervosa, 23, 54b
Bungee effect, 340
Burner mechanism of injury, 273f
Burners/stingers, 22, 29, 101–102
Burner syndrome, in transient quadriplegia, 101
Bursitis, 329–330, 329f
patellar, 399–400
Burst fractures, in lumbar spine injuries, 98
BW (Body weight), 182

C
CAD. See Coronary artery disease (CAD)
Caffeine, 41–42
Calcaneofibular ligament (CFL), 445

Calcific tendonitis
classification and pathophysiology of, 252–253
natural history of, 252t
progressive stages of, 253f
treatment of, 253
Calcium
in leg overuse injuries, 434
stress fractures and, 106–107, 113
Calcium channel blockers
for hypertension, 140
for Raynaud's phenomenon, 142
Calcaneal stress fractures, 107
CA ligament (Coracoacromial ligament), 255
Calluses, 162–163, 163f
Candida, 157
Cannabis saliva, 49
Cantu scale of concussions, 94
Capsular ligament, 263
Carbohydrate-protein combination (CHO/PRO), 46
Carbohydrates, 46
Carbonic anhydrase inhibitors, 38
Cardiac arrhythmias, 43
Cardiovascular concerns, 137–141
Cardiovascular condition
adverse effects of steroids on, 35b
clearance and, 28
medical history and, 21–22
physical examination and, 24
Cardiovascular system, steroids and, 35
Cast/casting
in Osgood-Schlatter syndrome, 75
in osteochondral lesions of talus, 458
in rupture of Achilles tendon, 454
Catheter-directed thrombolysis, in effort thrombosis, 211
Cauda equina syndrome (CES), 96
CC ligaments. See Coracoclavicular (CC) ligaments
Cellulitis, 159–160
Central nervous system
adverse effects of steroids on, 35b
stimulants, 32, 47–48
Cephalexin
for cellulitis, 159
for impetigo, 159t
Cervical spinal cord neurapraxia, 22
Cervical spine
evaluation in upper extremity nerve injury, 271
injuries, 100–103
Cervical stenosis, 102
CFL (Calcaneofibular ligament), 445
Chain reaction, in influenza, 166
Chest
pain, 21
tightness, 22
Chinese ephedra. See Ephedra
CHL (Coracohumeral ligament), 172f, 180, 232, 245
Cholesterol
screening in physical examination, 26
steroids and, 35

Chondral defects, 324
Chondral injury, 211
modified international cartilage repair society classification system for, 422t
Outerbridge classification of, 421t
Chondral lesions, 418, 424t
Chondroitin sulfate, 41t, 43, 423
CHO/PRO. See Carbohydrate-protein combination (CHO/PRO)
Chronic Achilles tendon ruptures, 123
Chronic ankle pain
ankle impingement in
anterolateral impingement and, 448
bony impingement and, 449–450, 449t
os trigonum syndrome and, 450–451
posterior impingement and, 448–449
syndesmotic impingement and, 449
instability in, 446–447
diagnosis of, 447
treatment of, 447–448
Chronic cocaine, 48
Chronic compartment syndrome, 10
Chronic distal biceps ruptures, 119–120
Chronic grade III PLC instability, in posterolateral corner injuries, 360
Chronic medial apophysitis, 298
Chronic olecranon bursitis
diagnosis of, 296–297
treatment of, 297
Chronic tears, in peroneal tendon injuries, 452
Chronology of instability, in the shoulder, 215
Ciprofloxacin, for travelers diarrhea, 143
CKC (Closed kinetic chain), 478–479
Clarithromycin, for impetigo, 155
Classic subacromial impingement, 208
Classification
of acromioclavicular (AC) joint, 256–257, 256f, 257t
of acute peroneal tendon dislocations, 453t
of ankle fractures, 459
of anterior cruciate ligament (ACL), 336
of articular cartilage injuries, 419–420, 419f, 421
of concussion, 91, 91t
of coronoid fractures, 292f, 292t
of elbow dislocation/terrible triad, 294–295, 294f
of instability of the shoulder, 214–215
of medial collateral ligament complex in the knee, 349
of meniscal tears, 406–407, 406f
of multiple ligament-injured knee, 378–379, 379t

Classification (*contd.*)
  of olecranon fractures, 286, 286*t*
  of osteochondral lesions of talus, 457, 457*t*
  of osteochondritis dissecans of capitellum, 300*t*
  of osteochondritis dissecans of the elbow, 300*t*
  of patellofemoral disorders, 392*b*
  of popliteal artery entrapment syndrome, 442*t*
  of posterolateral corner, 354
  of sports, 27, 27*b*, 28*b*
  of sternoclavicular (SC) joint, 264–266
Clavicle, 169, 171*f*, 262, 266
Clearance
  anemia and, 144
  barotrauma and, 148
  blood doping and, 144
  congenital coronary anomalies and, 139
  exercise-induced bronchospasm and, 137
  eye trauma and, 146
  hypertension and, 140
  hypertrophic cardiomyopathy and, 138
  long QT syndrome and, 139–140
  nasal injuries and, 146
  otitis media and, 148
  of patients after physical examination, 27
  Raynaud's phenomenon and, 142
  sickle cell anemia and, 144
  thalassemia and, 144
  travelers diarrhea and, 143
Clenbuterol, 36
Clindamycin, 160, 160*t*
Clomid (Clomiphene citrate), 37
Clomiphene citrate (Clomid), 37
Closed kinetic chain (CKC), 478–479
Clostridium tetani, 12
Cloxacillin, for impetigo, 155
Clunk test
  for glenoid labrum, 194
  for stressing anterior labrum, 64*f*
  for superior labral lesions, 204*t*
Cocaine, 35, 48
Cocking phase, 183, 183*f*, 201*t*
Congenital coronary anomalies, 139
Collagen, 11, 13, 14, 16
Collateral ligaments knee injury, 379
Committee on Head Injury nomenclature of the Congress of Neurological Surgeons, 88
Committee on Sports Medicine of the American Academy of Pediatrics, 55
Common clinical conditions, in skeletal muscles, 7–10
Common cold, 163
Communication with athletes, 27
Community-acquired MRSA, 160
Compartment syndrome
  acute, 9–10
  chronic, 10

Competition
  Olympic athletes and ban from, 32
  substances banned form use in, 49–50
Complete distal biceps ruptures, 119
Complete rupture, in partial ruptures of Achilles tendon, 454
Complex (degenerative) meniscal tears, 407, 407*t*
Complications
  in acromioclavicular joint disorder surgery, 262
  in ankle arthroscopy, 130–131
  in anterior cruciate ligament surgery, 345–346
  in biceps tendon rupture surgery, 307
  in elbow arthroscopy, 131–133
  in elbow dislocation/terrible triad, 295
  in elbow joint loose bodies surgery, 306
  in hyperextension valgus overload, 315
  interoperative, in anterior cruciate ligament, 345
  in knee arthroscopy, 127
  in olecranon fractures surgery, 289
  in osteoarthritis of the elbow surgery, 304
  in shoulder arthroscopy, 129
  in ulnar collateral ligament injury surgery, 318
Compression, in athletic pubalgia, 331
Compression Bankart lesion, 218
Compression-rotation test, for Glenoid labrum, 195
Compression stress fractures, 108
Compression test, for AC joint, 192
Computed tomography (CT)
  acetabular fractures and, 324
  anterior shoulder instability and, 220
  bony impingement and, 450
  brachial plexus injuries and, 274
  congenital coronary anomalies and, 139
  epidural hematoma and, 90*f*
  exertional compartment syndrome and, 439
  intra-articular disk ligament injury and, 266
  navicular fractures and, 110
  olecranon stress fractures and, 112
  os trigonum syndrome and, 451
  shoulder injury and, 205
  sternoclavicular (SC) joint and, 264
  upper extremity nerve injury and, 271
Concealed foreign body, in the eye, 145
Concussion. *See* Head injuries
Conditioning, in shoulder injury, 205
Congenital anomalies, 140, 103
Congress of Neurological Surgeons, 88
Conoid ligament, 255, 455*b*
"Conservative" therapy, 242
Contact, in sports, 27, 27*b*

Contact/collision, in classification of sports by contact, 27, 27*b*
Continuous passive motion (CPM), 478
Contraceptives, oral, 55
Contraindications
  in meniscal allograft transplantation, 416*b*
  in metallic radial head fractures, 292*b*
Contrast arteriography, in popliteal artery entrapment syndrome, 442–443
Contusion
  description of, 328–329
  hip pointer, 329
  as mechanism of tendon injury, 14
  in muscle injury, 8
  myositis ossificans, 329
  thigh, 329
Convulsive disorders, clearance and, 30
Coracoacromial (CA) ligament, 255
Coracoclavicular (CC) ligaments, 171, 185, 255, 260, 260*f*
Coracohumeral ligament (CHL), 172*f*, 180, 232, 245
Coracoid impingement, 209
Coracoid process fractures, in acromioclavicular (AC) joint, 262
Corneal abrasions, 145*f*, 146
Corns, 161–162, 162*f*
Coronary artery disease (CAD)
  androstenedione and, 36
  as medical issue, 141
  nicotine and, 48
Coronoid fractures
  classification of, 292*f*, 292*t*
  diagnosis of, 292–293
  indications and contraindications of, 293*b*
  pathophysiology of, 292
  treatment of, 293, 293*b*
Corticosteroid
  for infectious mononucleosis, 165
  injection
    for bursitis, 330
    for osteitis pubis, 327
  for otitis externa, 147
  for snapping iliotibial tract, 68
  for snapping psoas, 66
Cortisol, 34
Cosmetic deformity, in anterior dislocation, 266
Costoclavicular ligament, 170, 263
Cozen's test, 196–197, 197*f*
CP (Creatine phosphate), 6
CPM (Continuous passive motion), 478
C-protein, 1
Crackles, 24
Cramping, in muscle training, 7–8
Creatine, 39–41, 40*t*, 476
Creatine phosphate (CP), 6
Cromolyn sodium, in exercise-induced bronchospasm (EIB), 137

Crossover impingement test, for AC joint, 191, 191f
Cross-shoulder adduction test, in acromioclavicular joint disorder, 257
Cruciate knee injury, 379
Cryopreservation technique, in graft preparation, 116–117, 117f
Cryotherapy, in olecranon apophysitis, 302
C-17 alkylation, 34
CT. See Computed tomography (CT)
C tetani, 10
Cuboid stress fractures, 110
Cuneiform stress fractures, 110
Cycling, 34, 327
Cytadren. See Aminoglutethimide (Cytadren)

D

"Dancer's fracture," 111
Danis Weber classification of ankle fractures, 444, 459, 460f
Darbepoetin (Aranesp), 39
DDD (Degenerative disc disease), 98–99
DDH (Development dysplasia of the hip), 99
Debridement, in partial-thickness rotator cuff tears, 250
Deceleration phase, 183–184, 183f, 201t
Decision-making, in anterior shoulder instability surgery, 221
Deconate, 34
Decorin, 11
Deep medial collateral ligament, 349
Deep tendon reflexes, in spinal injuries, 97
Degenerative arthritis of sternoclavicular joint, 266
Degenerative conditions, 102–103
Degenerative disc disease (DDD), 98–99
Degree of shoulder instability, 215
Dehydration, 47
Dehydroepiandrosterone (DHEA), 33, 36, 476,
Delayed muscle soreness, 481
Delayed-onset muscle soreness (DOMS), 7
Dental mandible and skull injuries, 149–150
Dentoalveolar injuries, 149
Dermatologic conditions, 152–162, 160f. See also Skin
Developmental stenosis, 102
Development dysplasia of the hip (DDH), 108
DEXA (Dual-energy x-ray absorptiometry scan), 55
Dextroamphetamine (Dexedrine), 47
DHEA (Dehydroepiandrosterone), 33, 36, 476
Diagnosis. See specific injuries
Diagnostic and Statistical Manual of Mental Diseases, 4th edition (DSM IV), 53

Diagnostic failures, in posterior and multidirectional shoulder instability, 242
Diagnostic knee tests, 337t
Dial test
    for anterior cruciate ligament injury, 337t
    for posterolateral corner injuries, 356
Dianabol, 32–33, 35
Diarrhea, 23
Dicloxacillin
    for cellulitis, 159
    for folliculitis, 159t
    for impetigo, 155
Dietary Supplement Health and Education Act of 1924, 33, 50
Diltiazem, for Raynaud's phenomenon, 142
Dilutional pseudoanemia, 143
Direct immunofluorescence in influenza, 166
Direction of instability, in the shoulder, 215
Disc herniations, 98, 102
Discoid meniscus, 68–69
Disease transmission, in soft-tissue allografts, 116
Dislocation
    anterior shoulder instability and, 218
    hip, 325, 325f
    shoulder, 62–63
Displaced elbow fractures , treatment of, 287
Distal biceps ruptures, 119
Distal biceps tendon, soft-tissue allografts in, 119–120
Distal clavicle excision, in acromioclavicular joint disorder, 259, 261
Distal realignment, in patellar instability, 398–419
Distance training, 483
Distraction test, for AC joint, 191–192, 191f
Disuse atrophy, 482
Diuretics, 38–39
Docking technique, 119
Documentation of clearance, 27
DOMS (Delayed-onset muscle soreness), 7
Donor-site morbidity, allografts and, 115
Dorsal impaction, 66
Drilling, in osteochondral lesions of talus, 458
Drop arm sign, 203t
Drop sign test, 190
Drugs. See also Medications; Sports pharmacology
    banned or restricted, 37–39
    over-the-counter (OTC), 21
    recreational, 47–49
Drying agents, for herpes simplex, 153
Dual-chamber pacing, in hypertrophic cardiomyopathy (HCM), 138

Dual-energy x-ray absorptiometry scan (DEXA), 55
Duplex ultrasonography, in popliteal artery entrapment syndrome, 442
Dynamic muscle transfer, in acromioclavicular joint disorder, 259–260
Dynamic stability
    of long head of biceps, 181, 181f
    of rotator cuff, 175f, 178

E

Ears, in physical examination, 24
Eating disorders
    amenorrhea and, 53–56
    diagnostic criteria for, 54b
    medical complications of, 55b
    medical history and, 23
    premature osteoporosis and, 53–56
    warning signs and symptoms of, 55b
EBV (Epstein-Barr virus), 164
Eccentric exercise program, in multidirectional shoulder instability, 241
ECG. See Electrocardiogram (ECG)
ECM (Extracellular matrix), 402, 418–419, 419f
ECRB (Extensor carpi radials brevis), 309
ECRL (Extensor carpi radials longus), 309
ECS. See Exertional compartment syndrome (ECS)
Eden-Lange procedure, in spinal accessory nerve injury, 284
EIB (Exercise-induced bronchospasm), 135–137
Elastin, 16
Elbow. See also Elbow arthroscopy; Elbow injuries
    anterior view of the left elbow joint, 196f
    anterior view of the right elbow joint, 196f
    dislocation/terrible triad, 294–295
    flexion test for, 198–199
    history and physical examination of, 196
    of immature and adolescent athletes little league elbow in, 64
    instability in
        lateral pivot shift test for, 198, 198f
        milking test for, 198, 198f
        valgus stress test for, 197–198, 197f
        varus stress test for, 198, 198f
    lateral epicondylitis in
        Cozens test for, 196–197, 197f
        Golfer's elbow test for, 197, 197f
        passive tennis elbow test for, 197, 197f
    nerve compression and entrapment in
        elbow flexion test for, 198–199
        pinch grip test for, 199
        Tinel's test for, 199, 199f

Elbow arthroscopy
  complications in, 133–135
  portals in, 131–132, 131f
Elbow injuries
  adult lateral elbow and, 308–313
  adult medial elbow and, 313–315
  biceps tendon rupture and, 306–307
  biomechanics of, 285
  coronoid fractures and, 289–290
  hyperextension valgus overload and, 314–315
  little league elbow and, 297–302
  olecranon apophysitis and epiphyseal fracture and, 302–303
  olecranon bursitis and, 296–297
  olecranon fractures and, 285–289
  osteoarthritis and, 303–306
  radial head fractures and, 289–290
  triceps tendon rupture and, 307–308
  ulnar collateral ligament injury and, 315–318
Electrical muscle stimulation (EMS), 478
Electrocardiogram (ECG)
  cardiac problems and, 27
  hypertrophic cardiomyopathy and, 138
  screening structural abnormalities and, 27
Electrodesiccation, for Molluscum contagiosum, 154
Electromyogram (EMG)
  axillary nerve palsy and, 279
  medial epicondylitis and, 313
  musculocutaneous nerve injury and, 280
  spinal accessory nerve injury and, 283
  upper extremity nerve injury and, 272, 272b
Electromyography
  multiple ligament-injuries and, 383
  shoulders and, 178
Elevation of shoulders, 177–178, 177f
Emollient lotion, for blisters, 161
Embryology
  of skeletal muscles, 1
  of tendons, 10–11
EMG. See Electromyogram (EMG)
Empty can test, 187
EMS (Electrical muscle stimulation), 478
Endobutton, 340, 345
Endotracheal incubation, in anterior shoulder instability, 222–223
Endplate zone, 4
End-to-end repair technique, in rupture of Achilles tendon, 455
Endurance, 84–85
  training, 7, 483
Entheses, 12–13
Enthesopathies, 14
Environment
  anterior cruciate ligament injury and, 335

healing, creating of, 464
  pediatric sports injuries and, 62b
Enzyme immunoassay, in influenza, 166
Ephedra, 42–43, 476
Ephedra vulgaris, 42
Epidemiology
  of acromioclavicular (AC) joint, 255–256
  of aging athletes, 81–82
  of anterior cruciate ligament (ACL), 335
  of anterior shoulder instability, 218
  of articular cartilage injuries, 418
  of exertional compartment syndrome, 438
  of head injuries, 88–89
  of internal impingement, 248–249
  of medial collateral ligament (MCL) complex of the knee, 348
  of medial tibial stress syndrome, 436
  of meniscal tears, 405–406
  of multiple ligament-injured knee, 379
  of osteoarthritis of the elbow, 303
  of patellofemoral disorders, 391–392
  of popliteal artery entrapment syndrome, 441–442
  of posterior and multidirectional shoulder instability, 231–232
  of posterolateral corner, 354
  of sternoclavicular joint, 263
  of stress fractures, 430–431, 107
  of subacromial impingement, 246–247
  of upper extremity nerve injuries, 269
Epidural hematoma, 97f, 93–94
Epimysium, 1
EpiPen, 137
Epiphyseal fracture, 302–303
Epistaxis, 146
EPO. See Erythropoietin (EPO)
Epstein-Barr virus (EBV), 164
ERLS (External rotation lag sign), 189, 203t
Erythromycin
  for cellulitis, 159
  for otitis media, 148
  for streptococcal pharyngitis, 163, 164t
Erythropoietin (EPO), 33, 39, 144
Erythroxylum coca, 48
Estrogen replacement therapy, 53
Ethylene oxide, for sterilizing of graft, 117
Etiology
  of acromioclavicular (AC) joint, 256
  of anterior cruciate ligament (ACL), 335
  of anterior shoulder instability, 218
  of axillary nerve injury, 277–278
  of brachial plexus injuries, 273, 273f
  of exertional compartment syndrome, 438
  of head injuries, 88

of idiopathic brachial neuritis, 274–275
  of long thoracic nerve injury, 281, 281f
  of medial collateral ligament (MCL) complex of the knee, 348–349
  of medial tibial stress syndrome, 436
  of musculocutaneous nerve injury, 280
  of osteochondral lesions of the talus, 456–457, 457f
  of patellofemoral disorders, 391, 392f
  of popliteal artery entrapment syndrome, 441–442
  of posterolateral corner, 349t, 354
  of spinal accessory nerve injury, 282–283
  of stress fractures of tibia and fibula, 430–431
  of suprascapular nerve, 275f, 276
  of upper extremity nerve injuries, 268–269
EUA. See Examination under anesthesia (EUA)
Evaluation of shoulder injuries, 202–205
Examination under anesthesia (EUA), in posterior cruciate ligament injury, 367–368
Exercise
  muscular contraction and, 478–480
  and pregnancy in female athletes, 60
  protein and, 44
  stress fractures and, 107
  tendons and, 13
Exercise-induced anaphylaxis, 137
Exercise-induced asthma. See Exercise-induced bronchospasm (EIB)
Exercise-induced bronchospasm (EIB)
  background about, 135–137
  medical history and, 22
  physical examination and, 24, 27
Exercise-induced urticaria, 229
Exertional compartment syndrome (ECS)
  diagnosis of, 438–439
  etiology and epidemiology of, 437–438
  pathophysiology of, 438
  pressure criteria in, 440t
  treatment of, 439–441
Exertional dyspnea, 266–267
Extension of shoulders, 178
Extension of the anterior-labrum tear into superior labrum, surgical techniques in, 227
Extensor carpi radials brevis (ECRB), 309
Extensor carpi radials longus (ECRL), 309
External impingement
  concept of, 246
  in rotator cuff, 208
External rotation lag sign (ERLS), 189, 203t

External rotation of shoulders, 178, 203t
External rotation recurvatum test, for posterolateral corner injuries, 356–357
Extra-articular snapping of hip joint, 330
Extracellular matrix (ECM), 402, 418–419, 419f
Extracorporeal shock-wave therapy, in calcific tendonitis, 253
Extremity muscles, 3
Extrinsic risk factor
  ACL injuries and, 57–59
  stress fractures and, 105–106
Eye opening (E), in Glasgow coma scale, 92t
Eyes
  clearance and, 29
  medical history and, 22
  physical examination and, 24
  spinal injuries and, 96
  trauma, 144–146

F
FABER (Flexion-abduction-external rotation), 212
Facial flushing, 42
Famciclovir, for herpes simplex, 153
Fanelli PCL/ACL drill, 385f
Far medial portal, in knee arthroscopy, 127
Fasciodesis, in spinal accessory nerve injury, 284
"Fast-twitch" muscle fibers, 3
Fatigue fracture, 105. See also Stress fractures of the tibia and fibula
Fats, 46–47
FCL (Fibular collateral ligament), 355–356, 356f
FDA (U.S. Food and Drug Administration), 33, 56, 116
FDL (Flexor digitorum longus), 123
Feet, physical examination of, 26
Female athletes. See also Athletes; Women
  amenorrhea and, 28–29
  anterior cruciate ligament injuries in, 57–60
  history of participation of, 51
  lower-extremity alignment of, 52f
  male athletes vs., 51–52
  pregnancy and exercise in, 60
  stress fractures in, 57, 112, 430–431
  triad, 53–56, 53f, 107
Femoral diaphyseal fractures, 325
Femoral stress fractures, 108, 113, 327
Femoral tunnel, in anterior cruciate ligament injury, 342
Ferritin test, in physical examination, 26
FHL (Flexor hallucis longus), 123, 450
Fibrin clot technique, in meniscal injuries, 414–415

Fibroblastic phase, in tendon healing, 15
Fibroblasts, 16
Fibrocartilaginous entheses, 12
Fibrocartilaginous rim, 174, 175f
Fibrous entheses, 12
Fibula, in ankle anatomy, 444
Fibular collateral ligament (FCL), 355–356, 356f
Fibular stress fractures, 108–109
Fitness boom, 81
5α-Dihydrotestosterone (DHT), 33
5-Flourouracil, 16
Fixation across acromioclavicular joint, in acromioclavicular joint disorder, 260
Fixation between the clavicle and coracoid, in acromioclavicular joint disorder, 260
Fixation issues, in anterior cruciate ligament injury, 340
Flexion-abduction-external rotation (FABER), 212
Flexor digitorum longus (FDL), 123
Flexor hallucis longus (FHL), 123, 450
Flexor tendons, 11–12
Flu (Influenza), 164–165, 164t
Fluoroquinolones
  and tendinopathy, 14–15
  for travelers diarrhea, 143
Fluoxetine, for Raynaud's phenomenon, 142
Folliculitis, 156–157, 156f, 159t
Follow-through phase, 183f, 184, 201t
Foot
  of immature and adolescent athletes, 79
  stress fractures and, 106
Football players, posterior shoulder instability in, 233
Foot strike hemolysis, 143
Footwear, stress fractures and, 106, 106f
Fractures, 24. See also Stress fractures
  ankle, 459–462
  coronoid, 290–294
  dislocation, 380
  elbow dislocation/terrible triad, 294–295
  lumbar, 98
  olecranon, 285–290
  pelvis, 325
  radial head, 289–290, 289t
  sacral stress, 111
Frank knee dislocation, 380
Frank ruptures, 14
Free graft figure-of-eight technique, 386
Fresh-frozen technique, in graft preparation, 116
Full thickness injury, in articular cartilage, 420–421
Full-thickness rotator cuff tears, 250–252, 251f
Functional spinal stenosis, 103

Functional testing, for medial collateral ligament complex injuries, 352
Furosemide (Lasix), 38
Furuncle, 156

G
GAGs (Glycosaminoglycans), 14
Gamma irradiation technique, in graft preparation, 117
Ganglion cyst, 276, 277
Gastrointestinal conditions, 23, 142–143
Generalized examination, in musculoskeletal condition, 25
General physical examination, 24
Genetic-based therapy, in long QT syndrome, 139
Genitourinary condition
  medical history and, 23
  physical examination and, 25
GIRD (Glenohumeral internal rotation deficit), 125, 206
Glasgow coma scale, 92t, 96, 103
Glenohumeral abduction, 178f, 179
Glenohumeral internal rotation deficit (GIRD), 125, 209–211
Glenohumeral joint
  dynamic stability of
    long head of biceps and, 181, 181f
    periscapular muscles and, 182
    rotator cuff and, 178f, 181
  forces, 181–183, 182f
  motion of, 175–179
  rotator cuff and, 246
  static stability of, 179–180
    capsule and ligaments in, 195–196
    glenoid fossa in, 195
    humeral head in, 196
    intra-articular pressure in, 196
Glenohumeral ligaments, 185
Glenoid, scapula and, 174
Glenoid bone deficiency, 218, 218f, 232
Glenoid fossa, static stability of, 175f, 179
Glenoid hypoplasia, in the shoulder, 218
Glenoid labrum
  biceps load test for, 195
  biceps tension test for, 195
  clunk test for, 194
  compression-rotation test for, 195
  grind test for, 194
  O'Brien active compression test for, 195, 195f
  SLAP tests for, 195
Glenoid retroversion, in the shoulder, 218
Glucocorticoid, 45
Glucosamine, 40t, 43, 423
Glutamate, 45
Glutamine, 40t, 45
Glycosaminoglycans (GAGs), 16
Godfrey's test, for posterior cruciate ligament injury, 364

Golfers, stress fractures in, 112
Golfer's elbow test, 197, 197f
GORE-TEX® loop, 117
Gracilis tendon, 119
Graft
  in anterior cruciate ligament injury,
    342
  biomechanical properties of, 339t
  in bone-patellar tendon-bone, 340t
  in hamstring, 340t
  in multiple ligament-injured knee,
    387–388
  problems associated with, 339t
  sources of, 345t
  women athletes and selection of, 60
Greater tuberosity (GT), 172f, 172t
Grind test, for glenoid labrum, 194
Griseofulvin, 158
Growth factors, 18–19
Growth hormone, 6–7
GT (Greater tuberosity), 172f, 172t
Gymnast
  ankle of, 79
  stress fractures and, 112
  wrist of, 64, 66
Gynecomastia, 36

H
Haemophilus influenzae, 147
HAGL lesions (Humeral avulsion of
    glenohumeral ligament
    lesions), 216–217, 217f, 221
Hamstring grafts, 339–340, 340t
Hamstring Harvest, in anterior cruciate
    ligament surgery, 341–342
Hamstring syndrome, 331
Hawkins test
  for impingement, 26, 204, 204t
  for the rotator cuff, 188, 188f,
    247–248
hCG (Human chorionic gonadotropin),
    33, 37
HCM (Hypertrophic cardiomyopathy),
    137–138, 138f
HDL (High-density lipoprotein), 35
Head, in physical examination, 24
Headaches, 43
Head and neck area concerns,
    144–149
Head injuries
  classification of, 91
  diagnosis of, 91–93
  epidemiology of, 89–90
  etiology of, 88–89, 103–104
  evidence-based classification
    schemes for, 91t
  guidelines for return to play after,
    93t
  helmets and, 93b
  level of consciousness in, 103
  medical history and, 22
  1989–1998 NCAA surveillance
    system, 89t
  pathogenesis of, 88–89, 91
  pathophysiology of, 89, 91
  postconcussion signs and symptoms,
    91b

pupillary examination in, 103
  sports and, 29
  treatment of, 92–95
Healing
  of ligaments, 18
  of skeletal muscle clinical
    conditions, 7–9
  of tendons, 15–16
Heart murmur, 23, 24
Heart palpitations, 22, 42, 43
Heat capsulorrhaphy, in
    multidirectional shoulder
    instability, 239
Heat illness
  clearance and, 29
  in medical history, 22
Heat-related disorders, in medical
    history, 22
Heel lifts
  in bony impingement, 450
  in partial ruptures of Achilles
    tendon, 454
Helmets, head injuries and, 93b
Hematologic concerns, 143–144
Hemoglobin test, in physical
    examination, 26
Hepatitis
  clearance and, 28
  inhaled crack cocaine and, 48
  steroids and, 35b
Hepatomegaly, 29
Herbs, for enhancing athletic
    performance, 32
Herniated discs, 67
Herniated nucleus pulposus (HNP), 67
Herpes gladiatorum, 154
Herpes simplex (HSV1 and HSV2), 22,
    152–154, 153f, 159t
Heterophile lymphocytes, 164
Heterotopic ossification (HO), 295
Heterozygous state (carrier-HbS), 144
hGH. *See* Human growth hormone
    (hGH)
High-density lipoprotein (HDL), 35
High-impact collision sports, 27
High-to-moderate dynamic demands,
    28b
Hill-Sachs lesion, 180, 211, 217–218
Hip injuries
  anatomy of joints, 320–324, 322f
  athletic pubalgia and, 331–332
  bony injuries and, 325–327
  bursitis and, 329–330, 329f
  contusions and, 328–329
  differential diagnosis of, 325
  Hamstring syndrome and, 331
  hip replacement and, 86
  of immature and adolescent athletes,
    67–68
  muscle strains in, 328, 328f, 328t
  nerve entrapment syndromes and,
    330–331, 331f
  physical examinations in, 323–324
  radiologic examination in, 324
  snapping hip syndrome and, 330
  snapping iliotibial tract in, 68

snapping psoas in, 67–68
  soft-tissue injuries and, 327, 327f
Hirsutism, 35
Histopathology, of anterior cruciate
    ligament (ACL), 336
History and physical examination. *See*
    specific injuries
HIV. *See* Human immunodeficiency
    virus (HIV)
HMB (β-hydroxy-β- methylbutyrate),
    40t, 41–47
HNP (Herniated nucleus pulposus),
    67
HO (Heterotopic ossification), 295
Homozygous (disease HbS), 144
"Hoop stress concept," 402, 404f
Horizontal cleavage tears. *See*
    Horizontal meniscal tears
Horizontal meniscal tears, 406–407,
    407t
  management of, 411a
Hormonal risk factors, anterior cruciate
    ligament injuries and, 336
Hormones, skeletal muscles and, 6–8
Hornblower's sign, 203t
Horner syndrome, 274
Hospitalization and medical history, 21
Hot tub folliculitis, 156, 156f
HPO axis (Hypothalamic-pituitary-
    ovarian axis), 53
HSV1 and HSV2. *See* Herpes simplex
    (HSV1 and HSV2)
Human chorionic gonadotropin (hCG),
    33, 37
Human growth hormone (hGH), 33,
    37–38
Human immunodeficiency virus (HIV)
  clearance and, 28
  steroids and, 35, 35b
Humeral avulsion of glenohumeral
    ligament (HAGL) lesions,
    216–217, 217f, 221
Humeral bone deficiencies, 217–218
Humeral head, 180, 211
Humeral osteotomy, 237
Humerus stress fractures, 112
Hydration, 47, 144
Hydrochlorothiazide, 38
Hyperangulation of humerus, 209,
    210f
Hyperextension valgus overload,
    315–316
  diagnosis of, 315
  pathophysiology of, 315
  treatment of, 315–316
Hyperhydration, 47
Hyperreflexia, 97
Hypertension, 48–49, 140
Hyperthermia, 43
Hypertrophic cardiomyopathy (HCM),
    137–138, 138f
Hypertrophy, 481
Hyphema, 145
Hyponatremia, 47
Hyporeflexia, 97
Hypothalamic-pituitary-ovarian (HPO)
    axis, 53

I

I-band, 4
Ibuprofen, for viral upper respiratory
infections, 163
Ice
athletic pubalgia and, 331
muscle strain and, 85
stress fractures and, 112
subacromial impingement and, 248
tendinitis and, 451
tibial tubercle avulsion and, 70
valgus extension overload and, 305
Idiopathic brachial neuritis
diagnosis of, 275
etiology of, 274–275
treatment of, 275
IGHL. *See* Inferior glenohumeral
ligament (IGHL)
IKDC (International Knee
Documentation Committee),
115
Ilioinguinal nerve entrapment, 330
Iliopsoas bursa, 329, 330
Iliotibial band (ITB), 363
anatomy of, 354
graft, 340
syndrome, 330
Illicit drug use, 22, 23
Illness
acute, clearance and, 28
in medical history, 21
Imaging. *See* Computed tomography
(CT); Magnetic resonance
imaging (MRI); Ultrasound
Imidazoles, for tinea, 157
Immature athletes
about, 61
ankle injuries in, 76–49
elbow injuries in, 64
foot injuries in, 79
hip injuries in, 67–68
knee injuries in, 68–76
osteochondritis dissecans and, 298
shoulder injuries in, 61–64
spine injuries in, 66–67
wrist injuries in, 64–66
Immobilization
in chronic peroneal tendon injuries,
452
in medial collateral ligament complex
injuries, 351
in multidirectional shoulder
instability, 241
in os trigonum syndrome, 451
in posterior shoulder instability, 241
in stress fractures, 111
in tendinitis, 451
in tibial tubercle avulsion, 70
Immunizations, in medical history,
23–24
Immunologic, adverse effects of
steroids on, 35b
Impetigo, 22, 155–156, 155f, 159t
Impingement
ankle, 448–451
rotator cuff, 246–249

internal, 248–249
subacromial, 246–248, 247f, 249f
tests, 187
tests, 204t
Impression fracture, 218
Increased humeral retroversion, 211
Indications for meniscal allograft
transplantation, 416b
Infections, upper respiratory, 162–167
Infectious mononucleosis, 164–166,
165t
Inferior glenohumeral ligament
(IGHL), 172f, 180, 215, 215f
Inferior plication, in anterior shoulder
instability surgery, 224, 226f
Inflammatory phase
in ligaments injuries, 17
in tendon healing, 15
Inflammatory response of traumatic
brain injury, 89
Influenza (Flu), 165t, 166–167
Infraspinatus and teres minor gross
strength, 203t
Infraspinatus tendons
anatomy of, 244–245
layers of, 245t
transverse section of, 245f
Inguinal hernia, clearance and, 29
Inhaled crack cocaine, 48
Injectable steroids, 34
Inner epineurium, 268, 269f
Insertional activity, 272
Insertional tendinitis, 456
Inside-out technique, in meniscal
injuries, 415t
Instability
elbow
lateral pivot shift test for, 198,
198f
milking test for, 198, 198f
valgus stress test for, 197–198,
197f
varus stress test for, 198, 198f
shoulder
anterior drawer test for, 193
apprehension test for, 192
Jobe's apprehension-relocation test
for, 192, 193f
laxity and, 205–206
load and shift test for, 194
posterior drawer test for, 193–194
sulcus sign in, 192–193
Insufficiency fractures. *See* Stress
fractures of the tibia and
fibula
Insulin, 6
Interclavicular ligament, 170, 263
Internal impingement, 209–210, 209f,
246, 248–249
Internal rotation lag sign (IRLS), 189
Internal rotation of shoulders, 179
Internal rotation resistance stress test,
for the rotator cuff, 188, 188f
International Knee Documentation
Committee (IKDC), 115

International Olympic committee
(IOC), 33, 35, 42, 50, 137,
144
Interoperative complications, in
anterior cruciate ligament,
345
Interval training, 483
Intra-articular disc ligament, 262–263,
266
Intra-articular hip disorders, 323, 324,
330
Intra-articular pressure, 180
Intra-articular steroid injections, 84
Intrinsic risk factors
ACL injuries and, 57–58
in stress fractures, 105–106
IOC (International Olympic
committee), 33, 35, 42, 50,
137, 144
IRLS (Internal rotation lag sign), 189
Ischial tuberosity, 331
Ischiogluteal bursitis, 330
Isokinetic muscle contraction, 478f,
479, 482f
Isolated grade I and II instabilities, in
posterolateral corner injuries,
357–358
Isolated grade III instability, in
posterolateral corner injuries,
358
Isoleucine, 44–45
Isometric exercise, 479, 479f
Isometrics, in multidirectional shoulder
instability, 241
Isotonic muscle contraction, 479
ITB (Iliotibial band), 354, 355f, 363
Itraconazole, 158

J

"Jammed neck," 102
Jobe's apprehension-relocation test,
for shoulder instability, 192,
193f
Jobe's supraspinatus test, 187, 203t
Jock itch, 157–158, 158, 158f
Joint capsule knee injury, 379
Joint National Committee VII, 140
Joints, aging and changes in, 83
Joint-specific exam, 25
Jones-type fracture, 111
J-sign, in patellofemoral disorders, 394,
394b
Jumper knee, 399–400
Juvenile disc herniation, 67

K

Keratolytics, 160t
Ketoconazole, 158
Kidney abnormalities, clearance and,
29
"Kiesselbach's area," 146
Kinematics of shoulder injuries,
200–201
Kinetic chain, 483–485
Klippel-Feil syndrome, 103

Knee. *See also* Knee arthroscopic surgery; Multiple ligament-injured knee
  of immature and adolescent athletes, 68–76
  jumper, 399–400
  medial collateral ligament complex of
    anatomy of, 349, 349f
    classification of, 349
    diagnosis of, 349–351
    epidemiology of, 348
    etiology of, 348–349
    treatment of, 351–353
  physical examination of, 25–26
  posterolateral corner of
    anatomy of, 354–355
    classification of, 354
    diagnosis of, 356–357, 358f
    epidemiology of, 354
    etiology of, 349t, 354
    treatment of, 357–361
  replacement, 86
Knee arthroscopic surgery
  complications in, 127
  portals in, 125–127
Knee injury. *See* Meniscal injuries; Posterior cruciate ligament (PCL)
Kocher approach, in posterolateral rotator instability, 312
Krachow suture technique, 294f, 318

L

Laboratory investigations, in physical examination, 26
Labral tears, 324
Labrum, 174, 175f
Laceration, in muscle injury, 8, 14, 15f
Lachman test, 25, 337, 337t
Laser
  acne and, 160
  Molluscum contagiosum and, 154
  posterior shoulder instability and, 238
Lateral ankle ligament complex, 445, 445f
Lateral collateral ligament (LCL) complex of the knee, AMA guidelines for grading injuries in, 349t
Lateral compression elbow injuries
  diagnosis of, 299–300
  pathophysiology of, 299, 299f
  radiologic examination in, 290t, 300, 300f
  treatment of, 300–301
Lateral epicondylitis
  Cozen's test for, 196–197, 197f
  diagnosis of, 309
  golfer's elbow test for, 197, 197f
  passive tennis elbow test for, 197, 197f
  pathophysiology of, 308–309, 309t
"Lateral gutter syndrome," 448
Lateral meniscus, 403–404, 405f, 408
Lateral patellar compression syndrome, 395–396

Lateral pivot shift test, 198, 198f, 311
Lateral portal, in knee arthroscopy, 127
Lateral reconstruction, in multiple-ligament-injured knee, 385–386, 386f
Lateral ulnar collateral ligament (LUCL), 120, 290, 294, 310
Lauge-Hansen classification of ankle fractures, 459
Laxity testing
  for multiple ligament-injured knee, 380
  for shoulder injury, 205–206
LBM (Lean body mass), 33, 38, 40, 45
LCDC (Low contact dynamic compression), 288
LDL (Low-density lipoprotein), 35
Lean body mass (LBM), 33, 38, 40, 45
Legislation about sports pharmacology, 33
Leg overuse injuries. *See also* Stress fractures
  exertional compartment syndrome in, 437–441
  medial tibial stress syndrome in, 435–437
  popliteal artery entrapment syndrome in, 441–443
  stress fractures of the tibia and fibula in, 430–435
Lemos, Burbank, and Taniguchi technique, 261
Lesser tuberosity (LT), 172f
Leucine supplementation, 44–45
LFTs (Liver function tests), 32
Lift-off lag test, 203t
Lift-off test, 174f, 189, 190f, 203t, 251
Ligaments
  anatomy, structure, and biochemistry of, 16–17
  biomechanics of, 17–18
  grading of injuries, 17t
  healing of, 18
  static stability of, 172f, 179–180
Light touch sensation, in spinal injuries, 96
Limb buds, 1
Limited contact, in classification of sports by contact, 27b
Liquid nitrogen, for Molluscum contagiosum, 154
Little League elbow
  lateral compression injuries in
    diagnosis of, 299–300, 300f, 300t
    pathophysiology of, 298, 298f
    radiologic examination in, 290t, 299, 300f
    treatment of, 300–302, 302b
  management of, 65a
  medial tension injuries in
    diagnosis of, 298, 298f
    pathogenesis of, 64
    pathophysiology of, 298
    treatment of, 298–299
Little League shoulder
  diagnosis of, 61–62, 62f

  pathogenesis of, 61
  treatment of, 62, 62a
Liver
  adverse effects of steroids on, 35b
  steroids and, 363–35
Liver function tests (LFTs), 35
Load and shift test, 194, 194f
Load test, 26
Long head of biceps, dynamic stability of, 181, 181f
Longitudinal meniscal tears, 407, 407t
Long QT syndrome (LQTS), 139–140
Long thoracic nerve injury
  anatomy of, 281, 281f
  diagnosis of, 281, 281f
  treatment of, 282
Loop diuretics, 38
Loose bodies, in elbow joint, 304–306, 304f
Loperamide, 143
Low back pain, in lumbar spine injuries, 97
Low contact dynamic compression (LCDC), 288
Low-density lipoprotein (LDL), 35
Low dynamic demands, 28b
Lower extremity. *See also* Leg overuse injuries
  cellulitis in, 159
  physical examination of, 25–26
  soft-tissue allografts in, 120
Low-impact sports, 27
Low static demands, 28b
LQTS (Long QT syndrome), 139–140
LT (Lesser tuberosity), 172f
Lumbar spine injuries
  cauda equina syndrome and, 98
  description of, 97
  differential diagnoses of, 98b
  disc herniations and, 98
  fractures and, 98
  spondylolysis and, 99
  sprains and strains and, 98
Lymphadenopathy, 164

M

Macrolides, 160t
Macrotrauma injuries, 61
Magnetic resonance imaging (MRI), 22
  acute peroneal tendon injuries and, 452
  anterior cruciate ligament injury and, 337
  anterior shoulder instability and, 220–221, 221f
  athletic pubalgia and, 331
  congenital coronary anomalies and, 139
  full-thickness rotator cuff tears and, 251
  head injuries and, 92
  hip fracture and, 324
  idiopathic brachial neuritis and, 275
  lateral compression injuries and, 299, 300f
  lateral epicondylitis and, 309

medial collateral ligament complex and, 336*f*, 351
medial epicondylitis and, 313
medial tibial stress syndrome and, 436
meniscal injuries and, 410
navicular fractures and, 110
olecranon stress fractures and, 112
osteitis pubis and, 327
os trigonum syndrome and, 451
posterior and multidirectional shoulder instability and, 235, 236*f*
posterior cruciate ligament injury and, 365
posterolateral corner injuries and, 357, 358*f*
rupture of peroneal tendon and, 452
sciatic nerve inflammation and, 330
shoulder injury and, 205
stress fractures and, 108
subacromial impingement and, 248
suprascapular nerve palsy and, 276, 277*f*
triceps tendon rupture and, 308
upper extremity nerve injury and, 271
Ma Huang, 42
Major League Baseball (MLB), 35
Male athletes. *See also* Athletes
female athletes *vs.*, 52–53
lower-extremity alignment of, 52*f*
osteoarthritis of the elbow in, 303
stress fractures in, 431, 111*f*
Malignant hyperthermia, 9
Malalignment, in patellofemoral pathology, 392*b*
Management. *See also* Postoperative care/management
of anterior cruciate ligament (ACLs) tears, 69, 70*a*
of articular cartilage injuries, 84
of little league elbow, 64, 65*a*
of little league shoulder, 62, 62*a*
of muscle strains, 84–85
of osteochondritis dissecans, 76, 78*a*
of patellofemoral stress syndrome, 72, 73*a*
of shoulder dislocation, 62–63, 63*a*
of snapping psoas, 68, 68*a*
of spondylolysis, 66–67, 67*a*
of stress fractures, 112–113
of tibial spine avulsion, 69–70, 70*a*
of tibial tubercle avulsion, 70–71, 71*f*, 73*a*
Mannitol, 38
March fractures. *See* Stress fractures; Stress fractures of the tibia and fibula
Marfan syndrome, 141, 142*f*
Marijuana, 35, 49
Marrow-simulation technique for articular cartilage lesions, 395*b*
Marrow-stimulation technique for chondral lesions surgery, 424*t*
Massage, in athletic pubalgia, 331
Masses, abdominal, 24

Maturation phase, in ligaments injuries, 18
M-band, 2
McGuire, Mark, 36
MCL. *See* Medial collateral ligament (MCL)
McLaughlin lesion, 180
McMurray test, 26
in anterior cruciate ligament injury, 337*t*
in meniscal injuries, 408, 409*f*
MDI (Multidirectional instability), 231
Medial collateral ligament (MCL), 17, 119
AMA guidelines for grading injuries in, 349*t*
anatomy of, 349, 349*f*
classification of, 349
diagnosis of, 349–351
epidemiology of, 348
etiology of, 348–349
reconstruction of, 121–122, 122*f*
treatment of, 351–353
treatment results of, 353
Medial deltoid ligament, in leg anatomy, 445
Medial epicondyle avulsion, 64
Medial epicondylitis
anatomy of, 313–314
diagnosis of, 314
pathophysiology of, 313–314
treatment of, 314–315
Medial meniscus, 402–404, 408
Medial patellofemoral ligament (MPFL), 122–123, 391
Medial reconstruction, in multiple ligament-injured knee, 386–387
Medial tension injuries
diagnosis of, 298, 298*f*
pathophysiology of, 22w–14
treatment of, 298
Medial tibial stress syndrome (MTSS)
diagnosis of, 432*a*, 436
etiology and epidemiology of, 436
pathophysiology of, 436
treatment of, 437
Medical history
allergies and, 21
cardiovascular condition and, 21–22
eating disorders and, 23
eyes and vision and, 22
gastrointestinal and, 23
genitourinary and, 23
heat illness and, 22
hospitalizations and surgeries and, 21
immunizations and, 23–24
medications and, 21
menstrual history and, 24
musculoskeletal condition and, 22–23
neurologic condition and, 22
protective devices and, 23
psychosocial concerns and, 23
pulmonary conditions and, 22

recent or chronic injury/illness and, 21
skin conditions and, 22
Medications in medical history, 22
Medicolegal issues, 30
Men. *See also* Male athletes
adverse effects of steroids on, 35*b*
androstenedione and, 36
distal biceps disruptions in, 119
fibular stress fractures in, 109
steroids and, 35
stress fractures in, 106
Meniscal injuries
classification of, 406–407, 406*f*, 407*t*, 408*b*
diagnosis of, 408–410
epidemiology of meniscal tears, 405–406
meniscal allograft transplantation, 416*b*
meniscus replacement, 415–416
pathophysiology of meniscus, 404–405
structure and function of, 402–404, 403*f*, 404*f*, 405*f*
treatment of, 410–415
use of technology in, 416–417
Meniscal rasping and trephination techniques, 413
Meniscal repair
anterior cruciate ligament injury and, 341
techniques, 413–415
Meniscal resection techniques, 413
Menisci, 402–404
Meniscofemoral ligament, 363
Meniscus tears, 68–69
Menstrual disorders
clearance and, 28
in medical history, 24
Meralgia paresthetica, 330
Metabolism, skeletal muscles and, 6
Metabolites, 34
Metatarsal stress fractures, 110–111, 110*f*, 113
Methamphetamine (Desoxyn), 47
Methicillin-resistant staphylococcus aureus (MRSA), 159–160
Meyers and McKeever classification of tibial spine fractures, 70*f*
Microfracture technique
in articular cartilage injuries, 424–425, 426*t*
in osteochondral lesions of talus, 458–459
Microinstability of shoulder, 63–64
Middle glenohumeral ligament, 180
Midglenoid portal, in shoulder arthroscopy, 129
Midpatellar portal, in knee arthroscopy, 127
Midsubstance tears knee injury, 379
Military recruits, stress fractures in, 58, 105, 106
Milking test, 198, 198*f*
Miniopen technique, in full-thickness rotator cuff tears, 252

Minor traumatic brain injury, 91
MLB (Major League Baseball), 35
Mobilization of ligament, 18
Modulation of adhesion formation, in tendon healing, 16
Molluscum contagiosum, 22, 154–155, 154f, 159t
Moment arm, 182
Mononucleosis, 23
Monounsaturated fat, 47
Mood disorders, steroids and, 34
Moraxella catarrhalis, 147
Morgan-Burkhart model, 210
Mortality, in influenza, 166
Morton foot, metatarsal stress fractures and, 110–111
Motion
    at acromioclavicular joint, 171
    at glenohumeral and scapulothoracic, 175–179, 176f
    scapular, 176
    at sternoclavicular joint, 169–170, 170f
Motor endplate, 3, 4f
Motor neuron, 3–4
Motor unit, 2–3, 3f, 272
Motrin, for viral upper respiratory infection, 164t
MPFL (Medial patellofemoral ligament), 122–123, 391
M-protein, 1
MRI. *See* Magnetic resonance imaging (MRI)
MRSA (Methicillin-resistant staphylococcus aureus), 159–160
MTSS. *See* Medial tibial stress syndrome (MTSS)
Multidirectional instability (MDI), 231
Multiple ligament-injured knee
    anatomy and biomechanics of, 376–378, 377f
    associated injury of, 379–380
    description of, 376
    diagnosis of, 380–383
    epidemiology of, 379
    pitfalls of diagnosing and managing, 389b
    treatment of, 383–389
Multiple tears, management of, 411a
Mupirocin
    for folliculitis, 156
    for impetigo, 155
Murmur. *See* Heart murmur
Muscle contraction, 3–5, 57f
Muscle fibers, 1, 2f
    steroids and, 34
Muscle inhibition or weakness, 232
Muscle injury, 8–9
Muscle nerve root levels, in spinal injuries, 97t
Muscle-splitting approach, in ulnar collateral ligament injury, 318
Muscle soreness, 7, 481–482
Muscle strains
    in aging athletes, 84–85

grading of, 328f, 328t
    in hip and pelvis injuries, 328
    in muscle injury, 8
Muscle strength
    grading of, 97t
    in spinal injuries, 96
Muscle training, 7
Muscle twitch, 4
Muscular adaptation, 479–482
Muscular contraction, exercise and, 478–480
Musculocutaneous nerve injury
    anatomy of, 280, 280f
    diagnosis of, 280
    etiology of, 280
    treatment of, 280–281
Musculoskeletal condition
    in medical history, 22–23
    in physical examination, 25
Musculoskeletal effects, steroids and, 34, 35b
Myelopathy, 102–103
Myocardial infarction, nicotine and, 48
Myofibrils, 1
Myomectomy, in hypertrophic cardiomyopathy (HCM), 138
Myosin, 2, 44

N
Namath, Joe, 81
Nandrolone, 34
Nasal congestion, 163
Nasal injuries, 146–147
National Athletic Trainers' Association, 89
National Basketball Association (NBA), 35
National Collegiate Athletic Association (NCAA), 33, 35, 41, 100, 137, 23, 25, 475
National Football League (NFL), 35, 89, 335
National Hockey League (NHL), 35, 89
Navicular stress fractures, 110, 113
NBA (National Basketball Association), 35
NCAA (National Collegiate Athletic Association), 23, 25, 33, 35, 41, 100, 137, 476
NCS. *See* Nerve conduction study (NCS)
Neck pain, 102
Needle electrode examination, 272b
Neer's impingement test
    for the rotator cuff, 187–188, 187t, 188f, 204, 204t
    for subacromial space and supraspinatus muscle, 204t, 247–248
    for upper extremity, 26
Nerve compression and entrapment in elbow, 198–199
Nerve conduction study (NCS)
    axillary nerve palsy and, 279
    findings with nerve injury, 272b

musculocutaneous nerve injury and, 280
    with nerve injury, 272b
    spinal accessory nerve injury and, 283
    suprascapular nerve palsy and, 276
Nerve entrapment syndrome, 330–331
Nerve injuries
    in the knee, 382–383
    knee dislocation and, 380
Nerve lesions, in anterior shoulder instability, 219
Nervousness, 42, 43
Neuraminidase inhibitors, 166
Neurapraxia, 100–102
Neurological testing, in spinal injuries, 96
Neurologic condition
    in medical history, 22
    in physical examination, 26
Neuromuscular control, restoring, 483
Neurapraxia, 269
Neuropsychologic testing, head injuries and, 92
Neurotmesis, 269
Neurovascular conditions
    effort thrombosis in, 211–212
    thoracic outlet syndrome (TOC) in, 212, 212f
    vascular injuries in, 211
Neurovascular examination, in multiple ligament-injured knee, 380
Neviaser portal, in shoulder arthroscopy, 129
NFL (National Football League), 35, 89, 335
NHL (National Hockey League), 35, 89
Nicotine, 48–49
Nifedipine, for Raynaud's phenomenon, 142
Nitrogen balance, 44
Nitrogen (liquid), for Molluscum contagiosum, 154
No clearcut fracture line, in stress fracture, 108
Nolvadex. *See* Tamoxifen (Nolvadex)
Noncontact, in classification of sports by contact, 27b
Nondisplaced fractures of the elbow, treatment of, 286–287
Nonoperative treatment
    of lateral epicondylitis, 309
    of medial epicondylitis, 314
    of medial tibial stress syndrome, 437
    of shoulder injury, 205
Nonoutlet impingement. *See* Secondary impingement
Nonsteroidal anti-inflammatory drug (NSAID)
    for acute peroneal tendon injuries, 452
    for aging athlete, 84
    for anterolateral impingement, 449
    for articular cartilage injuries, 422–423
    for bursitis, 330

for calcific tendonitis, 253
for chronic peroneal tendon injuries, 452
for hyperextension valgus overload, 315
for infectious mononucleosis, 165
for lateral patellar compression syndrome, 395
for little league elbow, 65a
for medial epicondylitis, 314
for medial tension injuries, 298
for olecranon apophysitis, 302
for osteitis pubis, 327
for os trigonum syndrome, 451
for patellar tilt, 397
for spondylolysis, 99
for stress fractures, 112
for subacromial impingement, 248
for tendinitis, 451, 454
Nonsurgical treatment
    of acromioclavicular joint disorder, 258–259
    of acute peroneal tendon dislocations, 453
    of anterior cruciate ligament injury, 338
    of articular cartilage injuries, 422–423, 423a
    of chronic ankle pain, 447
    of elbow dislocation/terrible triad, 294–295
    of hyperextension valgus overload, 315
    of insertional tendinitis, 455–456
    of lateral epicondylitis, 309–310
    of leg overuse injuries, 434–435, 434t
    of long thoracic nerve injury, 282
    of medial collateral ligament complex injuries, 351–352
    of meniscal injuries, 411, 411a
    of multiple ligament-injured knee, 383
    of olecranon stress fractures, 296
    of osteoarthritis of the elbow, 303
    of osteochondral lesions of talus (OLT), 458
    of posterior cruciate ligament injury, 366
    of rupture of Achilles tendon, 454
    of spinal accessory nerve injury, 283
    of sternoclavicular joint injury, 266–267
    of suprascapular nerve injury, 286–277
    of tendinitis, 454
    of ulnar collateral ligament injury, 317–318
Non-weight bearing cast, in acute peroneal tendon dislocations, 453
Nose, in physical examination, 24
Notchplasty, in anterior cruciate ligament injury, 342
Notch width, 52f, 58
Nutrition

strengthening and conditioning and, 475–476
    stress fractures and, 106–107, 112
Nutritional supplements, 23, 25, 476
Nutrition Labeling and Education Act of, 1990, 33

O
OATS. See Osteochondral autograft transplant (OATS)
Ober test, for (ITB) in patellofemoral disorders, 393
Objectives, of preparticipation physical examination, 20
Oblique (flap or parrot beak) meniscal tears, 407, 407t
Oblique fractures with communication, 288
Oblique fractures without communication, 288
O'Brien's test (compression test)
    for acromioclavicular joint disorder, 257
    for glenoid labrum, 195, 195f
    for superior labral lesions, 204t
Observation, in shoulder injuries, 202
OCD. See Osteochondritis dissecans (OCD)
Office-based PPE, 21
OKC (Open kinetic chain), 478–479
Olecranon apophysitis
    diagnosis of, 302
    pathophysiology of, 302
    treatment of, 302–303
Olecranon bursitis
    diagnosis of, 296–297
    pathophysiology of, 296, 296f
    treatment of, 297
Olecranon fractures
    anatomy of, 285–286
    classification of, 286, 286t
    diagnosis of, 286
    pathophysiology of, 285–286
    stress, 113, 295–296
    treatment of, 286–289
OLT. See Osteochondral lesions of talus (OLT)
On-field evaluation, head injuries and, 92
On-field examination of spine, 96–97
Open approach surgery, in full-thickness rotator cuff tears, 252
Open kinetic chain (OKC), 478–479
Open physes, recommendations for, 302b
Open technique
    in adult lateral elbow, 309
    in anterior shoulder instability, 221–222, 230t
Oral contraceptives, 55
Oral steroids, 34
Organomegaly, 24, 29
Orthodontia, 23
Orthopaedics, soft tissue allografts and, 115

Orthosis, in chronic peroneal tendon injuries, 452
Orthotics, in tendinitis, 451, 454
"Os acromiale," 246–247
Oseltamivir (Tamiflu), 166
Osgood-Schlatter syndrome, 70, 74–76
Osmotic diuretics, 38
Osseous integrity, in knee dislocation, 380
Osseous lesions, in anterior shoulder instability, 219
Ossification, centers of, 320
Osteitis pubis, 327
Osteoarthritis, 262, 303–306
Osteochondral allograft
    in chondral lesions surgery, 424t, 428
    results of, 429t
Osteochondral autograft/mosaicplasty, in chondral lesions surgery, 424t, 426
Osteochondral autograft transplant (OATS), 395b
Osteochondral fractures, in articular cartilage, 421–422
Osteochondral lesions, 456–459
Osteochondral lesions of talus (OLT), 456–459
    classification of, 457–458
    diagnosis of, 458
    etiology of, 456, 457f
    treatment of, 458–459
Osteochondritis dissecans (OCD)
    classification of, 300t
    description of, 400–401, 401f, 78
    in immature athlete, 298
Osteoclast, 105
Osteopenic bone, 288, 288f
Osteoporosis, amenorrhea, eating disorders and, 53–56
Os trigonum syndrome, 450–451
OTC drugs. See Over-the-counter (OTC) drugs
Otitis externa (swimmer's ear), 147–148, 147f
Otitis media, 148
Outer epineurium, 269, 269f
Outside-in technique, in meniscal injuries, 415t
Over-the-counter (OTC) drugs, 21
Overweight, in physical examination, 24
Oxandrolone, 34
Oxymetholone, 34

P
PAES. See Popliteal artery entrapment syndrome (PAES)
Pain
    abdominal, 24
    decreasing, in rehabilitation, 464–466
    neck, 102
    posterior heel, 76, 78–79
    of posterior heel pain, 76, 78–79
Palliative treatment, in articular cartilage injuries, 424

Palpation
    of ankle, 25–26
    in patellofemoral disorders physical
        examination, 394b
    in shoulder injuries, 202
Panner's disease, 298
Papanicolaou testing, 24
Paratenon and blood supply, 11–12,
    12f
Paraxanthine, 41
Pars interarticularis stress fractures,
    111
Partial articular supraspinatus tendon
    avulsion(PASTA), 250
Partial distal biceps ruptures, 119
Partial rupture of Achilles tendon, 454
Partial thickness injury, in articular
    cartilage, 420
Partial-thickness rotator cuff tears
    (PTRCT), 249–250
Passive mechanisms, in glenohumeral
    joint, 215
Passive tennis elbow test, 197, 197f
PASTA (Partial articular supraspinatus
    tendon avulsion), 250
Patella, stress fractures of, 108
Patellar dislocation, acute, 397b, 399,
    400f
Patellar instability
    description of, 397–398, 74, 76
    distal realignment in, 398–399
    proximal realignment in, 398
Patellar mobility, in patellofemoral
    disorders, 394b
Patellar osteochondritis desiccans,
    400–401, 401f
Patellar tendinitis, 399–400
Patellar tendon reconstruction, 123
Patellar tilt, 397
Patellofemoral disorders
    acute patellar dislocation and, 399,
        400f
    classification of, 392b
    diagnosis of, 393–395, 393f, 407a
    epidemiology of, 391–392
    etiology of, 391, 392f
    lateral patellar compression
        syndrome and, 395–396
    patellar instability and, 397–399
    patellar tilt and, 397
    pathophysiology of, 392–393
    physical examination for, 394b
    structures of, 391b
    traumatic instability and, 396–397
Patellofemoral joint (PFJ), 391
Patellofemoral stress syndrome, 73–74
Pathogenesis
    of accessory navicular, 79
    of anterior cruciate ligament (ACLs)
        tears, 69
    of the anterior instability of the
        shoulder, 214–218
    of patellofemoral stress syndrome, 71
    of avascular necrosis, 79
    of gymnast ankle, 79
    of gymnast's wrist, 64, 66
    of juvenile disc herniation, 67

    of little league elbow, 64
    of little league shoulder, 61
    of medial epicondyle avulsion, 64
    of meniscus tears and discoid
        meniscus, 68
    of microinstability, 63
    of Osgood-Schlatter syndrome,
        74–75
    of osteochondritis dissecans, 76, 76f
    of patellar instability, 72, 73
    of posterior heel pain, 76, 78
    of shoulder dislocation, 62
    of snapping psoas, 67
    of spondylolysis, 66
    of stress fractures, 441
    of tibial spine avulsion, 69, 70f
    of tibial tubercle avulsion, 70, 72f
Pathology. See specific conditions
Pathophysiology
    of acromioclavicular (AC) joint,
        256–257
    of anterior cruciate ligament (ACL),
        335–336
    of the anterior shoulder instability,
        215–218
    of articular cartilage injuries,
        420–422
    of biceps tendon rupture, 306
    of calcific tendonitis, 252–253
    of coronoid fractures, 290–, 292
    of exertional compartment syndrome,
        438
    of hyperextension valgus overload,
        314–315
    of internal impingement, 248–249
    of lateral compression injuries, 298,
        299f
    of lateral epicondylitis, 308, 309t
    of medial epicondylitis, 313
    of medial tension injuries, 297–298
    of medial tibial stress syndrome, 436
    of meniscus, 404–405
    of olecranon bursitis, 296, 22ʂf
    of olecranon fractures, 285–286
    in olecranon stress fracture, 295
    of partial-thickness rotator cuff tears,
        249
    of patellofemoral disorders,
        392–393, 392f
    of popliteal artery entrapment
        syndrome, 442
    of posterolateral rotatory instability,
        310–311, 311f
    of radial head fractures, 289
    of rotator cuff tear arthropathy, 252
    of stress fractures, 431
    of subacromial impingement,
        246–247
    of triceps tendon rupture, 307
    of ulnar collateral ligament injury
        and, 315–316, 316f
    of upper extremity nerve injuries,
        269
PCL. See Posterior cruciate ligament
    (PCL)
PCL reconstruction. See Posterior
    cruciate ligament (PCL)

PCR (Polymerase chain reaction), 116
Pectoralis major, 174
Peel-back theory, 206, 207f
Peel-off knee injury, 379
Pelvis injuries
    anatomy of, 320–324, 321f
    anatomy of hip joints, 320–324,
        322f
    anatomy of pelvis, 321f
    athletic pubalgia and, 331–332
    bony injuries, 325–327
    bursitis and, 329–330, 330f
    contusions and, 329
    differential diagnosis of, 325
    muscle strains in, 328–329, 329f,
        328t
    nerve entrapment syndrome and,
        330–331, 331f
    pelvis fractures, 325
    physical examination in, 323–324
    radiologic examination of, 324
    snapping hip syndrome and, 330
    soft-tissue injuries, 327, 327f
Penicillin VK, for streptococcal
    pharyngitis, 163, 164t
"Pep pills." See Amphetamines
Percutaneous suture repair, in rupture
    of Achilles tendon, 455
Percutaneous technique, in adult
    lateral elbow, 309–310
Performance-enhancing agents, 23
Periscapular muscles, 182
Peritendinitis, 453
Peroneal tendon injuries
    acute tears and, 451–452
    chronic tears and, 32;9
    subluxation/dislocation and,
        452–453
    tears and, 451
    tendinitis and, 451
Peroneus longus and brevis, in leg
    anatomy, 446
PFJ (Patellofemoral joint), 391
PFL (Popliteofibular ligament), 355,
    355f
PFT (Pulmonary function testing), 27
Pharyngitis, 164
Photodynamic therapy with
    aminolevulinic acid, for acne,
        160
Physeal injuries
    in acromioclavicular (AC) joint, 262
    in sternoclavicular joint, 264
Physical activity
    for articular cartilage injuries, 84
    of seniors, 81–82
Physical examination. See specific
    diseases and conditions
Physical modifiers to tendon healing,
    16
Physical therapy
    acute peroneal tendon injuries and,
        452
    anterior cruciate ligament injury and,
        338
    anterolateral impingement and, 448
    arthritic joints and, 84
    articular cartilage injuries and, 422

bony impingement and, 450
chronic peroneal tendon injuries and, 452
degenerative disc disease and, 98
glenohumeral internal rotation deficit and, 210
hyperextension valgus overload, 315
idiopathic brachial neuritis and, 275
internal impingement and, 249
juvenile disc herniation and, 67
lateral epicondylitis and, 309
lateral patellar compression syndrome and, 395, 396
posterior heel pain and, 79
posterior shoulder instability and, 241
rib stress fracture and, 111
scapular dyskinesia and, 211
tendinitis and, 451, 454
Piano key sign, AC joint, 192
Pinched nerves, 22
Pinch grip test, 199
PIN (Posterior interosseous nerve), 309
Piriformis syndrome, 330
PITFL (Posterior-inferior tibiofibular ligament), 444, 445
Pivot shift test, for anterior cruciate ligament injury, 337t
Plantar fascitis, 76
Plantar wart (verrucae plantaris), 161, 161f
PLC. See Posterolateral corner (PLC)
PLRI. See Posterolateral rotatory instability (PLRI)
Plyometric training, 241, 479
PMB (Posteromedial bundle), 362–363, 363f
Pneumatic otoscopy, 12
PNF. See Proprioceptive neuromuscular facilitation (PNF)
POL (Posterior oblique ligament), 122, 349
Polymerase chain reaction (PCR), 116
Polymerase in influenza, 166
Polyunsaturated fat, 47
Popliteal artery entrapment syndrome (PAES)
classification of, 442t
diagnosis of, 432a, 442–443
etiology and epidemiology of, 441–442
treatment of, 443
Popliteofibular ligament (PFL), 355, 355f
Popliteus tendon, 355
Portals
in anterior shoulder instability, 222–224, 223f
in knee arthroscopy, 125–127
in shoulder arthroscopy, 128–129, 128f
Postconcussion, signs and symptoms of, 91b
Posterior impingement, 448–449

Posterior and multidirectional shoulder instability
bony deficiency of the glenoid in, 232
description of, 231
diagnosis of, 233–235
diagnostic and surgical failures in, 242
epidemiology in, 231–232
mechanism of injury in, 233
rotator interval in, 232
selective ligament-cutting in, 232
treatment of, 236–242
Posterior corner reconstruction, 120
Posterior cruciate ligament (PCL), 335f, 350
description of, 362
injury
anatomy and function of, 362–363, 363f
diagnosis of, 363–365
mechanism of, 363
treatment of, 366–374, 366a, 367a
reconstruction of, 120–121, 121f
Posterior drawer test
for anterior cruciate ligament injury, 337t
for posterior cruciate ligament injury, 364, 364f
for posterolateral corner injuries, 26, 356
for shoulder instability, 193–194, 194f
Posterior heel pain, 76, 78–79
Posterior hip dislocation, radiograph of, 325f
Posterior impingement, 448–449
Posterior-inferior glenohumeral ligament, 232
Posterior-inferior tibiofibular ligament (PITFL), 444, 445
Posterior interosseous nerve (PIN), 309
Posterior knee dislocation, 379–380
Posterior oblique ligament (POL), 122, 349
Posterior portal
in ankle arthroscopy, 130
in shoulder arthroscopy, 128
Posterior shoulder instability, 214
Posterior sternoclavicular (SC) joint dislocation, 265–266
Posterolateral corner (PLC)
anatomy of, 354–355
classification of, 354
diagnosis of, 356–357, 358f
etiology of, 354, 354t
pathogenesis of, 354
Posterolateral drawer test
for posterolateral corner injuries, 356
for posterolateral rotatory instability, 312
Posterolateral portal, in knee arthroscopy, 128–129

Posterolateral reconstruction, in multiple ligament-injured knee, 385–386, 386f
Posterolateral rotatory instability (PLRI)
diagnosis of, 311–312
pathophysiology of, 310–311, 311f
postoperative care of, 312–313
treatment of, 310–312
Posteromedial bundle (PMB), 362–363, 363f
Posteromedial portal, in knee arthroscopy, 128, 128f
Posteromedial reconstruction, in multiple ligament-injured knee, 386–387
Posterior sag test, for posterior cruciate ligament injury, 365
Postoperative care/management
adult lateral elbow and, 310
anterior shoulder instability and, 227–230
complications in, 229–230
chronic ankle pain and, 448
hyperextension valgus overload and, 315
lateral compression injuries and, 301–302, 302b
leg overuse injury and, 441
medial epicondylitis and, 314
medial tibial stress syndrome and, 31;8
multidirectional shoulder instability and, 241–242
olecranon apophysitis and, 303
olecranon fractures and, 288–289
osteochondral lesions of talus and, 459
popliteal artery entrapment syndrome and, 443
posterior and multidirectional shoulder instability and, 239–242, 241–242
posterior cruciate ligament injury and, 374–375
posterior shoulder instability and, 241
posterolateral corner injuries and, 359
posterolateral rotatory instability and, 312–313
surgery of elbow joint loose bodies and, 306
triceps tendon rupture and, 308
ulnar collateral ligament injury and, 318
Postsynaptic membrane, 3
PPE. See Preparticipation physical examination (PPE)
Prednisone, 165
Pregnancy
clearance and, 28
and exercise in female athletes, 60
guidelines for exercise during, 59b
and postpartum
guidelines for exercise during, 59b
Premature osteoporosis, 53–56

Preparticipation physical examination (PPE), 20–30
  clearance in, 27–30
  format of, 21
  laboratory investigations in, 26
  medical history in, 21–24
  medicolegal issues in, 30
  objectives of, 20
  physical examination in, 24–26
  special testing in, 26–27
  timing of, 20
Prepatellar bursitis, 399
Preseason practice, preparticipation physical examination and, 20
Pressure testing, for exertional compartment syndrome, 31f
Presynaptic membrane, 3
Presyncope, 21
Prevention
  of blood doping, 144
  of traveler's diarrhea, 143
Primary amenorrhea, 24, 55
Primary anterior shoulder instability, 215
Primary inferior shoulder instability, 215
Primary osteitis pubis, 327
Primary posterior instability, in the shoulder, 215
Primary Raynaud's phenomenon, 142
Primary traumatic brain injury, 89
Principles of repair, in meniscal injuries, 410
Principles of resection, in meniscal injuries, 410, 410f
Procurement, of soft-tissue allografts, 116
Prohormones, 33–37
Proliferative/repair phase, in ligaments injuries, 18
Propionibacterium acne, 160
Propranolol (Inderal), 39
Proprioceptive neuromuscular facilitation (PNF), 241
Protective devices, in medical history, 23
Protein, 43–44
Proteoglycans, 11, 16–17
Proven performance effects
  of amphetamines, 48
  of androstenedione, 36
  of β2-Agonists, 40
  of β-hydroxy-β- methylbutyrate, 41
  of branched-chain amino acids, 44–45
  of caffeine, 42
  of carbohydrate-protein combination, 46
  of carbohydrates, 46
  of chondroitin sulfate, 43
  of creatine, 39–40
  of dehydroepiandrosterone, 36
  of ephedra, 42
  of fats, 47
  of glucosamine, 43
  of glutamine, 45
  of human growth hormone, 37–38

  of steroids, 34
  of testosterone, 33
  of water and fluid replacement, 47
Provocative maneuvers, in patellofemoral disorders physical examination, 394f, 394b
Provocative tests, for shoulder injuries, 204
Proximal hamstring avulsions, 124
Proximal realignment, in patellar instability, 398
Pseudoephedrine, 163
Pseudomonas aeruginosa, 147, 156, 157
Psychosocial concerns, in medical history, 23
PTRCT (Partial-thickness rotator cuff tears), 249–250
Public rami stress fractures, 111
Pulmonary concerns, 135–137
Pulmonary condition
  in medical history, 22
  in physical examination, 24
Pulmonary dysfunction, clearance and, 29
Pulmonary function testing (PFT), 27
Pulsed electromagnetic field, in leg overuse injuries, 435
Pure knee dislocations, 380
Pyarthrosis, 323
Pyramiding, 34

Q
Q-angle measure, in patellofemoral disorders, 394, 394b, 394f
Quadriceps tendon, 340
Quadrilateral space syndrome, 212
Quinolones, 160

R
Radial collateral ligament (RCL), 310
Radial head fractures
  classification of, 289, 289t
  diagnosis of, 289
  pathophysiology of, 289
  treatment of, 289–290, 292b
Radial meniscal (transverse) tears, 407, 407t
Radio frequency-induced capsular shrinkage, in posterior shoulder instability, 238
Radiographs
  anterior shoulder instability and, 220
  brachial plexus injuries and, 274
  hip pain and, 324
  meniscal injuries and, 410
  musculocutaneous nerve injury and, 280
  posterolateral corner injuries and, 357
  shoulder injury and, 204–205
  stress fractures and, 107, 432, 433f
Radiologic examination
  Achilles tendinitis and, 454
  acromioclavicular joint disorder and, 258

acute peroneal tendon injuries and, 452, 453
ankle fractures and, 460–461, 461f
anterior cruciate ligament and, 337, 338f
anterior shoulder instability and, 220
anterolateral impingement and, 448
articular cartilage injuries and, 422
biceps tendon rupture and, 306–307
bony impingement and, 32;7, 450f
congenital coronary anomalies and, 139
elbow dislocation/terrible triad and, 294
exertional compartment syndrome and, 439, 439f
full-thickness rotator cuff tears and, 251
hypertrophic cardiomyopathy and, 138
lateral compression injuries and, 22–26t, 299–300, 300f
lateral epicondylitis and, 309
medial collateral ligament complex and, 350–351, 351f
medial tibial stress syndrome and, 436, 437f
meniscal injuries and, 410
multiple ligament-injured knee and, 380–381, 381f, 382f
olecranon apophysitis and, 302, 22f
olecranon fractures and, 286
osteoarthritis of the elbow and, 303
osteochondral lesions of talus and, 458
os trigonum syndrome and, 451
patellofemoral disorders and, 394–395, 396a
popliteal artery entrapment syndrome and, 442
posterior and multidirectional shoulder instability, 235
posterior cruciate ligament injury and, 365
posterolateral rotatory instability and, 312
radial head fractures and, 289
sternoclavicular (SC) joint and, 263–264
stress fractures and, 106, 432–434
subacromial impingement and, 248
triceps tendon rupture and, 308
ulnar collateral ligament injury and, 317
Radius stress fractures, 112
Raloxifene, 56
Range-of-motion (ROM) exercise
  assessment in brachial plexus injuries, 274
  exercises in osteitis pubis, 327
  lateral epicondylitis and, 309
  medial tension injuries and, 298
  shoulder injuries and, 202–203
  tendinitis and, 454
  testing, 25
  ulnar collateral ligament injury and, 317

Rapid antigen testing (RAT), 162–163
RAT (Rapid antigen testing), 162–163
Raynaud, Maurice, 141
Raynaud's phenomenon, 141–142, 142f
RCL (Radial collateral ligament), 310
RDAs. See Recommended daily allowances (RDAs)
Recalcitrant pain, 99, 99f
Recommended daily allowances (RDAs)
    for branched-chain amino acids, 44
    for carbohydrates, 46
    in labels, 33
    for proteins, 43
Reconstruction
    of medial patellofemoral ligament, 122–123
    in metallic radial head fractures, 292b
    of patellar tendon, 123, 123f
    of posterior cruciate ligament, 120–121, 121f, 367
    of posterolateral corner, 120, 121f
Recreational drugs, 47–49
Recreational sports, 81
"Recruitment," 4
Rectal tone, in spinal injuries, 96
Recurrence
    in anterior shoulder instability, 218
    in posterior and multidirectional shoulder instability, 242
Referrals, in articular cartilage injuries, 423b
Reflex sympathetic dystrophy, 127
Rehabilitation
    aging athletes and, 85
    anterior cruciate ligament and, 346–347
    apophyseal injuries and, 326b
    articular cartilage injuries and, 424
    avulsion fractures and, 326b
    biceps tendon rupture and, 307
    hyperextension valgus overload and, 315
    lateral epicondylitis and, 309
    little league elbow and, 65a
    medial epicondylitis and, 314
    medial tension injuries and, 298
    meniscal injuries and, 415
    multiple ligament-injured knee and, 389
    posterior and multidirectional shoulder instability and, 242
    posterior shoulder instability and, 241
    in sports medicine
        biology and, 465
        creating healing environment and, 473
        decrease pain and effusion and, 464–465
        emphasizing kinetic chain and, 471–472
        gradual reconditioning and, 472
        gradual return to functional activities and, 472–473

        normalizing soft-tissue balance and, 468
        preventing effects of immobilization and, 465–466
        principles of, 463–464
        restoring muscular strength and endurance and, 466–468
        restoring neuromuscular control and, 468–471
        retardation of muscular atrophy and, 466
    suprascapular nerve palsy and, 277
    ulnar collateral ligament injury and, 318
Rehabilitation Act of 1973, 30
Relocation test, 26, 188f, 204, 219
Remodeling phase
    in ligaments injuries, 18
    in tendon healing, 15
Repair, in meniscal injuries, 410, 411, 415t
Repair/proliferative phase, in ligaments injuries, 18
Repair/regeneration process, traumatic brain injury and, 89
Reparative treatment, in articular cartilage injuries, 424–425
Repetitive trauma, in patellofemoral pathology, 392b
Reproductive function and bone density, 56
Requirements of protein, 43
Resection, in meniscal injuries, 410, 410f, 411
Resistance training, stress fractures and, 107
Rest
    athletic pubalgia and, 331
    bony impingement and, 450
    bursitis and, 330
    infectious mononucleosis and, 165
    juvenile disc herniation and, 67
    Little League elbow and, 65a
    medial tibial stress syndrome and, 437
    musculocutaneous nerve injury and, 280
    osteitis pubis and, 327
    pelvis stress fracture and, 327
    shoulder injury and, 205
    spondylolysis and, 67
    strengthening and conditioning and, 482
    stress fractures and, 112
    subacromial impingement and, 248
    tendinitis and, 451, 453
    ulnar collateral ligament injury and, 317
    valgus extension overload and, 305
Restorative treatment, in articular cartilage injuries, 425–429, 426f
Resveratrol. See 3,4,5-trihydroxystilbene (Resveratrol)
Retard muscular atrophy, 478
Retinoids (topical), for acne, 160

Retraction bulb, 91
Reverse shift test, for posterior cruciate ligament injury, 365
Reverse pivot test
    for anterior cruciate ligament injury, 337t
    for posterolateral corner injuries, 357
Rhomboid ligament. See Costoclavicular ligament
Rhonchi, 24
Rib stress fractures, 111–112
Rimantadine, for influenza, 166
Ringworm, 157
Risk factors
    anterior cruciate ligament injury and, 57–58, 335–336
    immature and adolescent athletes and, 61
    noncontact ACL injuries and, 58
    pediatric sports injuries and, 62b
    stress fractures and, 57–58, 105–106
ROM exercise. See Range-of-motion (ROM) exercise
Rotator interval, 173
Rotator cuff. See also Rotator cuff disorders
    anatomy of, 244–245
    biomechanics of, 245–246
    disorders and impingement in, 208–210
        classic subacromial impingement in, 208
        coracoid impingement in, 209
        internal impingement in, 209–210, 209f
        secondary impingement in, 208
    dynamic stability of, 178f, 181
    function of, 185, 187
    Hawkins' test of the, 188, 188f
    impingement tests of, 187
    Internal rotation resistance stress test for, 188, 188f
    Jobe's supraspinatus test for, 187
    Neer's impingement test for, 187–188, 187t, 188f
    subcoracoid impingement test for, 188–189, 189f
    tendon degeneration in, 246
    tendons, 172–173, 172f
    tests for tears, 189–190
        belly press test in, 189–190, 190f
        drop sign in, 190
        external rotation lag sign in, 189
        internal rotation lag sign in, 189
        lift-off test for, 189, 190f
    Yocum's test for, 188
Rotator cuff disorders
    calcific tendonitis in, 252–253
    full-thickness rotator cuff tears in, 250–252, 251f
    impingement in, 246–249
    partial-thickness rotator cuff tears and, 249–250
    rotator cuff tear arthropathy in, 252
    tendon degeneration in, 246

Rotator cuff tear arthropathy, 252
Rotator interval
    anatomy of, 245
    in anterior shoulder instability
        surgery, 227, 228f
    in shoulder instability, 232, 233f
Running, stress fractures and, 58, 58f
Rupture
    of Achilles tendon, 454–455
    of peroneal tendon, 452

S
Sacral stress fractures, 111
Sagittal canal diameter, 102–103
Salbutamol, 38, 49
Salicylic acid, 160t
Salmeterol, 49
Sarcolemma, 1–2, 2f
Sarcoplasmic reticulum-transverse
        tubule system, 4
Saturated fat, 47
Sayers, Gayle, 81
Subacromial impingement, 208
Scapula, 173–174, 174f
Scapular dyskinesia, 211
Scapular instability, 232
Scapular pivoters, 175
Scapular winging, soft-tissue allografts
        in, 118–119, 118f
Scapulothoracic articulation, 175,
        176–177
Scapulothoracic bursa, 175
Scapulothoracic dyskinesia, 234f
Scapulothoracic fusion, in spinal
        accessory nerve injury, 284
Scapulothoracic motion, 172–179
SCFE. See Slipped capital femoral
        epiphysis (SCFE)
Schatzker classification of olecranon
        fractures, 286, 286f
Schwann cell, 268
Sciatic nerve, 330, 331f
SCIs. See Spinal cord injuries (SCIs)
Screening, of soft-tissue allografts, 116
SCUBA (Self-contained underwater
        breathing apparatus), 148
Secondary amenorrhea, 26, 57
Secondary impingement, 208
Secondary osteitis pubis, 327
Secondary Raynaud's phenomenon,
        142
Secondary traumatic brain injury, 89
Second impact syndrome, 88, 104
Seizures, 22, 30
Seldane-D (terfenadine plus
        pseudoephedrine), 49
Seldane (terfenadine), 49
Selective ligament-cutting studies, 232
Selective serotonin reuptake inhibitors,
        for Raynaud's phenomenon,
        142
Self-contained underwater breathing
        apparatus (SCUBA), 148
Self-testicular exam, 25
Semitendinosus-gracilis allograft, 117
Septal hematoma/deformity, 146
Septic olecranon bursitis, 297–298

Serology, in influenza, 166
Serratus anterior, 175
Sesamoid stress fracture, 111
Severe communication or osteopenic
        bone, in olecranon fracture,
        288
Sever's apophysitis, 76
Sexual arousal, steroids and, 34
SGHL (Superior glenohumeral
        ligament), 180, 232
Sharpey's fibers, 12
Shift test, 26
Shoe modification, in acute peroneal
        tendon injuries, 452
Shortness of breath, 21
Shoulder. See also Anterior shoulder
        instability; Shoulder
        arthroscopy; Shoulder girdle;
        Shoulder injuries
    acromioclavicular (AC) joint in
        anatomy of, 171, 171f
        compression test for, 192
        crossover impingement test for,
            191, 191f
        distraction test for, 191–192, 191f
        motion of, 171
        piano key sign, 192
        stability of, 171–172
    anterior instability of
        categories of, 214–215
        description of, 214
        diagnosis of, 218–221
        etiology and epidemiology, 218
        management of, 221a
        mechanisms of, 215–218
        pathogenesis of, 215–218
        pathophysiology in, 215–218
        postoperative management in,
            227–230
        sulcus sign in repair of, 235f
        treatment of, 221–230
    biceps tendon (BT) in, 172t, 190
        speed's test for, 190, 190f
        Yergason's test for, 191, 191f
    complex, integrated motion of, 177,
        177f
    dislocation of, 62–63, 62f, 63a
    glenohumeral joint in, 179, 183
        anatomy of, 172–175, 172f, 173f,
            174f, 175f
        dynamic stability of, 1480
        motion of, 175–179
        static stability, 179–180
    glenoid labrum in, 194–195
        Adson's maneuver for, 195, 195f
        biceps load test for, 195
        biceps tension test for, 195
        brachial plexus stretch test for,
            195
        clunk test for, 194
        compression-rotation test for, 195
        grind test for, 194
        O'Brien active compression test
            for, 195, 195f
        SLAP tests for, 195
    of immature and adolescent athletes,
        61–64

    instability of, 192–194
        anterior drawer test for, 193, 193f
        apprehension test for, 192, 192f
        Jobe's apprehension-relocation test
            for, 192, 193f
        load and shift test for, 194, 194f
        posterior drawer test for,
            193–194, 194f
        sulcus sign in, 192–193, 193f
    joint (right anterior view), 186f
    microinstability of, 63–64
    physical examination of, 187
    posterior, muscles of, 186f
    posterior and multidirectional
        instability in
        bony deficiency of the glenoid in,
            232
        description of, 231
        diagnosis of, 233–235
        diagnostic and surgical failures in,
            236–242
        epidemiology in, 231–232
        mechanism of injury in, 233
        rotator interval in, 232
        selective ligament-cutting in, 232
        treatment of, 236–242
    rotator cuff in
        function of, 185, 187
        Hawkins' test for, 188, 188f
        impingement tests for, 187
        internal rotation resistance stress
            test for, 188, 188f
        Jobe's supraspinatus test for, 187
        Neer's impingement test for,
            187–188, 187t, 188f
        subcoracoid impingement test for,
            188–189, 189f
        tests for tears, 189–190
    structure of, 185
Shoulder arthroscopy, portals in,
        128–129, 128f
Shoulder girdle
    groupings of muscles of, 179b
    muscles of, 174–175
Shoulder injuries
    adaptation, 201–202
    biomechanics and kinematics,
        200–201
    conditioning of, 205
    conditions and surgical
        considerations of, 205–212
        Bennett lesion in, 211
        chondral injuries in, 211
        glenohumeral internal rotation
            deficit in, 210, 210f
        increased humeral retroversion in,
            210–211
        laxity and instability in, 205–206
        neurovascular conditions in, 1412
        rotator cuff disorders and
            impingement in, 208–210
        scapular dyskinesia in, 211
        superior labrum anterior-posterior
            lesions in, 206, 206–208,
            207f, 207t
    description of, 200
    evaluation of

history of, 202
physical examination of, 202–204
functional tests for, 203t
nonoperative treatment of, 205
training of, 205
Shoulder translation, grading system for, 220t
Sickle cell anemia, 144
Sideline examination, head injuries and, 92
Silver sulfadiazine cream, for folliculitis, 157
Simple compression fractures, in lumbar spine injuries, 99
Simple transverse fractures, 287, 287f
Single-and double-bundle technique, in posterior cruciate ligament injury, 368–373, 369f, 370f, 371f, 372f
Single-leg hop test, 431
Single motor neuron, 3
Single-photon emission computed tomography (SPECT), 111
Single physician assembly line, 23
Single-stage arthroscopic ACL/PCL reconstruction, 384
Skeletal muscles
biomechanics of, 4–6
common clinical conditions in, 7–10
embryology of, 1
energy metabolism of, 6
motor unit in, 2–3, 3f
muscle contraction and, 3–4
normal structure of, 1–2, 2f
response to hormones and, 6–7
Skin
adverse effects of steroids on, 35b
clearance and, 28
lesions, 153
in medical history, 22
in physical examination, 25
steroids and, 34
SLAC (Superior labrum anterior cuff), 216
SLAP lesion (Superior labrum anterior and posterior), 181, 206–208, 206f, 207, 207t, 216, 216f, 235, 249
SLAP test, for glenoid labrum, 195
Sling, in acromioclavicular joint disorder, 258
Slipped capital femoral epiphysis (SCFE), 108, 326
Smokeless tobacco, 23, 48–49
Snapping hip syndrome, 330
Snapping psoas, 67–68
Soft-tissue allografts
advantages of, 115–116, 116b
biological incorporation of, 117
disadvantages of, 115–116, 116b
disease transmission of, 116
graft preparation and storage, 116–117
procurement of, 116
screening of, 116
surgical techniques in, 117–124
use of, 115

Soft-tissue injuries, 327–328, 327–332, 327f
Soft-tissue lesions, in anterior shoulder instability, 219
Soft-tissue mobility and flexibility, 480
Soft-tissue procedures, in posterior shoulder instability, 237
Soft tissues knee injury, 379
Somatotropes. See Human growth hormone (hGH)
Somatotropin, 37
Soreness, muscle, 7, 481–482
Sore throat, 162
Special situations, team physicians and, 149–150
SPECT (Single-photon emission computed tomography), 111
Speed's test, 176f, 190, 190f, 203t
Spina bifida occulta, 103
Spinal accessory nerve injury
anatomy of, 282, 283f
diagnosis of, 283
etiology of, 282–284
treatment of, 283–284
Spinal contribution to shoulder motion, 179
Spinal cord injuries (SCIs), 100
Spinal injuries
cervical, 100–103
head injuries and concussion in, 103–104
lumbar spine injuries, 97–99
spinal examination, 96–97
Spinal stenosis, 102
Spine. See also Spinal injuries
of immature and adolescent athletes, 66–67
in physical examination, 25
range-of-motion testing of, 25
Spirometry, in exercise-induced bronchospasm (EIB), 136
Spironolactone, 38
Spleen, infectious mononucleosis and, 165
Splenomegaly, 29
Split biceps tendon transfer, 385–386
Spondylolysis, 66–67
management of, 67a
Sporting activities, in United States, 88–89
Sports by contact, classification of, 27b
Sportsmetrics, 57
Sports pharmacology
antiestrogens in, 35
banned or restricted drugs in, 37–39
β-hydroxy-β- methylbutyrate in, 41–47
future of, 50
history of, 32–33
international Olympic committee and, 33
legislation about, 33
recreational drugs in, 47–49
sports supplements in, 39–41
steroids and prohormones in, 33–37
substances banned from use in competition, 49–50

Sports-specific conditions, 100–102
Sports supplements, 39–41, 40t
Sprains, 30
lumbar, 98
sternoclavicular, 278
in transient quadriplegia, 102
Spurling's test, for brachial plexus injury, 271
SSP (Supraspinatus), 172f
Stability
of acromioclavicular joint, 171–172
glenohumeral joint, 179–182, 204
scapular, 6f, 12, 176–177
of sternoclavicular joint, 170
Stabilization, in posterior shoulder instability, 241
Stable tears, 408b
Stacking, 34
Staging of osteochondral lesions of the talus, 457, 457t
Standard throat culture, for streptococcal pharyngitis, 162–163
Stanozolol, 34
Staphylococcal scalded skin syndrome, 155
Staphylococcus aureus, 147, 155, 156
Staphylococcus auricularis, 147
Staphylococcus epidermidis, 147
Static demands, 28b
Static posterior subluxation, 232, 232f
Static stability, glenoid fossa, 175f, 179
Station-based PPE, 21
Stenosis, 101–102
Stereophotogrammetry, for shoulders, 178
Sterilization technique, in graft preparation, 117
Sternoclavicular articulation, 185
Sternoclavicular (SC) joint
anatomy of, 169–170, 170f, 262–263, 263f
biomechanics of, 262–263
classification and treatment, 264–266
diagnosis of, 263–264
epidemiology, mechanism, and history of, 263
motion of, 170, 170f
stability of, 170
Sternoclavicular sprain or subluxation, 264
Sternum stress fractures, 112
Steroids
anabolic/androgenic, 476
for exercise-induced anaphylaxis, 137
injection
for acne, 160t
in anterolateral impingement, 448
in juvenile disc herniation, 67
in the subacromial impingement, 248
oral, 34
and prohormones, 33–37
androstenedione, 36
dehydroepiandrosterone, 36
steroids, 32, 34–36

Steroids (*contd.*)
  testosterone, 33–34
  Tribulus terrestris, 36–37
Stiffness, 17
Stingers, 101–102
Strain curve, stress, 13f
Strains, 8, 22, 30
  lumber, 98
  in sternoclavicular (SC) joint, 264
  in transient quadriplegia, 102
Strength and conditioning, 475
  in medial collateral ligament complex injuries, 351
  nutrition and, 475–476
  in patellar tilt, 397
  physical training effects on muscle, 477–482
  physiology and, 477
  in posterior shoulder instability, 241
  in shoulder injury, 205
  in snapping iliotibial tract, 68
  in subacromial impingement, 248
  supplements and, 42
  testing for shoulder injuries, 203
  training, 7, 476–477
  in ulnar collateral ligament injury, 317–318
Strenuousness, in sports, 27, 28b
Strenuousness, classification of sports by, 27, 28b
Streptococcal pharyngitis, 162–163
Streptococcus pneumoniae, 147
Streptococcus pyogenes, 155, 159
Stress fractures, 296, 326–327. *See also* Stress fractures of the tibia and fibula
  bone remodeling in, 105
  calcaneal, 109
  cuboid and cuneiform, 110
  description of, 105
  diagnosis of, 107
    magnetic resonance imaging in, 108
    physical examination in, 107
    prevention of, 112–113
    public rami, 111
    radiologic examination and, 107
    radius, 112
    rib, 111–112
    risk factors in
      exercise and resistance training and, 107
      female athlete triad and, 107
      nutrition and, 105–107
      triple-phase bone scans in, 107–108
  epidemiology of, 105, 430–431
  in female athletes, 56–57, 107
  femur, 108
  fibular, 109
  humerus, 112
  in male athlete, 109f
  management of, 112–113
  metatarsal, 110–111, 110f
  navicular, 110
  olecranon, 112

pars interarticularis, 111
  patellar, 109
  pubic ramus, 111
  sesamoid, 111
  of the spine, 99
  sternum, 112
  talar, 109–110
  tibial, 109
Stress fractures of the tibia and fibula, 430–435
  diagnosis of, 432a, 454
  etiology and epidemiology of, 430–431
  pathophysiology of, 431
  treatment of, 434–435
Stress response (no clearcut fracture line), in stress fracture, 108
Stress strain curve, 13f
Stretching
  bursitis and, 330
  lateral epicondylitis and, 309
  medial epicondylitis and, 314
  medial tension injuries and, 298
  muscle, 8
  posterior shoulder instability and, 241
  shoulder injury and, 205
  snapping iliotibial tract and, 68
  stress fractures and, 112
Structure
  of ligaments, 16–17
  of meniscus, 402–404, 403f, 404f, 405f
  of patellofemoral disorders, 391b
  of skeletal muscles, 1–2, 2f
  of tendons, 11–13, 11f
Strychnine, 32
Stryker notch, 204, 211, 235
Subacromial access, in shoulder arthroscopy, 129
Subacromial decompression, in partial-thickness rotator cuff tears, 250
Subacromial impingement, 246–248, 247f, 249f
Subacromial injections, in calcific tendonitis, 253
Subclavian artery compression, 266
Subconjunctival hemorrhage, 145
Subcoracoid impingement test, for the rotator cuff, 188–189, 189f
Subluxation/dislocation
  peroneal tendon, 452–453, 453t
  sternoclavicular, 278
  sternoclavicular joint, 264
Subscapularis gross strength, 203t
Subscapularis muscle, 244–245, 246
Subscapularis testing, in full-thickness rotator cuff tears, 251
Substances banned from use in competition, 49–50
Sulcus sign, 26
  in anterior instability repair, 235f
  anterior shoulder instability repair and, 235f
  grading in multidimensional instability, 235t

grading of, 220t
  in shoulders instability, 192–193, 193f
Superficial corneal foreign body, 145
Superficial medial collateral ligament, 349
Superior glenohumeral ligament (SGHL), 180, 232
Superior labral lesions, tests for, 204t
Superior labrum anterior and posterior (SLAP lesion), 181, 206–208, 206f, 207, 207t, 216, 216f, 235, 249
Superior labrum anterior cuff (SLAC), 216
Superior labrum extension, 216–217
Superolateral portal, in knee arthroscopy, 126
Supplement industry, 33
Suprascapular nerve
  anatomy of, 275–276, 275f
  diagnosis of, 276
  etiology of, 275f, 276
  treatment of, 276–277
Supraspinatus portal, in shoulder arthroscopy, 129
Supraspinatus (SSP), 172f
Supraspinatus tendons, 203t
  anatomy of, 244–245
  layers of, 245t
  transverse section of, 245f
Surgery
  acromioclavicular joint disorder and, 259
  acute peroneal tendon injuries and, 452, 453
  adult lateral elbow and, 309–310
  aging athletes and, 86
  anterior cruciate ligament injury and, 337–339
  anterior shoulder instability and, 221–227
  articular cartilage injuries and, 423–429
  athletic pubalgia and, 332
  cauda equina syndrome and, 98
  chronic ankle pain and, 489
  elbow dislocation/terrible triad and, 295
  elbow joint loose bodies and, 305
  exertional compartment syndrome and, 31f–12
  full-thickness rotator cuff tears and, 252
  head injuries and, 93–95
  hyperextension valgus overload and, 315
  insertional tendinitis and, 455–456
  leg overuse injuries and, 435, 435f
  long thoracic nerve injury and, 282
  medial collateral ligament complex injuries and, 352
  medial epicondylitis and, 314
  medial tibial stress syndrome and, 437
  medical history and, 22

meniscal injuries and, 411–413, 412*a*

multidirectional shoulder instability and, 239, 239*t*, 240*f*

multiple ligament-injured knee and, 383–388

nerve entrapment syndrome and, 330

olecranon stress fractures and, 112, 296

osteitis pubis and, 327

osteoarthritis of the elbow and, 303–304

osteochondral lesions of talus (OLT) and, 458

osteochondritis dissecans and, 77

popliteal artery entrapment syndrome and, 443

posterior cruciate ligament injury and, 366–374

posterior shoulder instability and, 236–239, 237*t*, 238*f*

posterolateral corner injuries and, 360–361, 361*f*

recalcitrant cases and, 99, 99*f*

rupture of Achilles tendon and, 454

scapular dyskinesia and, 211

spinal accessory nerve injury and, 283–284

sternoclavicular joint (SC) dislocation and, 267

stress fractures and, 112

subacromial impingement and, 248

suprascapular nerve palsy and, 277

tendinitis and, 453

triceps tendon rupture and, 308

ulnar collateral ligament injury and, 318

Surgical failures

anterior cruciate ligament injury and, 343–345, 343*f*

posterior and multidirectional shoulder instability and, 242

Surgical techniques

in anterior cruciate ligament injury

graft sources and selection principles in, 339–341

in anterior shoulder instability, 222, 222*f*

Bankart repair with suture anchors in, 224

extension of the anterior-labrum tear into superior labrum in, 227

inferior plication in, 224, 226*f*

patient position and portal placement in, 222–224, 222*f*, 223*f*

preparation in, 224, 224*f*

rotator interval in, 227, 228*f*

suture first technique in, 217*f*, 226–227, 226*f*

in multiple ligament-injured knee, 384–385, 384*f*, 385*f*

Suture first technique, in anterior shoulder instability surgery, 217*f*, 226–227, 226*f*

Swimmer's ear (Otitis externa), 147

Swimming, in pelvis stress fracture, 327

Syncope, 21

Syndesmotic impingement, 449

Syndesmotic ligament complex, 445–446

T

Talar stress fractures, 111–112

Talus, in ankle anatomy, 444–445

Tamoxifen (Nolvadex), 37, 56

Tanner staging, 23

Taping

for lateral patellar compression syndrome, 395, 396

for tendinitis, 451

Tazarotene gel, for acne, 160

Team physician, medical concerns of, 135–149

Tear patterns

and repair potential, 407*t*

stable *versus* unstable, 408*b*

Technology use, in meniscal injuries, 416–417

Tendinitis, 451

patellar, 399–400

Tendinopathy, fluoroquinolones and, 14–15

Tendinosis, 14, 453, 454

Tendon degeneration, in rotator cuff, 246

Tendonitis, 14

Tendons, 10–16

biomechanical effects of aging, 14

biomechanics of, 13

embryology of, 10–11

exercise and, 13

healing, 15–16

healing of, 15–16

injuries of, 14–15

structure of, 11–13, 11*f*

Tendon-to-bone fixation, in anterior cruciate ligament injury, 341

Tennis elbow, 308–310

Tenosynovectomy, in chronic peroneal tendon injuries, 452

Tenosynovectomy, in tendinitis, 451

Tensile overload, 14

Tension stress fractures, 108

T:E ratio. *See* Testosterone to epitestosterone ratio (T:E ratio)

Terbinafine, 158

Terbutaline, 38, 49

Teres minor muscle, 244

Terfenadine. *See* Seldane (terfenadine)

Terfenadine plus pseudoephedrine. *See* Seldane-D (terfenadine plus pseudoephedrine)

Testicular disorders

clearance and, 29

exam in, 23

Testosterone, 7, 33–34, 36

Testosterone to epitestosterone ratio (T:E ratio), 33–34, 35–36

Tests/testing. *See* specific injuries

Tetanus, 10

Tetracycline, 160, 160*t*

Thalassemia, 144–145

Theophylline, in exercise-induced bronchospasm (EIB), 137

Thermal capsulorrhaphy, for microinstability, 64

Thermal chondroplasty, in chondral lesions surgery, 424*t*

Thiazide, 38

Thiazide diuretics, for hypertension, 140

Thick filaments, 2, 4

Thigh injuries

anatomy of, 320, 321*f*

athletic pubalgia, 331–332

bony injuries, 325–327

bursitis and, 329–330, 329*f*

contusions and, 328–329

differential diagnosis of, 324–325

Hamstring syndrome and, 331

of immature and adolescent athletes, 69–70

muscle strains in, 328, 328*f*, 328*t*

nerve entrapment syndrome and, 330–331, 331*f*

physical examinations and, 323–324

radiologic examination and, 324

snapping hip syndrome and, 330

soft-tissue injuries, 327, 327*f*

Thoracic outlet syndrome (TOS), 211–212, 212*f*, 266

3,4,5-Trihydroxystilbene (Resveratrol), 37

3-Norandrosterone, 34

Throat, in physical examination, 24

Throwing

biomechanics of, 183–184, 199*f*

cycle, differential diagnosis of, 202*t*

phases of baseball pitch, 201*t*

program in shoulder injury, 205

Tibial collateral ligament, 349

Tibial external rotation test, for posterior cruciate ligament injury, 365, 365*f*

Tibial inlay technique, in posterior cruciate ligament injury, 371–373, 373*f*

Tibialis anterior allograft preparation, in anterior cruciate ligament injury, 342

Tibialis anterior tendon allograft, in acromioclavicular joint disorder, 261

Tibial plateau fractures, 380

Tibial spine avulsion, 69–70, 70*f*

Tibial stress fractures, 108, 109*f*, 113

Tibial tubercle avulsion, 70–71

Tibial tunnel, in anterior cruciate ligament injury, 342

Tibiotalar articulation, in leg anatomy, 446

Tidemark, 12

Timing of preparticipation physical examination, 20
Tinea, 157–159, 159t
Tinea capitis, 158
Tinea corporis, 157f
Tinea cruris, 158, 158f
Tinea pedis, 157–158, 158f
Tinel's test, 199, 199f
Tissue harvesting, 116
Titin, 1
Tobacco, 23, 35
Torg ratio, 103, 103f
Torque, 182
TOS. See Thoracic outlet syndrome (TOS)
Training
  basics, 482–483
    endurance, 483
    interval, 483
    resistance
      stress fractures and, 107
    in shoulder injury, 205
    strength, 476–477
    stress fractures and errors in, 106
Transient quadriplegia, 100–102
Transmalleolar portal, in ankle arthroscopy, 130
Transpatellar tendon portal, in knee arthroscopy, 127
Transtalar portal, in ankle arthroscopy, 130
Transtibial tunnel reconstruction, in posterior cruciate ligament injury, 368–373
Transverse fractures with communication, 288, 288f
Trapezius, 174–175
Trapezoid, 255, 255b
Traumatic bone deficiency, 217–218
Traumatic brain injury, pathophysiology of, 89–90
Traumatic instability, 396–397, 397b
Traumatic osteitis pubis, 327
Traumatic anterior shoulder instability, 214
Traveler's diarrhea, 143
Treatment. See specific diseases
Trembling, 42
Trendelenburg test, 323, 324
Tretinoin (topical), for acne, 160
Triad Consensus Conference of 1992, 53
Tribulus terrestris, 36–37
Triceps tendon rupture
  diagnosis of, 308
  pathophysiology of, 307–308
  treatment of, 308
Trichophyton, 157
Triple-phase bone scans, 107–108
  with angiogram, 433
Trochanteric bursa, 329–330
Tryptophan, 44
T-tubule system, 4
Tubercle-sulcus angle, in patellofemoral disorders, 394, 394b
Talus, in ankle anatomy, 445

Two-incision approach, in biceps tendon rupture, 307
2-Boretiocholanolone, 34
Toxicity, caffeine, 42
Tylenol, 164t
Type 1 a lesion treatment, in lateral compression injuries, 301
Type 1b lesion treatment , in lateral compression injuries, 301
Type II A motor units, 3
Type II B motor units, 3
Type II lesion treatment, in lateral compression injuries, 301
Type II motor units, 3
Type I motor units, 3
Tzanck smear, 153

U
UCL injury. See Ulnar collateral ligament (UCL) injury
Ulnar collateral ligament (UCL) injury
  diagnosis of, 316–317, 318f
  pathophysiology of, 316–317, 461f
  treatment of, 318–319
Ulnar (medial) collateral ligament, soft-tissue allografts in, 119
Ulnohumeral arthroplasty, in osteoarthritis of the elbow surgery, 304
UltraSling (DJ Orthor, Vista, CA) device, 241
Ultrasonography (duplex), in popliteal artery entrapment syndrome, 442
Ultrasound
  calcific tendonitis and, 253
  exertional compartment syndrome and, 439
  full-thickness rotator cuff tears and, 251
Underweight, in physical examination, 24
United States, sporting activities in, 88–89
United States Olympic Committee (USOC), 23
University of Connecticut, postoperative protocol for anterior-inferior shoulder instability, 227–228
Unstable patterns, 408b
Upper extremity. See also Upper extremity nerve injuries
  physical examination of, 26
  soft-tissue allografts in, 117–120
  stress fractures in, 112
Upper extremity nerve injuries, 268–284
  anatomy of, 268, 269f, 270f
  axillary nerve and, 277–280
  brachial plexus injuries, 272–274
  diagnosis of, 271–272
  epidemiology of, 269
  etiology of, 268–269

  idiopathic brachial neuritis in, 274–275
  long thoracic nerve and, 281–282
  musculocutaneous nerve and, 280–281
  pathophysiology of, 269
  spinal accessory nerve and, 282–284
  study findings with, 272b
  suprascapular nerve and, 275–277
  treatment of, 272
Upper respiratory infections, 162–167
"Uppers." See Amphetamines
Urinalysis, in physical examination, 26
U.S. Food and Drug Administration (FDA), 35, 58, 116
U.S. Olympic Committee (USOC), 23

V
Vaccinations, 23, 166
Valacyclovir, for herpes simplex, 153
Valgus extension overload of the elbow, 304f, 305–306
Valgus stress test
  for anterior cruciate ligament injury, 337t
  of knee, 350f
  for shoulder instability, 197–198, 197f
Valine, 44, 45
Valvular heart disease, 140–141
Vancomycin, 160
Varus stress test
  for anterior cruciate ligament injury, 337t
  for elbow instability, 198, 198f
  for isolated posterolateral corner injuries, 357–359
Vascular compromise in knee dislocation, 379–380
Vascular concerns, 141–142
Vascular injuries in the knee, 382
Vasodilator, for Raynaud's phenomenon, 142
Vastus medialis obliquus (VMO), 123, 349, 391, 392
Velpeau axillary, 63f
Venography, in effort thrombosis, 211
Verapamil, for hypertrophic cardiomyopathy (HCM), 138
Verbal response (V), in Glasgow coma scale, 92t
Verrucae vulgaris, 161, 161f
Vertical longitudinal tears
  management of, 412a
  in meniscal injuries, 407, 407t
Viral culture, in influenza, 166
Viral upper respiratory infections, 164, 165t
Viscosupplementation, for joint pain, 84
Vision
  clearance and, 29
  in medical history, 22
  in physical examination, 24
Vitamin C/zinc, for viral upper respiratory infection, 164t

Vitamin D, in stress fractures, 107, 113
VMO. *See* Vastus medialis obliquus (VMO)
Voice deepening, steroids and, 35
VO$_{2max}$, 39, 43, 52, 82
Vomiting, 23

W
Wallerian degeneration, 269
Warts, 161–162, 161*f*, 162*f*
Water
  and fluid replacement, 47
  in traveler's diarrhea, 143
Weaver-Dunn technique, in acromioclavicular joint disorder, 20;7, 260*f*
Weight lifting, posterior shoulder instability in, 233

Weight loss, in articular cartilage injuries, 422
West Point view, for shoulder injury, 205
Wheezing, 22, 24
White individuals, stress fractures in, 106
"White" muscle fibers, 3
Windshield wiper effect, 340
Windup phase, 183, 183*f*, 201*t*
Wissinger rod, 129
Women. *See also* Athletes; Female athletes
  adverse effects of steroids in, 35*b*
  androstenedione and, 36
  fibular stress fractures in, 109
  osteoarthritis of the elbow in, 303
  public rami stress fractures in, 111
  steroids and, 35
  stress fractures in, 106, 112

Wrestlers, stress fractures in, 112
Wrist
  in gymnast's wrist, 64, 66
  of immature and adolescent athletes, 64, 66

Y
Yergason's test, 191, 191*f*
Yocum's test, of the rotator cuff, 188
Yttrium-aluminum-garnet laser, in posterior shoulder instability, 239

Z
Zanamivir, 166
Zanca anteroposterior (AP) view, in acromioclavicular joint disorder, 258
Z-band, 1–2
Ziegler, J., 32–33